Smart Sensors for Healthcare and Medical Applications

Smart Sensors for Healthcare and Medical Applications

Editors

Domenico Formica
Emiliano Schena

MDPI • Basel • Beijing • Wuhan • Barcelona • Belgrade • Manchester • Tokyo • Cluj • Tianjin

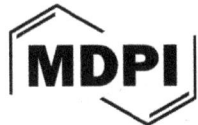

Editors
Domenico Formica
Università Campus Bio-Medico di Roma
Italy

Emiliano Schena
Università Campus Bio-Medico di Roma
Italy

Editorial Office
MDPI
St. Alban-Anlage 66
4052 Basel, Switzerland

This is a reprint of articles from the Special Issue published online in the open access journal *Sensors* (ISSN 1424-8220) (available at: https://www.mdpi.com/journal/sensors/special_issues/sensor_for_healthcare).

For citation purposes, cite each article independently as indicated on the article page online and as indicated below:

LastName, A.A.; LastName, B.B.; LastName, C.C. Article Title. *Journal Name* **Year**, *Volume Number*, Page Range.

ISBN 978-3-0365-0650-0 (Hbk)
ISBN 978-3-0365-0651-7 (PDF)

© 2021 by the authors. Articles in this book are Open Access and distributed under the Creative Commons Attribution (CC BY) license, which allows users to download, copy and build upon published articles, as long as the author and publisher are properly credited, which ensures maximum dissemination and a wider impact of our publications.

The book as a whole is distributed by MDPI under the terms and conditions of the Creative Commons license CC BY-NC-ND.

Contents

About the Editors ix

Preface to "Smart Sensors for Healthcare and Medical Applications" xi

Domenico Formica and Emiliano Schena
Smart Sensors for Healthcare and Medical Applications
Reprinted from: *Sensors* **2021**, *21*, 543, doi:10.3390/s21020543 1

Edrine Damulira, Muhammad Nur Salihin Yusoff, Ahmad Fairuz Omar and Nur Hartini Mohd Taib
A Review: Photonic Devices Used for Dosimetry in Medical Radiation
Reprinted from: *Sensors* **2019**, *19*, 2226, doi:10.3390/s19102226 7

Prasara Jakkaew and Takao Onoye
Non-Contact Respiration Monitoring and Body Movements Detection for Sleep Using Thermal Imaging
Reprinted from: *Sensors* **2020**, *20*, 6307, doi:10.3390/s20216307 35

Hung-Chi Chang, Hau-Tieng Wu, Po-Chiun Huang, Hsi-Pin Ma and Yu-Lun Lo and Yuan-Hao Huang
Portable Sleep Apnea Syndrome Screening and Event Detection Using Long Short-Term Memory Recurrent Neural Network
Reprinted from: *Sensors* **2020**, *20*, 6067, doi:10.3390/s20216067 49

Carlo Massaroni, Daniela Lo Presti, Domenico Formica, Sergio Silvestri and Emiliano Schena
Non-Contact Monitoring of Breathing Pattern and Respiratory Rate via RGB Signal Measurement
Reprinted from: *Sensors* **2019**, *19*, 2758, doi:10.3390/s19122758 65

Daniela Lo Presti, Chiara Romano, Carlo Massaroni, Jessica D'Abbraccio, Luca Massari, Michele Arturo Caponero, Calogero Maria Oddo, Domenico Formica and Emiliano Schena
Cardio-Respiratory Monitoring in Archery Using a Smart Textile Based on Flexible Fiber Bragg Grating Sensors
Reprinted from: *Sensors* **2019**, *19*, 3581, doi:10.3390/s19163581 81

Yuki Haseda, Julien Bonefacino, Hwa-Yaw Tam, Shun Chino, Shouhei Koyama and Hiroaki Ishizawa
Measurement of Pulse Wave Signals and Blood Pressure by a Plastic Optical Fiber FBG Sensor
Reprinted from: *Sensors* **2019**, *19*, 5088, doi:10.3390/s19235088 95

Kang-Ho Lee, Yeong-Eun Kwon, Hyukjin Lee, Yongkoo Lee, Joonho Seo, Ohwon Kwon, Shin-Won Kang and Dongkyu Lee
Active Body Pressure Relief System with Time-of-Flight Optical Pressure Sensors for Pressure Ulcer Prevention
Reprinted from: *Sensors* **2019**, *19*, 3862, doi:10.3390/s19183862 107

Paloma Massó, Antonio Callejas, Juan Melchor, Francisca S. Molina and Guillermo Rus
In Vivo Measurement of Cervical Elasticity on Pregnant Women by Torsional Wave Technique: A Preliminary Study
Reprinted from: *Sensors* **2019**, *19*, 3249, doi:10.3390/s19153249 119

Daniela Lo Presti, Sofia Dall'Orso, Silvia Muceli, Tomoki Arichi, Sara Neumane, Anna Lukens, Riccardo Sabbadini, Carlo Massaroni, Michele Arturo Caponero, Domenico Formica, Etienne Burdet and Emiliano Schena
An fMRI Compatible Smart Device for Measuring Palmar Grasping Actions in Newborns
Reprinted from: *Sensors* **2020**, *20*, 6040, doi:10.3390/s20216040 . . . . **133**

Raluca Maria Aileni, Sever Pasca and Adriana Florescu
EEG-Brain Activity Monitoring and Predictive Analysis of Signals Using Artificial Neural Networks
Reprinted from: *Sensors* **2020**, *20*, 3346, doi:10.3390/s20123346 . . . . **149**

Yuan-Pin Lin, Ting-Yu Chen and Wei-Jen Chen
Cost-efficient and Custom Electrode-holder Assembly Infrastructure for EEG Recordings
Reprinted from: *Sensors* **2019**, *19*, 4273, doi:10.3390/s19194273 . . . . **171**

Shanshan Tian, Mengxuan Li, Yifei Wang and Xi Chen
Application of an Improved Correlation Method in Electrostatic Gait Recognition of Hemiparetic Patients
Reprinted from: *Sensors* **2019**, *19*, 2529, doi:10.3390/s19112529 . . . . **183**

Filippo Colombo Zefinetti, Andrea Vitali, Daniele Regazzoni, Caterina Rizzi and Guido Molinero
Tracking and Characterization of Spinal Cord-Injured Patients by Means of RGB-D Sensors
Reprinted from: *Sensors* **2020**, *20*, 6273, doi:10.3390/s20216273 . . . . **195**

Mohammad I. Daoud, Abdullah Alhusseini, Mostafa Z. Ali and Rami Alazrai
A Game-Based Rehabilitation System for Upper-Limb Cerebral Palsy: A Feasibility Study
Reprinted from: *Sensors* **2020**, *20*, 2416, doi:10.3390/s20082416 . . . . **215**

Antonio Cobo, Elena Villalba-Mora, Rodrigo Pérez-Rodríguez, Xavier Ferre, Walter Escalante, Cristian Moral and Leocadio Rodriguez-Mañas
Automatic and Real-Time Computation of the 30-Seconds Chair-Stand Test without Professional Supervision for Community-Dwelling Older Adults
Reprinted from: *Sensors* **2020**, *20*, 5813, doi:10.3390/s20205813 . . . . **239**

Su-Chun Huang, Gloria Dalla Costa, Marco Pisa, Lorenzo Gregoris, Giulia Leccabue, Martina Congiu, Giancarlo Comi and Letizia Leocani
The Danger of Walking with Socks: Evidence from Kinematic Analysis in People with Progressive Multiple Sclerosis
Reprinted from: *Sensors* **2020**, *20*, 6160, doi:10.3390/s20216160 . . . . **263**

Enrico Piovanelli, Davide Piovesan, Shouhei Shirafuji, Becky Su, Natsue Yoshimura, Yousuke Ogata and Jun Ota
Towards a Simplified Estimation of Muscle Activation Pattern from MRI and EMG Using Electrical Network and Graph Theory
Reprinted from: *Sensors* **2020**, *20*, 724, doi:10.3390/s20030724 . . . . **275**

Daniel Sanchez-Morillo, Pilar Muñoz-Zara, Alejandro Lara-Doña and Antonio Leon-Jimenez
Automated Home Oxygen Delivery for Patients with COPD and Respiratory Failure: A New Approach
Reprinted from: *Sensors* **2020**, *20*, 1178, doi:10.3390/s20041178 . . . . **295**

Wonki Hong, Jungmin Lee and Won Gu Lee
A Dual-Padded, Protrusion-Incorporated, Ring-Type Sensor for the Measurement of Food Mass and Intake
Reprinted from: *Sensors* **2020**, *20*, 5623, doi:10.3390/s20195623 319

Roman Gabl and Florian Stummer
Development of a Sensor to Measure Physician Consultation Times
Reprinted from: *Sensors* **2019**, *19*, 5359, doi:10.3390/s19245359 331

Luca Massari, Andrea Bulletti, Sahana Prasanna, Marina Mazzoni, Francesco Frosini, Elena Vicari, Marcello Pantano, Fabio Staderini, Gastone Ciuti, Fabio Cianchi, Luca Messerini, Lorenzo Capineri, Arianna Menciassi and Calogero Maria Oddo
A Mechatronic Platform for Computer Aided Detection of Nodules in Anatomopathological Analyses via Stiffness and Ultrasound Measurements
Reprinted from: *Sensors* **2019**, *19*, 2512, doi:10.3390/s19112512 345

Chakaveh Ahmadizadeh and Carlo Menon
Investigation of Regression Methods for Reduction of Errors Caused by Bending of FSR-Based Pressure Sensing Systems Used for Prosthetic Applications
Reprinted from: *Sensors* **2019**, *19*, 5519, doi:10.3390/s19245519 359

Vessela Krasteva, Irena Jekova and Ramun Schmid
Simulating Arbitrary Electrode Reversals in Standard 12-Lead ECG
Reprinted from: *Sensors* **2019**, *19*, 2920, doi:10.3390/s19132920 379

Abhishek Kumar Ghosh, Sonny F. Burniston, Daniel Krentzel, Abhishek Roy, Adil Shoaib Sheikh, Talha Siddiq, Paula Mai Phuong Trinh, Marta Mambrilla Velazquez, Hei-Ting Vielle, Niamh C. Nowlan and Ravi Vaidyanathan
A Novel Fetal Movement Simulator for the Performance Evaluation of Vibration Sensors for Wearable Fetal Movement Monitors
Reprinted from: *Sensors* **2020**, *20*, 6020, doi:10.3390/s20216020 399

About the Editors

Domenico Formica received his Ph.D. degree in biomedical engineering from the Università Campus Bio-Medico di Roma, Italy, in 2008. Since 2011, he has been working as faculty staff at the Università Campus Bio-Medico di Roma, where he is currently an associate professor in Industrial Bioengineering. In 2016, he co-founded the NEXT: Neurophysiology and Neuroengineering of Human–Technology Interaction research unit, a multidisciplinary research group with a focus on the study of motor neuroscience in both healthy subjects and neurological patients. In 2007, he was a visiting student at the Department of Mechanical Engineering of the Massachusetts Institute of Technology, and from 2014 to 2018, he was a visiting scientist at the Nanyang Technological University of Singapore. He has been awarded two national grants for young researchers, by the Italian Ministry of Education, University and Research, and by the Italian Ministry of Health. Currently, he is the European coordinator of the EU project CONBOTS and the PI of the EU project NIMA. He has published more than 120 peer-reviewed scientific papers in international journals and conference proceedings.

Emiliano Schena (Ph.D. 2009) is currently an associate professor at the Department of Engineering of the Università Campus Bio-Medico di Roma (UCBM), Rome, Italy. He received a Laurea Degree (B.Sc. + M.Sc.) and a Ph.D. in Biomedical Engineering from UCBM in 2003, 2006, and 2009, respectively. He has been a visiting researcher/professor at many international and highly renowned universities, including: the Division of Molecular Medicine, Department of Surgery and Department of Developmental & Stem Cell Biology of The City of Hope, Duarte—California (2014, 2015, 2016, 2018 and 2019, respectively); School of Mechanical Engineering & SAINT of Sungkyunkwan University, Seoul—Republic of Korea (2017); and School of Biomedical Engineering of Technion, Israel Institute of Technology, Haifa—Israel (2018).

His current research interests include the design, development and assessment of wearable systems for monitoring physiological parameters (e.g., cardiac activities, respiratory activities, human joints movements, and patients' motion). Currently, his research is mainly devoted to the design and assessment of wearable systems in different scenarios, instrumented with sensors based on different technologies. He has been involved as a coordinator/principal investigator/WP responsible in many national and international research projects. He currently serves on several journals' editorial boards, such as that of *Sensors* MDPI and IEEE *Sensors Journal*. He has participated in several international conferences/workshops as the general chair, technical program chair, organizer of special session, chair of session, technical program committee member, and international program committee member. He is an IEEE senior member and chair of the Italy Chapter of the IEEE *Sensors* Council. He is currently the UCBM rector's delegate to the Third Mission. Since 2018, he has been one of the three members of the committee to assess the research quality at the Department of Engineering of UCBM. Since 2018, he has been a member of the scientific board of the Ph.D. Program in "Science and Engineering for Humans and the Environment" of the UCBM. Since 2013, he has been a responsible of the Educational Laboratory of Engineering at UCBM. Regarding international activities, since 2016 he has been a responsible of the Erasmus plus EU program at UCBM (School of Engineering), Italy. He is also the responsible of Erasmus + project for the school of Industrial Engineering.

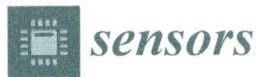

Editorial

Smart Sensors for Healthcare and Medical Applications

Domenico Formica [1],* and Emiliano Schena [2]

1. Unit of Neurophysiology and Neuroengineering of Human Technology Interaction (NeXT), Università Campus Bio-Medico di Roma, 00128 Rome, Italy
2. Laboratory of Measurements and Biomedical Instrumentation, Università Campus Bio-Medico di Roma, 00128 Rome, Italy; e.schena@unicampus.it
* Correspondence: D.Formica@unicampus.it

Received: 5 January 2021; Accepted: 8 January 2021; Published: 14 January 2021

This special issue on "Smart Sensors for Healthcare and Medical Applications" focuses on new sensing technologies, measurement techniques, and their applications in medicine and healthcare. We proposed this topic, being aware of the pivotal role that smart sensors can play for the improvement of healthcare services in both acute and chronic conditions as well as for prevention towards a healthy life and active aging. In this editorial we shortly describe the potential of smart sensors in the aforementioned applications, before moving on providing a general overview of the 24 articles selected and published in this special issue.

Recent advances in mechatronics, Internet of Things, wearable devices, and the miniaturization of sensors and electronics have significantly increased the capabilities of smart sensors enlarging the range of their applications. Among others, healthcare and medical fields have been strongly influenced by the evolution of these technologies, which are providing substantial contributions in several applications in the field [1–4]. In fact, smart sensors are increasingly offering novel solutions to several relevant challenges in healthcare, such as early detection of pathologies, or minimally invasive management and prevention of high-burden diseases (e.g., cardiovascular diseases and cancer) [5]. Furthermore, the development of miniaturized and lightweight smart sensors-based systems may be a key player in enabling a more rapid growth of unobtrusive and unsupervised approaches to home-rehabilitation and continuous monitoring of patients' status.

The 24 articles (i.e., 1 review paper, 22 articles, and 1 letter) selected in this special issue cover a variety of topics related to the design, validation, and application of smart sensors to healthcare. Indeed, the accepted papers report on different technologies exploited to develop smart sensors, several applications in diagnostic and/or therapeutic processes, new systems to assess the performance of smart sensors, wearable systems, and new approaches to analyze biomedical signals.

The only review paper published in this special issue focuses on the principles of work and technologies used to develop systems for estimating the radiation dose in medical applications [6]. In fact, the use of radiation is crucial in many radiotherapeutic or imaging procedures, but the absorbed dose could cause secondary malignancies [7]. Therefore, the accurate monitoring of the exposure to radiation is mandatory for both patients and clinicians. This work [6] allows the reader to have a global vision of the current landscape of photonic instruments used for dosimetry.

Five articles investigate new measuring systems and data analysis techniques for monitoring cardiac and/or respiratory activities, as well as syndromes related to their deficiencies [8–12]. In [8], the respiratory activity has been investigated as a parameter related to sleep disorders; the authors analyzed respiration and body movements by a non-contact technique, based on thermal imaging cameras, without disturbing human sleep. Their analysis was performed on 16 volunteers showing good performances in terms of respiratory rate estimation. In [9], a multi-sensor module to monitor the presence of breath by accelerometers, ECG, and SpO2 was proposed for monitoring patients affected by obstructive sleep apnea-hypopnea syndrome. The hardware solution was combined with novel neural network classification techniques for identifying obstructive sleep apnea. A further non-contact method for estimating the respiratory rate has been proposed in [10]. The system, consisting of a laptop's built-in RGB camera and a custom algorithm, was assessed on 12 healthy volunteers by comparing the results with a gold standard. The agreement between the proposed method, and the reference one was promising. The importance of cardio-respiratory monitoring was also investigated in precision sports [11]. The system was proposed to monitor respiratory rate and heart rate on archers, since the breathing and heartbeat can influence the stability and, thus, athlete's performance. A custom wearable system based on fiber optic sensors (i.e., fiber Bragg grating, FBG, sensors) was assessed on both 9 volunteers and in a real-life scenario on an archer during shooting session. The use of FBGs was also exploited for detecting pulse wave and estimating blood pressure in [12] and assessed on four healthy volunteers. The authors highlighted the importance of their solution to improve accuracy and repeatability in terms of pulse wave signal.

A second group of five papers propose methods to assess or predict patients' conditions by monitoring different parameters (e.g., physiological parameters, physiological behaviors, and motion behaviors) [13–17]. The first article explores the use of optical sensors for pressure ulcer prevention [13]. Data collected by the system were used as feedback of an active pressure relief system by regulating the air flow. The authors demonstrated that the proposed system is able to reduce the pressure in a scenario mimicking the real condition. The second article focuses on a torsional wave sensor for estimating the cervical elasticity on pregnant women [14]. This novel technique was evaluated on 18 single-pregnant women showing that it is safe and allows quantifying cervical shear stiffness. Moreover, results proved that cervical stiffness can be considered a valuable predictor of gestational age at the moment of evaluation. The third article proposes a measurement system based on fiber optic sensors to detect grasping actions in newborns [15]. The authors focused on fiber optic technology since it allowed developing an MR compatible system. This feature is important because the use of the proposed system during functional magnetic resonance imaging (fMRI) helps to relate the brain activity to the grasping actions. The combination of these two analyses may provide important insights on how functional outcomes can be improved following cerebral injury. In [16], authors proposed a novel method based on artificial neural networks to detect epileptic seizures using data of 30 subjects from a public database. EEG, submentalis and bilateral anterior tibialis EMG, and an earlobe PPG were used showing promising results in terms of detection of epileptic seizures. A custom EEG-electrode holder infrastructure is presented in [17]. A low-end consumer 3D printer was used to manufacture all the elements (e.g., sensor-positioning ring, inter-ring bridge, and bridge shield), and the practicability of the assembled headset was validated on fifteen volunteers demonstrating the potential of a cost-efficient electrode-holder assembly infrastructure.

Seven articles focused on patients' motor functions for potential application in rehabilitation or in the assessment of their functional impairment [18–23]. The first article proposes a novel contactless method, based on electrostatic field, for extracting gait features of hemiplegic patients [18], together with an improved version of the traditional detrended cross-correlation analysis to analyze the signal collected on 10 hemiparetic patients and 10 healthy volunteers. The authors found that the proposed method can quantify the gait difference between the hemiparetic patients and the healthy controls. The second paper proposes a solution to support medical personnel in the assessment of patients with spinal cord injury [19]. The authors present a system based on 3 RGB-D cameras (Microsoft Kinect v2) to assess patients' movements using a wheelchair. The system allows analyzing the pushing cycle, and other key movements useful to evaluate the patient's performance, thus, capable of supporting the clinician in the definition of the rehabilitation process. The system was assessed on patients for a total of 138 acquisitions showing promising results, also considering the low cost of the proposed system compared to the more expensive motion capture systems often used in similar applications. The third article finds its motivation in the development of a game-based system for upper-limb cerebral palsy [20]. The authors highlighted the importance of an accurate estimation of patient motor performance in order to have an effective game-based rehabilitation system. They used a Kinect sensor to monitor arm movements, focusing on the shoulder joint. The system was assessed on two groups of cerebral palsy and typically developing children showing good results in the movements evaluation of the right arm during the proposed rehabilitation sessions. The fourth article investigates a system for monitoring a medical exam (i.e., 30 s chair stand test) used to assess the functional status of elderly people [21]. The aim was to develop a system able to achieve the counts of sit-to-stand transitions without the supervision of a physician, and to guide the people through the whole exam via a home care application. The abovementioned count was performed by a simple wearable system based on an elastic band worn around the subject's leg. The system was assessed on seven elderly subjects showing the capability of the system to identify all the sit-to-stand transitions. The fifth work proposes a wearable system for monitoring body acceleration and electromyography on patients affected by multiple sclerosis [22]. The system was tested on 40 patients and 15 healthy volunteers during the timed 10 min walking test under three different conditions: standard (i.e., wearing shoes), reduced grip (i.e., wearing socks), and increased cognitive load (i.e., backward-counting dual-task). The knowledge of both muscle activity and kinematics during walking may be beneficial to monitor the disease progression and the efficiency of rehabilitation for multiple sclerosis patients. In addition, results showed that walking tests wearing socks should be discouraged to prevent falls for these patients. The sixth article of this group focuses on the impact that the simultaneous knowledge of morphology and muscle activation can have in understanding the impairment status, thus providing a targeted rehabilitation treatment [23]. The study investigates a method that uses the morphological information contained in the MRI scan to build an electrical lumped model of the conductive volume to provide an estimation of all muscles' activation. The last research paper of this group focuses on monitoring patients' activity by a wearable system based on three-axis accelerometer and a triple-axis gyroscope [24]. Data collected on the patients are intended to be used to adjust the oxygen flow delivered by portable oxygen concentrator in patients with COPD and respiratory failure. The system was assessed on 18 patients showing a significant reduction of the number of desaturation events.

A solution for dietary monitoring in terms of food mass and intake (FMI) based on a ring-type sensor has been proposed in [25]. This evaluation is important since the knowledge of FMI can be important to assess the physical condition of a person. The proposed solutions allowed the wearable system to optimize its sensitivity. The authors highlighted the potential of this solution to support the prevention of obesity and metabolic syndrome.

The development of a system based on multiple sensors (i.e., a magnetic door sensor, a motion detection sensor, and two time of flight sensors) to estimate the duration of patient-physician contact (consultation time) is the focus of [26]. The knowledge of this parameter may help in the optimization of the treatment processes and on the healthcare service. The system was assessed in two scenarios with preliminary experiments to evaluate the quality of the estimated time.

A mechatronic platform for detection of cancer nodules has been proposed in [27]. The system uses multi-sensors data providing mechanical stiffness and Ultrasound impedance of the tissue under exam. The system was assessed using phantoms mimicking diseased tissues showing promising results (the system correctly identified the tissue in the 90.3% of the cases).

The study reported in [28] grounds its motivation in the reduction of measurements error of a type of force/pressure sensor (i.e., force sensitive resistors, FSR) largely used in applications related to the pressure map at the interface of a prosthetic socket and a residual limb. Authors reported a regression-based method to calibrate these sensors considering different surfaces of contact (i.e., flat or curved surfaces). Different algorithms were assessed to improve the accuracy of this type of sensor.

The relevant problem in clinical practice of errors in the placement of ECG electrodes, that can cause significant signal changes, has been faced in [29]. The study proposed a method to simulate all possible ECG reversals and applied the proposed novel algebraic transformation in the standard 12-lead ECG setup.

The unique research paper with a novel system to assess the performance of sensors is reported in [30]. The study explores the development of a novel movement simulator devoted to assessing the performance of wearable systems for monitoring fetal movements. The rationale behind this study is motivated by the clinical importance of fetal movements to assess the fetal health and the difficulty of assessing the performance of the proposed system in preclinical stage.

In summary, the special issue "Smart Sensors for Healthcare and Medical Applications" reports a wide collection of articles focused on smart sensors and their applications in healthcare. The large part of the contributions is expected to consolidate the use of smart sensors in medicine and healthcare in order to support physiological monitoring, to assist rehabilitation processes, to validate medical devices, and to optimize performance of measuring systems in a variety of fields.

Author Contributions: D.F. and E.S. wrote and proofread the manuscript. All authors have read and agreed to the published version of the manuscript.

Funding: This research received no external funding.

Acknowledgments: Special thanks to all reviewers, anonymous servitors of science, and to all the contributors of the articles selected in this special session.

Conflicts of Interest: The authors declare no conflict of interest.

References

1. Bellagente, P.; Bona, M.; Gorni, D. The Use of Smart Sensors in Healthcare Applications: Review. *Appl. Mech. Mater.* **2015**, *783*, 29–41. [CrossRef]
2. Pramanik, P.K.D.; Upadhyaya, B.K.; Pal, S.; Pal, T. Internet of things, smart sensors, and pervasive systems: Ena-bling connected and pervasive healthcare. In *Healthcare Data Analytics and Management*; Academic Press: Cambridge, MA, USA, 2019; pp. 1–58.
3. Kim, J.; Campbell, A.S.; De Ávila, B.E.-F.; Wang, J. Wearable biosensors for healthcare monitoring. *Nat. Biotechnol.* **2019**, *37*, 389–406. [CrossRef]
4. Kenry; Yeo, J.C.; Lim, C.T. Emerging flexible and wearable physical sensing platforms for healthcare and biomedical applications. *Microsyst. Nanoeng.* **2016**, *2*, 16043. [CrossRef]
5. Andreu-Perez, J.; Leff, D.R.; Ip, H.M.D.; Yang, G.-Z. From Wearable Sensors to Smart Implants—Toward Pervasive and Personalized Healthcare. *IEEE Trans. Biomed. Eng.* **2015**, *62*, 2750–2762. [CrossRef] [PubMed]
6. Damulira, E.; Yusoff, M.N.S.; Omar, A.F.; Taib, N.H.M. A Review: Photonic Devices Used for Dosimetry in Medical Radiation. *Sensors* **2019**, *19*, 2226. [CrossRef] [PubMed]
7. Kron, T.; Lehmann, J.; Greer, P.B. Dosimetry of ionising radiation in modern radiation oncology. *Phys. Med. Biol.* **2016**, *61*, R167–R205. [CrossRef] [PubMed]
8. Jakkaew, P.; Onoye, T. Non-Contact Respiration Monitoring and Body Movements Detection for Sleep Using Thermal Imaging. *Sensors* **2020**, *20*, 6307. [CrossRef] [PubMed]
9. Chang, H.-C.; Wu, H.-T.; Huang, P.-C.; Ma, H.-P.; Lo, Y.-L.; Huang, Y.-H. Portable Sleep Apnea Syndrome Screening and Event Detection Using Long Short-Term Memory Recurrent Neural Network. *Sensors* **2020**, *20*, 6067. [CrossRef] [PubMed]
10. Massaroni, C.; Presti, D.L.; Formica, D.; Silvestri, S.; Schena, E. Non-Contact Monitoring of Breathing Pattern and Respiratory Rate via RGB Signal Measurement. *Sensors* **2019**, *19*, 2758. [CrossRef]
11. Lo Presti, D.; Romano, C.; Massaroni, C.; D'Abbraccio, J.; Massari, L.; Caponero, M.A.; Schena, E. Car-dio-respiratory monitoring in archery using a smart textile based on flexible fiber Bragg grating sensors. *Sensors* **2019**, *19*, 3581. [CrossRef]

12. Haseda, Y.; Bonefacino, J.; Tam, H.-Y.; Chino, S.; Koyama, S.; Ishizawa, H. Measurement of Pulse Wave Signals and Blood Pressure by a Plastic Optical Fiber FBG Sensor. *Sensors* **2019**, *19*, 5088. [CrossRef] [PubMed]
13. Lee, K.-H.; Kwon, Y.-E.; Lee, H.; Lee, Y.; Seo, J.; Kwon, O.; Kang, S.-W.; Lee, D. Active Body Pressure Relief System with Time-of-Flight Optical Pressure Sensors for Pressure Ulcer Prevention. *Sensors* **2019**, *19*, 3862. [CrossRef] [PubMed]
14. Massó, P.; Callejas, A.; Melchor, J.; Molina, F.S.; Rus, G. In Vivo Measurement of Cervical Elasticity on Pregnant Women by Torsional Wave Technique: A Preliminary Study. *Sensors* **2019**, *19*, 3249. [CrossRef] [PubMed]
15. Presti, D.L.; Dall'Orso, S.; Muceli, S.; Arichi, T.; Neumane, S.; Lukens, A.; Sabbadini, R.; Massaroni, C.; Caponero, M.A.; Formica, D.; et al. An fMRI Compatible Smart Device for Measuring Palmar Grasping Actions in Newborns. *Sensors* **2020**, *20*, 6040. [CrossRef]
16. Aileni, R.M.; Pasca, S.; Florescu, A. EEG-Brain Activity Monitoring and Predictive Analysis of Signals Using Arti-ficial Neural Networks. *Sensors* **2020**, *20*, 3346. [CrossRef] [PubMed]
17. Lin, Y.-P.; Chen, T.-Y.; Chen, W.-J. Cost-efficient and Custom Electrode-holder Assembly Infrastructure for EEG Recordings. *Sensors* **2019**, *19*, 4273. [CrossRef]
18. Tian, S.; Li, M.; Wang, Y.; Chen, X. Application of an Improved Correlation Method in Electrostatic Gait Recognition of Hemiparetic Patients. *Sensors* **2019**, *19*, 2529. [CrossRef]
19. Zefinetti, F.C.; Vitali, A.; Regazzoni, D.; Rizzi, C.; Molinero, G. Tracking and Characterization of Spinal Cord-Injured Patients by Means of RGB-D Sensors. *Sensors* **2020**, *20*, 6273. [CrossRef]
20. Daoud, M.I.; Alhusseini, A.; Ali, M.Z.; Alazrai, R. A Game-Based Rehabilitation System for Upper-Limb Cerebral Palsy: A Feasibility Study. *Sensors* **2020**, *20*, 2416. [CrossRef]
21. Cobo, A.; Villalba-Mora, E.; Pérez-Rodríguez, R.; Ferre, X.; Escalante, W.; Moral, C.; Rodriguez-Mañas, L. Auto-matic and Real-Time Computation of the 30-Seconds Chair-Stand Test without Professional Supervision for Communi-ty-Dwelling Older Adults. *Sensors* **2020**, *20*, 5813. [CrossRef]
22. Huang, S.-C.; Costa, G.D.; Pisa, M.; Gregoris, L.; Leccabue, G.; Congiu, M.; Comi, G.; Leocani, L. The Danger of Walking with Socks: Evidence from Kinematic Analysis in People with Progressive Multiple Sclerosis. *Sensors* **2020**, *20*, 6160. [CrossRef] [PubMed]
23. Piovanelli, E.; Piovesan, D.; Shirafuji, S.; Su, B.; Yoshimura, N.; Ogata, Y.; Ota, J. Towards a Simplified Estimation of Muscle Activation Pattern from MRI and EMG Using Electrical Network and Graph Theory. *Sensors* **2020**, *20*, 724. [CrossRef] [PubMed]
24. Sanchez-Morillo, D.; Muñoz-Zara, P.; Lara-Doña, A.; Leon-Jimenez, A. Automated Home Oxygen Delivery for Pa-tients with COPD and Respiratory Failure: A New Approach. *Sensors* **2020**, *20*, 1178. [CrossRef] [PubMed]
25. Hong, W.; Lee, J.; Lee, W.G. A Dual-Padded, Protrusion-Incorporated, Ring-Type Sensor for the Measurement of Food Mass and Intake. *Sensors* **2020**, *20*, 5623. [CrossRef]
26. Gabl, R.; Stummer, F. Development of a Sensor to Measure Physician Consultation Times. *Sensors* **2019**, *19*, 5359. [CrossRef]
27. Massari, L.; Bulletti, A.; Prasanna, S.; Mazzoni, M.; Frosini, F.; Vicari, E.; Messerini, L. A Mechatronic Platform for Computer Aided Detection of Nodules in Anatomopathological Analyses via Stiffness and Ultrasound Measure-ments. *Sensors* **2019**, *19*, 2512. [CrossRef]
28. Ahmadizadeh, C.; Menon, C. Investigation of Regression Methods for Reduction of Errors Caused by Bending of FSR-Based Pressure Sensing Systems Used for Prosthetic Applications. *Sensors* **2019**, *19*, 5519. [CrossRef]
29. Krasteva, V.; Jekova, I.; Schmid, R. Simulating Arbitrary Electrode Reversals in Standard 12-lead ECG. *Sensors* **2019**, *19*, 2920. [CrossRef]
30. Ghosh, A.K.; Burniston, S.F.; Krentzel, D.; Roy, A.; Sheikh, A.S.; Siddiq, T.; Trinh, P.M.P.; Velazquez, M.M.; Vielle, H.-T.; Nowlan, N.C.; et al. A Novel Fetal Movement Simulator for the Performance Evaluation of Vibration Sensors for Wearable Fetal Movement Monitors. *Sensors* **2020**, *20*, 6020. [CrossRef]

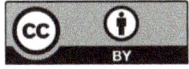

© 2021 by the authors. Licensee MDPI, Basel, Switzerland. This article is an open access article distributed under the terms and conditions of the Creative Commons Attribution (CC BY) license (http://creativecommons.org/licenses/by/4.0/).

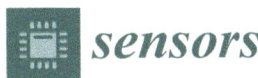

Review

A Review: Photonic Devices Used for Dosimetry in Medical Radiation

Edrine Damulira [1,*], Muhammad Nur Salihin Yusoff [1,*], Ahmad Fairuz Omar [2] and Nur Hartini Mohd Taib [3]

1. Medical Radiation Programme, School of Health Sciences, Universiti Sains Malaysia, Kubang Kerian 16150, Malaysia
2. Engineering Physics Laboratory, School of Physics, Universiti Sains Malaysia, Penang 11800, Malaysia; fairuz_omar@usm.my
3. Department of Radiology, School of Medical Sciences, Universiti Sains Malaysia, Kubang Kerian 16150, Malaysia; nhartini@usm.my
* Corresponding: edudam@outlook.com (E.D.); mnsalihin@usm.my (M.N.S.Y.)

Received: 9 March 2019; Accepted: 9 May 2019; Published: 14 May 2019

Abstract: Numerous instruments such as ionization chambers, hand-held and pocket dosimeters of various types, film badges, thermoluminescent dosimeters (TLDs) and optically stimulated luminescence dosimeters (OSLDs) are used to measure and monitor radiation in medical applications. Of recent, photonic devices have also been adopted. This article evaluates recent research and advancements in the applications of photonic devices in medical radiation detection primarily focusing on four types; photodiodes – including light-emitting diodes (LEDs), phototransistors—including metal oxide semiconductor field effect transistors (MOSFETs), photovoltaic sensors/solar cells, and charge coupled devices/charge metal oxide semiconductors (CCD/CMOS) cameras. A comprehensive analysis of the operating principles and recent technologies of these devices is performed. Further, critical evaluation and comparison of their benefits and limitations as dosimeters is done based on the available studies. Common factors barring photonic devices from being used as radiation detectors are also discussed; with suggestions on possible solutions to overcome these barriers. Finally, the potentials of these devices and the challenges of realizing their applications as quintessential dosimeters are highlighted for future research and improvements.

Keywords: radiation-induced current; dosimetry; photodiodes; phototransistors (MOSFETs); photovoltaic sensor; CCD/CMOS

1. Introduction

Radiation can be classified into mainly two, i.e., charged particle radiation that consists of fast electrons and heavy charged particles, and uncharged radiation that comprises electromagnetic radiation and neutrons [1]. In radiation spectroscopy, both these radiation types interact with matter in different ways, hence, the need for radiation measurement and monitoring in order to control its effects in the matter accordingly. Today, radiation is used for carrying out radiotherapeutic or imaging procedures like Computed Tomography (CT)—in the field of medicine [2]. However, during its applications, there has to be precaution since excessive radiation attenuation by human tissue may result into high absorbed dose values [3,4]. This could be a root cause of secondary malignancies [4]. Therefore, stringent measures to control and manage both intentional and unintentional radiation exposures through radiation dosimetry is necessary.

Medical radiation dosimetry involves measurement, calculation, and assessment of the quantity and quality of ionizing radiation exposed to and attenuated by the human body. Various gas, liquid and solid-state dosimeters are used to quantify radiation; these are predominantly grouped under the ionization chamber, semiconductor and diamond detector types [5,6]. These detectors are used to measure radiation delivered internally (in-vivo)—by ingesting or inhaling radioactive substances, and externally using external beam radiation therapy.

X-rays are electromagnetic waves with a wavelength shorter than that of ultra violet light but longer than that of gamma rays. X-rays, and other electromagnetic waves such as visible light, are also discrete energy packets known as photons/quanta. Quantization of X-rays could therefore make X-ray photons show characteristics of high-energy particles. In X-ray radiation detection, detection efficiency is the ratio of the number of counts in the detector's spectrum to the number of photons emitted by the radiation source [7]. High density and the atomic number of a radiation detector material imply higher sensitivity of the detector [8]. Comparing silicon's density; 2.3 gcm^{-3} to that of air; 1.3×10^{-3}gcm^{-3}, Romei et al. [9] state that solid-state detectors avail the same overall detection efficiency as that of gas detectors; for instance, semiconductor detectors need less energy to form an electron-hole pair compared to ionization chambers [9]. This way, applications of solid-state dosimeters in radiation detection has become recurrent in recent technologies. At an atomic level, atoms in the solid state are close to each other. On the other hand, atoms are fairly far apart from each other in gases and liquids. This makes solids to be with a higher density when compared to liquids and gases. During radiation detection, if a radiation photon strikes an atom, electrons are excited into the conduction band-hence a detectable current signal. On the other hand, when the radiation photon strikes the interatomic spacing, there will be less/no energy absorbed by the atomic electrons, hence low/no electron excitations. Consequently, there is a low detectable current signal. Therefore, a radiation photon strikes more atoms in solids than in liquids and gases. This way, solid-state detectors provide a higher resolution and sensitivity during radiation detection, i.e., if compared to liquid-state detectors and ionization chambers [2].

In particular, the semiconductor solid-state detectors mainly comprise photonic devices; circuit board components of electronic gadgets that are used for production and detection of electromagnetic radiation. Photodiodes, phototransistors, and CCDs are some of the semiconductor-based photonic devices that have profoundly been used for producing, detecting and manipulating light. Light has a wavelength range of 440–800 nm [10,11]. Nevertheless, these photonic devices are also sensitive to other ranges of the electromagnetic spectrum. Therefore, current researches aim to exploit this capability. For instance, silicon photodiodes can detect radiations having wavelengths shorter than 1.2 µm, i.e., visible and ultraviolet light, and some wavelengths near infrared radiation [12].

Using equations, schematics, and graphs, a detailed explication of the photonic device structure and physics is presented in the form of benefits and limitations as dosimeters. Further, factors such as minimum and maximum measurable dose, ability to give real-time measurements, reduction in sensitivity after radiation exposure, and price among others are examined. This is aimed at providing a comparative analysis of these photonic devices as medical radiation detectors since there is currently no study that has addressed this type of contradistinction.

This article, therefore, benchmarks; photodiodes, phototransistors/ MOSFETs, solar cells, and CCDs for accurate and effective medical radiation detection and measurement. This work is based on previous and current researches by different authors and ultimately aims at facilitating the development of alternative dosimeters to improvise for the conventional medical radiation dosimeters that are quite costly.

2. Photodiodes/LEDs

A photodiode is a semiconductor-based electrical device that converts photonic energy, in the form of electromagnetic radiation, to a detectable electrical signal in the form of current or voltage (Figure 1a). LEDs are also semiconductor-based devices. However, LEDs convert electrical energy—in the form of current, to light (photons); through the electroluminescence process [13]. To a greater extent, most of the semiconductor-based photodiodes and LEDs consist of silicon PN junctions. Today, photodiodes are typically used for signal detection [9,14–16] while LEDs are principally used for luminescence [13]. However, some novel studies have directly manipulated LEDs for electromagnetic radiation detection (sensing) [11,17–20].

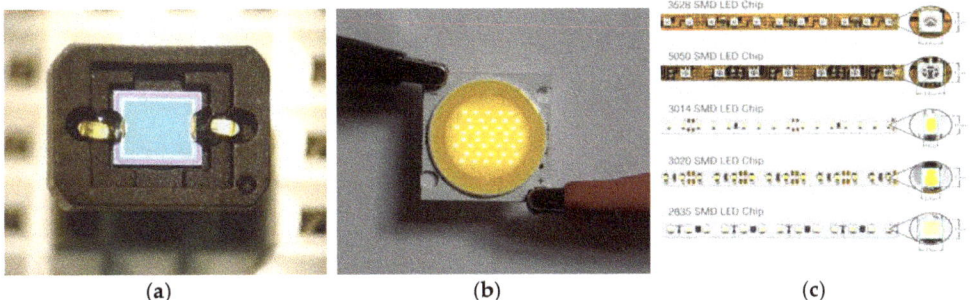

Figure 1. Images of some of the semiconductor-based photonic devices (**a**) Photodiode [21]; (**b**) chip on board light-emitting diode (COB LED) [22]; (**c**) surface mount diodes light-emitting diode (SMD LED) [23].

Photodiodes can be broadly classified into four, i.e., PN photodiodes; consisting of a heavily positive semiconductor (P) affixed to a heavily negative semiconductor (N) to form a junction, PIN photodiodes; comprising a PN junction with an intrinsic region sandwiched between the P and N semiconductors in order to increase detection volume [14], Avalanche photodiodes (APDs): Photodiodes that are very sensitive to relatively low intensity electromagnetic radiation due to their high precision and gain capability [24], and Schottky photodiodes: Photodiodes associated with appreciably low operational capacitance [25].

Recent technologies deploy surface mount diodes (SMDs) and chip on board LEDs (COB LEDs). SMDs and COBs are multiple sole LEDs adhered onto a printed circuit board to form one compatible unit as shown in Figure 1b,c. COBs have more chips/LEDs, hence, provide more luminescence than SMDs; they also consume less energy [26].

2.1. Structure

Silicon being a group four element, comprises of four valence electrons in its outer most shell. This way, a silicon atom makes covalent bonds by sharing electrons with the neighbouring atoms. The sharing could be among the silicon atoms themselves or even atoms of a different element - through the doping process [13]. Therefore, pure/intrinsic silicon is almost incapable of conducting current naturally [13,27]. It has gotten few/no free electrons in the conduction band but has gotten more holes in the valence band as shown by Figure 2a [13]. Nonetheless, conduction could still occur due to crystal defects or thermal excitation [27]. Current electronic applications mostly deploy doped silicon. In doped silicon, the sharing atoms are from either group 3 or group 5. During the bonding process, electron sharing creates an electron deficiency; if the sharing atoms are from group 3, or an excess of electrons; if the sharing atoms are from group 5 [13,27]. A deficiency creates holes [13] which are free and move around just like the excess electrons. After the bonding process, the loss of excess electrons leaves a positive charge on the impurity atoms while the gain of an electron leaves a negative charge on the impurity atoms. Therefore, a region where there is an excess of the negatively charged electrons becomes an N region: N-type doped semiconductor, while a region with an excess of positively charged holes becomes the P region: P-type doped semiconductor [13,27].

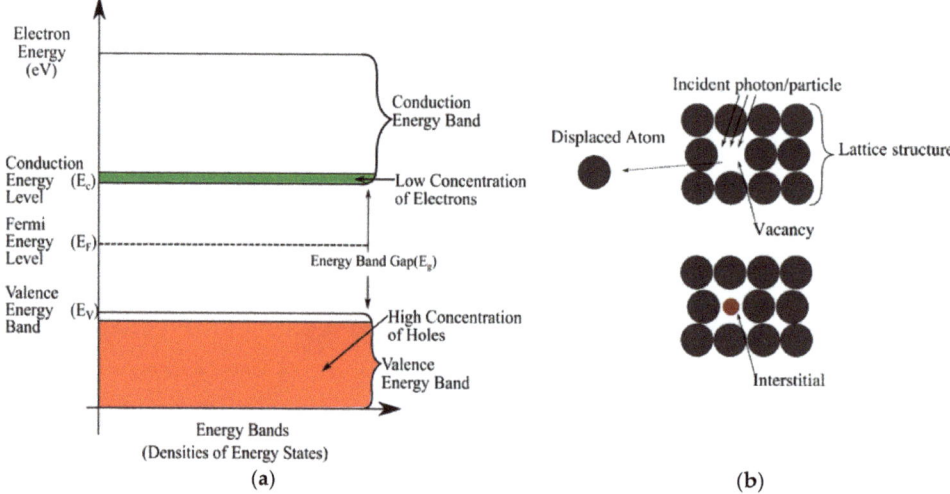

Figure 2. (**a**) Semiconductor Energy Bands; (**b**) lattice structure Vacancies and Interstitials.

When the P and N types are in contact, electrons in the N region move across to the P region to make recombinations with the holes [13]. At this junction, the impurity atoms get depleted of charges that results in an electric field due to their positive and negative polarization. The electric field has an associated electric potential that ceases further charge flow across the junction. Therefore, this results in a necessity for an external potential, bias, for charges to travel across the junction [28]. This applied potential should be in opposition to the intrinsic region's electric field potential. Charges are not only stimulated electrically with the potential bias [13] but also thermally [10,29], and optically [30]. PN junctions are the main components of semiconductor devices as shown in Figure 3a.

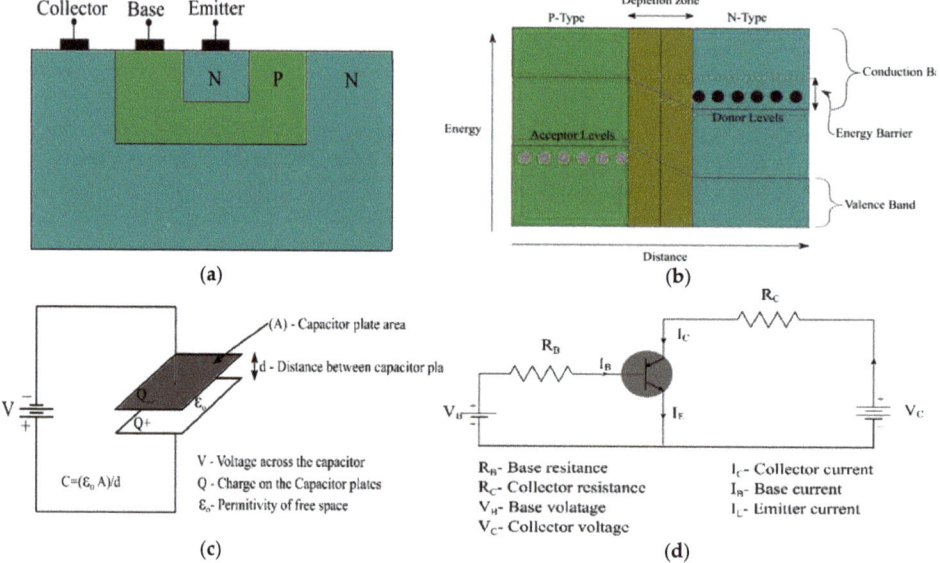

Figure 3. (**a**) Cross-section of an NPN transistor (similar to that of a photodiode); (**b**) an unbiased PN Junction; (**c**) a parallel plate capacitor; (**d**) an NPN transistor circuit diagram.

2.2. Functionality and Operational Principle

The operation of LEDs is based on electrical stimulation/ electroluminescence; electrons gain electrical energy and drift towards holes that results into recombinations [13]. During these recombinations, energy equivalent to the semiconductor material's energy band gap is dissipated off in the form of light photons [13]. There is also a direct proportionality between the electrical energy applied and the photonic light produced by LEDs, i.e., more current leads to more charge recombinations, hence, the production of more light and vice versa [13]. Transposition of these processes explains the working principle of photodiodes. Here, the charges receive energy in the form of electromagnetic radiation that makes electrons drift towards the holes.

This charge flow creates an internal electric field that ceases the further flow of charge, hence, establishing an equilibrium in the depletion region of the PN junction. Therefore, an external positive or negative potential has to be applied against the newly-present internal potential; so that electrons and holes move across the junction again. This positive or negative potential is also termed as forward or reverse biasing depending on its orientation. In the forward biasing of a PN junction, the positive bias voltage repels the holes on the P side. Similarly, the negative bias voltage repels the electrons on the N side. These repulsions from both the negative and positive bias voltages make the charges overcome the internal electric field potential in the depletion zone (Figure 3b). This makes charges eventually flow over the junction, hence, the operation of a PN junction. In contrast, during the reverse bias, the positive bias voltage attracts the electrons from the N side while the negative bias voltage also attracts the holes from the P side; that results in no charge flow across the junction.

Despite the reverse bias, some random charges can still overcome the electric field potential in the depletion zone. This random charge flow over the junction leads to a current flow termed as a leakage/dark current. This dark current flow during the reverse bias gives a clue to the intuition of radiation detection by a PN junction, i.e., medical radiation detection using a reversely biased PN junction. When photons fall on a reversely biased PN junction, their energy is absorbed by the electrons in the N region. Due to this energy absorption, electrons overcome the depletion region's electric field potential thus formulation of recombinations. From Equation (1) [16], an electrical current *(I)* is a result of summing up (integrating) all the small charges, *(dq)*, flowing per unit time *(dt)*. The current *(I)* can also be defined as the rate of charge flow. An induced measurable photocurrent [31] can be used to depict the nature of photonic energy that induced it. The generated electrical signal may be of small magnitude or incompatible to the measuring device (ammeter/ multimeter). Therefore, a photocurrent may not be directly sensed by a detector device. In this case, amplification has to be done to produce a measurable electrical current [25,32,33]. Medical radiation detection using PN junction-based dosimeters exploits this principle to measure and characterize the quality and quantity of radiation striking the dosimeter; the characterization is based on the induced photocurrent.

$$I = \frac{dq}{dt} \quad (1)$$

2.3. Present Literature

The ability of PIN photodiodes to detect mammography and radiology clinical beams are examined in a study by Romei et al. [9]. Here, reproducible linearity, system sensitivity, diode batch-to-batch reproducibility, and the correlation between diode read-out and absorbed dose are investigated using an S2506-02 photodiode [9]. A Monte Carlo simulation was also performed to investigate the effect of the photodiode casing during the measurement of low energy radiations. As highlighted in Section 2.2, there was a need for an amplification stage in order to acquire the signal in the current mode [9].

PIN diodes were also evaluated for detection of diagnostic radiology clinical beams while using a standard reference as calibration [34]. A linear correlation between the PIN photodiode read-out and the dose measured with standard dosimeters was observed [34]. In this study, satisfactory sensitivity;

in accordance with the read-out dose values, small size, and being cost effective are highlighted as the advantages of using PIN photodiodes [34].

Further, a BPW34FS photodiode was benchmarked for; angular dependence-variation of the output signal according to the radiation beam angle of incidence, energy dependence, dose linearity, and sensitivity degradation (due to accumulated dose) using computed tomography X-rays [35]. Its response was then compared to those of the OP520 and OP521 phototransistors [35]. Air kerma/energy dependence response for all of the three devices implied the need for calibration for each device. All the three device signals were also highly dependent on the angle of incidence of the radiation beam [35]. The photodiode had low sensitivity that was unaffected by increased X-ray exposure [35]. The transistors' high sensitivity also considerably plummets with an increased absorbed dose; this presented a need for calibration in order to obtain accurate results following continued exposures [35].

SFH206, BPW34, SFH205, and BPX90F PIN photodiodes were also examined for application as radio-protection detectors in radiology [14]. The examination was based on the minimum sensitive area (5 mm^2), half angle (60°), and low-cost as comparison criteria [14]. This was because these devices are inexpensive and have a small volume [14]. Photodiodes are also defined as direct-reading real-time dosimeters, and their responsiveness to x and gamma rays, air kerma/absorbed dose linearity, and repeatability were analysed [14].

In addition, current mode S1223, BPW34, and PS100-6-CER2 PIN photodiodes were also appraised as real-time gamma radiation detectors while using photodiodes of different active areas and varying the number of diodes connected in parallel [15]. The assessment was done by deducing the photocurrent-dose rate, and accumulated charge-absorbed dose relationship [15]. A customized computer-based electrometer, that could measure photoinduced currents as low as 50 pA with considerably low errors, was also used. In this study, the photodiode's induced current was linear with the dose rate while the accumulated charge was also linear with the absorbed dose [15]. The current response of the devices could be estimated with a function that is based on the dose rate and the photodiode's detection volume, i.e., the product of the active area and depletion layer width [15].

2.4. Benefits, Limitations and Challenges as Potential dosimeters

Accurate detection and measurement of radiation-induced photocurrent is paramount and the ability to perform this is termed as sensitivity. Photodiode sensitivity can be enhanced by increasing the device's sensitive area; to ensure more accurate results in medical radiation applications. However, this is related to an adverse effect of increasing the capacitance [14]. From Equation (2) [16], while assuming a parallel plate capacitor [18] with constant charge, the capacitance is inversely proportional to the applied voltage. It can also be observed from Equation (3) [15,16] that area-A (sensitive area) is directly proportional to the capacitance thus an increase in the area increases the capacitance. Therefore, due to the inverse proportionality between the capacitance and the voltage, there is an output signal-voltage amplitude drop associated with an increase in the area [14]. In other words, the parameter that affects the PIN photodiode's photocurrent most is the active detection volume [28]. The detection volume is a product of the active area and the depletion region's width [15]. While the active area is constant, the depletion layer can be varied by the amount of the reverse bias voltage [15]. This however increases the leakage/dark current that eventually affects the minimum dose rate (current) that can be measured [15]. A study by authors [14] also suggests combining the photodiodes in parallel (tiling) to increase the detection area. However, they further explicate that increasing the sensitivity this way has a cost of increasing the capacitance; hence a low voltage output signal.

$$Q = CV \quad (2)$$

Q-Charge on capacitor plates, C- Capacitance of the capacitor, V-Voltage across the capacitor plates

$$C = \frac{\varepsilon A}{d} \quad (3)$$

C-Capacitance, ε-Dielectric constant, d-Distance between the capacitor plates, A-Area of the capacitor plates

PIN photodiodes have a higher quantum efficiency over other current read-out sensors [15]. This infers that a higher fraction of the incident photon beam contributes to the photocurrent [14,36]. The PIN photodiode's wide intrinsic region has high charge densities [37] that implies many charge carriers per photon that strikes this region [14]. There are no electrons filling the outermost energy bands in this intrinsic region, hence charges prefer filling up these empty energy bands; a phenomenon that results in a high charge concentration in this region.

Compared to ionization chambers, semiconductor detectors also have a higher signal-to-noise ratio, i.e., they require lower average energy to create a pair of charge carriers [9]. This could also imply high sensitivity to low energy radiation thus increase in the measurable range. Although photodiodes may give a small signal to radiation exposure, they are preferred because accuracy is crucial in dosimetry; photodiodes produce a pure signal with less noise [35].

Some attributes of an efficient medical radiation dosimeter include; having a wide dose-measurement range, high accuracy levels, giving a real-time response to radiation exposure, and being user-friendly [9]. The radiation-induced current of photodiodes only flows during radiation exposure, thus giving a direct measurement/output electric signal [14]. This implies that photodiodes are active and real-time dosimeters [15]. Therefore, photodiodes are preferred to passive dosimeters like the TLDs [15]. This is because the absorbed dose of the TLDs could be affected by fading during the time between radiation exposure and measurement; that leads to inaccuracy in measurements.

Photodiodes can be termed as hard dosimeters because their loss of sensitivity after radiation exposure is negligible [35]. In other words, they have higher repeatability [15]. In dosimetry, repeatability refers to the extent to which the dosimeter gives stable/constant results following successive/consecutive radiation exposures - keeping all parameters constant [16]. This is a key feature for dosimeters since they are repeatedly used for dose measurements in different sessions. Therefore, the ability to give unwavering readings is pivotal.

Since dosimeters measure the radiation received by the body, their structural composition relative to the human body should be taken into consideration. Silicon's atomic number-14 is different from that of human tissue-approximately 7.4 [9]; therefore, both silicon and human tissue are associated with different chemical interactions. However, silicon may still be used for dosimetry of x and gamma rays, interacting with human tissue, by applying calibration factors [9].

PINs are vulnerable to atomic displacements in their lattice structure [38]. These displacements are due to absorbed dose/ photon energy of the incident beam as shown in Figure 2b. Increase in displacements could imply an increase in dark currents [15], but these damages in the PIN's structure may be negligible. For instance, the lowest measurable photocurrent level for each sample in [15]'s study was more than two orders of magnitude higher than the nominal dark current before radiation exposure [15]. Considerably high dark current levels could, however, limit the minimum measurable level of radiation-induced photocurrent [15]. This is because the low energy radiations won't be able to stimulate electrons and holes from the dosimetric traps [30]. Eventually, the post-recombination current signal will be weaker/lower than the pre-existing dark current signal: Unmeasurable.

Since an increase in the dark currents leads to a decrease in the photocurrent, periodic recalibration has to be carried out to ensure long term stability and accuracy. This is supported by the finding that states that the level of sensitivity loss as a function of radiation damage depends on the photodiode's characteristics, the energy of the source, and the total absorbed dose [15].

Increase in ambient temperature also leads to a relative increase in the leakage current; the charge drift is stimulated by the heat energy. Yukihara [30] also observes a significant charge concentration (signal) decrease at room temperature. This is because the heat energy could easily stimulate the charges out of shallow traps. Recombinations of these charges from shallow traps produce dark currents; shallow traps are situated close to energy levels at the edge of the conduction and valence bands [30].

3. Phototransistors

Since photonic devices emit, detect, and manipulate light, devices such as metal–oxide–semiconductor field-effect transistors (MOSFETs), bipolar joint transistor (BJT), vertical double-diffused MOSFETs (VDMOSFETs), and transistors are not considered as photonic devices. Although this paper mainly focuses on photonic devices, this section also includes MOSFETs, BJT, VDMOSFET, RADFETs and transistors because they have the same structure, operation principles, and are often compared to photonic devices during medical radiation detection.

3.1. Structure

Phototransistors consist of a PN junction in the NPN format (Figure 3a)-similar to photodiodes and transistors. The only difference between photodiodes and phototransistors is that the phototransistor base section (P) is sensitive to the photons of light that strike it [11]. Since transistors are fundamentally amplifiers, they multiply the base current with a gain factor giving rise to an amplified collector current. Therefore, if the base of the transistor is photosensitive, amplified photocurrent signals will be produced as collector currents. Phototransistors are therefore defined as optoelectronic devices commonly constituting two relatively thick N-type sandwiching a thin P-type semiconductor material layer [39]. The NPN junction sections are emitter, base, and collector, respectively [16]. These sections are named according to the roles they play in electron transmission across the junction. In reference to Figure 3a, both the base and the collector are bigger than the emitter. The base inputs charge into the junction and on the other hand, the collector gathers charge out of the junction. Further, the collector is bigger than the base thus collects and takes into account all of the emitted charge without omitting any; this implies high sensitivity. Andjelković and Ristić also state that the base-collector junction is the sensitive volume of the phototransistor and is deliberately made longer than the base-emitter to achieve high sensitivity to the incident radiation [16].

3.2. Functionality and Operational Principle

Exposure of phototransistors to radiation stimulates the flow of a charge/photocurrent in them. This charge/photocurrent is a record of the type of radiation that induced it. Therefore, accurate quantification, evaluation and measurement of all collected charge guarantees accurate backtracking to the radiation that induces this charge/photocurrent. The product of the photocurrent and the time taken to collect this photocurrent is equivalent to the charge collected by the sensor during this time. This accumulated charge is proportional to the absorbed dose [15]. In addition, if there is a linear relationship between the intensity of the radiation-induced current and the dose rate, the intensity of the radiation-induced current is equivalent to the dose rate [15]. The radiation-induced photocurrent will be stable and proportional to the dose rate as long as the incident radiation dose rate is high enough during exposure [16].

3.3. Present Literature

Gamma radiation from a Co-60 source was detected with a collector-emitter biased NPN phototransistor [16]. The accumulated charge-absorbed dose relationship, dose rate effect on the induced current, short term repeatability, and stability of induced current were assessed. The radiation-induced current was stable with a less than 5% uncertainty and the induced charge was considerably good with a less than 3% uncertainty [16]. A notable current fall after an absorbed dose of 20 Gy was however observed; this was attributed to the radiation-induced lattice structural damages [16,38]. A non-linear relationship between the absorbed dose and the accumulated charge was also noticed; this was similarly due to the current gain damages [16]. The results of this study recommended the use of an NPN phototransistor because of its high sensitivity, linear induced current-dose rate relationship, and minimal dose rate dependence on charge sensitivity [16].

Radiation Field Effect Transistors (RADFETs) are p-channel metal oxide semiconductor transistors purposely manufactured for radiation detection. RADFETs were compared to a p-channel VDMOSFETs for radiation detection by analysing the radiation-induced threshold voltage alteration; the threshold voltages change after radiation exposure [40]. Here, the threshold voltage shift and radiation dose exhibited a linear dependence on each other when a +10v gate bias was applied [40]. The p-channel power VDMOSFETs responded more to radiation exposures than the RADFETs – there was a higher threshold voltage shift. This was attributed to more fixed traps that are induced by gamma radiation [40]. Fading was also examined at room temperature and it was more eminent in VDMOSFETs than in RADFETs [40].

In breast cancer radiotherapy treatment, bipolar junction transistors were tested as radiation detectors despite the fact that they are affected by accumulated dose structural damages [39]. Similar to the threshold voltage shift technique used in VDMOSFETs, this study uses the current amplification factor (β) shift to determine the absorbed dose – radiation absorption alters the value of β. Therefore, radiation is quantified and characterized according to the change in the value of β. In particular, a Darlington type BJT was used since it has a higher gain compared to other BJTs; its gain is a product of two BJTs-$\beta_1 \beta_2$ [41]. This high gain ultimately implies a high response/sensitivity to low energy radiations [39].

Another study also tested the accuracy of MOSFETs in the detection of radiotherapy absorbed dose [42]. The MOSFET dose calculations were ascertained by referring to the Monaco and MasterPlan pre-treatment plans of different anatomical regions; this was aimed at ensuring synchrony between the planned and actual absorbed dose [42].

RADFETs can't provide real-time/ online dose information using conventional methods. Therefore, they were configured as a PN junction, i.e., the gate, drain and source terminals (Figure 4) were inactivated /grounded. Co-60 gamma radiation-induced current was thereafter measured from the bulk terminal [28]. The radiation induced-currents were stable and progressively increased with the increase in the bias voltage of up to 30V [41]. While the current increased with the dose rate in accordance with the power law, its read-out sensitivity was linear to the applied bias voltage [38,41]. This led to an overall performance that is relatively similar to that of the PN photodiodes; additionally, the device is unsusceptible to radiation-induced lattice structural damages [38,41].

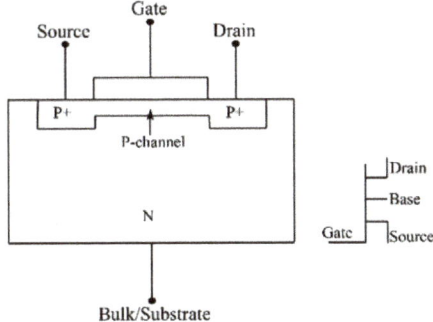

Figure 4. Depletion mode p-channel MOSFET.

While examining reproducibility, dose linearity, energy dependence, and fading, MOSFETs were investigated for in-vivo applications using an Alderson phantom [43]. The radiation-induced current signal was linear with applied doses between 0.2 and 2 Gy of the absorbed dose [43]. From the attained results, there was minimal temperature dependence between 22 and 40 °C, and the beam angle variation was within 5% [43]. The MOSFET's in-vivo dosimetry was applicable in the 80 kV–250 kV range, and reproducibility was observed as a function of the absorbed dose [43]. The measured signal also faded/reduced as the time between radiation exposure and measurement increased [43].

3.4. Benefits, Limitations and Challenges as Potential Dosimeters

Santos et al. [44] demonstrated that phototransistors have good read-out stability for low energy radiation (Diagnostic range) [44]. However, they exhibit a high sensitivity loss during high energy radiation exposure; doses up to 100 Gy [16]. Furthermore, phototransistors have a higher current gain/higher sensitivity in comparison to PIN photodiodes, but they experience faster sensitivity loss with respect to the absorbed dose; this is due to the gain degradation [44]. In Figure 3d, the small base current I_B is amplified by the gain factor of the phototransistor-β; β is the ratio of the collector current I_C to the base current I_B. Typical current gains for phototransistors range from a hundred to several thousands [16]. A higher transistor gain factor, therefore, corresponds to the multiplication of the base current with a bigger value in order to obtain the collector current. This way, the phototransistor amplifies the small radiation-induced photocurrent, I_B, to a greater value, I_C, hence, higher sensitivity and good read-out stability for low energy radiation [44]. The main advantage of phototransistors over the photodiodes is this inherent current gain which brings the benefit of higher sensitivity to incident radiation [16].

This sensitivity can even be further augmented by increasing the bias voltage [45], i.e., the collector-emitter voltage. This consequently enhances the collection efficiency [16]. For investigating the emitter-collector capacitance, a parallel plate capacitor will be analogized. Since the emitter-base junction is considerably smaller than the collector-base junction, the emitter-collector capacitance will be assumed to be the collector-base junction capacitance [16]. The total charge on the parallel plate capacitor plates in Figure 3c is given by Equation (2) [16].

In Equation (3) [15,16], ε is the dielectric constant of the material between the capacitor plates. ε is equivalent to ε_0 if the dielectric material between the capacitor plates is air. Substitution of Equation (3) [15,16] in Equation (2) [16] makes the distance d between the capacitor plates directly proportional to the applied voltage V; with ($\varepsilon A/Q$) as the proportionality constant. An increase in the voltage across the capacitor, therefore, implies that d increases relatively. This thickness-d is related to the depletion layer of the capacitor - as stated by Anđelković [16]. In a study by Oliveira [14], this depletion layer implies the intrinsic region in PIN diodes [14]. Therefore, a wide intrinsic region implies many charge carriers per photon; this optimizes the device's sensitivity. However, an increment in the depletion layer by increasing the voltage [45,46] is associated with an increase in dark currents; Figure 3 of Anđelković [16] clearly elaborates the dark current increment of various transistors [16]. Despite the fact that the transistors are of different brands, the dark current effects showed the same trend they appreciably increased with the increase in the collector-emitter voltage. Therefore, the increase in the bias voltage and structural damages increase dark currents.

Similar to photodiodes, dark currents of phototransistors determine their minimum measurable dose rate [16]. For higher precision during dose rate and absorbed dose rate measurements, the difference between the measured current and dark currents should be as large as possible. This is because the induced current is the difference between the measured and dark currents [16]. Therefore, if the radiation-induced current is low, effectively differentiating it from the already existing dark currents will involve some inaccuracies. This implies that a phototransistor will measure only radiations that can produce photocurrents with values above the dark currents. Therefore, low energy radiations producing photocurrents below the dark current can't be measured by the device; the induced currents are calculated by subtracting the dark current from the measured current [16]. Therefore, the difference between the measured and dark currents should be reasonably large to enhance precise current measurements [16]. A dark current can hence be termed as the "phototransistor's induced-current threshold value" since only radiations that can produce currents above the threshold value can be measured. A phototransistor with a high threshold value has a limited measurable dose range, i.e., only radiations with enough energy to induce currents above the high threshold value will be detectable [37]. On the other hand, transistors with a low threshold value have a wide measurable dose range (high sensitivity). This is because low energy radiations can also induce currents above the relatively low threshold value, hence, being measurable. In practice, [16] states that the photovoltaic mode is preferred since it ensures a low dark current [16]. The low dark currents imply a low threshold value that increases detectable and measurable energy ranges, hence, high sensitivity.

In comparison to photodiodes, phototransistors are more susceptible to radiation damage. Therefore, phototransistors have a faster sensitivity degradation with respect to an absorbed dose; this is because of radiation-induced displacement defects in the Si bulk [16]. A displacement effect is when an incident radiation or particle dislodges a lattice atom from its normal location through the Rutherford/nuclear elastic and nuclear inelastic scattering processes. This results into a vacancy; non-existence of an atom in its lattice vicinity, and an interstitial; the existence of an atom in a lattice structure vicinity where it is not meant to be (Figure 2b) [36,47]. An increase in these defects implies an increase in the density of the recombination centres; this reduces the minority carrier lifetime [36,46]—time taken by a minority carrier to recombine. Consequently, there is a decrease of the current gain [16] because there was an increase in the leakage current; resulting from an increase in the density of the generation-recombination centres [48]. In other words, the creation of more recombination centres in the form of isolated and clustered defects [47] could be assumed to be diluting the charge concentration. This is because an increase in these centres will make the constant charges numbers to be less compared to the newly increased number of recombination centres. Therefore, charges will have more room to easily recombine from anywhere thus reduced minor carrier lifetime; this finally results into low currents. Despite this degradation due to the absorbed dose, phototransistors could still be used as dosimeters while applying a correction factor; because they have a higher sensitivity to radiation [35].

MOSFETs also consist of a PN junction, but they have a metal oxide layer as their sensitive/radiation detection region [28]. Therefore, MOSFETs with a thick metal oxide layer have more hole-trapping centres; this implies higher responsivity [49]. When both the MOSFET source and drain terminals are grounded, the radiation sensitive field effect transistor version of MOSFETs could be considered as two P^+/N junctions connected in parallel [28]. MOSFETs are used in radiation detection, but the p-channel MOSFETs (RADFETs) are preferred over current mode dosimeters. This is because they are portable compared to diodes and photodiodes, and their sensitivity could be boosted with bias voltage applications – just like for diodes and photodiodes [28]. Similar to PN junctions [28], incident radiation on the metal oxide layer of the MOSFET immediately leads to the formation of electron-hole pairs [45]. This is followed by the attraction of all the electrons to the aluminium gate plate by the positive voltage bias; a condition that leads to a high hole concentration [40]. This ultimately makes the volume density of electrons in the inversion layer to be different from that in the substrate layer. The voltage obtained by application of the charge conservation principle between the gate and substrate semiconductor interface is termed as threshold voltage-V_{th} [50]. This voltage can also be defined as the voltage at which the device operation commences [51]. After radiation exposure, a new equilibrium is established; this corresponds to a new threshold voltage value. A proper analysis of this threshold voltage shift could, therefore, be used to investigate the quality and quantity of radiation attenuated in the metal oxide hence this voltage shift. Applying the same principle, Sedra [52] uses the radiation-induced lattice damages as a parameter for dosimetry [39]; these damages reduce the gain factor of a transistor. A BJT Darlington transistor is used in particular due to its higher gain compared to other transistor types [52]. Here, the limitation of transistors-having high post-radiation exposure lattice structural damages is a benefit. This is because this limitation is used to depict the amount of radiation that led to the transistor gain factor drop. Therefore, higher gain drop implies more damages, hence, more absorbed dose and a low gain factor drop, on the other hand, implies less damage, hence, less absorbed dose.

4. Photovoltaic sensors/Solar Cells

Photovoltaic sensors are devices whose operating principle is based on the photovoltaic effect. The photovoltaic effect is a process where incident photons of light excite valence electrons to higher energy levels/ conduction bands. The flow of these electrons in the conduction bands implies induction of a voltage and current in the device [36,53]. In medical radiation applications, it's not only the light section of the electromagnetic radiation spectrum that excites these electrons to the conduction bands; the X-ray section can also stimulate electrons.

4.1. Structure and Operational Principle

In reference to Section 2.1 of this paper, Gallium Nitride (GaN) and Cadmium Telluride (CdTe) are semiconductor materials. They are deployed in solar cells (Figure 5) to convert sunlight (electromagnetic radiation) to a current/charge which is stored as an electrical potential difference (voltage). Upon radiation exposure, semiconductor material electrons absorb the incident radiation energy and are excited to the conducting band (Figure 2a). Considering an unbiased PN junction of the semiconductor material in Figure 3b, these excited electrons could be localized in the N region. Therefore, their possession of radiation-gained energy enables them to drift towards the P section in order to recombine with the holes. In photovoltaic films, there is a non-equilibrium (free carrier concentration) created by illumination. This reduces the total volume of the depletion region while increasing the effective volume of the material where charges can be transported [2]. Photocurrents are also monitored with an application of a small bias voltage across the terminals of the device [2]. The drift of electrons implying a flow of a radiation-induced electric current, there is a conversion of radiation to a radiation-induced current. Therefore, a solar cell converts solar energy (radiation) to a storable form of electrical energy (charge).

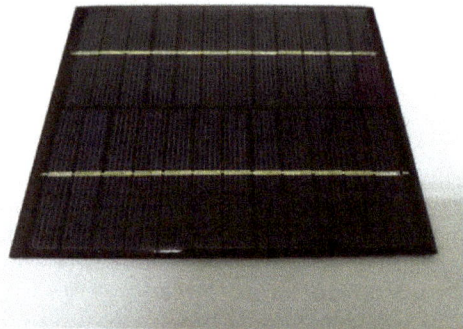

Figure 5. Solar Cell.

A flow of 6.2×10^{18} electrons in one second implies one unit of current-Ampere. This can also be defined as the flow of one Coulomb of charge per second. The quantity of induced current being directly proportional to the amount of radiation induce it, we can depict the type and quantity of the radiation that is inducing a photocurrent in solar cells – during medical applications today. Solar cells are grouped into three subgroups, i.e., first-generation wafer-based silicon; consisting of monocrystalline and polycrystalline solar cells, second-generation thin films; composed of amorphous silicon and CdTe thin film solar cells, and third-generation new emerging technology; including nanocrystal, polymer, and perovskite-based solar cells, dye-sensitized, and concentrated solar cells [54].

4.2. Present Literature

A GaN thin film was adopted in the detection of 40–300 kV Bremsstrahlung sourced X-rays while simulating the X-ray imaging of the index finger and wrist of the human phantom [2]. The film showed a high current gain, minimal radiation angular dependence, high sensitivity to X-ray intensity and had a linear total dose response [2]. It could also measure the 1 µGy s^{-1}–10 mGy s^{-1} air kerma range with a signal stability of 1% [2]. Additionally, there was no need for geometry/ energy recalibration because the results varied with only a percentage of 2 – within the measured range of energy in the study [2]. Further, in this study, the solar cell executed high-resolution X-ray imaging since solar cells normally have a detection volume smaller than 10^{-6} cm^3 [2]. With some more enhancements, they would also be used in vivo biosensing [2].

A semiconductor monocrystalline silicon solar cell's response to cobalt-60 gamma radiation dose was also studied using the thermal luminescence glow peak technique [10]. To navigate the sources of errors in gamma radiation dose measurements, both the solar cell and TLDs were used for radiation detection. According to the results, gamma dose measurements were more accurate while using solar cells [10].

Because of their low operational power and low cost, thin film sensors connected to data acquisition electronics and wireless data transmissions were used in kV and MV photon beam detections [33]. Their sensitivity per unit area was compared to that of normal photodiodes, and to that of an Electronic Portal Image Device (EPID) [33]. The thin films were placed under block sheets of a solid water slab phantom, and radiation exposures were made while varying parameters such as beam energies, dose rates, total doses, depths, and radiation exposure angles [33]. Further, IMRT sensitivity and precision tests like closed Multi-Leaf Collimator (MLC) were performed [33]. The detector's performance was not dependent on the amount of the absorbed dose and the dose rate. The sensor's sensitivity was also sufficient, i.e., a stable and accurate read-out signal was detected during the radiation exposures; hence, being a possible quality assurance tool [33].

Photovoltaic CdTe semiconducting thin films were also used for detecting diagnostic radiology and radiotherapy keV and MeV energies – imaging dosimetry energies associated with image-guided radiotherapy techniques (IGRT) [8]. The films provided real-time tracking of the tumours in IGRT treatment delivery [8]. The films further facilitated noise reduction and better image resolution compared to the commercially available indirect electronic portal imaging devices (EPIDs); these EPIDs are mainly made of amorphous/non-structured silicon [8,54].

4.3. Benefits, Limitations and Challenges as Potential Dosimeters

GaN thin films are almost independent of the angle of radiation exposure. This implies that the films will be able to give accurate dose measurements independent of the beam direction; thus, a wide range of geometric applicability [2]. Therefore, the application of GaN films in radiotherapeutic beam fields is feasible; the angles of these fields are selected while ensuring maximum dose delivery to the targets, and at the same time sparing the organs at risk (OAR) [4,55]. Therefore, the ability to efficiently measure the absorbed dose at all angles doesn't present a need to alter the radiation field angles in order to suit the measurable dosimetry angle of the thin film dosimeter. In case beam alteration is done to suit the film's dosimetric range, there may be increased radiation exposure to the OARs. These films could, hence, stage a better performance when compared to ionization chambers that are associated with a large angular dependence [56]. However, considering the geometrical shape of these films, they aren't symmetrical like the ionization chambers. Therefore, there may be a variation in the results displayed from the different angles and positions of radiation exposure [33].

Even after frequent consecutive radiation exposures, the GaN thin film-based dosimeter's radiation-induced current varied within only a 2-percentage range – hence, consistent results. Therefore, there is no need for GaN film recalibration; a procedure that is normally applicable to dosimeters in medical radiation [2]. This consistency may be due to fewer vacancies and interstitials [10,47,57] created in the GaN lattice structure – hence, insusceptibility to radiation-induced damages [58]. In other words, the films 'accumulated-dose related errors are minimum, i.e., they produce consistent results. Due to the radiation hardness of GaN, its usage in tracking detectors affected by luminosity has also been suggested in space science and astronomical applications [59]. This radiation hardness is eminent in Figure 3a of Hofstetter [2]. In Hofstetter's study [2], the photocurrents before and after radiation exposure are equivalent when plotted on the same graph. This implies that there were trivial photocurrent degradations due to radiation exposures [2].

GaN thin films with detection volumes of smaller than $10^{-6} cm^3$ imply a high spatial precision [2]. These films could be further developed for not only X-ray detection but also other radiotherapy treatment modalities such as the Stereotactic Body Radiation Therapy/Stereotactic Radiosurgery (SBRT/SRS) and Intensity Modulated Radiation Therapy (IMRT). These treatment modalities involve the delivery of high doses to relatively small dynamic fields in a short period of time [4]. SBRT and SRS volumes are normally small and therefore a correspondingly small volume dosimeter would be vital in the replication and simulation of these treatment fields during dosimetry. Since these films are relatively thinner and more flexible than present dosimetric films, they could also be easily applied in dosimetry applications that involve curved surfaces where normal dosimeters cannot easily be applied [33].

The band gap energy is proportional to the amount of energy of a photon released after recombination of an electron and a hole [13]. CdTe's bandgap being in the 1.44–1.47eV range [8,54], and that of GaN being 3.4 eV [60], CdTe and GaN-based films can be operated at room temperature [60,61]. Therefore, CdTe-based dosimeters will have less temperature dependence because the room temperature's heat energy may not excite electrons from the valence band to the conduction band; the excitation consequently results into a photocurrent. Therefore, a fairly huge proportion of the induced current would be as a result of the electromagnetic radiation incident on the detector. This implies higher accuracy and quantum efficiency levels of the dosimeter. Nevertheless, a large band gap also insinuates that only radiation whose energy is above this band gap will be measured. This is because the band gap energy is required to pluck an electron from the valence band to the conduction band; so that an electron drift occurs in the conduction band, i.e., a photocurrent (Figure 2a). Therefore, low energy radiation whose energy is below the band gap will have less probability of being accurately detected. This may limit the dosimeters from measuring low energy radiations that affects their sensitivities. Contrarily, some studies have reported the detection of some photocurrents induced by radiations whose energy is below the band gap [60]. For incident radiations whose energies are above the band gap, 10^3–10^4 range gains were observed [60]. In addition, since shallow and deep traps are situated between the valence and conduction energy bands, a wider band gap may also imply higher sensitivity because charges will get easily stuck in these multitudinous traps. The magnitude of the radiation energy used to free these charges is proportional to the number of freed charges; this is proportional to the induced photocurrent [10]. Presence of these numerous traps could also lead to fading where the charges can easily be stimulated out of these traps. The stimulations could be by, for example, heat energy at room temperature. There will thus be inaccuracies in the signal detected. This is because all the trapped charges are a "record" of the energy used to trap them [10]. Due to the numerous traps containing charge, less energy would be required to stimulate charge out of any of these traps. Ultimately, there will be inaccurate backtracking of the amount of energy that was involved in the trapping of these charges.

GaN thin films are associated with large charge gains where free charge carriers are generated due to incident radiation. This increases the number of free charge carriers available to transport charge; a phenomenon known as photoconductivity [60]. Photoconductivity leads to more charge flow and a high non-linear photocurrent flow [60]. This results into an amplified radiation-induced current produced by the detector; a slight change in the kerma can readily be observed under typical operational conditions [2]. This photoconductive model could also be referred to as conductivity modulation (carrier density) because of the photogenerated carriers [60]. This model produces more photoconductive gains that are in the order of $10^3 - 10^4$ for GaN sensors [60]. These gains are high compared to the detection process where there is direct charge extraction [2]. In addition, there is a linear relationship between these current gains and the amount of radiation incident on the dosimeter-thus being linear for the 0.5–2 Gy dose range [10]. Despite blockage of all the ambient light and operation of the detector at room temperature, photoconductivity produces dark currents, i.e., a signal will be detected even before any radiation strikes the dosimeter [2].

CdTe films are cost-effective [54] and are associated with a direct detection method–thus low noise effects [8]. GaN films also have a high sensitivity to noise ratio and they are nearly independent of the air kerma rate [2]. A GaN film detector produced direct signals that were not processed using any configuration formula/measurements; hence, faster and simpler read-out compared to traditional detectors [2]. In addition, the induced photocurrent is stable with a standard deviation of ±0.028 µA; the current varied within a range of 1% during 10 min of radiation exposure [2]. This is as a result of very slow non-exponential photoconductance decays; these decays are associated with carriers being trapped in shallow and deep traps [30,60]. The stability of this current could also imply reproducibility; repeated series of experiments produce the same results while maintaining a constant set-up. GaN sensors were observed to be reproducible, i.e., there was an average standard deviation of 1.3% in five repeated series of measurements carried out by Hofstetter [2]. In another study [33], the variation of results of the individual photocells in a solar cell array-based prototype was within a percentage of one [33]. However, the reproducibility of the solar cells cannot be compared to that of diodes used in dosimetry; this could be attributed to errors during manufacturing [33].

5. Charge Couple Devices (CCD)/Charge Metal Oxide Semiconductors (CMOS)

When a capacitor is fully charged, charge flow ceases and there is a static charge stored on the capacitor plates and in the dielectric material. The capacitor is then referred to as fully charged because this trapped charge in the dielectric material, and on the capacitor plates, doesn't flow unless a complete circuit is connected to it. For the capacitor in Figure 3c, the dielectric material is air, but any other material could be placed between these plates. This could boost the capacitor's capacitance since the dielectric constant is dependent on the dielectric material. The dielectric constant is also directly proportional to the capacitance as seen in Equation (3) [15,16]. Capacitors, therefore, are energy-banks since they store charge equivalent to the voltage potential connected across them as observed in Equation (2) [16]. When the capacitor plates are metal, and the dielectric material is a metal oxide, a capacitor with a PN junction is formed. Therefore, electromagnetic radiation striking the surface of the capacitor plate induces an electron-hole pair; thus, conversion of the incident electromagnetic radiation energy to charge. A Charge Coupled Device (CCDs) is an array of single and independent metal oxide semiconductor capacitors closely packed in a sole block. The charge on each capacitor is transferable from one-unit cell/pixel/photo site of this block to another. Ultimately, the Analog to Digital Converter (ADC) transforms this analog current signal (charge) to digital format [62].

5.1. Structure and Operational Principle

In a CCD, the actual charge transfer takes place in potential energy wells situated in *n* or *p* substrates that are found below electrodes; these electrodes are connected to a multiphase pulsed clock voltage [62] (Figure 6). Biasing one gate electrode with a positive step potential leaves the adjacent electrodes at a lower voltage [62]. This, therefore, creates a deep potential well below the biased electrode [62]. In this potential well, the electron charge is trapped and stored as seen in the first-time phase t_1 of Figure 6 [62]. However, if these adjacent electrodes are also consequently biased with a higher positive potential, there will be deeper potential wells below the adjacent gate electrode [62]. Since electrode charge carriers prefer lower energy for stability, there will be a drift of charge to the newly created deeper wells as illustrated in the second time phase t_2 of Figure 6 [62]. These wells could also be filled with electrons, which are not induced by radiation—heat induced electrons. Therefore, the charge signal can be stored for a short time; this time is much shorter than the thermal relaxation times for metal oxide capacitors [62]. This time normally ranges from 1 s to several minutes at room temperature; varies depending on the structure and fabrication process [62].

When the pixels are exposed to electromagnetic radiation, a charge; whose amount is a linear function of the illumination intensity, is accumulated from the electron-hole pair [62]. This charge is transferred and converted to a small voltage that is amplified in order to be compatible for analog to digital conversion by the ADC [62]. The amplified voltage is still susceptible to noise such as heat energy that also contributes to the electron-hole pair stimulations [62]. Complementary Metal Oxide Semiconductor Devices (CMOS) similarly operates under the same principle as the CDDs but their accumulated charge is amplified at each cell unit/pixel by multiple chip amplifiers, respectively [62]. Advantages of CMOS over CCD include; low power consumption, being inexpensive and easy to manufacture [63]. On the other hand, CCDs merits have; fast speeds, high dynamic ranges, greater light sensitivity and produce high-quality low noise images [63]. Factors such as camera size and noise [64,65] could also be a device preference and selection criteria.

CCD pixel numbers range from 128–16 million [62] and it's selected by the manufacturer and hence, they determine the level of sensitivity of the device.

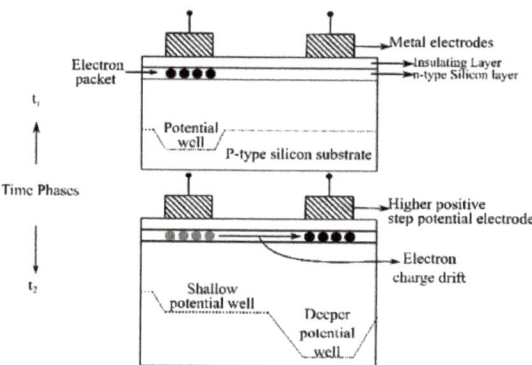

Figure 6. Electron Drift to deeper wells.

5.2. Present Literature

Radioactive tracers such as Iondine-131 (^{131}I), Yttrium(^{90}Y), and Fluorodeoxyglucose (FDG)–(^{18}F), are radionuclides that decay by emitting charged particles like electrons(β^-), positrons(β^+) [57,66], and gamma rays at speeds surpassing the speed of light in that particular medium/tissue [66–71]. This phenomenon polarizes the medium, and photons are emitted after a molecule retains its normal/stable position [68,69]. In other words, the excited electrons fall back to their ground states due to the fading of the polarization effect [66,68,69]. The photons are emitted as an electromagnetic radiation wave front [69]–Cherenkov radiation (λmax ~180 nm; water [68,72]). When Cherenkov radiation is accurately quantified and detected using CCD detectors [70], it depicts information regarding its source. For instance, the Cherenkov radiation could be emitted by anatomical structures, tissues or even cells [57,73]. The speed at which light travels through a medium is proportional to the refractive index of the traversed medium; Cherenkov Luminescence (CL) emissions increase as the refractive index increases [69]. Therefore, different media will produce different CL emissions. The solid state of matter has particles closely packed together and therefore if radiation or a particle is travelling through it, there will be more interactions between the photons of the radiation/particle and the solid particles. Therefore, there are more interactions in solids than in liquids and gases; the speed of light in fluids is higher than that and in solids. However minimal these interactions may seem, they reduce the velocity of the light; the reduction in the speed of light has a positive correlation with the refractive index, η, of the medium [69]. With the η of water being 1.33 [66] and that of biological tissue being ~1.36–1.45 [66,74], the velocity of light, v_m, in these media is ~0.75 c and ~0.7 c, respectively (Equation (4) [69,71]) [69].

$$v_m = \frac{c}{\eta} \qquad (4)$$

v_m Velocity of light in a medium, η refractive index of the medium, c Speed of light in a vacuum

When a body moves with a speed relatively close to that of light, its kinetic energy will not be be given by the classical mechanics formula $-E = 1/2mv^2$. The kinetic energy will be given by Equation (5) [69,71].

$$E = mc^2 \left[\frac{1}{\sqrt{(1 - \frac{v^2}{c^2})}} - 1 \right] \quad (5)$$

E Energy of a particle moving at a speed close to that of light, c speed of light, m mass of the particle, v velocity of the particle

If this energy exceeds a certain threshold energy value [75], the Cherenkov radiation will be produced [69]. We can substitute the threshold kinetic energy (0.511 Mev) [66] into Equation (5) [69,71] in order to calculate the minimum velocity that has to be possessed by a particle to stimulate Cherenkov Emissions (CEs). CEs increase with an increase in the refractive index of a medium (Equation (7) [71,75]); the threshold energy to induce the Cherenkov radiation is inversely proportional to the refractive index. However, CEs don't solely depend on the refractive index but rather many other factors such as the density and geometry of the medium, and the type of radioisotope [66,71]. During radiation-tissue particle interactions, there may be some Bremsstrahlung radiation. Bremsstrahlung is the radiation that is dissipated after deceleration of a particle cutting through the Coulomb field of an atomic nucleus [66]. Bremsstrahlung would, however, have no effect on the refractive index of the medium during particle interactions [69].

The Cherenkov radiation principle has its applications in both diagnostic radiology; Cherenkov Luminescence Imaging (CLI), and radiotherapy; thyroid and the liver radiotherapy [57,66,68–71]. Despite the use of the Cherenkov radiation in the measurement of beta-emitting radionuclides starting as early as 1968 [76], CLI is a new modality in the nuclear medicine arena – it was recently initiated in 2009 [69]. Therefore, literature pertaining to CL in medicine is not much compared to other photonic devices, but it is progressively emerging.

In one study [68], the CLI of β emitters and imaging agents characterized with both radioactive and a fluorescence emission were examined. First, the medical imaging applications of β emitters and imaging agents were each investigated separately. Later on, both the β emitters and imaging agents were combined in a hybrid technology during image-guided surgery [68]. Application of β emitters and imaging agents separately is associated with both some advantages and disadvantages. However, in a hybrid technology combining a β emitter and an imaging agent, the shortcomings of one technique could be compensated by the other. Nonetheless, further research still has to be done to ensure the accuracy and sensitivity of the attained signal.

Radiotracers emitting high-energy positrons via post-decays were also used to detect CLI. Radiotracer elements are radioactive and their quantity and number of particles they emit reduce with time –according to Equation (6) [69]. In this study, CLI in vivo application was validated by investigating the signal/Cherenkov light emitted by radiotracers injected in mice [69].

$$t_{\frac{1}{2}} = \left[\frac{ln(2)}{\tau} \right] \quad (6)$$

$t_{\frac{1}{2}}$ Half-life (Time for half the quantity of the radioactive nuclei to decay), τ Decay constant

The viability of Cherenkov Emission (CE)-based portal imagers in dynamic and stationary CyberKnife radiotherapy treatment fields was investigated [70]. Using a half-full water tank and a circular radiation beam with a diameter of 60 mm, CEs were stimulated in tissue equivalent materials [70]. CCDs placed behind the tissue equivalent materials were then used to detect CEs stimulated by both dynamic and stationary radiation [70]. A comparison with the results from an onboard linac portal imager was done to reveal potential resolution and contrast limits [70]. Results showed that the CE-based technique's contrast percentages through both air and water were lower than those of the linac-based portal imaging system [70]. In all the above applications, Cherenkov Luminescence was emitted after a particle(s) travelled through a medium. From Equation (5) [69,71], the velocity of the particle must exceed the velocity of light in a given medium. Let's now assume a particle whose velocity v is just equivalent to the speed of light v_m in a particular medium. To attain its kinetic energy, we shall substitute Equation (4) [69,71] into Equation (5) [69,71] that will give rise to;

$$E' = mc^2 \left[\frac{1}{\sqrt{(1-\frac{1}{n^2})}} - 1 \right] \quad (7)$$

Equation (7) [71,75] therefore represents the amount of kinetic energy the particle has if it is traversing the medium at a speed of light in the medium. Since the particle velocity has to surpass that of light in the same medium, the particle with energy E' will not produce the Cherenkov radiation. This is because the light photons also have this same energy while travelling through the medium. Therefore, a Cherenkov particle has a velocity v greater than v_m i.e., $v > v_m$. Thus, the Cherenkov particle's energy $E_{Cherenkov}$ is greater than E' ($E_{Cherenkov} > E'$). With this, we could now define E' as the minimum energy that a particle must be having above which it will emit Cherenkov radiation. Hence, $E' = E_{Threshold}$ which is the minimum energy that a particle is supposed to attain before it emits a Cherenkov radiation. With the refractive index of water being 1.33, $E_{Threshold}$ is 0.264 MeV and if the refractive index of tissue is assumed to be 1.4, $E_{Threshold}$ is 0.219 MeV [71].

5.3. Benefits, Limitations and Challenges as Potential Dosimeters

Since CCDs are luminescence-based detectors, they can yield inaccurate results from the luminescence emitted by the used fluorophore [66,68,71]; the fluorophore brightness affects the signal intensity. The CE brightness is affected by several signal depletion factors such as excessive luminescence attenuation by tissues that have chromophore absorbers like hemoglobin; tissues are also heterogeneous in regard to their refractive indices [66,68,71]. Scattering effects, ambient light, electrical noise by camera dark currents, and surface reflections could also affect the signal [66,68,71]. All these factors consequently reduce the final signal magnitude and the image resolution. This signal could, however, be boosted by using liquid scintillators in conjunction with CLI imaging; as one hybrid technique [66].

CDDs or CMOSs detect the wavelength of CLs close to that of visible light (Ultra Violet (UV)). This implies that other light sources produce noise effects; CLI should be performed in total darkness to increase the detection efficiency of CCDs [66,68]. Ambient signal detection could also be eliminated by synchronizing the linac pulses with the CCD camera capturing time intervals [71].

The signal detected by the CCDs is directly proportional to the CL intensity. Further, the CL intensity is also directly proportional to the half-life (Equation (6) [69]) of the radioisotopes that stimulate the luminescence [68]. CLs measured by CCDs are, therefore, of low spatial resolutions compared to fluorescence luminescence. This is because CL is an indirect (secondary) luminescence; high-speed moving charged particles polarize molecules of a material–primary CL stimulation stage [68]. Since different radioisotopes emit decay particles with varying magnitudes of energy, there will also be a variation in the CEs generated; the radiation intensity reduces due to the half-life effects [66]. Further, with reference to Equation (7) [71,75] CE luminescence is refractive index dependent. Therefore, CEs will fluctuate according to the tissue refractive index variation [71]. This implies that there will be no homogeneity in the intensity of the signals attained. In turn, some regions in the image will appear brighter and clearer than the others due to more luminescence. Similarly, other regions will appear darker due to less luminescence in those regions. However, studies have been carried out and results have shown that CLI imaging could be used to increase the spatial resolution of SPECT images [71].

CCDs have high quantum efficiencies in the ~570–720 nm spectral range [68]. This makes CCDs feasible in the imaging of common luminescent molecules [68]. However, CCD efficiency declines to half when the imaged wavelength is less than 350 nm; yet this is a region where CL is highly concentrated [68]. Despite the fact that the efficiency decline effect is less in near-infrared dyes, there is consequently deterioration of the CCD signal [68].

CCDs are also less likely to take real-time measurements since they involve the use of visible light [69]. Visible light has a low penetration power because its wavelength is more than 450 nm. This implies the need for proper exposure of the areas of interest before any imaging is done. This way, image acquisition could take approximately 5 min [68,69]. However, this operation time is still quite short compared to other imaging modalities like Positron Emission Tomography (PET) where it takes about 20 min to acquire the same images [69]. Longer treatment times/data acquisition times could, however, increase susceptibility to errors resulting from patient movements; hence, the need for additional patient immobilization procedures. This extra immobilization process is likely to cause fatigue in patients.

When CE-based images were compared to EPID images [70], CE demonstrated an almost similar contrast for imaging of an air-water inter-surface lining [70]. On the other hand, EPIDs had a higher image contrast for the air and water media inter-surface lining—during a real-time video [70]. Cherenkov luminescence-based video imaging during a breast cancer intra-surgery also increased precision in the patient positioning [71].

Novel techniques like CE-based imaging could also improvise for lack of EPIDs on devices like CyberKnife®. This would improve patient immobilization/positioning in radiation therapy; hence, accurate tracking of the targets (tumours)—conventionally achieved using portal imaging (EPIDs) [66,70]. CE-based imaging would be moderately cheaper compared to the normal imaging tools that are currently used in medical radiation imaging [66,71].

CL intensity depends on the speed of the particle; this speed is determined by the half-life ($t_{\frac{1}{2}}$) of the radioisotope [69]. When the quantity of a radioisotope reduces to half its initial amount (after the half-life), the CCD signal intensity will similarly dwindle [68]. To ensure a low patient absorbed dose, radionuclides with short half-lives are commonly used. However, larger quantities of radioisotopes having short half-lives could be administered in order to attain a prolonged stable signal. This ultimately leads to excessive radiation attenuation by tissues [3,4] and high diagnostic patient doses [68]. Lack of sensitivity stability over a prolonged duration could limit the application of the CLI imaging technique to procedures like total body tomography; imaging of the whole body is done—not only a specific region of interest [69].

Although Cherenkov luminescence emits a very weak signal, if a highly sensitive camera is used, higher quality images may be obtained; this could be an alternative to the PET and SPECT scanners [57]. In addition, PET and SPECT scanners are relatively less efficient in the imaging of some radionuclides like yttrium-90 [66] that are used in radiotherapy [57]. Development of modalities such as radio-immunotherapy could also be facilitated; these modalities use radionuclides like yttrium-90 [57]. In addition, CLI could be used to validate SPECT images because it has a better spatial resolution compared to PET; during imaging/ display of positron-sourced proton distributions [66,71]. CLI is also currently a basis for the development of other novel techniques such as the Integrated Monte Carlo code; manipulates principles of both ionizing radiation and optical photons, Cherenkov Luminescence Tomography (CLT), and Cherenkov Luminescence Endoscopy [57,71].

Scatter radiation particles move at slow speeds, i.e., they have low kinetic energies. Therefore, they do not satisfy Equation (5) [69,71]; hence no CE illuminations will arise from stray particles [70]. This implies less need for noise filtration procedures [70]. In other words, there would be low noise signals when the radiation source is due to the Cherenkov luminescence since it doesn't involve external optical stimulation [68].

With the promising CCD camera benchmark results as detectors for Cherenkov imaging in Table 1, we could further expound this phenomenon to estimate the absorbed dose. Cherenkov emissions were observed during radiotherapeutic radiation exposure of a human phantom with X-ray beams—a procedure that involved an absorbed dose of 5 Gy [77]. In this case, a specific Cherenkov image resolution would be correlated to a particular absorbed dose quantity involved in the production of the Cherenkov image (Table 2). Therefore, CCDs would be applied as indirect dosimeters where an image resolution would be calibrated to imply an absorbed dose value.

Table 1. Comparison of the devices based on some dosimetry parameters and benchmarks.

Dosimetric Parameter	Dosimetric Device				
	Photodiodes	Phototransistors/ MOSFETs	Photovoltaic Sensors/Solar cells	CCD/CMOS (In relation to CLI)
Susceptibility to post-radiation lattice structural damages	Low [35]	High [16,35,38]	Negligible [2,10,59]	Not Applicable
Post-radiation dark currents/Noise	Low [35]	High [16]	Low [2,8]	Low-noise [68,70]
Post-radiation sensitivity loss	Negligible [15]	High [16,35,44]	Negligible [33,58,59]	Radioactive half-life leads to signal loss [68]
Quantum efficiency	High [14,15,78]	Adjustable [16]	High [33]	High [68]
Angular dependence	High [35]	High [35]	Almost independent [2,33]	Not applicable
Reproducibility/Repeatability	High [9,15]	Varies with absorbed dose [16]	Feasible [2,33]	Low [66,70]
Sensitivity to radiation	Low/varies with energy [35]	High [16,45]	High	Low [69]
Read-out type	Real-time [14,15]	Indirect/passive [28]	Direct [8,54]	Indirect [68,69]

Table 2. Medical Photonic Device Dosimetric Ranges.

Medical Procedure Analysed			Tested/Reviewed Dose Range (cGy)			
	Radiation Type	Dose Type	Photodiodes/LEDs	Phototransistors/ MOSFETs	Photovoltaic sensors/Solar cells	CCD/CMOS
Diagnostic Radiology	X-rays	Air Kerma	0.003–0.450 [9]	–	–	–
	X-rays	Air Kerma	0.001–0.043 [34]	–	–	–
	X & Gamma rays	Air Kerma	0.006–0.400 [14]	–	–	–
Computed Tomography	X-rays	Air Kerma	0.340–8.30 [35]	0.340–8.30 [35]	–	–
Not specified	Gamma rays	Air Kerma	47.2–330 [15]	–	–	–
Not specified	Gamma rays	Air Kerma	–	10,000–50,000 [40]	–	–
Breast Cancer Radiotherapy	X-rays	Alderson Rando Absorbed Dose	–	200 [39]	–	–
Radiotherapy	X-rays	Anthropomorphic phantom Absorbed Dose	–	4,000–18,500 [42]	–	–
Imaging	X-rays	Human wrist and index finger phantom (one pixel)	–	–	0.086 [2]	–
Radiotherapy	Gamma rays	Air Kerma	–	–	50–200 [10]	–
General Medical Dosimetry	X-rays	Solid Water Phantom	–	–	0.1–500 [33]	–
Radiotherapy	X-rays	Human Body phantom	–	–	–	500 [77]

6. Summary

Although there may be a multitude of photonic devices applied in medical radiation dosimetry, this paper has focused on mainly photodiodes, phototransistors, photovoltaic sensors and CCD cameras. This is because they are; currently the most commonly applied in medical radiation detection based on the literature available, relatively low-cost devices, and there are no complex systems associated with their applications. CCDs have been in implementation for approximately a decade [69,71]. Therefore, CCDs could have more medical application deficiencies and less literature pertaining to their usage compared to other photonic devices. Such new technologies: Cherenkov imaging using CCD cameras, and the margining of fluorescence dyes and Cherenkov radiation exposure as a hybrid technology (in form of a single-imaging modality) present better results. However, further studies have to be carried out to increase CCD efficiency while minimizing their related hazardous effects. This would facilitate a quicker approval by governing and implementation bodies; hence, more animal and preclinical trials [57]. This will stimulate more clinical trials that will finally improve the results of these applications [57].

As a discrete analysis, photodiodes and phototransistors have relatively more frequent applications compared to the CCDs and solar cells; based on the present literature and studies. Photodiodes like the BPW34 have been associated with more pros as medical radiation detectors in this review-Table 1. They have a high quantum efficiency, low dark currents, and low radiation-induced structural damages. These characteristics could be considered to be some of the cornerstone characteristics of ideal dosimeters [15]. These features further suggest that these devices are durable when applied as radiation dosimeters. This is because there is less need for correctional/calibrations while using the BPW34 [35]. This implies that they cannot easily wear out due to repeated usage. Being resistant to radiation-induced damages is an essential feature in radiation dosimetry that may guarantee accurate and stable results even after repeated usage; the long-life span of a dosimeter could also imply durability [35].

On the other hand, phototransistors are susceptible to radiation-induced damages despite having a relatively high amplification capability [35]. Therefore, calibration and correction procedures will have to be carried out to maintain the device accuracy; this implies a short lifespan for these devices since there is degradation and wear out with increased radiation exposure [35]. Users will have to consequently buy new devices after numerous calibrations on old ones. On the other hand, photodiodes can be used for quite long durations with less or negligible wear out. Durability could thus also be considered a key characteristic of dosimeters associated with accurate results even preceding multiple applications.

This presents photodiodes as fairly more robust compared to phototransistors, solar cells and CCDs. This is because they produce low dark currents, have fairly higher insusceptibility to radiation-induced structural damages and are negligible post-radiation sensitivity loss [15]. However, more studies have to be carried out to further resolve their flaws like low sensitivity to radiation and having a narrow measurable range. Alternatively, applying a solid-state scintillator in front of the photodiode could resolve its low sensitivity to the detected radiation [79]. This may perhaps make them to be more quintessential dosimeters in medical radiation.

The displacement effects of these photonic devices take place in the lattice structure as illustrated in Figure 2b. Therefore, phototransistors could be fabricated using elements more resistant to radiation-induced displacements – such as those of solar cells or even better ones. More research on how to make the lattice structure of semiconductor devices more radiation hard will resolve this setback. Radiation-induced displacements occur in almost all photonic devices used for radiation detection; the magnitude of these damages could vary from one device to another. Photodiodes with inbuilt gains/amplification could also be fabricated. Alternatively, better amplification techniques could be applied to photodiodes in order to improve their signal magnitude and quality. In Hofstetter's Figure 3b [2], solar cells are shown to be radiation-hard. Therefore, further exploitation of this characteristic may also make them ideal radiation detectors. During photonic-device based radiation detections, ambient light and temperature/heat buffers should be applied; an appreciably high spurious signal may be detected due to these factors.

In medicine, radiation is mainly used in diagnostic radiology and radiation oncology. Diagnostic procedures such as bone densitometry use significantly low radiation doses to produce X-ray images. On the other hand, high dose radiotherapeutic treatment modalities such as stereotactic radiosurgery (SRS) could impart absorbed doses of approximately 8–18 Gy [80,81] in one fraction. This implies that the photonic devices to be used for medical radiation detection should measure radiation doses from about 0 to 18 Gy in one exposure/fraction. Table 2, therefore, shows the dosimetric ranges of photonic devices in order to determine their feasibility for medical radiation dosimetry applications.

From Table 2, photodiodes could measure minimum and maximum air kerma doses of approximately 0.001 cGy and 8.3 cGy, respectively. In addition, the table illustrates that photodiodes could be implemented in diagnostic radiology procedures like CT scans and X-ray imaging since their relative absorbed doses lie in the photodiode's measurable range. Therefore, radiotherapy dosimetric procedures involving relatively higher absorbed doses may not be effectively implemented with photodiodes. Instead, phototransistors (MOSFETS) and photovoltaic sensors could be preferred since their reviewed dose range is 0.340–18,500 cGy; which is suitable for radiotherapeutic dose measurements. For a Cherenkov emission to take place, the threshold particle energy ($E_{Threshold}$) has to be surpassed. This threshold energy could perhaps be surpassed in applications involving higher energies and doses. In other words, CLI does not involve low absorbed dosages and energies. CCD cameras could, therefore, be calibrated and developed to measure absorbed doses in relation to a specific CLI image resolution. In this aspect, CCDs can be possibly designed to measure high radiotherapeutic doses.

Solar cells are reasonably hard to absorbed dose-related wearing [2] in addition to their fairly broad dosimetric range of 0.086–500 cGy as observed in Table 2. Therefore, it would be more appropriate for dosimetry compared to the phototransistor that are greatly affected by radiation-induced damages. The phototransistors (MOSFETs) would have been the optimum choice due to their wide measurable dose of 0.340–18,500 cGy but are impaired by their appreciable displacement damage effects.

Since cost also determines the application/preference of a specific device, Table 3 gives an insight into the probable prices of some of the photonic devices reviewed in this study.

Fabricating phototransistors using elements more resistant to radiation-induced displacements would be the principal solution to their radiation-induced damages. This solution can, however, be implemented by only the device manufacturers. Since signal amplification using scintillators would perhaps resolve the photodiode's low measurable dose range, photonic device users/researchers may resort to using photodiodes for diagnostic radiation detection. Similarly, researchers may enhance the solar cell's measurable dose range using scintillators/signal amplifiers. Photodiodes and solar cells are therefore the most promising devices for detecting diagnostic and radiotherapeutic radiation, respectively. In nuclear medicine, CLI would be enhanced by mitigating light, heat and other ambient signals. Alternatively, higher resolution/sensitive cameras would also be used for CLI. However, as shown in Table 3, these cameras may be costly.

Photonic devices are generally promising radiation detectors, but more research has to be carried out to resolve or alleviate grave flaws like lattice structure displacements that mainly hinder their reproducibility and repeatability dosimetric parameters. Execution of more successful studies addressing the various drawbacks highlighted in this review presents a potential for providing more resilient, reliable and accurate photonic dosimeters.

In general, these research/development trends could be focused on mainly improving the photonic device sensitivity to radiation. This is because the photonic devices are purposely fabricated for light applications. While enhancing the sensitivity of these devices, their measurable dose ranges could also be expanded. This would, hence, make the photonic devices applicable for both low and high radiation dose measurements.

Table 3. Some Photonic Device Retail Price Ranges.

Photonic Device	Approximate Unit-Price (USD-$)	Online Store
Photodiodes		
S2506-02	0.0001–1.5	Alibaba
BPW34	1.6–2.45	Amazon
BPW34FS	1.98	Amazon
SFH206	1.6	Mouser Electronics
SFH205	0.79–1.92	Amazon
BPX90F	0.1–10	Alibaba
S1223	0.1–9.9	Alibaba
PS100-6-CER2PIN	78.38	Mouser Electronics
Phototransistors		
OP501	0.10–9.80	Alibaba
OP505A (Optek)	0.84–2.02	Amazon
BPW85 (Vishay)	0.10–18.80	Alibaba
OP521	0.001–10.00	Alibaba
Transistors		
BCV47 Darlington type BJT	0.20–0.23	Alibaba
MOSFETs	0.12–113	Mouser Electronics
Photovoltaic Sensors		
Solar cell	0.46–1.20	Alibaba
Cameras		
CCD	8.42–7000	Amazon
CMOS	9.99–6500	Amazon

Author Contributions: M.N.S.Y. and E.D. conceived, designed, and conceptualised the research study. E.D. wrote the original, revised, and the accepted manuscript versions. E.D., M.N.S.Y., A.F.O. and N.H.M.T. reviewed and edited the manuscript. M.N.S.Y., A.F.O. and N.H.M.T. supervised the research study. M.N.S.Y. administered and acquired funding for the project.

Funding: This research was funded by the Short-Term Grant, Universiti Sains Malaysia, Grant no.: 304/PPSK/6315117.

Conflicts of Interest: The authors declare no conflict of interest.

References

1. Knoll, G.F. *Radiation Detection and Measurement*; John Wiley and Sons: Hoboken, NJ, USA, 2010; ISBN 0-471-07338-5.
2. Hofstetter, M.; Howgate, J.; Sharp, I.D.; Stutzmann, M.; Thalhammer, S. Development and evaluation of gallium nitride-based thin films for x-ray dosimetry. *Phys. Med. Biol.* **2011**, *56*, 3215. [CrossRef]
3. Rivera-Montalvo, T. Radiation therapy dosimetry system. *Appl. Radiat. Isot.* **2014**, *83*, 204–209. [CrossRef]
4. Kron, T.; Lehmann, J.; Greer, P.B. Dosimetry of ionising radiation in modern radiation oncology. *Phys. Med. Biol.* **2016**, *61*, R167. [CrossRef] [PubMed]
5. Ptw. Ionising Radiation Detectors Including Codes of Practice Freiburg, Germany: PTW. 2018. [2018/2019, [PTW Detector Mannual]. Available online: https://www.ptw.de/fileadmin/data/download/catalogviewer/DETECTORS_Cat_en_16522900_11/blaetterkatalog/blaetterkatalog/pdf/complete.pdf (accessed on 30 November 2018).
6. Vatnitsky, S.; Jarvinen, H. Application of a natural diamond detector for the measurement of relative dose distributions in radiotherapy. *Phys. Med. Biol.* **1993**, *38*, 173. [CrossRef] [PubMed]
7. Lépy, M.C. Detection Efficiency. Laboratoire National Henri Becquerel, CEA Saclay, F-91191 Gif-sur-Yvette Cedex, France. 2010. Available online: http://www.nucleide.org/ICRM_GSWG/Training/Efficiency.pdf (accessed on 7 May 2019).
8. Kang, J.; Parsai, E.; Albin, D.; Karpov, V.; Shvydka, D. From photovoltaics to medical imaging: Applications of thin-film CdTe in x-ray detection. *Appl. Phys. Lett.* **2008**, *93*, 223507. [CrossRef]

9. Romei, C.; Di Fulvio, A.; Traino, C.A.; Ciolini, R.; d'Errico, F. Characterization of a low-cost PIN photodiode for dosimetry in diagnostic radiology. *Phys. Med.* **2015**, *31*, 112–116. [CrossRef]
10. Diab, H.; Ibrahim, A.; El-Mallawany, R. Silicon solar cells as a gamma ray dosimeter. *Measurement* **2013**, *46*, 3635–3639. [CrossRef]
11. Bryant, J. Photodiodes and Other Light Sensors. Analog Com. 2014. Available online: https://wiki.analog.com/university/courses/electronics/text/light-sensors-photodiodes (accessed on 27 March 2019).
12. Soref, R. The past, present, and future of silicon photonics. *IEEE J. Sel. Top. Quantum Electron.* **2006**, *12*, 1678–1687. [CrossRef]
13. Gayral, B. LEDs for lighting: Basic physics and prospects for energy savings. *Comptes Rendus Phys.* **2017**, *18*, 453–461. [CrossRef]
14. Oliveira, C.N.; Khoury, H.J.; Santos, E.J. PiN photodiode performance comparison for dosimetry in radiology applications. *Phys. Med.* **2016**, *32*, 1495–1501. [CrossRef] [PubMed]
15. Anđelković, M.S.; Ristić, G.S. Feasibility study of a current mode gamma radiation dosimeter based on a commercial PIN photodiode and a custom made auto-ranging electrometer. *Nucl. Technol. Radiat. Prot.* **2013**, *28*, 73–83. [CrossRef]
16. Andjelković, M.S.; Ristić, G.S. Current mode response of phototransistors to gamma radiation. *Radiation Measurements* **2015**, *75*, 29–38. [CrossRef]
17. Bryant, J. LEDs are Photodiodes Too. 2014. Available online: https://www.analog.com/en/analog-dialogue/raqs/raq-issue-108.html (accessed on 27 March 2019).
18. Pandharipande, A.; Li, S. (Eds.) Illumination and light sensing for daylight adaptation with an LED array: Proof-of-principle. Industrial Electronics Society. In Proceedings of the 39th Annual Conference of the IEEE IECON, Vienna, Austria, 10–13 November 2013. [CrossRef]
19. O'Toole, M.; Diamond, D. Absorbance based light emitting diode optical sensors and sensing devices. *Sensors* **2008**, *8*, 2453–2479. [CrossRef]
20. Bui, D.A.; Hauser, P.C. Absorbance measurements with light-emitting diodes as sources: Silicon photodiodes or light-emitting diodes as detectors? *Talanta* **2013**, *116*, 1073–1078. [CrossRef]
21. Morcheeba. Photodiode-Closeup2.jpg. 2006. Available online: https://en.wikipedia.org/wiki/File:Photodiode-closeup2.jpg (accessed on 4 December 2018).
22. wdwd. High Power COB-LED with Low Current at 5pct.JPG 2015 [High Power COB LEDs Supplied at a Low Current Level with 5% of Maximum Current. Showing 40 Single Blue Power LEDs below the Yellow Surface]. Available online: https://commons.wikimedia.org/wiki/File:High_Power_COB-LED_with_low_current_at_5pct.JPG (accessed on 4 December 2018).
23. BrentMauriello. SMD-LED-Comparison-5050-2835-3528-3014-Flexfireleds.jpg 2015 [Comparison of SMD LED Modules on Strip Lights]. Available online: https://commons.wikimedia.org/wiki/File:SMD-LED-comparison-5050-2835-3528-3014-Flexfireleds.jpg (accessed on 12 February 2019).
24. Vilella Figueras, E.; Vilà i Arbonès, A.M.; Palacio, F.; López de Miguel, M.; Diéguez Barrientos, À. Characterization of linear-mode avalanche photodiodes in standard CMOS. *Procedia Eng.* **2014**, *87*, 728–731. [CrossRef]
25. Zhao, S.; Lioliou, G.; Barnett, A. Temperature dependence of commercial 4H-SiC UV Schottky photodiodes for X-ray detection and spectroscopy. *Nucl. Instrum. Methods Phys. Res. Sect. A Accel. SpectrometersDetect. Assoc. Equip.* **2017**, *859*, 76–82. [CrossRef]
26. Manufacturer, S.M.S.L. Difference between LED Light: COB and SMD Dongyang Street—Jinhua City—Zhejiang China. 2018 [Product Manufacturer Website]. Available online: https://www.solarlightsmanufacturer.com/cob-led-smd-led/ (accessed on 3 December 2018).
27. Singh, Y. *Semiconductor Devices*; IK International Pvt Ltd.: Delhi, India, 2010; ISBN 10 9380026129.
28. Andjelković, M.S.; Ristić, G.S.; Jakšić, A.B. Using RADFET for the real-time measurement of gamma radiation dose rate. *Meas. Sci. Technol.* **2015**, *26*, 025004. [CrossRef]
29. Singh, R.; Kainth, H.S. Effect of heating rate on thermoluminescence output of LiF: Mg, Ti (TLD-100) in dosimetric applications. *Nucl. Instrum. Methods Phys. Res. Sect. B Beam Interact. Mater. At.* **2018**, *426*, 22–29. [CrossRef]
30. Yukihara, E.; McKeever, S. Optically stimulated luminescence (OSL) dosimetry in medicine. *Phys. Med. Biol.* **2008**, *53*, R351. [CrossRef] [PubMed]

31. Van Zeghbroeck, B. Principles of semiconductor devices. 2004. Available online: http://ecee.colorado.edu/~bart/book/ (accessed on 13 May 2019).
32. Kester, W.; Bryant, J.; Jung, W.; Wurcer, S.; Kitchin, C. Sensor signal conditioning. *Sens. Technol. Handb.* **1999**, *2*, 31–136.
33. Zygmanski, P.; Abkai, C.; Han, Z.; Shulevich, Y.; Menichelli, D.; Hesser, J. Low-cost flexible thin-film detector for medical dosimetry applications. *J. Appl. Clin. Med. Phys.* **2014**, *15*, 311–326. [CrossRef] [PubMed]
34. Nazififard, M.; Suh, K.Y.; Mahmoudieh, A. Experimental analysis of a novel and low-cost pin photodiode dosimetry system for diagnostic radiology. *Rev. Sci. Instrum.* **2016**, *87*, 073502. [CrossRef]
35. Paschoal, C.M.M.; Souza, D.d.N.; Santo, L.A.P. Characterization of three photo detector types for computed tomography dosimetry. *World Acad. Sci. Eng. Technol.* **2011**, *56*, 92–95. [CrossRef]
36. Nikolić, D.; Vasić-Milovanović, A. Comparative study of gamma and neutron irradiation effects on the silicon solar cells parameters. *FME Trans.* **2016**, *44*, 99–105. [CrossRef]
37. Lischka, H.; Henschel, H.; Kohn, O.; Lennartz, W.; Schmidt, H. (Eds.) Radiation effects in light emitting diodes, laser diodes, photodiodes, and optocouplers. Radiation and its Effects on Components and Systems, 1993, RADECS 93. In Proceedings of the 2th IEEE European Conference on RADECS, Saint-Malo, France, 13–16 September 1993. [CrossRef]
38. Omar, N.I.C.; Hasbullah, N.F.; Rashid, N.K.A.M.; Abdullah, J. (Eds.) Effects on electrical characteristics of commercially available Si and GaAs diodes exposed to californium-252 radiation. Computer and Communication Engineering (ICCCE). In Proceedings of the IEEE International Conference on ICCCE, Kuala Lumpur, Malaysia, 3–5 July 2012. [CrossRef]
39. Santos, L.A.; Araujo, G.G.; Oliveira, F.L.; Silva, E.F., Jr.; Santos, M.A. An alternative method for using bipolar junction transistors as a radiation dosimetry detector in breast cancer treatment. *Radiat. Meas.* **2014**, *71*, 407–411. [CrossRef]
40. Pejovic, M.M. Application of p-channel power VDMOSFET as a high radiation doses sensor. *IEEE Trans. Nucl. Sci.* **2015**, *62*, 1905–1910. [CrossRef]
41. Sedra, A.S.; Smith, K.C. *Microelectronic Circuits*, 7th ed.; Oxford University Press: New York, NY, USA, 2014; ISBN 9780199339136.
42. Dybek, M.; Kozłowska, B. Evaluation of the applicability of MOSFET detectors in radiotherapy. *Radiat. Meas.* **2014**, *71*, 412–415. [CrossRef]
43. Ehringfeld, C.; Schmid, S.; Poljanc, K.; Kirisits, C.; Aiginger, H.; Georg, D. Application of commercial MOSFET detectors for in vivo dosimetry in the therapeutic x-ray range from 80 kV to 250 kV. *Phys. Med. Biol.* **2005**, *50*, 289. [CrossRef] [PubMed]
44. Santos, L.; Barros, F.; Filho, J.; da Silva Jr, E. Precise dose evaluation using a commercial phototransistor as a radiation detector. *Radiat. Prot. Dosim.* **2006**, *120*, 60–63. [CrossRef]
45. Knoll, G. *Radiation Detection and Measurement*; John Willey and Sons Inc.: New York, NY, USA, 2000; ISBN 978-0-470-13148-0.
46. Dixon, R.L.; Ekstrand, K.E. Gold and platinum doped radiation resistant silicon diode detectors. *Radiat. Prot. Dosim.* **1986**, *17*, 527–530. [CrossRef]
47. Srour, J.; Palko, J. Displacement damage effects in irradiated semiconductor devices. *IEEE Trans. Nucl. Sci.* **2013**, *60*, 1740–1766. [CrossRef]
48. Omar, N.I.C.; Hasbullah, N.F.; Rashid, N.K.A.M.; Abdullah, J. (Eds.) Electrical properties of neutron-irradiated silicon and GaAs commercial diodes. Industrial Electronics and Applications (ISIEA). In Proceedings of the IEEE Symposium on ISIEA, Bandung, Indonesia, 23–26 September 2012. [CrossRef]
49. Holmes-Siedle, A.; Adams, L. RADFET: A review of the use of metal-oxide-silicon devices as integrating dosimeters. *Int. J. Radiat. Appl. Instrum. Part. C Radiat. Phys. Chem.* **1986**, *28*, 235–244. [CrossRef]
50. Yau, L. A simple theory to predict the threshold voltage of short-channel IGFET's. *Solid-State Electron.* **1974**, *17*, 1059–1063. [CrossRef]
51. Arora, N. *MOSFET Models for VLSI Circuit Simulation: Theory and Practice*; Springer: Berlin, Germany, 1993; pp. 230–324. ISBN 978-3-7091-9247-4.
52. Sedra, A.S.; Smith, K.C. *Microelectronic Circuit*, 5th ed.; Oxford University Press: New York, NY, USA, 2004. Available online: http://fuuu.be/polytech/ELECH402/Microelectronic%20Circuits%20by%20Sedra%20Smith,%205th%20edition.pdf (accessed on 13 May 2019).

53. Yadav, A.; Kumar, P.; RPSGOI. Enhancement in efficiency of PV Cell through P&O algorithm. *Int. J. Technol. Res. Eng.* **2015**, *2*, 2642–2644.
54. Sharma, S.; Jain, K.K.; Sharma, A. Solar cells: In research and applications—A review. *Mater. Sci. Appl.* **2015**, *6*, 1145. [CrossRef]
55. Brahme, A. Development of radiation therapy optimization. *Acta Oncol.* **2000**, *39*, 579–595. [CrossRef]
56. Lambert, J.; Yin, Y.; McKenzie, D.R.; Law, S.H.; Ralston, A.; Suchowerska, N. A prototype scintillation dosimeter customized for small and dynamic megavoltage radiation fields. *Phys. Med. Biol.* **2010**, *55*, 1115. [CrossRef]
57. Nordstrom, R.; Cherry, S.; Azhdarinia, A.; Sevick-Muraca, E.; VanBrocklin, H. Photons across medicine: Relating optical and nuclear imaging. *Biomed. Opt. Express* **2013**, *4*, 2751–2762. [CrossRef]
58. Shvydka, D.; Parsai, E.; Kang, J. Radiation hardness studies of CdTe thin films for clinical high-energy photon beam detectors. *Nucl. Instrum. Methods Phys. Res. Sect. A Accel. Spectrometers Detect. Assoc. Equip.* **2008**, *586*, 169–173. [CrossRef]
59. Sellin, P.J. Recent advances in compound semiconductor radiation detectors. *Nucl. Instrum. Methods Phys. Res. Sect. A Accel. Spectrometers Detect. Assoc. Equip.* **2003**, *513*, 332–339. [CrossRef]
60. Garrido, J.; Monroy, E.; Izpura, I.; Munoz, E. Photoconductive gain modelling of GaN photodetectors. *Semicond. Sci. Technol.* **1998**, *13*, 563. [CrossRef]
61. Abbene, L.; Del Sordo, S. CdTe detectors. *Compr. Biomed. Phys.* **2014**, 285–314.
62. Pallas-Areny, R.; Webster, J.G. *Sensors and Signal. Conditioning*; John Wiley and Sons: New York, NY, USA, 2012; ISBN 0-471-33232-1.
63. Mehta, S.; Patel, A.; Mehta, J. (Eds.) CCD or CMOS Image sensor for photography. In Proceedings of the IEEE International Conference on Communications and Signal Processing (ICCSP), Melmaruvathur, India, 2–4 April 2015. [CrossRef]
64. Chang, H.-C.; Chung, C.-K. The Development of Fluorescence Imaging Systems for Clinical Applications-Part I, Broad-Field Fluorescence Imaging. *Int. J. Instrum. Sci.* **2012**, *1*, 16–20. [CrossRef]
65. Reibel, Y.; Jung, M.; Bouhifd, M.; Cunin, B.; Draman, C. CCD or CMOS camera noise characterisation. *Eur. Phys. J. Phys.* **2003**, *21*, 75–80. [CrossRef]
66. Ciarrocchi, E.; Belcari, N. Cerenkov luminescence imaging: Physics principles and potential applications in biomedical sciences. *Ejnmmi Phys.* **2017**, *4*, 14. [CrossRef]
67. Čerenkov, P. Visible radiation produced by electrons moving in a medium with velocities exceeding that of light. *Phys. Rev.* **1937**, *52*, 378. [CrossRef]
68. Chin, P.T.; Welling, M.M.; Meskers, S.C.; Olmos, R.A.V.; Tanke, H.; van Leeuwen, F.W. Optical imaging as an expansion of nuclear medicine: Cerenkov-based luminescence vs fluorescence-based luminescence. *Eur. J. Nucl. Med. Mol. Imaging* **2013**, *40*, 1283–1291. [CrossRef]
69. Robertson, R.; Germanos, M.S.; Li, C.; Mitchell, G.S.; Cherry, S.R.; Silva, M.D. Optical imaging of Cerenkov light generation from positron-emitting radiotracers. *Phys. Med. Biol.* **2009**, *54*, N355. [CrossRef] [PubMed]
70. Roussakis, Y.; Zhang, R.; Heyes, G.; Webster, G.; Mason, S.; Green, S.; Pogue, B.; Dehghani, H. Real-time Cherenkov emission portal imaging during CyberKnife® radiotherapy. *Phys. Med. Biol.* **2015**, *60*, N419. [CrossRef]
71. Tanha, K.; Pashazadeh, A.M.; Pogue, B.W. Review of biomedical Čerenkov luminescence imaging applications. *Biomed. Opt. Express* **2015**, *6*, 3053–3065. [CrossRef]
72. Cho, J.S.; Taschereau, R.; Olma, S.; Liu, K.; Chen, Y.-C.; Shen, C.K.; Dam, R.M.; Chatziioannou, A.F. Cerenkov radiation imaging as a method for quantitative measurements of beta particles in a microfluidic chip. *Phys. Med. Biol.* **2009**, *54*, 6757. [CrossRef]
73. Miao, T.; Bruza, P.; Pogue, B.W.; Jermyn, M.; Krishnaswamy, V.; Ware, W.; Rafie, F.; Gladstone, D.J.; Williams, B.B. Cherenkov imaging for linac beam shape analysis as a remote electronic quality assessment verification tool. *Med Phys.* **2019**, *46*, 811–821. [CrossRef]
74. Mobley, J.; Vo-Dinh, T. Optical properties of tissue. *Biomed. Photonics Handb.* **2003**, *2*, 1–2.
75. Jelley, J. Cerenkov radiation and its applications. *Br. J. Appl. Phys.* **1955**, *6*, 227. [CrossRef]
76. Elrick, R.; Parker, R. The use of Cerenkov radiation in the measurement of β-emitting radionuclides. *Int. J. Appl. Radiat. Isot.* **1968**, *19*, 263–271. [CrossRef]

77. Ahmed, S.R.; Jia, J.M.; Bruza, P.; Vinogradov, S.; Jiang, S.; Gladstone, D.J.; Jarvis, L.A.; Pogue, B.W. Radiotherapy-induced Cherenkov luminescence imaging in a human body phantom. *J. Biomed. Opt.* **2018**, *23*, 030504. [CrossRef]
78. Orlova, K.; Gradoboev, A.; Asanov, I. (Eds.) Gamma degradation of light-emitting diodes based on heterostructures AlGaInP. Strategic Technology (IFOST). In Proceedings of the 7th IEEE International Forum on IFOST, Tomsk, Russia, 18–21 September 2012. [CrossRef]
79. Bateman, J. A solid state scintillation detector for high-energy charged particles. *Nucl. Instrum. Methods* **1969**, *71*, 261–268. [CrossRef]
80. Andolino, D.L.; Johnson, C.S.; Maluccio, M.; Kwo, P.; Tector, A.J.; Zook, J.; Johnstone, P.A.S.; Cardenes, H.R. Stereotactic body radiotherapy for primary hepatocellular carcinoma. *Int. J. Radiat. Oncol. Biol. Phys.* **2011**, *81*, e447–e453. [CrossRef]
81. Schipani, S.; Wen, W.; Jin, J.-Y.; Kim, J.K.; Ryu, S. Spine radiosurgery: A dosimetric analysis in 124 patients who received 18 Gy. *Int. J. Radiat. Oncol. Biol. Phys.* **2012**, *84*, e571–e576. [CrossRef]

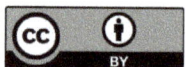

© 2019 by the authors. Licensee MDPI, Basel, Switzerland. This article is an open access article distributed under the terms and conditions of the Creative Commons Attribution (CC BY) license (http://creativecommons.org/licenses/by/4.0/).

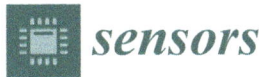

Article

Non-Contact Respiration Monitoring and Body Movements Detection for Sleep Using Thermal Imaging

Prasara Jakkaew [1,2,*,†] **and Takao Onoye** [1,†]

1. Information Systems Synthesis Laboratory, Department of Information Systems Engineering, Graduate School of Information Science and Technology, Osaka University, 1-5 Yamadaoka, Suita, Osaka 565-0871, Japan; onoye@ist.osaka-u.ac.jp
2. School of Information Technology, Mae Fah Luang University, 333-1 Thasud, Muang, Chiang Rai 57100, Thailand
* Correspondence: prasara.jak@ist.osaka-u.ac.jp
† These authors contributed equally to this work.

Received: 15 September 2020; Accepted: 2 November 2020; Published: 5 November 2020

Abstract: Monitoring of respiration and body movements during sleep is a part of screening sleep disorders related to health status. Nowadays, thermal-based methods are presented to monitor the sleeping person without any sensors attached to the body to protect privacy. A non-contact respiration monitoring based on thermal videos requires visible facial landmarks like nostril and mouth. The limitation of these techniques is the failure of face detection while sleeping with a fixed camera position. This study presents the non-contact respiration monitoring approach that does not require facial landmark visibility under the natural sleep environment, which implies an uncontrolled sleep posture, darkness, and subjects covered with a blanket. The automatic region of interest (ROI) extraction by temperature detection and breathing motion detection is based on image processing integrated to obtain the respiration signals. A signal processing technique was used to estimate respiration and body movements information from a sequence of thermal video. The proposed approach has been tested on 16 volunteers, for which video recordings were carried out by themselves. The participants were also asked to wear the Go Direct respiratory belt for capturing reference data. The result revealed that our proposed measuring respiratory rate obtains root mean square error (RMSE) of 1.82 ± 0.75 bpm. The advantage of this approach lies in its simplicity and accessibility to serve users who require monitoring the respiration during sleep without direct contact by themselves.

Keywords: respiration monitoring; non-contact monitoring; body movements detection; thermal imaging; natural sleep environments

---

1. Introduction

The respiratory rate is one of the critical vital signs that indicate health problems. The respiratory system is the gas exchange process to take in oxygen and expel carbon dioxide, as breathing moves air in and out of the lungs. The frequency of breaths is defined as a respiratory rate (RR) that is usually measured by counting the number of breaths a person takes per minute. A clinical staff member can count the number of times the chest moves up and down for a full minute. In general, the regular respiratory rate for healthy individuals is 12–20 bpm [1]. A change as little as three to five bpm may indicate a change in the patient's condition [2]. A patient suffering a severe adverse event on the general wards, such as a cardiac arrest or ICU admission, shows an increase in RR of up until 24 h before the severe events with high specificity [3]. For that reason, respiration monitoring should be performed continuously for a long time without impressing the patient's burden.

Owing to the fact that humans spend almost 30% of the time in sleeping, the respiration monitoring during sleep, which accurately reflects one's health condition is an appropriate and reasonable option. It is generally known that poor sleep significantly affects work productivity, cognitive performance, and overall life quality. Sleep monitoring can detect sleep disorders associated with cardiovascular disease, including heart failure, hypertension, and increased arrhythmia [4]. The breathing patterns during sleeping are utilized to identify the sleep disorder as sleep apnea, including obstructive sleep apnea (OSA), central sleep apnea, and complex sleep apnea syndrome. Sleep apnea is a cessation of the airflow that occurs when breathing repeatedly stops and starts during sleep, resulting in decreased oxygen flow to the brain and the rest of the body. Sleep apnea is generally characterized by cessation of breath for at least 10 s during sleep [5]. The well-known index used to indicate the severity of sleep apnea is Apnea–Hypopnoea Index (AHI), which counts the number of apnea events per hour. Harvard Medical School [6] classifies the severity of OSA as:

- None/Minimal: AHI < 5 per hour
- Mild: AHI ≥ 5, but < 15 per hour
- Moderate: AHI ≥ 15, but < 30 per hour
- Severe: AHI ≥ 30 per hour

Besides, sleep monitoring can detect periodic limb movement disorder (PLMD), which is repetitive cramping or jerking of the legs during sleep. Patients with PLMD may suffer from daytime sleepiness, daytime fatigue, trouble falling asleep at night, and difficulty staying asleep throughout the night [7]. Usually, patients with PLMD are unaware of their leg movements unless their bed partner tells them. It is also reported that movements are repetitive and rhythmic and occur every 20–40 s [8].

It has been demanded for long years to develop a novel technology to monitor respiratory and body movements without disturbing human sleeping. In recent years, non-contact respiration monitoring solutions have been proposed, like camera imaging [9], thermal imaging [10], and microwave Doppler radar [11]. As for camera imaging, a simple camera like a CCD camera, webcam, digital camera, or smartphone camera is used to detect the respiratory rate from the breathing motion, whereas for thermal imaging, a thermal camera or infrared camera is used to detect the temperature changes due to breaths. Respiratory rate often relies on visual observation of chest movement at periodic intervals [1]; a small movement that is hard to see with the naked eye. A motion magnification technique was proposed to magnify a baby's respiratory chest movements from a digital video camera [12]. Several researchers have analyzed video and image sequences to detect breath motions and extract vital signs in sleeping positions. For example, Nakajima et al. and Frigola et al. apply an optical flow technique to image data from a CCD camera and a remote TV camera, respectively [13,14]. Wiesner et al. monitor respiratory by tracking the motion of a fiducial marker placed on the patient's abdomen with a single webcam [15]. However, there are still some limitations of disturbing the natural sleep environment, such as visible light and privacy issues.

Thermal imaging is a rapidly evolving technology, now turning up in hospitals, airports, and even smartphones. Respiratory can be monitored through thermal imaging [16–21]. Thermal imaging cameras rely on microelectromechanical sensors to produce an image from heat; the human body stands out from the surrounding field because it gives off more heat. The thermal image-based method has an advantage under conditions of varying illumination and can reduce privacy issues. Previously, several approaches have been proposed to monitor respiration with a thermal camera by detecting the temperature change around the nostrils [18,21–28] or the airflow [19,20,29] in seated positions. They set the nose or the mouth as the region of interest (ROI) that can be defined manually or automatically by using anatomical features integrated with tracking algorithms [18,21–23,25]. They performed by simulated breathing following scenarios that the researcher designed, i.e., regular breathing, fast breathing, and hold breathing [18,21,24–26]. The excellent result showed when they took the experiments in a controlled room like temperature, humidity, and light. However, the nose detection during sleep is still unsuccessful at all monitoring times.

In the sleeping position, the thermal-based method is an effective technique to measure the nasal airflow patterns [16] and has been utilized to detect sleep apnea [30,31], analyze sleep activity [32], classify body posture [33] during sleep to assist the diagnosis of sleep disorders or evaluation of the quality of sleep. The studies using thermal imaging to monitor the respiration in sleeping position are reviewed in Table 1. Usman et al. [30] adopted thermal imaging to detect sleep apnea and study in a variety of breathing patterns. They used the Kanade–Lucas–Tomasi tracking algorithm to track the manual selected nose region. The result has shown that 16% of a subject's head position did not allow correct identification of the region of interest at nostrils. Therefore, this method was only possible with minor head movement without changing position. The automatic ROI selection was used to locate the nostrils, the tip of the nose, and mouth area [31,34,35]. That ROI requires a tracking algorithm and works well without large head movement under a controlled environment. Abbas et al. [16] developed respiration monitoring for neonatal intensive care units by manually select the ROI around the nostrils of infant. Most techniques work well when the nose is clearly visible in the image. The measurement was not feasible when the nose is outside the camera's field of view, a blanket blocks the nose, or the subject has large head movements. Recent works from Pereira et al. and Lorato et al. [36,37] detected the respiration signal without the use of anatomical features. They selected the ROI containing the respiration information by using the Signal Quality Index to analyze the ROIs. However, they took an experiment in a controlled environment with a short period that is not a real environment. Moreover, the motion artifacts are still a significant drawback of the proposed algorithm. It was suitable for monitoring infants in neonatal care who did not have large movements.

The present study aims to develop the measuring system capable of non-contact monitoring of respiration and body movements in natural sleep environments using a thermal video. The natural sleep environments imply an uncontrolled sleep posture, darkness, and covered subjects with a blanket. In the study, the different approaches based on temperature detection and motion detection were investigated to extract the respiration signal, and then the suitable approach is selected. Our main contributions of this paper are to present: (1) the respiration monitoring based on ROI detection combined with breathing motion, which does not require facial landmarks' visibility; (2) body movement detection to estimate the numbers of movement during sleeping that affect sleep quality. We validated the proposed approach by comparing it with the signal obtained from the respiratory belt.

Table 1. A research review of the thermal imaging-based method for respiration monitoring of sleeping position.

Authors	Subjects	Exp Duration	Controlled Env	Simulated Breathing	Selection/ Detection	ROI Localization Area	Tracking
Usman et al. [30]	Adult	5 min	Yes	Yes	M	Nostrils	Yes
Fei et al. [31]	Adult	60 min	Yes	No	A-S	Nostrils	Yes
Al-Khalidi et al. [34]	Children	2 min	Yes	No	A-S	Tip of the nose	Yes
Hu et al. [35]	Adult	10 min	Yes	Yes	A-S	Nose, mouth	Yes
Abbas et al. [16]	Infant	2 min	Yes	No	M	Nostrils	No
Pereira et al. [36]	Infant	5 min	No	No	A-D	N/A	No
Lorato et al. [37]	Adult	2 min	Yes	Yes	A-D	N/A	No
Our proposed	Adult	60–90 min	No	No	A-D	N/A	No

M: Manually, A-S: Automatically Selection, A-D: Automatically Detection.

2. Proposed Method

In this section, the proposed method for respiration monitoring and body movements detection is described. An overview of the proposed method is depicted in Figure 1. The input of the proposed method is the thermal video obtained under darkness light. The Gaussian filter is applied to the input images as the pre-processing so as to remove noises from the input. The main part of the proposed method is composed of respiration monitoring and body movements detection, each of which utilizes image processing and signal processing techniques in order. Details of these processes will be written below.

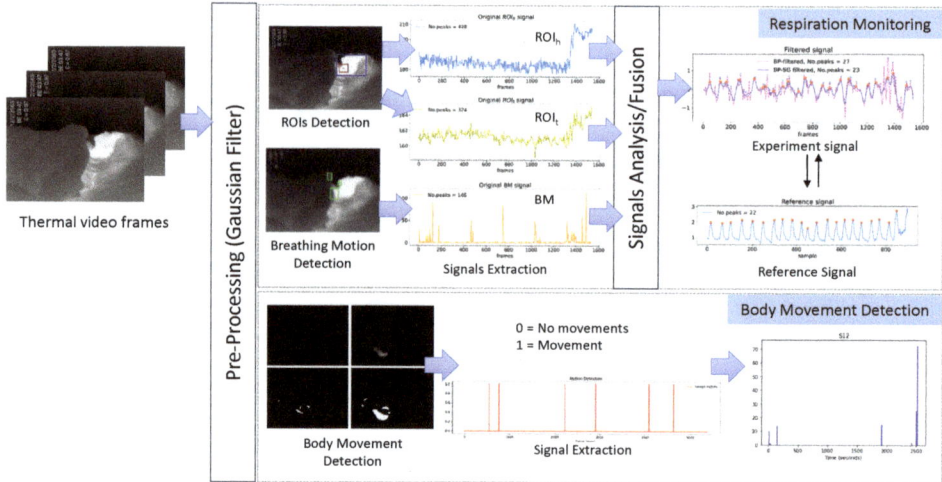

Figure 1. Proposed method.

2.1. Respiration Monitoring

The respiration monitoring method contains an automatic detection of ROIs by finding the highest temperature point and the largest portion of the high-temperature area and a breathing motion detection. The respiration signals extracted by automatic ROI detection and breathing motion detection are integrated. Then the signal processing is applied to calculate the respiratory rate.

2.1.1. Automatic ROI Detection

We employ the ROI detection to limit the observation area, extracting important information to raise the accuracy of the respiratory estimation. Determining a suitable ROI position with proper size is also important. In the sleep monitoring environment, it is not easy to detect a face or nostrils as an ROI because of the uncontrolled sleep posture, and the fixed camera position may mean that they could make a face that does not appear in the camera view on some occasions. Besides, when the subject changes the sleep posture, ROI should be updated to the new location for which some research applied a tracking algorithm, as summarized in Section 1. The tracking algorithm works well with an apparent object, but sometimes fails to track the nose or mouth in a sleeping posture. In this work, we propose an ROI detection on the thermal image in a sleeping position that does not require a tracking algorithm. Two different ROI detections are considered: (1) The highest temperature point detection and (2) The largest portion of high-temperature area detection.

(1) The highest temperature point is detected by using minMaxLoc. The minMaxLoc function is one of the OpenCV [38] libraries that returns minimum and maximum intensities found in an image with their (x,y) coordinates. It is assumed that the maximum pixel intensities of the thermal image refer to a human's heat signature that is not covered by a blanket. The maximum pixel intensities found in the image correspond to the highest temperature of the body. We set the pixel to the center of the observation area. Then we draw a rectangle around the pixel, with the size of the square $N \times N$ pixels depending on original frame resolution. In [39], the authors compared the ROI size of 10×10, 25×25, 50×50, 100×100, and 150×150 pixels. They found that the size of the ROIs for respiratory rate estimation is usually smaller than that for heart rate estimation. Therefore, in this study, we consider the three different ROI_h sizes as 10×10, 25×25, and 50×50, as shown in Figure 2. The result in empirical research has shown that the 50×50 pixels provided the highest accuracy in accordance with the original frame resolution of 640×480.

(2) The largest portion of the high-temperature area is detected by using the thresholding method. Thresholding is the method of segmenting the object from the background. The threshold image $g(x,y)$ can be defined as (1) [40]:

$$g(x,y) = \begin{cases} 1 & if \quad I(x,y) \geq T_R \\ 0 & if \quad I(x,y) < T_R \end{cases} \qquad (1)$$

This operation replaces each pixel values in an image with a white pixel if the pixel intensity $I(x,y)$ is greater than or equal to the threshold value (T_R), assigned to a black pixel if the pixel intensity is less than T_R. In this work, the white pixels are considered to represent the human skin area.

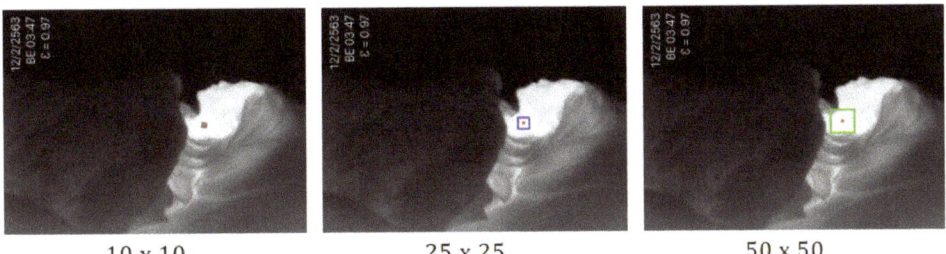

Figure 2. The sample of three different ROI_h sizes as 10×10, 25×25, and 50×50 (red point indicates the highest temperature point).

To determine the threshold value T_R, we coordinated empirical research with varying the value among 128, 144, 160, 176, 192, 208 and 224. It was confirmed that the T_R value 176 is the one that yielded the best results in all the performed tests.

Figure 3a shows the segmentation of the input image with the thresholding method. Then, we used the findContours function to find the location of white regions that return the outlines corresponding to each of the white blobs on the binary image. The bounding box is drawn around those contours (see Figure 3b). Finally, we find the most prominent contour and bounding box around that contour, as shown in Figure 3c. In this study, we selected the biggest box as ROI_t.

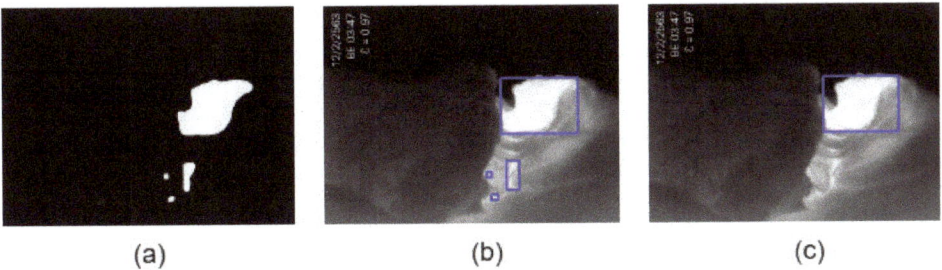

Figure 3. (a) All contours, (b) bounding rectangles around all contours, and (c) bounding rectangle around the most prominent contour.

Then ROI_h and ROI_t are cropped for extract signals $\tilde{S}_h(f)$ and $\tilde{S}_t(f)$ by computing the average of pixel values (2) within each ROI of each frame, where $S(x,y,f)$ is the pixel values of the thermal image at pixel (x,y) in the video frame f, N_* is the vector of pixel coordinates in ROI_h or ROI_t, and n_* is its number.

$$\tilde{S}_*(f) = \frac{1}{n_*} \sum_{x,y \in N_*} S(x,y,f) \qquad (2)$$

2.1.2. Breathing Motion Detection

Breathing motion detection applies, in the background, a subtraction method for detecting the motion by calculating the difference between the current frame and previous frame. Specifically, absolute difference for all pixels between the current frame $I(x, y, f)$ and the frame one second before $I(x, y, f - s)$ is calculated (3):

$$B(x, y, f) = |I(x, y, f) - I(x, y, f - s)|, \qquad (3)$$

where s is the frame rate.

Then, we extract portions of moved area by using thresholding, erosion, and dilation operations. Parameters used in these operations are 5 for thresholding pixel value difference is less than 5 and 5×5 kernel for opening (i.e., erosion and dilation). Next, bounding boxes are determined by finding contours with filtering out small movement as noise. Finally, the number of bounding boxes are counted as the metric of breathing motion (BM).

2.1.3. Respiration Signal Analysis

There are three respiration signals extracted by ROIs detection based on temperature detection and breathing motion detection. The following are the steps to estimate the respiration signals.

(1) The respiration can be extracted by detecting the chest movements, the breaths airflow, and the temperature change around the nostrils. However, the detection in a specific method cannot be guaranteed in the sleep monitoring because of the fixed camera position, and an independent subject posture may make the region out from the camera view. In such a case, an alternative method for respiration detection is required. It is reasonable to assume that the respiration can be detected by blending the temperature change of ROIs and breathing motion. Therefore, we combine three signals by employing the root mean square (RMS) to calculate the average of the respiration signals as (4).

$$Respiration\ signals = \sqrt{ROI_t^2 + ROI_h^2 + BM^2} \qquad (4)$$

(2) The 3rd order of Butterworth bandpass filter [41] with a lower cutoff frequency of 0.05 Hz and a higher cutoff frequency of 1.5 Hz was applied. The frequency bound is equivalent to 3–90 bpm, based on the typical RR for an adult person (12–20 bpm) and monitoring the abnormal RR that is less than 12 bpm and higher than 20 bpm.

(3) The Savitzky–Golay (SG) filter is a least-square polynomial filter that reduces noises while retaining the shape and height of waveform peaks [42]. Here, the SG filter was used to smooth the signal after the bandpass filter. The SG filter's output increased the precision of the data without distorting the signal tendency. There are two parameters of the SG filter, including window length and the filter order, which closely relates to the performance of the filter. In this study, we tested the parameters and selected the optimal values to get the best-filtered signal, i.e., the window length of 51 and the polynomial order at 3rd were used. The result of SG filter still includes the small peaks, and thus a moving average is calculated to detect only the desired peaks and ignore small ones.

(4) The fusion signal in Figure 4a was smoothed by the SG filter and moving average (see Figure 4b), and then the number of peaks is counted. Figure 4c depicted the peaks detection of the experiment signal, followed by the peaks detection of the reference signal in Figure 4d, which are assumed to correspond to the number of breaths. The findpeaks function is used with adjusting the width as 10 based on empirical research.

(5) The number of peaks is calculated as breaths per minute (bpm) for each 60 s slice of input video (1020 samples at 17 fps) and was compared with the reference RR. For performance comparison, the accuracy of the RR estimation was tested using the RMSE defined as (5)

$$RMSE = \sqrt{\frac{1}{N}\sum_{i=1}^{N}\left(x_i^{exp} - x_i^{ref}\right)^2} \qquad (5)$$

where N is the total number of the slices, and x_i^{exp} and x_i^{ref} represent the experimented and reference RR values obtained for slice.

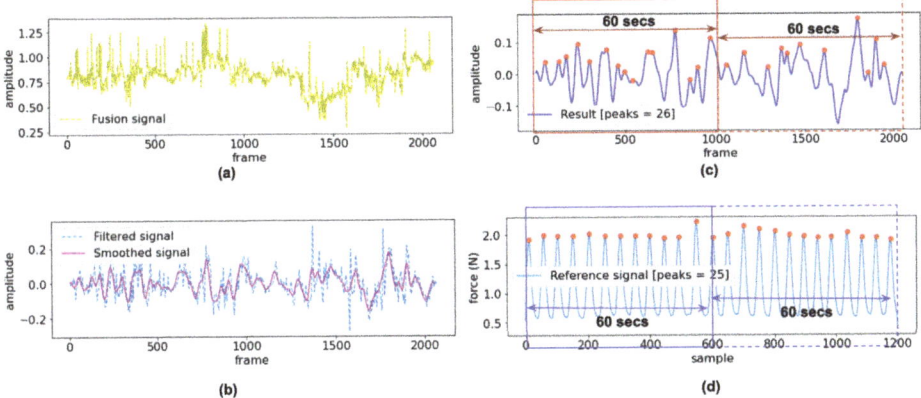

Figure 4. (**a**) Sample of fusion signal, (**b**) filtered and smoothed signals, (**c**) peak detection of experiment signal, and (**d**) peak detection of the reference signal.

2.2. Body Movements Detection

This process aims to determine the more significant action than the respiration representing the big movement like limb movement, head movement, and full position change during sleep. First, an absolute difference image $B'(x,y,f)$ between adjust two thermal images ($I(x,y,f)$ and $I(x,y,f-1)$) is obtained by $B'(x,y,f) = |I(x,y,f) - I(x,y,f-1)|$. Then, we binarize the difference image by thresholding method.

In the same manner as the breathing motion detection, we extract portions of the moved area by erosion and dilation operations. While using 35 for thresholding in order to detect large body movements, the same parameters are used for erosion and dilation. Then, we apply the findContour function to examine whether those are a portion of moved area. If any contour is found, the body movement signal is set to 1. An example output of the body movement is shown in Figure 5, where the left panel is the movement detection, and the right panel plots the movement signal.

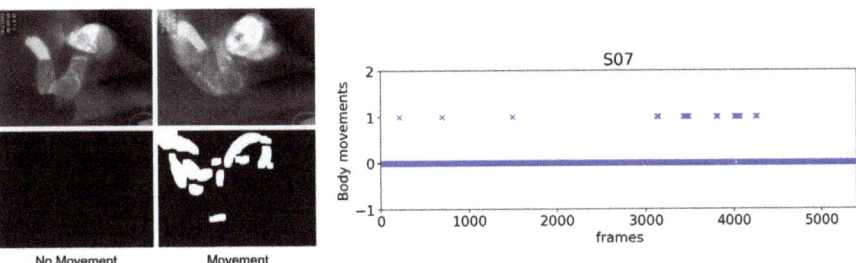

Figure 5. Sample output of the body movements detection.

3. Experimental Results

This section analyzes the signal gathered in two experiments. Experiment (1) the respiration monitoring, and experiment (2) the body movements detection during sleep. The results were compared with the reference signals obtained by the Go Direct Respiration Belt.

3.1. Experimental Setup

We assessed the performance of our proposed non-contact monitoring of respiration and body movement detection under natural sleep environments. During the experiments, the thermal videos were captured using a portable thermal camera (Seek Thermal Compact PRO for iPhone) attached to a smartphone and fixed on a tripod in front of a participant located at approximately 100 cm. The camera was set at the proper position so that the upper body of a participant was apparent in the camera's field of view. The Seek Thermal Compact PRO is a highly portable thermal imaging camera with a wide, 32-degree field of view. This thermal camera has a resolution of 640 × 480 pixels and detects infrared wavelengths in the spectral range of 7.5 to 14 Microns. The camera's emissivity was set to 0.97, as this is suitable for human skin temperature measurement [43]. Besides, the videos were recorded at 17 frames per second (fps). The Go Direct Respiration Belt [44] was used as a reference to collect human respiratory effort and respiratory rate from a force sensor and an adjustable nylon strap around the chest during respiration. The measuring parameters were set to 10 samples/s, and the duration is approximately 5400 s.

The data were collected on different days, from multiple camera positions with volunteers wearing different clothing. The experiments were conducted on real-life conditions, and volunteers were invited to record in their room while they were sleeping. They placed a respiratory belt around their ribs and mounted a thermal camera on a tripod by themselves before they go to bed. Figure 6 illustrates an environment setup. Sixteen healthy volunteers with ages between 25 years old and 37 years old (29.88 ± 3.26 years old), ten females and six males, with height between 151 cm and 180 cm (162.63 ± 7.37 cm), weight between 47 kg and 78 kg (57.38 ± 9.28 kg) and body mass index (BMI) between 18.65 kg/m^2 and 27.64 kg/m^2 (21.64 ± 2.98 kg/m^2) volunteered for this experiment. Table 2 shows the participants' data.

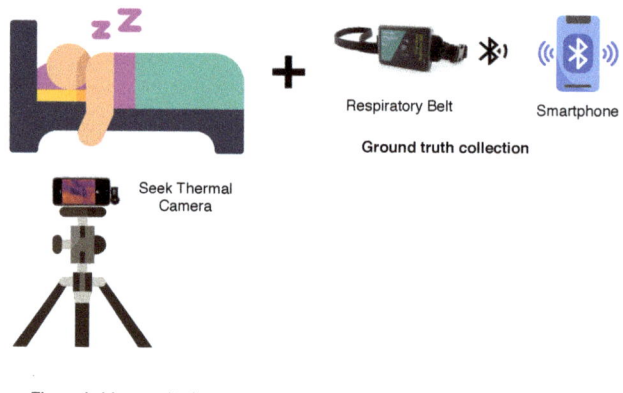

Figure 6. Data collection setup.

3.2. Respiratory Rate Estimation and Body Movements Detection

Table 3 contains the results obtained for all subjects, including respiratory rate estimation and body movement detection. The respiratory rate estimated by our proposed method was compared with the reference signal obtained by the respiratory belt. The RMSE was calculated by considering all the breaths in each signal collected during the experiment minute-by-minute. The average respiratory rate in the overall subjects is 14.78 ± 1.93 bpm for the reference signal and 14.47 ± 0.60 bpm for the proposed approach. The standard deviation of RMSE for the respiratory rate of all subjects is 0.75 bpm, and the average is 1.82 bpm. The small RMSE indicates that the proposed approach is robust for subjects variation. As for body movements detection, we counted the number of movement, the number of frames including body movement, and the total duration of body movements as summarized in Table 3.

Table 2. Participants Data.

Subjects	Gender	Age (years)	Height (cm)	Weight (kg)	BMI (kg/m^2)
S01	F	28	162	56	21.34
S02	F	36	167	52	18.65
S03	F	31	162	50	19.05
S04	F	29	163	53	19.95
S05	F	32	158	54	21.63
S06	M	25	161	70	27.01
S07	F	31	151	47	20.61
S08	F	29	160	50	19.53
S09	M	30	168	55	19.49
S10	F	28	159	58	22.94
S11	M	28	180	75	23.15
S12	M	26	169	58	20.31
S13	M	27	168	59	20.90
S14	M	29	168	78	27.64
S15	F	32	153	56	23.92
S16	F	37	153	47	20.08

Table 3. The result of respiratory rate estimation and body movements detection.

Subjects	Respiratory Rate (bpm)				Body Movements			
	Duration (s)	Reference	Experiment	RMSE	#Movements	#Frames	Duration (s)	Degree
S01	5371.05	12.71	14.05	1.56	14	269	15.69	1.12
S02	5397.54	13.69	14.22	1.11	15	199	11.65	0.78
S03	5379.37	16.75	14.78	2.20	7	63	3.69	0.53
S04	5192.31	12.23	13.37	2.00	35	642	37.86	1.08
S05	5212.78	17.62	14.39	3.32	9	200	11.72	1.30
S06	5200.51	16.45	14.48	2.23	9	214	12.53	1.39
S07	5332.39	14.38	14.36	1.47	16	218	12.80	0.80
S08	3495.39	14.65	14.29	1.18	15	749	43.48	2.90
S09	5407.22	12.17	14.60	2.68	0	3	0.17	0.00
S10	4520.26	14.91	14.79	0.75	5	91	5.33	1.07
S11	5346.70	13.12	13.76	1.25	16	417	24.42	1.53
S12	5361.45	13.25	15.37	2.35	7	140	8.20	1.17
S13	5399.74	18.61	15.99	2.79	5	20	1.17	0.23
S14	5380.52	15.15	14.32	1.49	16	535	31.14	1.95
S15	5315.23	16.32	14.40	1.99	12	225	13.19	1.10
S16	4287.12	14.43	14.41	0.72	6	250	14.51	2.42
Mean	5100.00	14.78	14.47	1.82				1.21
STD	537.63	1.93	0.60	0.75				0.74

The histogram of the number of body movements in every 40 s is also calculated to check the symptoms of PLMD. A small movement like a limb or head movement while sleeping takes a short duration, while significant movements or position changes can take a long time. Therefore, we calculated the degree of body movements by dividing the movement period with the number of movements, which is assumed to be closely related to sleep quality. Figure 7 shows the respiratory rate and body movements of S01–S16. The blue bar represents an occurred body movement. Several times in the event, in the beginning, refer to difficulty falling asleep like subject 4 and subject 8. The reference and experiment's respiratory rates were plotted 'x' and 'o', respectively. The blue column represents the histogram of body movements every 40 s. From this table, we can confirm that there was no regular and repetitive body movements for all subjects during experiments, which is the typical phenomenon of PLMD.

Our proposed approach provides respiration and body movements monitoring, which no existing thermal image based sleep monitoring system presents. We believe that body movement detection would characterize abnormal movements and behaviors during sleep, and is more comfortable for the users and completely unobtrusive.

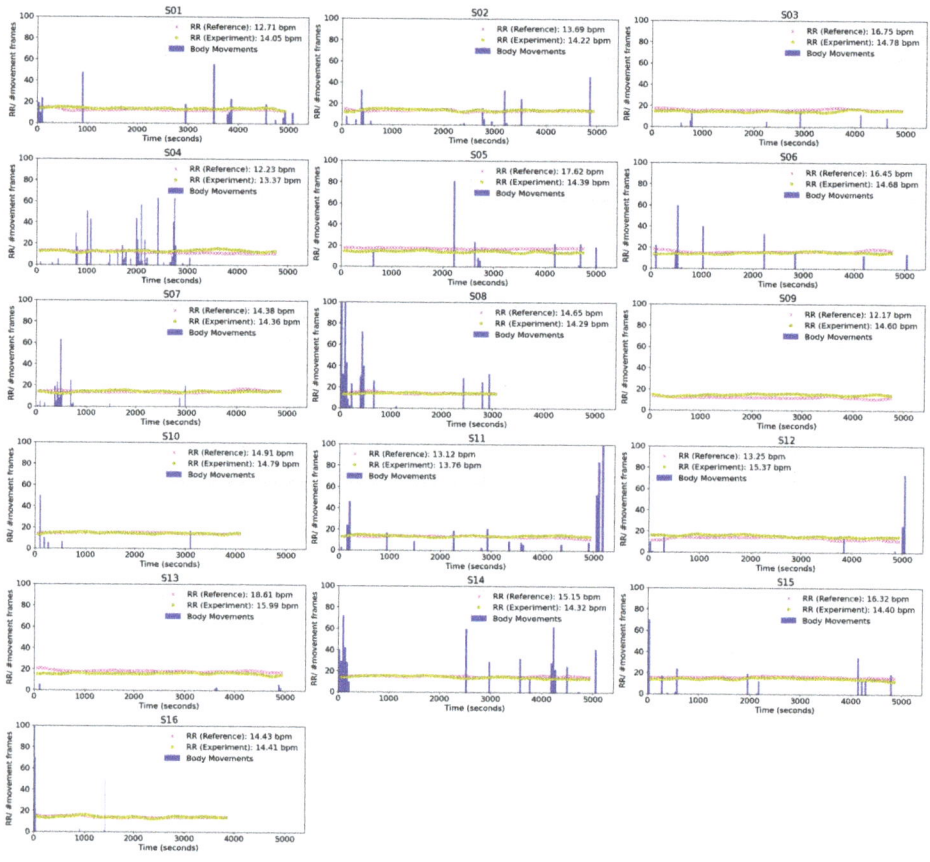

Figure 7. The result of the RMSE (respiratory rate) and body movements of S01–S16.

4. Conclusions

This paper proposed an approach for non-contact respiration monitoring and body movements detection in a natural sleep environment using a thermal camera. The thermal camera can handle many viewing angles, which makes installation in the bedroom easy. We have to overcome specific challenges to acquire non-contact respiration data from participants in their natural sleep environment when the lights were turned off and they were covered by a blanket. The thermal video sleep monitoring can be performed in a dark environment to settle privacy concerns. The participants were asked to set up the system and perform a recording by themselves at their home. This approach aims to use for screening the irregular respiration before going to the hospital.

The proposed approach consists of automatically computing the ROIs that it can use to acquire the respiration signal and detecting the body movements of the participant by employing an image processing on the continuous thermal image. The signals were obtained in each frame process with normalizing and smoothing signals. Then, we computed the number of breathing and counted the number of body movements. The approach has been validated using a respiratory belt as a reference signal. We evaluate respiration monitoring performance and body movements detection in different rooms with 16 participants who have independent sleep postures. Our results show that the proposed approach successfully estimated that the RR was obtaining an RMSE of 1.82 ± 0.75 bpm. The performed experiments confirmed that a thermal camera is easy to use for respiration monitoring and body movements during sleeping within various environments. In future work, we will focus on monitoring a patient who has irregular breathing. Another element of our work that could be improved is the automatic optimization of the thresholding value. The other limitations of the proposed method, such as a variation of room temperature, the type of bed cover, blanket, and night sweats (neck or face) in subjects, rapid eye movement (REM) stage, and heart rate, provide ideas for addressing these issues in future studies.

Author Contributions: Conceptualization, T.O. and P.J.; methodology, P.J.; software, P.J.; validation, P.J.; formal analysis, P.J.; investigation, P.J.; resources, T.O.; data curation, P.J.; writing—original draft preparation, P.J.; writing—review and editing, T.O. and P.J.; visualization, P.J.; supervision, T.O.; project administration, P.J.; funding acquisition, T.O. All authors have read and agreed to the published version of the manuscript.

Funding: This research received no external funding.

Conflicts of Interest: The authors declare no conflict of interest.

References

1. Wheatley, I. Respiratory rate 3: How to take an accurate measurement. Available online: https://www.nursingtimes.net/clinical-archive/respiratory-clinical-archive/respiratory-rate-3-how-to-take-an-accurate-measurement-25-06-2018/ (accessed on 30 January 2020)
2. Sheppard, M.; Wright, M.W. *Principles and Practice of High Dependency Nursing*; Elsevier Health Sciences: Amsterdam, The Netherlands, 2006.
3. Cretikos, M.; Chen, J.; Hillman, K.; Bellomo, R.; Finfer, S.; Flabouris, A.; Investigators, M.S. The objective medical emergency team activation criteria: A case–control study. *Resuscitation* **2007**, *73*, 62–72. [CrossRef] [PubMed]
4. Somers, V. American Heart Association Council for High Blood Pressure Research Professional Education Committee, Council on Clinical Cardiology. American Heart Association Stroke Council. American Heart Association Council on Cardiovascular Nursing. American College of Cardiology Foundation. Sleep apnea and cardiovascular disease: An American Heart Association/American College Of Cardiology Foundation Scientific Statement from the American Heart Association Council for High Blood Pressure Research Professional Education Committee, Council on Clinical Cardiology, Stroke Council, and Council On Cardiovascular Nursing. In collaboration with the National Heart, Lung, and Blood Institute National Center on Sleep Disorders Research (National Institutes of Health). *Circulation* **2008**, *118*, 1080–1111. [PubMed]
5. Meoli, A.L.; Casey, K.R.; Clark, R.W.; Coleman, J.A.; Fayle, R.W.; Troell, R.J.; Iber, C.; Clinical Practice Review Committee. Hypopnea in sleep-disordered breathing in adults. *Sleep* **2001**, *24*, 469–70. [PubMed]
6. Harvard Medical School, H.U. Understanding the Results: Sleep Apnea. Available online: http://healthysleep.med.harvard.edu/sleep-apnea/diagnosing-osa/understanding-results (accessed on 20 February 2020).
7. Zagaria, M.A.E. Periodic Limb Movement Disorder, Restless Legs Syndrome, and Pain. *US Pharm.* **2015**, *40*, 19–21.
8. Madhushri, P.; Ahmed, B.; Penzel, T.; Jovanov, E. Periodic leg movement (PLM) monitoring using a distributed body sensor network. In Proceedings of the 2015 37th Annual International Conference of the IEEE Engineering in Medicine and Biology Society (EMBC), Milan, Italy, 25–29 August 2015; pp. 1837–1840.
9. Koolen, N.; Decroupet, O.; Dereymaeker, A.; Jansen, K.; Vervisch, J.; Matic, V.; Vanrumste, B.; Naulaers, G.; Van Huffel, S.; De Vos, M. Automated Respiration Detection from Neonatal Video Data. In Proceedings of the International Conference on Pattern Recognition Applications and Methods (ICPRAM-2015), Lisbon, Portugal, 10–12 January 2015; pp. 164–169.

10. AL-Khalidi, F.Q.; Saatchi, R.; Burke, D.; Elphick, H. Tracking human face features in thermal images for respiration monitoring. In Proceedings of the ACS/IEEE International Conference on Computer Systems and Applications-AICCSA 2010, Hammamet, Tunisia, 16–19 May 2010; pp. 1–6. [CrossRef]
11. Lee, Y.S.; Pathirana, P.N.; Steinfort, C.L.; Caelli, T. Monitoring and analysis of respiratory patterns using microwave doppler radar. *IEEE J. Transl. Eng. Health Med.* **2014**, *2*, 1–12. [CrossRef] [PubMed]
12. Al-Naji, A.; Chahl, J. Remote respiratory monitoring system based on developing motion magnification technique. *Biomed. Signal Process. Control* **2016**, *29*, 1–10. [CrossRef]
13. Nakajima, K.; Matsumoto, Y.; Tamura, T. A monitor for posture changes and respiration in bed using real time image sequence analysis. In Proceedings of the 22nd Annual International Conference of the IEEE Engineering in Medicine and Biology Society (Cat. No. 00CH37143), Chicago, IL, USA, 23–28 July 2000; Volume 1, pp. 51–54.
14. Frigola, M.; Amat, J.; Pagès, J. Vision based respiratory monitoring system. In Proceedings of the 10th Mediterranean Conference on Control and Automation (MED 2002), Lisbon, Portugal, 9–12 July 2002; pp. 9–13.
15. Wiesner, S.; Yaniv, Z. Monitoring patient respiration using a single optical camera. In 2007 29th Annual International Conference of the IEEE Engineering in Medicine and Biology Society, Lyon, France, 22–26 August 2007; pp. 2740–2743.
16. Abbas, A.K.; Heimann, K.; Jergus, K.; Orlikowsky, T.; Leonhardt, S. Neonatal non-contact respiratory monitoring based on real-time infrared thermography. *Biomed. Eng. Online* **2011**, *10*, 93. [CrossRef]
17. Fei, J.; Pavlidis, I. Thermistor at a distance: unobtrusive measurement of breathing. *IEEE Trans. Biomed. Eng.* **2009**, *57*, 988–998.
18. Lewis, G.F.; Gatto, R.G.; Porges, S.W. A novel method for extracting respiration rate and relative tidal volume from infrared thermography. *Psychophysiology* **2011**, *48*, 877–887. [CrossRef]
19. Murthy, R.; Pavlidis, I. Noncontact measurement of breathing function. *IEEE Eng. Med. Biol. Mag.* **2006**, *25*, 57–67. [CrossRef] [PubMed]
20. Murthy, R.; Pavlidis, I.; Tsiamyrtzis, P. Touchless monitoring of breathing function. In Proceedings of the 26th Annual International Conference of the IEEE Engineering in Medicine and Biology Society, San Francisco, CA, USA, 1–5 September 2004; Volume 1, pp. 1196–1199.
21. Pereira, C.B.; Yu, X.; Czaplik, M.; Rossaint, R.; Blazek, V.; Leonhardt, S. Remote monitoring of breathing dynamics using infrared thermography. *Biomed. Opt. Express* **2015**, *6*, 4378–4394. [CrossRef] [PubMed]
22. Alkali, A.H.; Saatchi, R.; Elphick, H.; Burke, D. Facial tracking in thermal images for real-time noncontact respiration rate monitoring. In Proceedings of the 2013 European Modelling Symposium, Manchester, UK, 20–22 November 2013; pp. 265–270.
23. Alkali, A.H.; Saatchi, R.; Elphick, H.; Burke, D. Thermal image processing for real-time non-contact respiration rate monitoring. *IET Circuits Devices Syst.* **2017**, *11*, 142–148. [CrossRef]
24. Bennett, S.L.; Goubran, R.; Knoefel, F. The detection of breathing behavior using Eulerian-enhanced thermal video. In Proceedings of the 2015 37th Annual International Conference of the IEEE Engineering in Medicine and Biology Society (EMBC), Milan, Italy, 25–29 August 2015; pp. 7474–7477. [CrossRef]
25. Pereira, C.B.; Yu, X.; Czaplik, M.; Blazek, V.; Venema, B.; Leonhardt, S. Estimation of breathing rate in thermal imaging videos: A pilot study on healthy human subjects. *J. Clin. Monit. Comput.* **2017**, *31*, 1241–1254. [CrossRef]
26. Kwasniewska, A.; Szankin, M.; Ruminski, J.; Kaczmarek, M. Evaluating Accuracy of Respiratory Rate Estimation from Super Resolved Thermal Imagery. In Proceedings of the 2019 41st Annual International Conference of the IEEE Engineering in Medicine and Biology Society (EMBC), Berlin, Germany, 23–27 July 2019; pp. 2744–2747.
27. Jagadev, P.; Giri, L.I. Non-contact monitoring of human respiration using infrared thermography and machine learning. *Infrared Phys. Technol.* **2020**, *104*, 103117. [CrossRef]
28. Al-khalidi, D.F.; Saatchi, R.; Elphick, H.; Burke, D. Tracing the Region of Interest in Thermal Human Face for Respiration Monitoring. *Int. J. Comput. Appl.* **2015**, *119*, 42–46. [CrossRef]
29. Fei, J.; Pavlidis, I. Analysis of breathing air flow patterns in thermal imaging. In Proceedings of the 2006 International Conference of the IEEE Engineering in Medicine and Biology Society, New York, NY, USA, 30 August–3 September 2006; pp. 946–952.

30. Usman, M.; Evans, R.; Saatchi, R.; Kingshott, R.; Elphick, H. Non-invasive respiration monitoring by thermal imaging to detect sleep apnoea. submitted.
31. Fei, J.; Pavlidis, I.; Murthy, J. Thermal vision for sleep apnea monitoring. In Proceedings of the International Conference on Medical Image Computing and Computer-Assisted Intervention, London, UK, 20–24 September 2009; Springer: Berlin/Heidelberg, Germany, 2009; pp. 1084–1091.
32. Seba, A.; Istrate, D.; Guettari, T.; Ugon, A.; Pinna, A.; Garda, P. Thermal-Signature-Based Sleep Analysis Sensor. *Informatics* **2017**, *4*, 37.
33. Chen, Z.; Wang, Y. Sleep monitoring using an infrared thermal array sensor. In *Sensors and Smart Structures Technologies for Civil, Mechanical, and Aerospace Systems*; International Society for Optics and Photonics: Bellingham, WA, USA, 2019; Volume 10970, p. 109701D.
34. Al-Kalidi, F.; Elphick, H.; Saatchi, R.; Burke, D. Respiratory rate measurement in children using a thermal camera. *Int. J. Sci. Eng. Res.* **2015**, *6*, 1748–1756.
35. Hu, M.; Zhai, G.; Li, D.; Fan, Y.; Duan, H.; Zhu, W.; Yang, X. Combination of near-infrared and thermal imaging techniques for the remote and simultaneous measurements of breathing and heart rates under sleep situation. *PLoS ONE* **2018**, *13*, e0190466. [CrossRef]
36. Pereira, C.B.; Yu, X.; Goos, T.; Reiss, I.; Orlikowsky, T.; Heimann, K.; Venema, B.; Blazek, V.; Leonhardt, S.; Teichmann, D. Noncontact monitoring of respiratory rate in newborn infants using thermal imaging. *IEEE Trans. Biomed. Eng.* **2018**, *66*, 1105–1114. [CrossRef]
37. Lorato, I.; Bakkes, T.; Stuijk, S.; Meftah, M.; De Haan, G. Unobtrusive respiratory flow monitoring using a thermopile array: A feasibility study. *Appl. Sci.* **2019**, *9*, 2449. [CrossRef]
38. Opencv dev team. Operations on Arrays. 2019. Available online: https://docs.opencv.org/3.4/d2/de8/group__core__array.html (accessed on 20 February 2020).
39. Tarassenko, L.; Villarroel, M.; Guazzi, A.; Jorge, J.; Clifton, D.A.; Pugh, C. Non-contact video-based vital sign monitoring using ambient light and auto-regressive models. *Physiol. Meas.* **2014**. [CrossRef]
40. Kumbhar, P.G.; Holambe, S.N. A Review of Image Thresholding Techniques. *Int. J. Adv. Res. Comput. Sci. Softw. Eng.* **2015**, *5*, 160–163.
41. Virtanen, P.; Gommers, R.; Oliphant, T.E.; Haberland, M.; Reddy, T.; Cournapeau, D.; Burovski, E.; Peterson, P.; Weckesser, W.; Bright, J.; et al. SciPy 1.0: Fundamental Algorithms for Scientific Computing in Python. *Nat. Methods* **2020**, *17*, 261–272. [CrossRef]
42. Schafer, R.W. What is a Savitzky-Golay filter? [lecture notes]. *IEEE Signal Process. Mag.* **2011**, *28*, 111–117. [CrossRef]
43. Sanchez-Marin, F.J.; Calixto-Carrera, S.; Villaseñor-Mora, C. Novel approach to assess the emissivity of the human skin. *J. Biomed. Opt.* **2009**, *14*, 024006. [CrossRef]
44. Vernier. Go Direct® Respiration Belt. Available online: https://www.vernier.com/manuals/gdx-rb/ (accessed on 20 March 2020).

Publisher's Note: MDPI stays neutral with regard to jurisdictional claims in published maps and institutional affiliations.

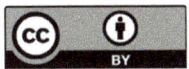

© 2020 by the authors. Licensee MDPI, Basel, Switzerland. This article is an open access article distributed under the terms and conditions of the Creative Commons Attribution (CC BY) license (http://creativecommons.org/licenses/by/4.0/).

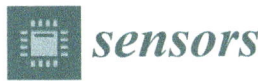 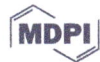

Article

Portable Sleep Apnea Syndrome Screening and Event Detection Using Long Short-Term Memory Recurrent Neural Network

Hung-Chi Chang [1], Hau-Tieng Wu [2], Po-Chiun Huang [1], Hsi-Pin Ma [1] and Yu-Lun Lo [3,*] and Yuan-Hao Huang [1,*]

1. Department of Electrical Engineering, National Tsing Hua University, Hsinchu 30013, Taiwan; Scott_Chang@asus.com (H.-C.C.); pchuang@ee.nthu.edu.tw (P.-C.H.); hp@ee.nthu.edu.tw (H.-P.M.)
2. Department of Mathematics and Department of Statistical Science, Duke University, Durham, NC 27708, USA; hauwu@math.duke.edu
3. Department of Thoracic Medicine, Healthcare Center, Chang Gung Memorial Hospital, School of Medicine, Chang Gung University, Taipei 33302, Taiwan
* Correspondence: lo3043@cgmh.org.tw (Y.-L.L.); yhhuang@ee.nthu.edu.tw (Y.-H.H.)

Received: 15 September 2020; Accepted: 22 October 2020; Published: 25 October 2020

Abstract: Obstructive sleep apnea/hypopnea syndrome (OSAHS) is characterized by repeated airflow partial reduction or complete cessation due to upper airway collapse during sleep. OSAHS can induce frequent awake and intermittent hypoxia that is associated with hypertension and cardiovascular events. Full-channel Polysomnography (PSG) is the gold standard for diagnosing OSAHS; however, this PSG evaluation process is unsuitable for home screening. To solve this problem, a measuring module integrating abdominal and thoracic triaxial accelerometers, a pulsed oximeter (SpO_2) and an electrocardiogram sensor was devised in this study. Moreover, a long short-term memory recurrent neural network model is proposed to classify four types of sleep breathing patterns, namely obstructive sleep apnea (OSA), central sleep apnea (CSA), hypopnea (HYP) events and normal breathing (NOR). The proposed algorithm not only reports the apnea-hypopnea index (AHI) through the acquired overnight signals but also identifies the occurrences of OSA, CSA, HYP and NOR, which assists in OSAHS diagnosis. In the clinical experiment with 115 participants, the performances of the proposed system and algorithm were compared with those of traditional expert interpretation based on PSG signals. The accuracy of AHI severity group classification was 89.3%, and the AHI difference for PSG expert interpretation was 5.0 ± 4.5. The overall accuracy of detecting abnormal OSA, CSA and HYP events was 92.3%.

Keywords: abdominal movement signal; hypopnea; LSTM-RNN; neural network; oxygen saturation; sleep apnea syndrome; sleep–wake detection; synchrosqueezing transform; triaxial accelerometer; thoracic movement signal

1. Introduction

According to a recent report [1], 13% men and 6% women between the ages of 30 and 70 years are affected by obstructive sleep apnea-hypopnea syndrome (OSAHS). Patients suffering from OSAHS have symptoms such as excessive daytime sleepiness, morning headache, hypertension and decreased libido [2]. However, people are often unaware of OSAHS because apnea/hypopnea events only occur during sleep. According to the American Academy of Sleep Medicine scoring manual [3], an apnea event is identified when a drop of 90% respiratory airflow lasts for at least 10 s. Moreover, a hypopnea event is defined when a drop of over 30% respiratory airflow lasts for at least 10 s with at least 3% associated decrease in oxygen saturation (SpO_2) or arousal from sleep. The apnea-hypopnea index (AHI), which is defined as the total number of apnea and hypopnea events per hour of sleep, is a vital metric to quantize the severity of sleep breathing disorder. Although AHI is recently criticized and other phenotype information of sleep breathing problems should be considered in clinical diagnosis [4], it still is a reliable metric for SDB screening at home before the patients are recommended for other decent testing or diagnosis in hospital. Full-channel polysomnography (PSG) is the traditional method of diagnosing OSAHS. In PSG, various physical and biological signals containing sleep information are comprehensively recorded. Although PSG is the standard for diagnosing OSAHS, it has several drawbacks. Subjects are required to wear numerous sensors (more than 20 channels) for monitoring the condition of the body during sleep. The PSG examination can be performed only in the hospital and the sleep quality of the patients can be influenced by several external constraints. Moreover, to diagnose an OSAHS patient, it usually requires more than 6 h for a doctor or sleep technician to observe multichannel and overnight PSG signals and to label the sleep breathing events accordingly. Therefore, PSG measurement and diagnosis are expensive, time consuming and unsuitable for large-scale home-based screening. Several solutions have been proposed to alleviate this difficulty. A common solution is reducing the number of sensors. Several issues on the ambulatory monitoring for obstructive sleep apnea syndrome were raised by [5], and guidelines of using critical channels were also provided for sleep disorder diagnosis and management. In general, these solutions are classified into four classes [6]. A Level-III or Level-IV solution is considered in this paper.

In the past decade, several reduced-channel technologies have been developed to evaluate OSAHS severity. Multiple biological signals, such as electrocardiogram (ECG) [7], ballistocardiography [8], SpO_2 [9], respiratory efforts [10] and snoring sounds [11], have been used to derive statistical or instantaneous signal features that are highly related with apnea events for sleep event identification. With the derived features from the selected sensors, various automatic annotation algorithms have been developed for sleep apnea events. Classification levels are of two types—the AHI level and event level. At the AHI level, the AHI of the whole night sleep is estimated for diagnosis. At the event level, each single apnea and hypopnea event is identified and classified and hence the AHI is accordingly calculated for the diagnosis. For the classification, various machine learning techniques such as support vector machine (SVM) [12], ensemble classifiers [13], and Bayesian network-based classifier [14] have been used to identify the sleep apnea events. Recently, a convolutional-neural-network-based deep learning framework [15] was proposed to detect obstructive sleep apnea events. In another study [7], the hidden-Markov-model-based deep neural network was used for detecting sleep apnea based on ECG signals. Raw biological signals without feature extraction have been used in several studies for detecting sleep apnea events through deep learning [9]. Quiceno-Manrique [16], Mendez [17], De Chazal [13] and Novak [18] used ECG signal for diagnosing OSAHS. In [10,19], abdominal (ABD) and thoracic (THO) movements were proven to be excellent parameters for diagnosing OSA occurrence. In [20], multiple channels, SpO_2 and photoplethysmography (PPG) were used to estimate the blood volume changes for OSA prediction. For other literature works, refer to [21,22]. The primary differences and contributions of this study are presented as follows:

- This study is the first work to apply two triaxial accelerometers, a single-lead ECG and a finger oximeter for portable sleep apnea syndrome screening. The clinic experiments were performed by recording overnight signals of suspected patients under the approval of Institutional Review Board of hospital. Most works designed new sensing devices without clinic experiments or developed new detection algorithms by using public database.
- This work proposes a complete systematic framework of sensing devices and algorithms to detect and identify OSA, central sleep apnea (CSA) and hypopnea (HYP) events. This system can not only evaluate AHI values but also provide reliable event-level classification results of various sleep apnea events. Except our previous work [23] based on piezo-electronic bands, most works can only detect OSA events and evaluate AHI only.

In this study, a hardware solution was combined with a novel neural-network-based classification technique for identifying OSA, CSA and HYP events and NOR breathing by using two triaxial accelerometers (TAA), a pulsed oximeter and ECG. The proposed classification algorithm performs event level prediction but not the AHI level prediction. The features of the abdominal TAA (ABD-TAA), thoracic TAA (THO-TAA) and SpO$_2$ signals were extracted from the recorded signals. Then, a modified long short-term memory recurrent neural network (LSTM-RNN) was proposed to classify the OSA, CSA and HYP events and NOR breathing in the overnight recorded signals. To avoid underestimation of the AHI from the predicted apnea and hypopnea events, the sleep–wake status was predicted by analyzing the ECG signal with a CNN classifier. The AHI severity group classification, AHI difference and OSA/CSA/HYP event and normal breathing classification were also analyzed to demonstrate the superiority of the proposed OSAHS screening system.

This study aimed to develop an unattended sleep apnea screening system that can be incorporated in the personal healthcare services with less labeling labor. The proposed screening system can be applied to evaluate the long-term sleep breathing performance of the potential subjects. These devices should be used in patients with a high pretest probability for obstructive sleep apnea/hypopnea syndrome according to 2007 AASM guideline (Reference 4) for the home-base diagnosis test. Patients suspected with respiratory, cardiologic and neurologic disorders should be excluded in this test. Primary care physician or sleep specialist would be the one who arranges this test.

2. Material and Methods

2.1. Material

The THO and ABD movements were recorded using piezo-electric bands at a sampling rate of 100 Hz on the Alice 5 PSG acquisition system (Philips Respironics, Murrysville, PA, USA). The SpO$_2$ signals were also recorded at a sampling rate of 1 Hz in the PSG signals. The OSA, CSA and HYP events and NOR breathing were identified and labeled by sleep experts in the PSG signals as the reference classifier. At the same time as the PSG recoding process, the proposed THO-TAA, ABD-TAA and ECG sensing devices were also attached to the chest and abdomen of the participant for capturing the signals required for the proposed AHI evaluation system. Polysomnography (Alice 5, Respironics) was performed on all patients using standard techniques. Sleep stages and arousals were scored according to the AASM criteria [3]. Respiratory efforts were measured by piezo-electric bands, and arterial oxygen saturation was measured by pulse oximetry.

Established criteria were used to score respiratory events such as hypopnea, obstructive apnea, central apnea and mixed type apnea [3] during sleeping time. Apnea was defined as nasal flow cessation for more than 10 s. It was scored as obstructive (OSA) if the paradoxical respiratory and abdominal efforts were observed. It was scored as central (CSA) if none of these excursions were observed. It was scored as mixed if this effort is resumed toward the end of the period of apnea. The mixed type apnea was classified as OSA in this work because of its similar contribution factors to OSA. Hypopnea (HYP) was defined as a 30% reduction in nasal pressure transducer followed by an arousal or more than 3% decrease in SpO$_2$. In this work, a segment signal was scored as normal if none of the above-mentioned events was identified.

2.2. Integrated Sensing System

Figure 1a depicts the proposed integrated sensing system that captures biomedical signals for sleep event detection/classification and AHI evaluation. A 27-g sensing device was devised and fabricated with a nine-axis accelerometer, an ECG sensor, a Bluetooth module and a microcontroller (Figure 1b). The sensing device included an ultra-low-power microcontroller (MSP430) that controlled MPU9250 to capture TAA signals, which were then delivered to a mobile device, such as smartphone or tablet, through Bluetooth module CC2541. The integrated sensing system could continuously sense and record signals for 34 h with a 300 mAh battery. The signal word-length and sampling rate are 12 bits/500 Hz and 16 bits/50 Hz for the ECG and accelerator, respectively. The transmission baud rate from a sensor device to iOS device is 115,200 bps. The bandwidth and reliability was verified to be sufficient for continuous transmission of the overnight ECG and acceleration signals. The reconnection procedure was also implemented in the Bluetooth link in case that patients might wake up and leave the transmission coverage, for example to go to restroom at night.

In the clinical experiment, two integrated TAA/ECG sensing devices were attached on the chest and abdomen of the participants and the ECG electrode was attached to the chest (Figure 1c). To record respiratory information, one sensing device was placed from the left parasternal line, 4th or 5th intercostal space to the mid-clavicle line to measure the maximal thoracic movement. The other sensing device was placed from the left subcostal anterior axillary line to the umbilical area to measure the maximal abdomen movement. In this way, we not only obtained strong thoracic and abdomen movement signal but also strong EKG signal. In the proposed recording and storage system, a prototype app software with graphic user interface on iOS device was built to control the progress of the data recording. All the sensed physiological signals were transmitted from the sensing devices to the iOS device through Bluetooth. Then, they were uploaded to the Dropbox cloud data server for the following data analysis.

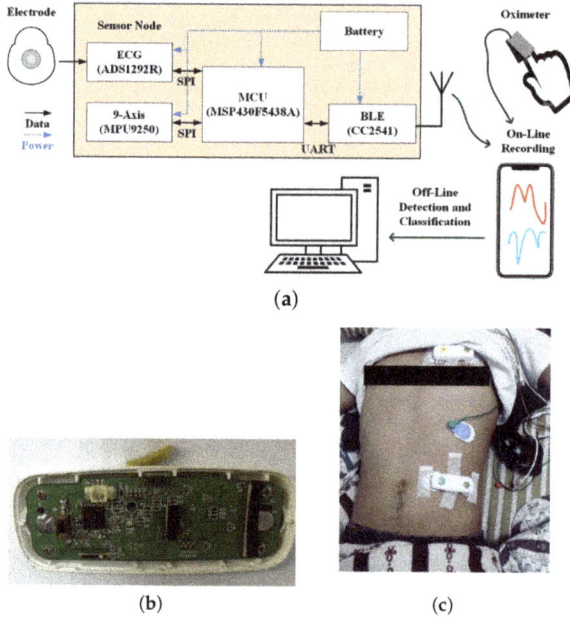

Figure 1. (a) Block diagram of the integrated sensing device and system; (b) photo of the sensing device; and (c) devices worn for sensing the ABD-TAA, THO-TAA and ECG signals.

2.3. Signal Preprocessing

Figure 2 displays the processing diagram of the proposed AHI evaluation system. Six channels of the ABD-TAA and THO-TAA signals were passed through six-order low-pass filters with a 0.8-Hz cut-off frequency and then converted into two respiratory motion signals, namely THO and ABD. Subsequently, the THO and ABD signals were segmented by a 10-s window and the SpO_2 signal was segmented by a 20-s window. Nine features in each segment were generated. These features were used to classify four types of sleep breathing events with an LSTM-RNN classifier. SpO_2 desaturation and sleep–wake detectors were used to improve the results of the LSTM-RNN classifier for the AHI evaluation. The algorithm is detailed step by step as follows.

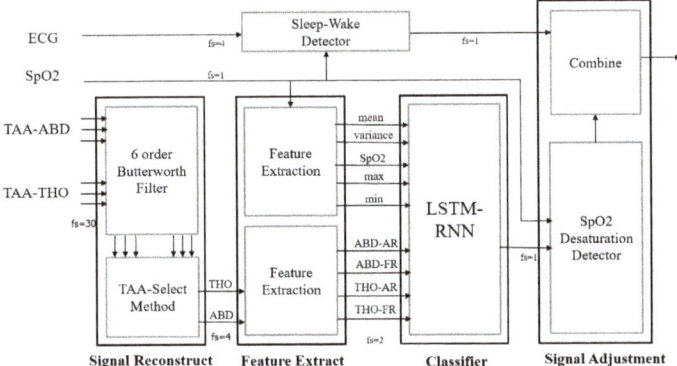

Figure 2. Processing diagram of the proposed AHI evaluation system.

Each TAA sensor sampled a three-axis acceleration vector at a time. Typically, principle component analysis (PCA) is used to combine the three-dimensional (3D) acceleration vector into 1D signal for the following analysis. Although PCA is suitable when the recording time is short, this approach is insufficient for overnight recording. The PCA could possibly distort the useful information of sleep breathing features because of the nonstationarity, particularly when the selected axis is switched frequently because of change in the sleep position. Thus, a TAA selection method was proposed to avoid this problem as shown in Figure 3. Three-dimensional TAA signals were first segmented by 30-s window with a 10-s time step. The number of periodic peaks was counted in a segment of an axis. Then, the axis with the most similar number of peaks to the human average respiration rate (6–9 peaks per 30 s) was selected as the output axis. After determining the selected axes of five successive segments, the most frequent axis in the previous five segments was selected as the output signal for the following analysis, as depicted in Figure 3a. If two axes had equal appearances, the axis with the larger magnitude was selected, as depicted in Figure 3b.

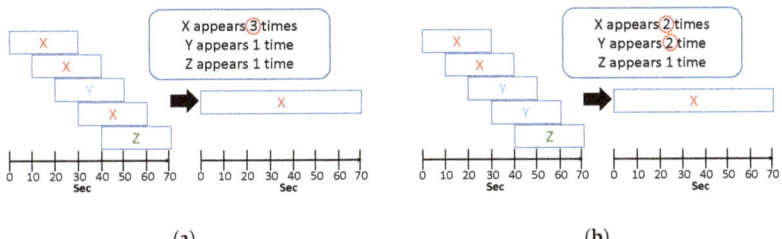

(a)   (b)

Figure 3. (a) TAA selection with the most appearances of one axis; and (b) TAA selection with equal appearances of two axes.

2.4. Feature Extraction

The preprocessed 1D THO and ABD signals were used to generate the features for sleep breathing event classification. The most obvious feature of the OSA event is the paradox between the THO and ABD signals. For the CSA event, the signal strengths of the THO and ABD signals are extremely small and exhibit small frequency deviation (e.g., the cardiogenic artifact). Because distinguishing HYP events in the ABD and THO signals is difficult, SpO_2 is incorporated to detect the HYP events.

2.4.1. Features of the THO and ABD signals

The THO and ABD signals are denoted as Y_{tho} and Y_{abd}, respectively. The THO and ABD signals were segmented using a 10-s window with a step of 0.5 s for feature extraction. According to the aforementioned physiological properties of the OSA, CSA and HYP events, the amplitude ratios (ARs) and the frequency ratios (FRs) [23] were considered as follows:

$$AR_{tho}(n) = \frac{Q_{95}(\tilde{A}_{tho}(t)\chi_{CW(n)})}{Q_{95}(\tilde{A}_{tho}(t)\chi_{PW(n)})}$$
$$AR_{abd}(n) = \frac{Q_{95}(\tilde{A}_{abd}(t)\chi_{CW(n)})}{Q_{95}(\tilde{A}_{abd}(t)\chi_{PW(n)})}. \qquad (1)$$

$$FR_{tho}(n) = \log_{10}\left(\frac{\int_{0.8}^{1.5}|\mathcal{F}(Y_{tho}(t)\chi_{CW(n)})(\xi)|^2 d\xi}{\int_{0.1}^{0.8}|\mathcal{F}(Y_{tho}(t)\chi_{CW(n)})(\xi)|^2 d\xi}\right)$$
$$FR_{abd}(n) = \log_{10}\left(\frac{\int_{0.8}^{1.5}|\mathcal{F}(Y_{abd}(t)\chi_{CW(n)})(\xi)|^2 d\xi}{\int_{0.1}^{0.8}|\mathcal{F}(Y_{abd}(t)\chi_{CW(n)})(\xi)|^2 d\xi}\right) \qquad (2)$$

where χ is the indicator function (1 or 0) for the windowing segmentation of input signals; Q_{95} represents the 95% quantile of the given function; $\tilde{A}_{tho}(t)$ and $\tilde{A}_{abd}(t)$ are the amplitudes of the THO and ABD signals, respectively, which were determined using the synchrosqueezing transform; and $\mathcal{F}$ represents the Fourier transform. CW represents the current window, that is, the nth CW is denoted as $CW(n) \subset \mathbb{R}$, where n is the index of segment. PW is the previous 60-s windowed signal before the current window. PW contains the baseline amplitude for AR. The nth PW associated with the nth CW is denoted as $PW(n) \subset \mathbb{R}$. Consequently, $AR_{tho}(n)$ and $AR_{abd}(n)$ represent the ARs and $FR_{tho}(n)$ and $FR_{abd}(n)$ represent the FRs of the THO and ABD signals, respectively, over the nth CW.

Synchrosqueezing transform (SST) is a novel nonlinear-type time–frequency analysis technique aiming to analyze complicated and nonstationary time series. It has been theoretically proved to enjoy several nice properties [24,25]. For our application, the main benefit of SST is an accurate estimation of the instantaneous frequency and the amplitude modulation of the respiratory signal. Moreover, the estimation does not depend on whether or not the oscillatory patter or wave-shape function is sinusoidal [26]. In addition, the SST is robust to various kinds of noise, including colored or even nonstationary random process [25].

The AR features were determined from the estimated amplitudes of the THO and ABD signals, which are denoted as $\tilde{A}_{tho}(t)$ and $\tilde{A}_{abd}(t)$, respectively, by using the synchrosqueezing transform. This step is critical because it suppresses the artifacts caused by the sudden change of body posture. The FR indicates the frequency distributions of the respiration and probably the cardiogenic artifact caused by heart beats. The integration range from 0.8 to 1.5 Hz in the numerator in (2) is the average range of heart beat rate. In our algorithm, the heart beat information was taken into account and the cardiogenic artifact indicates how silent the respiratory signal is. The detailed properties of the ARs and FRs of the THO and ABD signals can be obtained from [23].

2.4.2. Features of SpO$_2$ signal

SpO$_2$ is the percentage of oxyhemoglobin in hemoglobin. When sleep apnea and hypopnea events occur, SpO$_2$ decreases gradually until the subject breathes again. According to our data, the average delay time between an apnea (hypopnea) event and the 3% drop of SpO$_2$ was 19.3 ± 9.6 s. The average event duration is 20.2 ± 3.4. Figure 4a,b displays the distributions of the desaturation delay times of all events for the patients with AHI $>$ 30 and AHI $<$ 30, respectively. For patients with severe symptoms (AHI $>$ 30), the desaturation distribution exhibits a high probability of error in which the previous respiratory event related to desaturation is labeled as the current event, that is, the desaturation drop of the previous respiratory event is almost adjacent to the current event. Therefore, features of SpO$_2$ were generated for every 20-s segment with a 20-s delay from the sampling point, as depicted in Figure 5. The minimum, maximum, mean and variance of the first derivative were used as the four features, and the original SpO$_2$ signal was also reserved as the baseline. To eliminate the variation of subjects, the SpO$_2$ signal was normalized by subtracting it by its median and dividing the obtained value by its standard deviation.

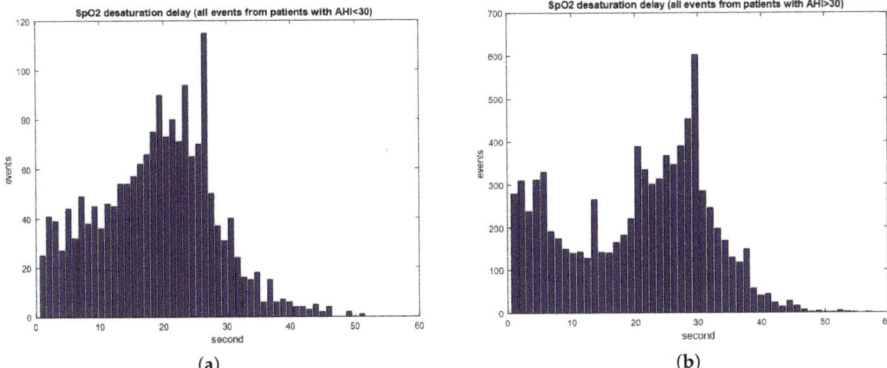

Figure 4. (**a**) SpO$_2$ desaturation time of patients with AHI lower than 30; and (**b**) SpO$_2$ delay time of patients with AHI higher than 30.

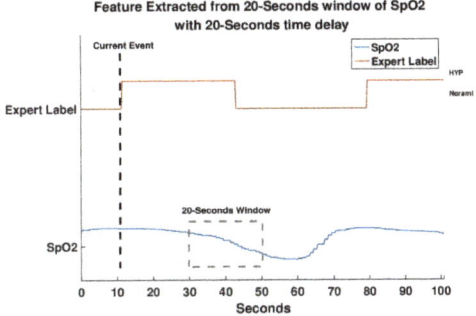

Figure 5. The decline of the SpO$_2$ signal occurs 20–40 s after abnormal events according to the physiological phenomenon.

2.5. Neutral Network Model, Event Classification and AHI Evaluation

2.5.1. Neural Network Model Classifier

The RNN based on the LSTM model, which was first presented by Hochreiter [27], was instrumental in solving many sequence problems with long-term dependency, such as language translation, speech recognition, image captioning and genomic information learning [28–31]. The features of the sleep breathing events based on THO/ABD and SpO$_2$ signals are time-varying and have long-term dependency. Therefore, an LSTM-RNN model was used to classify the sleep breathing events. The LSTM-RNN is an extension of the RNN and has more complex memory neurons than the RNN (Figure 6a). Unlike the original neuron with a simple loop in the RNN, every neuron in the RNN is replaced with an LSTM cell. An LSTM cell has three gates, namely the input, output and forget gates. These gates are scalars that are trained in every iteration to control the input, output and memory of every cell. Furthermore, the computation of output is reserved in the LSTM and combined with the new input. With the aforementioned design, the LSTM can thus deal with the long-term dependency problem, various desaturation times and many other subject variations for sleep breathing event classification.

Figure 6b illustrates the LSTM-RNN architecture, which has three layers, namely the input, LSTM-cell hidden and output layer. The input layer consists of nine neurons corresponding to nine extracted features from the THO/ABD and SpO$_2$ signals. The output layer contains four neurons representing four types of events, namely the OSA, CSA and HYP events and NOR breathing. The output of the network was normalized by using the softmax function. In total, 80 LSTM cells were utilized in the hidden layer according to the thumb of rule. The upper bound of the hidden neuron number was calculated by dividing the number of cases in the training dataset by the sum of the numbers of input and output layers in the network. The LSTM-RNN model was trained with 500 epochs of 500 batches of Adam gradient descents and a learning rate of 0.001. The activation function used in each layers was the rectified linear unit (ReLU) because of the benefit of sparsity and its capability of reducing the vanishing gradient. The loss function was used to compute the sum of cross entropy and L2 regularization with $\beta = 0.05$. Moreover, gradient clipping was added to the loss function to avoid the exploding gradient. Figure 7 illustrates the event detection results of 1-h segment for a patient. The PSG labeling results obtained from experts are displayed in the top panel of Figure 7. The middle panel displays the softmax output results of the LSTM-RNN classifier. In this panel, the four curves represent the probabilities of the four types of events. The decision rule of the LSTM-RNN classifier involves selecting the event with the highest probability in every time step, as depicted in the red line in the bottom panel. The LSTM-RNN classifier generates almost the same event states as PSG labeling does.

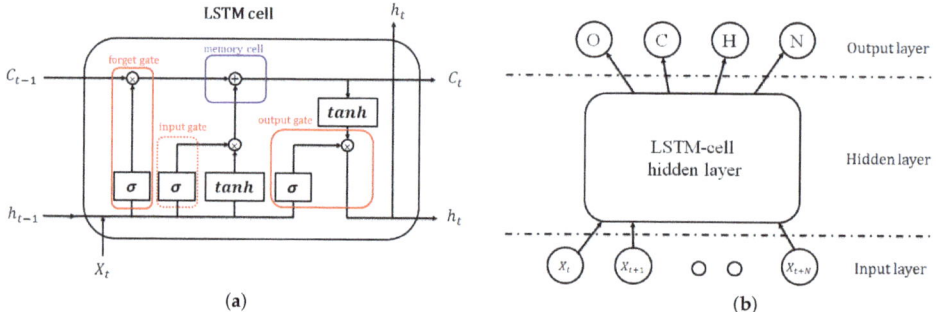

Figure 6. (a) X_t is the tth input feature, where $t = 1, 2, \ldots, N$. N is the total number of data points; C_t is the tth memory; h_t is the tth output; and σ and $tanh$ represent the sigmoid and hyperbolic tangent function, respectively [27]. (b) LSTM-RNN architecture with the input layer, hidden layer and four-neuron output layer for classifying CSA, OSA, HYP and NOR states in every N seconds.

2.5.2. Oxygen Desaturation Detection

According to the 2014 guidelines from the American Academy of Sleep Medicine [3], a 3% drop of SpO$_2$ is considered as a potential sleep apnea and hypopnea event. Therefore, the proposed sleep breathing event classifier incorporates a SpO$_2$ desaturation detection scheme to capture every 3% drop in the SpO$_2$ signal (Figure 8). First, the difference of SpO$_2$ saturation signal was calculated and then convolved with a 20-s unity window to accumulate the difference. Afterwards, every desaturation with over 3% drop can be marked as an HYP event, which may not easily be detected using the LSTM-RNN classifier because limited CSA or OSA features can be extracted for the hypopnea event. Finally, the remarked signal was moved 20-s forward to compensate the delay of SpO$_2$ desaturation. Figure 9 illustrates the 1-h classification results of PSG labeling, the softmax outputs of the RNN and the outputs of the LSTM-RNN classifier with desaturation detection. By adding SpO$_2$ desaturation, the HYP softmax output exhibits higher probability than the NOR state. Therefore, the HYP events can be easily (see HYP softmax output) detected.

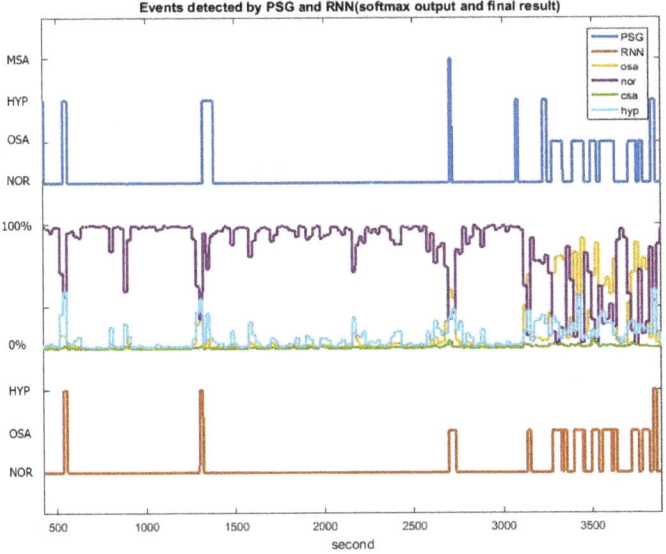

Figure 7. Event classification results of the PSG labeling, LSTM-RNN softmax outputs and final results of the LSTM-RNN classifier during 1-h sleep of a patient.

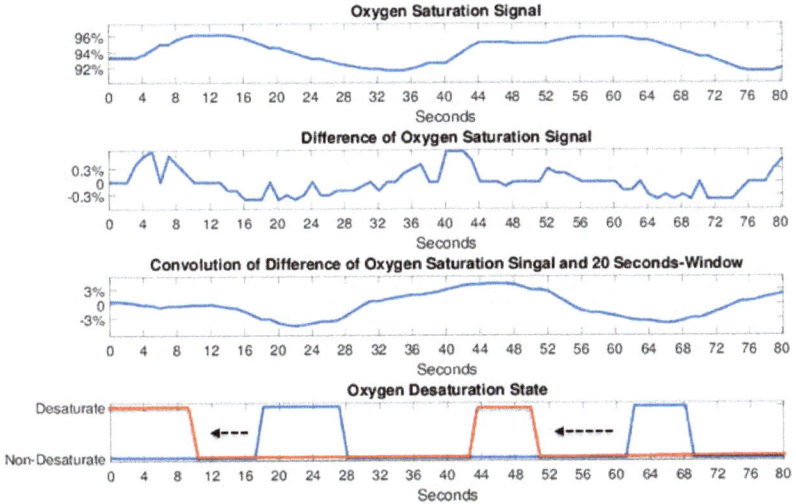

Figure 8. Processing steps for the oxygen desaturation detection.

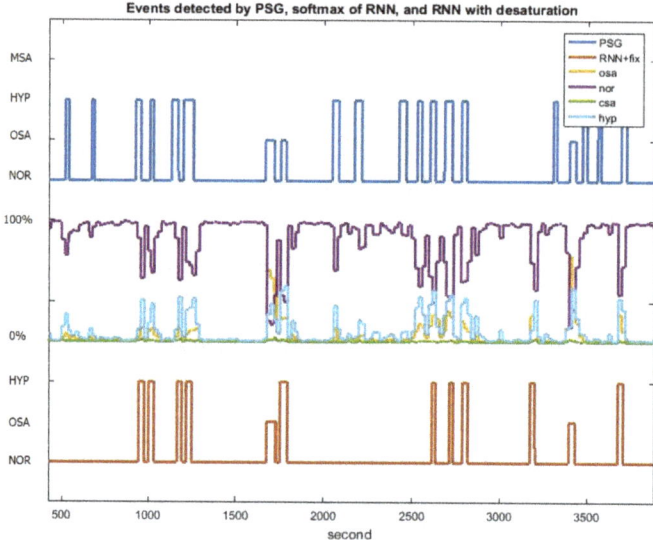

Figure 9. Event classification results of PSG labeling, the LSTM-RNN softmax outputs and the final results of the LSTM-RNN classifier with desaturation detection during 1-h sleep of a subject.

2.5.3. Sleep–Wake Classification

Because AHI is defined as the number of apnea and hypopnea events that occur during sleep, heart rate variability (HRV) was used in this study to detect the sleep and wake status during overnight sleep [32]. According to a previous study [33], a CNN was used to classify the sleep and wake status by using the instantaneous heart rate (IHR) signal converted from the ECG signal and SpO_2. Finally, the LSTM-RNN classification results and the sleep–wake state are combined to remove false positive events during the wake state. HRV is quantified by the intervals between successive heartbeats of ECG signals. HRV is estimated as the IHR per minute as follows:

$$\text{IHR}(r_i) = \frac{60}{r_i - r_{i-1}} \quad i = 2, \ldots, n, \qquad (3)$$

where r_i denotes time instants in seconds when the ith R peak is detected. The unit of IHR is then beats per minute (bpm). Subsequently, the IHR signal along with the 20-s-delayed SpO_2 signal was segmented into 30-s epochs for the CNN network.

Figure 10a displays the CNN network used to classify the sleep and wake state. The input is first passed through five convolution layers and then two fully connected layers. Figure 10b illustrates each convolution layer. A single convolution layer has ten filters with a kernel size 8, and the stride is equal to 1 and 2. Each fully connected layer has 20 nodes, and every node is associated with a bias and ReLU activation function. Finally, a softmax function is applied before the output layer. Five minutes of the IHR and SpO_2 signals were used as inputs, which were normalized by subtracting the median value. The output was a 2D one-hot code for the sleep and wake states. L2 regularization was applied with $\beta = 0.3$. The CNN network was trained using the Adam gradient descent with a learning rate of 10^{-3}, a batch size of 100 and cross entropy as the loss function.

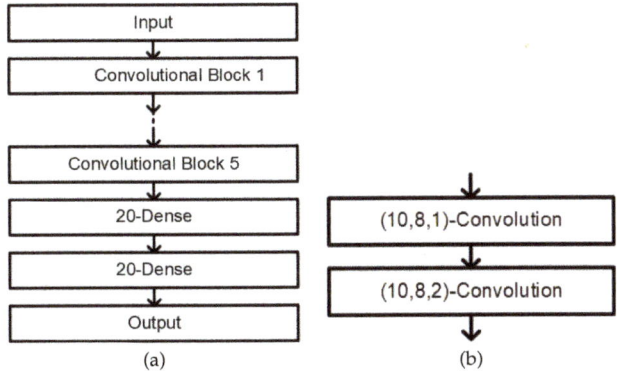

Figure 10. (a) Architecture of the one-dimensional CNN. The notation 20-Dense denotes that the fully connected layer possesses 20 nodes. For 5-min input signals, we used five convolution blocks [33]. (b) Architecture of a single convolution block. The notation (f, k, s)-convolution denotes that the convolutional layer has f filters with a kernel size k and stride s. The output of the block is half the size of the input [33]. A bias is added to the output of each filter, and the result is fed into a rectified linear unit (ReLU) activation function. A dropout with probability 0.5 is applied to the last layer and both fully-connected layers. The output of the network is normalized by the softmax function. An epoch is predicted to be wake if the output of the wake node is greater than or equal to that of the sleep node. We refer readers to Section 2.3 of [33] for more details.

3. Results

The clinic experiments were approved by the Institutional Review Board of the Chang Gung Memorial Hospital (CGMH: No. 201601576B0). Clinical patients at the sleep center in CGMH, Linkou, Taoyuan, Taiwan who were suspected of having sleep apnea were considered for this study. In total, 115 participants were examined in the clinical experiments. The demographic details of the participants are summarized in Table 1. The sleep experts identified the OSA, CSA, mixed sleep apnea (MSA) and HYP events from the overnight PSG signals of all patients. The remaining signals were NOR states. The MSA was regarded as the OSA in this study because of the similarity of physiological features. The training and testing databases had nearly the same distribution over various severity levels, as presented in Table 2.

Table 1. Demographic details of the 115 participants.

Severity	Gender	AHI (times/hr)	BMI (kg/m^2)	Age (year)	* TST (min)	** SE (%)	*** REM (%)	**** NREM (%)
Normal	all (9) male (6) female (3)	1.8 ± 1.6	23.2 ± 3.3	30.0 ± 8.2	312.9 ± 37.2	84.4 ± 9.9	15.4 ± 5.7	84.6 ± 5.7
Mild	all (17) male (13) female (4)	9.4 ± 2.4	25.6 ± 3.7	49.0 ± 11.3	313.4 ± 28.0	84.3 ± 7.3	17.8 ± 5.8	82.2 ± 5.8
Moderate	all (28) male (21) female (7)	21.7 ± 4.1	25.4 ± 2.7	48.5 ± 12.9	311.0 ± 40.7	83.9 ± 11.1	14.9 ± 5.6	85.1 ± 5.6
Severe	all (61) male (50) female (11)	61.1 ± 24.0	30.2 ± 6.0	50.3 ± 12.3	291.0 ± 52.6	79.4 ± 13.8	11.0 ± 6.2	89.0 ± 6.2

* TST, Total Sleep Time; ** SE, Sleep Efficiency; *** REM, Rapid Eye Movement Percentage; *** NREM, None Rapid Eye Movement Percentage.

Table 2. Distribution of the training and testing participants.

Level of Severity	Training Subjects	Testing Subjects	Total Subjects
Normal	6	3	9
Mild	9	8	17
Moderate	14	14	28
Severe	30	31	61
All levels	59	56	115

In our previous studies [23,34], SVM was used and followed by a state machine for screening OSAHS. The SVM model is divided into three types. First, the original SVM uses 50% of participants for training and 50% of participants for testing. Second, in the phenotype-based SVM [34], $K = 15$ nearest subjects of all data are selected according to gender, BMI and age with weights of 4, 2 and 1, respectively. Third, in the phenotype-based SVM with comorbidity information, the most similar 20 subjects are first selected and then the nearest 15 subjects are selected from these candidates using the K-nearest neighborhood method. For the LSTM-RNN model, the time step N was first evaluated for screening OSAHS. The detection performances of various Ns are presented in Table 3. When N was 20, the largest F_1 score was 0.72 ± 0.22 and the AHI difference was 8.1 ± 7.3. As the time step increased, the performance declined because the average duration of all events (apnea and hypopnea) was approximately 20 s (Figure 3).

Table 3. Sensitivity, precision, F_1 score and AHI difference of LSTM-RNN with different time steps (N).

Time Step (N)	Precision	Sensitivity	F_1 Score	AHI Difference
10 s	0.59 ± 0.25	0.88 ± 0.16	0.68 ± 0.24	9.7 ± 7.2
15 s	0.67 ± 0.23	0.74 ± 0.22	0.68 ± 0.21	8.8 ± 6.6
20 s	0.74 ± 0.22	0.73 ± 0.22	0.72 ± 0.22	8.1 ± 7.3
25 s	0.72 ± 0.22	0.75 ± 0.21	0.71 ± 0.21	8.7 ± 6.3
30 s	0.71 ± 0.21	0.77 ± 0.2	0.71 ± 0.2	8.6 ± 6.5

Precision = # of True Positive/(# of True Positive + # of False Positive); Sensitivity = # of True Positive/(# of True Positive + # of False Negative); F_1 Score = (2 × Precision · Sensitivity)/(Precision + Sensitivity).

LSTM-RNN with Oxygen Desaturation and Sleep–Wake Detection

Using the sleep–wake information of the overnight sleep, the classified sleep breathing events occurring when subjects were awake were eliminated. Thus, highly accurate sleeping hours for AHI evaluation could also be obtained in the experiment. Table 4 lists the sensitivity, precision, F_1 score and AHI difference for all subjects at various severity levels. We observed that sensitivity, precision and F_1 increased with the severity. The primary reason for this result was that the database size of the sleep breathing events for the severe group was considerably larger than that for the normal, mild and moderate groups. Compared with the generic SVM (F_1 score of 65% ± 26%) in Table 5, the proposed LSTM-RNN with oxygen desaturation and sleep–wake detection had a higher F_1 score (71% ± 22%) with respect to the PSG labeling of the sleep experts. The average AHI difference of the proposed LSTM-RNN model was 5.0 ± 4.5, which is smaller than that of the generic SVM model. Table 6 lists the confusion matrix of the classification of the proposed LSTM-RNN model with oxygen desaturation and sleep–wake detection for different severity levels. The severity classification achieved an accuracy of 89.3%.

Table 7 presents the confusion matrix of the classification of OSA, CSA and HYP events and NOR breathing. The overall event-by-event classification accuracy was 83.3%. The NOR breathing and OSA events could be well identified, whereas the identification of HYP events was difficult because of the lack of obvious information for HYP events. Some CSA events were classified as OSA events mainly because the OSA events had more than twice the CSA events in the database. However, the accuracy of distinguishing abnormal events was still 92.3%. This detection accuracy approximates the recommended intra-class correlation (95%) for the reliability of different scorers by [35]. This difference is very close to traditional subjective interpretation. Therefore, the proposed portable sensing system and OSAHS event identification algorithm can be reliable for the OSAHS screening in the home environment.

Table 4. Sensitivities, precisions, F_1 scores and AHI differences of LSTM-RNN with oxygen desaturation and sleep–wake detection for different severity groups.

LSTM-RNN Model	Sensitivity	Precision	F_1 Score	AHI Difference
Normal	0.62 ± 0.44	0.16 ± 0.15	0.23 ± 0.2	4.9 ± 4.4
Mild	0.62 ± 0.16	0.48 ± 0.14	0.54 ± 0.13	2.4 ± 1.7
Moderate	0.64 ± 0.2	0.77 ± 0.15	0.68 ± 0.16	5.8 ± 5.7
Severe	0.81 ± 0.13	0.86 ± 0.07	0.83 ± 0.09	5.7 ± 4.0
All levels	0.73 ± 0.2	0.74 ± 0.23	0.71 ± 0.22	5.0 ± 4.5

Table 5. Comparison of the LSTM-RNN and SVM models with oxygen desaturation.

Model + Oxygen Desaturation	Original SVM [23]	Phenotype SVM [34]	Phenotype SVM+ Comoribidity [34]	LSTM-RNN
Precision	0.77 ± 0.25	0.74 ± 0.27	0.74 ± 0.28	0.72 ± 0.22
Sensitivity	0.63 ± 0.27	0.64 ± 0.27	0.65 ± 0.27	0.81 ± 0.2
F1 score	0.65 ± 0.26	0.65 ± 0.26	0.65 ± 0.29	0.72 ± 0.22
AHI difference	10.6 ± 13.4	9.8 ± 10.0	9.0 ± 11.8	6.0 ± 5.2

Table 6. Confusion matrix of the LSTM-RNN model with oxygen desaturation and sleep–wake detection.

LSTM-RNN with Desaturation and Awake Detection		Expert Label			
		Normal	Mild	Moderate	Severe
RNN Label	Normal	3	0	0	0
	Mild	0	8	3	0
	Moderate	0	0	11	3
	Severe	0	0	0	28
Accuracy			89.28%		

Table 7. Confusion matrix of the OSA, CSA and HYP events and NOR breathing for the LSTM-RNN model with oxygen desaturation and sleep–wake detection.

Four Events Types Classification in LSTM-RNN		Expert Label			
		Normal	OSA	CSA	HYP
RNN Label	Normal	37,788	232	470	1824
	OSA	1391	7485	2132	1213
	CSA	21	35	1855	32
	HYP	556	1703	149	2138
Accuracy			83.34%		

4. Discussion

From the clinical perspective, through the proposed LSTM-RNN classifier with the TAA, ECG and SpO$_2$ signals, the respiratory events (apnea vs. hypopnea) and pattern (obstructive vs. central) can be effectively detected by the proposed system. Moreover, sleep–wake status be identified by using a CNN algorithm with instantaneous heart rate derived from ECG and SpO$_2$ signals. According to the heat rate and rhythm information in the ECG signal, our sensing devices and algorithm fully meet the requirements of AASM "SCOPER" (sleep, cardiovascular, oximetry, position, effort and respiratory) criteria for the home-base OSAHS detection. Compared with other Level 3 home-base equipments for sleep event screening using fewer sensors and channels for reducing sleep interference, the proposed sensing system and classification algorithm can provide better sleep quality and higher accuracy without sacrificing any useful information. The proposed system and algorithm can also support an effective early diagnosis and early treatment possibility for a clinically vital disease with high prevalence and low diagnostic and treatment rates.

From the hardware perspective, as suggested by a preliminary result provided in [33], the sleep–wake classification can be conducted accurately through PPG. This indicates that the ECG signal can be replaced by the PPG signal. Because only the partial information SpO_2 of the PPG signal was considered, one channel can be reduced in the next-generation sensing device.

From the algorithmic perspective, the following aspects should be considered to further improve the algorithm. The signal quality was considered in this study. The robustness properties of the feature extraction algorithm was simply focused on avoiding the impact of the inevitable noise and artifact. In addition to using the existing signal quality index (SQI) for the ECG or PPG signal, a suitable SQI should be developed for the ABD-TAA and THO-TAA signals. By incorporating these indices into the algorithm, the algorithm performance should be improved. This possibility will be explored in future study.

Limitation

This discussion is not complete without mentioning its limitation. First, the data were collected in a hospital environment designed for type I sleep screening. Additional data should be collected at the home-base environment to further confirm the applicability of the proposed model and algorithm. Another limitation is the database size. According to the encouraging positive results provided by the phenotype-based SVM, we expect to achieve a superior result if the database size increases. Specifically, with a larger database, we can have more cases with similar phenotype to build up an accurate model for each new-arriving patient.

5. Conclusions

In this study, a series of classification and detection algorithms was developed for screening sleep apnea patients by using a pulse oximeter and a wireless sensing system with TAA and ECG sensors. The features were extracted from the THO/ABD and SpO_2 signals and then used for training the LSTM-RNN classifier. The proposed system incorporates an SpO_2 desaturation detector and an ECG-based sleep–wake detector to improve the overall classification performance of the LSTM-RNN classifier. The severity group classification based on the AHI evaluation results of the proposed algorithm achieved an accuracy of 89.3%, and the sleep breathing event classification achieved an accuracy of 92.3%. Thus, we believe that the proposed screening system and classification algorithms can establish a solid foundation for the clinical screening of OSAHS.

This study has some potential future works. The proposed LSTM-based neural network has been proven to be effective in identifying several sleep apnea event types in this work. Since the proposed portable sensing system was designed for a homecare screening system, the LSTM-based neural network can be customized for individual person by using distributed learning techniques, which can be achieved by adopting phenotype information such as gender, weight, age and other personal physical information so as to enhance the personalized and high-accuracy sleep disorder screening system. Moreover, the proposed sensing system and APP software on a smartphone can record overnight data. To realize home-based screening or monitoring, the off-line data analysis (detection and event classification algorithms) on the PC can be further replaced by cloud-based analysis. That is, the user can upload the data by smartphone to a cloud server, and the data are then analyzed on the cloud server. Accordingly, the results can be easily viewed by the remote users such as doctors or caregivers.

Author Contributions: Conceptualization, Y.-L.L. and Y.-H.H.; methodology, Y.-H.H., P.-C.H., H.-P.M. and H.-T.W.; software, H.-C.C.; validation, H.-C.C., H.-T.W. and Y.-H.H.; formal analysis, I I.-C.C.; investigation, H.-T.W.; data curation, Y.-L.L., P.-C.H. and H.-P.M.; writing—original draft preparation, Y.-H.H. and H.-C.C.;

writing—review and editing, Y.-L.L. and H.-T.W.; supervision, Y.-H.H.; and funding acquisition, Y.-L.L. and Y.-H.H. All authors have read and agreed to the published version of the manuscript.

Funding: This work was supported by Chang Gung University and National Tsing Hua University Joint Project under grant numbers CMRPG3H0251 (Chang Gung University) and 107Q2516E1 (National Tsing Hua University).

Conflicts of Interest: The authors declare no conflict of interest.

References

1. Peppard, P.E.; Young, T.; Barnet, J.H.; Palta, M.; Hagen, E.W.; Hla, K.M. Increased prevalence of sleep-disordered breathing in adults. *Am. J. Epidemiol.* **2013**, *177*, 1006–1014. [CrossRef] [PubMed]
2. Kapur, V.K.; Auckley, D.H.; Chowdhuri, S.; Kuhlmann, D.C.; Mehra, R.; Ramar, K.; Harrod, C.G. Clinical Practice Guideline for Diagnostic Testing for Adult Obstructive Sleep Apnea: An American Academy of Sleep Medicine Clinical Practice Guideline. *J. Clin. Sleep Med.* **2017**, *15*, 479–504. [CrossRef] [PubMed]
3. Berry, R.B. The AASM Manual for the Scoring of Sleep and Associated Events. Available online: http://aasm.org/clinical-resources/scoring-manual/ (accessed on 25 October 2020).
4. Pevernagie, D.A.; Gnidovec–Strazisar, B.; Grote, L.; Heinzer, R.; McNicholas, W.T.; Penzel, T.; Randerath, W.; Schiza, S.; Verbraecken, J.; Arnardottir, E. S. On the rise and fall of the apnea–hypopnea index: A historical review and critical appraisal. *J. Sleep Res.* **2020**. [CrossRef] [PubMed]
5. Corral-Peñafiel, J.; Pepin, J.-L.; Barbe, F. Ambulatory monitoring in the diagnosis and management of obstructive sleep apnoea syndrome. *Eur. Respir. Rev.* **2013**, *22*, 312-324. [CrossRef]
6. Collop, N.A.; Anderson, W.M.; Boehlecke, B.; Claman, D.; Goldberg, R.; Gottlieb, D.J.; Hudgel, D.; Sateia, M.; Schwab, R. Clinical guidelines for the use of unattended portable monitors in the diagnosis of obstructive sleep apnea in adult patients. *J. Clin. Sleep Med.* **2007**, *3*, 737–747.
7. Li, K.; Pan, W.; Li, Y.; Jiang, Q.; Liu, G. A method to detect sleep apnea based on deep neural network and hidden Markov model using single-lead ECG signal. *Neurocomputing* **2018**, *294*, 94–101. [CrossRef]
8. Jung, D.W.; Hwang, S.H.; Yoon, H.N.; Lee, Y.J.G; Jeong, D.U.; Park, K.S. Nocturnal Awakening and Sleep Efficiency Estimation Using Unobtrusively Measured Ballistocardiogram. *IEEE Trans. Biomed. Eng.* **2014**, *61*, 131–1138. [CrossRef] [PubMed]
9. Almazaydeh, L.; Faezipour, M.; Elleithy, K. A neural network system for detection of obstructive sleep apnea through SpO_2 signal features. *Int. J. Adv. Comput. Sci. Appl.* **2012**, *3*, 7–11. [CrossRef]
10. Avci, C.; Akba, A. Sleep apnea classification based on respiration signals by using ensemble methods. *Bio-Med. Mater. Eng.* **2015**, *26*, S1703–S1710. [CrossRef]
11. Jane, R.; Fiz, J.A.; Solà-Soler; Mesquita, J.; Morera, J. Snoring Analysis for the Screening of Sleep Apnea Hypopnea Syndrome with a Single-Channel Device Developed using Polysomnographic and Snoring Databases. In Proceeding of 33rd Annual International Conference of the IEEE Engineering in Medicine an Biology Society (EMBC), Boston, MA, USA, 30 August–3 September 2011; pp. 8331–8333.
12. Eiseman, N.A.; Westover, M.B.; Mietus, J.E.; Thomas, R.J.; Bianchi, M.T. Classification algorithms for predicting sleepiness and sleep apnea severity. *J. Sleep Res.* **2012**, *21*, 101–112. [CrossRef]
13. De Chazal, P.; Sadr, N. Sleep apnoea classification using heart rate variability, ECG derived respiration and cardiopulmonary coupling parameters. In Proceeding of 38th Annual International Conference of the IEEE Engineering in Medicine and Biology Society (EMBC), Orlando, FL, USA, 16–20 August 2016; pp. 3203–3206.
14. Rodrigues, P.P.; Santos, D.F.; Leite, L. Obstructive sleep apnoea diagnosis: The Bayesian network model revisited. In Proceeding of 28th International Symposium on Computer-Based Medical Systems, Sao Carlos, Brazil, 22–25 June 2015; pp. 115–120.
15. Dey, D; Chaudhuri, S.; Munshi, S. Obstructive sleep apnoea detection using convolutional neural network based deep learning framework. *Biomed. Eng. Lett.* **2018**, *8*, 95–100. [CrossRef] [PubMed]
16. Quiceno-Manrique, A.; Alonso-Hernandez, J.; Travieso-Gonzalez, C.; Ferrer-Ballester, M.; Castellanos-Dominguez, G. Detection of obstructive sleep apnea in ECG recordings using time-frequency distributions and dynamic features. In Proceeding of 31st IEEE Annual International Conference of the IEEE Engineering in Medicine and Biology Society (EMBS), Minneapolis, MN, USA, 3–6 September 2009; pp. 5559–5562.
17. Mendez, M.; Ruini, D.; Villantieri, O.; Matteucci, M.; Penzel, T.; Bianchi, A. Detection of sleep apnea from surface ECG based on features extracted by an autoregressive model. In Proceeding of 29th IEEE International Conference on Engineering in Medicine and Biology Society (EMBS), Lyon, France, 22–26 August 2007; pp. 6105–6108.

18. Novak, D.; Mucha, K.; Al-Ani, T. Long short-term memory for apnea detection based on heart rate variability. In Proceeding of 30th IEEE Annual International Conference of the IEEE Engineering in Medicine and Biology Society (EMBS), Vancouver, BC, Canada, 20–25 August 2008; pp. 5234–5237.
19. Ng, A.; Chung, J.; Gohel, M.; Yu, W.; Fan, K.; Wong, T. Evaluation of the performance of using mean absolute amplitude analysis of thoracic and abdominal signals for immediate indication of sleep apnoea events. *J. Clin. Nursing* **2008**, *17*, 2360–2366. [CrossRef] [PubMed]
20. Garde, A.; Dekhordi, P.; Ansermino, J. M.; Dumont, G. A. Identifying individual sleep apnea/hypoapnea epochs using smartphone-based pulse oximetry. In Proceeding of 38th IEEE Annual International Conference of the IEEE Engineering in Medicine and Biology Society (EMBS), Orlando, FL, USA, 16–20 August 2016; pp. 3195–3198.
21. Mendonca, F.; Mostafa, S.S.; Ravelo-Garcia, A.G.; Morgado-Dias, F.; Penzel, T. A Review of Obstructive Sleep Apnea Detection Approaches. *IEEE J. Biomed. Health Inf.* **2019**, *23*, 825–837. [CrossRef] [PubMed]
22. Collop, N.A.; Tracy, S.L.; Kapur, V.; Mehra, R.; Kuhlmann, D.; Fleishman, S.A.; Ojile, J.M. Obstructive sleep apnea devices for out-of-center (OOC) testing: Technology evaluation. *J. Clin. Sleep Med.* **2011** *7*, 531–548. [CrossRef]
23. Lin, Y.Y.; Wu, H.T.; Hsu, C.A.; Huang, P.C.; Huang, Y.H.; Lo, Y.L. Sleep apnea detection based on thoracic and abdominal movement signals of wearable piezo-electric bands. *IEEE J. Biomed. Health Inf.* **2017**, *21*, 1533–1545. [CrossRef]
24. Daubechies, I.; Lu, J.; Wu, H.-T. Synchrosqueezed Wavelet Transforms: An empirical mode decomposition-like tool. *Appl. Comput. Harmon. Anal.* **2011**, *30*, 243–261. [CrossRef]
25. Chen, Y.-C.; Cheng, M.-Y.; Wu, H.-T. Nonparametric and adaptive modeling of dynamic seasonality and trend with heteroscedastic and dependent errors. *J. R. Stat. S.* **2014**, *76*, 651–782. [CrossRef]
26. Wu, H.-T. Instantaneous frequency and wave shape function (I). *Appl. Comput. Harmon. Anal.* **2013**, *35*, 181–199. [CrossRef]
27. Hochreiter, S.; Schmidhuber, J. Long short-term memory. *Neural Comput.* **1997**, *9*, 1735–1780. [CrossRef]
28. Auli, M.; Galley, M.; Quirk, C.; Zweig, G. Joint language and translation modeling with recurrent neural networks. In Proceedings of Conference on Empirical Methods in Natural Language Processing, Seattle, WA, USA, 18–21 October 2013; pp.1044–1054.
29. Sutskever, I.; Vinyals, O.; Le, Q.V. Sequence to sequence learning with neural networks. In Proceeding of Advances in Neural Information Processing Systems (NIPS), Montreal, QC, Canada, 8–13 December 2014; pp. 3104–3112.
30. Vinyals, O.; Toshev, A.; Bengio, S.; Erhan, D. Show and tell: A neural image caption generator. In Proceedings of the IEEE Conference on Computer Version and Pattern recognition, Boston, MA, USA, 7–12 June 2015; pp. 3156–3164.
31. Lipton, Z.C.; Kale, D.C.; Elkan, C.; Wetzel, R. Learning to Diagnose with LSTM Recurrent Neural Networks. Available online: https://arxiv.org/abs/1511.03677 (accessed on 25 October 2020)
32. Snyder, F.; Hobson, J.A.; Morrison, D.F.; Goldfrank, F. Changes in respiration, heart rate, and systolic blood pressure in human sleep. *Eur. J. Appl. Physiol.* **1964**, *19*, 417–422. [CrossRef]
33. Malik, J.; Lo, Y.L.; Wu, H.T. Sleep-wake classification via quantifying heart rate variability by convolutional neural network. *Physiol. Meas.* **2018**, *39*, 085004. [CrossRef] [PubMed]
34. Wu, H.T.; Wu, J.C.; Huang, P. C.; Lin, T.Y.; Wang, T.; Huang, Y.H.; Lo, Y.L. Phenotype-based and self-learning inter-individual sleep apnea screening with a level IV-like monitoring system. *Front. Physiol.* **2018**, *9*, 723. [CrossRef]
35. Whitney, C.W.; Gottlieb, D.J.; Redline, S.; Norman, R.G.; Dodge, R.R.; Shahar, E.; Surovec, S.; Nieto, F.J. Reliability of scoring respiratory disturbance indices and sleep staging. *Sleep* **1998**, *21*, 749–757. [CrossRef]

Publisher's Note: MDPI stays neutral with regard to jurisdictional claims in published maps and institutional affiliations.

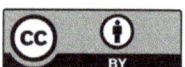

© 2020 by the authors. Licensee MDPI, Basel, Switzerland. This article is an open access article distributed under the terms and conditions of the Creative Commons Attribution (CC BY) license (http://creativecommons.org/licenses/by/4.0/).

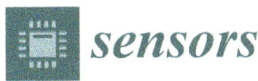

Article

Non-Contact Monitoring of Breathing Pattern and Respiratory Rate via RGB Signal Measurement

Carlo Massaroni [1,*], Daniela Lo Presti [1], Domenico Formica [2], Sergio Silvestri [1] and Emiliano Schena [1]

[1] Unit of Measurements and Biomedical Instrumentation, Department of Engineering, Università Campus Bio-Medico di Roma, 00128 Rome, Italy; d.lopresti@unicampus.it (D.L.P.); s.silvestri@unicampus.it (S.S.); e.schena@unicampus.it (E.S.)

[2] Unit of Neurophysiology and Neuroengineering of Human-Technology Interaction, Department of Engineering, Università Campus Bio-Medico di Roma, 00128 Rome, Italy; d.formica@unicampus.it

* Correspondence: c.massaroni@unicampus.it; Tel.: +39-06225419650

Received: 12 April 2019; Accepted: 18 June 2019; Published: 19 June 2019

Abstract: Among all the vital signs, respiratory rate remains the least measured in several scenarios, mainly due to the intrusiveness of the sensors usually adopted. For this reason, all contactless monitoring systems are gaining increasing attention in this field. In this paper, we present a measuring system for contactless measurement of the respiratory pattern and the extraction of breath-by-breath respiratory rate. The system consists of a laptop's built-in RGB camera and an algorithm for post-processing of acquired video data. From the recording of the chest movements of a subject, the analysis of the pixel intensity changes yields a waveform indicating respiratory pattern. The proposed system has been tested on 12 volunteers, both males and females seated in front of the webcam, wearing both slim-fit and loose-fit t-shirts. The pressure-drop signal recorded at the level of nostrils with a head-mounted wearable device was used as reference respiratory pattern. The two methods have been compared in terms of mean of absolute error, standard error, and percentage error. Additionally, a Bland–Altman plot was used to investigate the bias between methods. Results show the ability of the system to record accurate values of respiratory rate, with both slim-fit and loose-fit clothing. The measuring system shows better performance on females. Bland–Altman analysis showed a bias of -0.01 breaths·min^{-1}, with respiratory rate values between 10 and 43 breaths·min^{-1}. Promising performance has been found in the preliminary tests simulating tachypnea.

Keywords: measuring system; measurements; contactless; respiratory rate; breathing pattern

---

1. Introduction

Accurate measurement of vital signs and physiological parameters, such as body temperature, pulse rate, blood pressure, and respiratory rate, plays a pivotal role in the healthcare sector and management of patients. Among these, the respiratory rate (f_R) is still considered the neglected vital sign in both the clinical practice and sports activity monitoring [1,2]. Temporal changes in the respiratory rate may indicate relevant variations of the physiological status of the subject, even better than other vital signs (e.g., pulse rate) [2] and it is found to be more discriminatory between stable and unstable patients than pulse rate [1].

In a clinical setting, the respiratory rate is an early indicator of physiological deterioration [3] and a predictor of potentially dangerous adverse events [1]. Indeed, respiratory rate is an important predictor of cardiac arrest and of unplanned intensive care unit admission [1], as well as an independent prognostic marker for risk assessment after acute myocardial infarction [4]. Besides, it is fundamental in the early detection and diagnosis of dangerous conditions such as sleep apnea [5], sudden infant death syndrome, chronic obstructive pulmonary disease, and respiratory depression in post-surgical patients [6]. In intensive care units, the respiratory waveform and f_R are typically recorded. In mechanically ventilated patients, such data can be obtained directly by the mechanical ventilator traces [7] or retrieved by pulse oximetry sensors [8]. However, f_R is typically collected at regular interval by operators (i.e., every 8–10 h) in the clinical setting outside this ward, while is often neglected in home monitored people and patient [1].

Conventional methods for measuring respiratory parameters require sensing elements in contact with the patient [9]. These methods are mainly based on the analysis of several parameters sampled from the inspiratory and/or expiratory flow. Differently, approaches based on the measurement of respiratory-related chest and abdominal movements have been also adopted [10]. Sensors may be directly attached on the torso [11] or integrated into clothing fibers. Several sensors have been used as resistive sensors, capacitive sensors, inductive sensors. Such monitoring systems must be worn and powered [11]. Additionally, they may cause undesirable skin irritation and discomfort, especially when long-term monitoring is required or during sleep. Substantial evidence indicates all these contact-based measurement techniques may influence the underlying physiological parameters being measured [12].

Contactless monitoring systems may overcome these issues related to placing sensors on patients and influence the measurand [13]. Mainly, solutions based on the analysis of depth changes of the torso using time-of-flight sensors [14] during breathing, low-power ultra wideband impulse radio radar [15,16], and laser Doppler vibrometers [17–19] have been designed and tested. Principal limitations of such solutions are related to the high cost of the instrumentation, need for specialized operators, and, in some cases, a low signal-to-noise ratio. Contactless monitoring systems based on the use of optical sensors are gaining preeminence in the field of respiratory monitoring mainly because of recent progress in video technology. Commercial and industrial cameras may be exciting solutions as they provide low-cost and easy-to-use non-contact approaches for measuring and monitoring physiological signals [4]. Some attempts have been made to record respiratory parameters from breathing-related movements of thoraco-abdominal area, face area, area at the edge of the shoulder, pit of the neck [20–25]. Then, different approaches have been also used to post-process the video to extract the respiratory-related signal mainly based on image subtraction [26], optical flow analysis [27], Eulerian Video Magnification [24] and Independent Component Analysis (ICA) applied to pixel intensity changes [28]. By the review of the literature, there is a lack of results about accuracy of such methods in the monitoring of eupneic respiratory pattern and f_R monitoring, since the majority of the cited studies present proof of concepts and preliminary tests, but accuracy evaluation is not performed. When available, typically a frequency-domain analysis is carried out to extract the frequency content of the respiratory-related video signal and to measure the average respiratory rate. Since analysis with these techniques requires the recording of the torso movement, clothing can influence the data quality and validity of the methods. However, no studies have focused on such potential influences on respiratory pattern and f_R measurement. Only a preliminary study of our research group tried to investigate this influencing factor in [29].

In this paper, we present a measuring system capable of non-contact monitoring of respiratory pattern by using RGB video signal acquired from a single built-in high-definition webcam. The aim of this study is three-fold: (i) the development of the measuring system and the related algorithm for the extraction of breath-by-breath f_R values; (ii) the evaluation of the error between the breath-by-breath f_R values retrieved by using the proposed measuring system and those recorded with a reference instrument; and (iii) the analysis of influence of clothing (i.e., slim-fit and loose-fit) and sex on the performance of the proposed method.

2. Measuring System

The proposed measuring system is composed of a hardware module (i.e., a built-in webcam) for video recording and an algorithm for (i) preprocessing of the video to obtain a respiratory signal, and (ii) event detection, segmentation and extraction of breath-by-breath f_R values. The working principle of the method used to extract respiratory information from a video is explained in the following section.

2.1. Light Intensity Changes Caused by Respiration

Each video can be considered a series of f frames (i.e., polychromatic images), where f is the number of the frames collected. Each frame is an image composed of three images in the red (R), green (G) and blue (B) channels. Each image in the R, G and B channels is a matrix composed of pixels. The size of the matrix (of dimensions x along the x-axis, and y along the y-axis) depends on the resolution of the camera used for the data collection. Each pixel assumes a value representing the color light intensity: the value 0 means black, whereas the maximum value is the white. The numerical values of each pixel depend on the number of bytes used to represent a given R, G, B channel. When considering commercial 8-bit/channel cameras (24-bit for RGB colors), the maximum value is 2^8 (i.e., 255 colors including zero).

When an object is recorded by a video, the pixel of each frame of the video assume an intensity level caused by the light reflected from the object over a two-dimensional grid of pixels. In the RGB color model separate intensity signals corresponding to each channel—$V_R(x,y,f), V_G(x,y,f), V_B(x,y,f)$—can be recorded at each frame f. The measured intensity of any reflected light (V) can be decomposed into two components: (i) intensity of illumination (I), and (ii) reflectance of the surface (R):

$$V(x,y,f) = I(x,y,f) \cdot R(x,y,f). \tag{1}$$

The respiratory activity causes the periodic movement of the chest wall. During inspiration, the ribcage widens: it results in an upward movement of the thorax; during expiration, the opposite occurs. By considering the chest wall covered by clothing as the surface framed by the camera, and the intensity of illumination almost constant, the changes of intensity of reflected light between two consecutive frames can be considered caused by the movement of the chest surface. Breathing-related chest movements are transmitted to the clothing (e.g., t-shirts, sweaters), so the subsequent changes of V can be used to collect respiratory patterns and events indirectly. Loose- or slim-fit clothing differently adhere to the skin. In the case of slim-fit clothing, we can hypothesize the complete transfer of chest wall movement to the side of the t-shirt framed by the camera, whereas only a partial transfer in the case of loose-fit clothing.

2.2. Hardware for Video Data Recording

The proposed system needs to collect a video of a person seated in front of the camera (Figure 1). The hardware module consists of a built-in CCD RGB webcam (iSight camera) integrated into a MacBook Pro laptop (by Apple Inc., California, USA). This camera is used to collect video with a resolution of 1280·720 pixel. Video images are recorded at 24-bit RGB with three channels, 8 bits per channel. A bespoke interface was developed in MATLAB (MathWorks, Massachusetts, USA) to record the video and pre-process the data (i.e., images) collected with the camera. The video is collected for 120 s at a frame rate of 30 Hz, which is enough to register the breathing movements.

2.3. Algorithm for the Preprocessing of the Video

The preprocessing of the recorded video is performed off-line via a bespoke algorithm developed in MATLAB, which is an upgraded version of the algorithm presented in our previous papers [29,30]. Several steps must be followed as shown in Figure 1.

Basically, after the video is loaded, the user (i.e., the one who is designated to analyze the data) is asked to select one pixel (with coordinates x_P, y_P) at the level of the jugular notch (i.e., the anatomical point near the suprasternal notch) in the first frame of the video. This anatomical marker has been chosen because it is easily identifiable (see Figure 1).

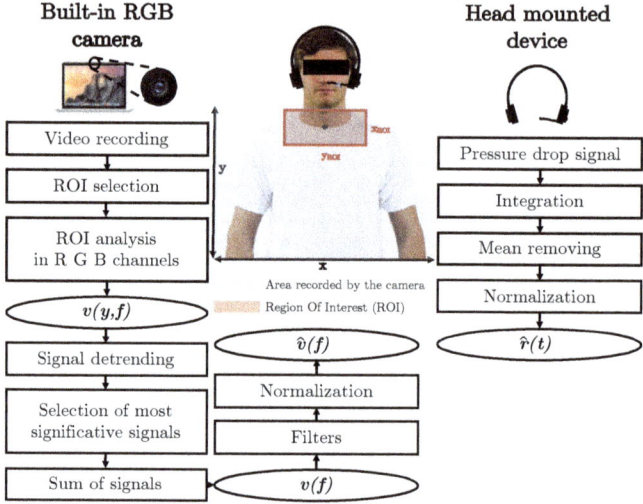

Figure 1. Flowchart presenting all the steps carried out to extract the respiratory pattern from video recorded with the built-in camera (on the left) and from the pressure-drop signal collected at the level of nostrils with the reference device (on the right). Region Of Interest (ROI) is the red rectangle; the area recorded by the camera is highlighted with the blue rectangle, the black point is the pixel (with coordinates x_P, y_P) at the level of the jugular notch.

Automatically a rectangular region of interest (in short ROI) is delineated, with dimensions $x_{ROI} \times y_{ROI}$:

$$x_{ROI} = [x_P - \tfrac{1}{100} \cdot 15 \cdot x, x_P + \tfrac{1}{100} \cdot 15 \cdot x],$$
$$y_{ROI} = [y_P - \tfrac{1}{100} \cdot 15 \cdot y, y_P + \tfrac{1}{100} \cdot 15 \cdot y], \quad (2)$$

where x and y are the x-axis and y-axis frame dimensions (related to camera resolution), respectively.

The selected ROI is then split into three same-size images corresponding to the red, green, and blue channels. At each frame f, the intensity components of each channel $I(x, y, c, f)$ are obtained, where c is the color channel (i.e., red (R), green (G), and blue (B)). Then, the intensity components are averaged for each line y of the ROI according to Equation (3):

$$v(y, f) = \frac{1}{x_{ROI}} \cdot \sum_{x=1}^{x_{ROI}} \left(\sum_{c=R,G,B} I(x, y, c, f) \right), \quad (3)$$

where $y \in y_{ROI}$.

From each $v(y, f)$, the mean of the signal is removed from the signal itself (i.e., the signal is detrended). The standard deviation of each $v(y, f)$ signal is then calculated. The 5% of the $v(y, f)$ with the higher standard deviations are selected. The 5% value was selected with an empirical approach using data from previous experiments carried out on volunteers aimed at calibrating the algorithm. The 5% of the $v(y, f)$ are used to calculate the mean value considering the selected lines at each frame. The $v(f)$ signal is obtained with this procedure. At that point, filters were applied to the $v(f)$ signal. For filtering the signal and to emphasize the respiratory content, adequate cut-off frequencies and bandwidth need to be defined. A bandpass configuration was chosen, by fixing the low cut-off frequency around 0.05 Hz, to avoid the slow signal variations unrelated to respiratory movements and a high cut-off frequency around 2 Hz. In this way, the changes generated by the respiratory movements recorded to the webcam sensor can be adequately isolated and relayed to the subsequent elaboration stages. A third order Butterworth digital filter was employed. Finally, the $v(f)$ signal is normalized to obtain $\hat{v}(f)$ as reported in the following Equation (4):

$$\hat{v}(f) = \frac{v(f) - \mu(v(f))}{\sigma(v(f))} \quad (4)$$

where $\mu(v(f))$ and $\sigma(v(f))$ are the mean and standard deviation of signal $v(f)$, respectively.

The signal $\hat{v}(f)$ is used for extracting respiratory temporal information (i.e., period duration—T_R and respiratory rate—f_R) since $\hat{v}(f)$ would be proportional to the changes in the intensity component, and thus to the underlying respiratory signal of interest (Figure 2). A window of 60 s is shown in Figure 2B. In this figure the apnea phase of about 5 s used for synchronizing reference signal and video-derived signal in the experimental trials is not shown (see Section 3.1).

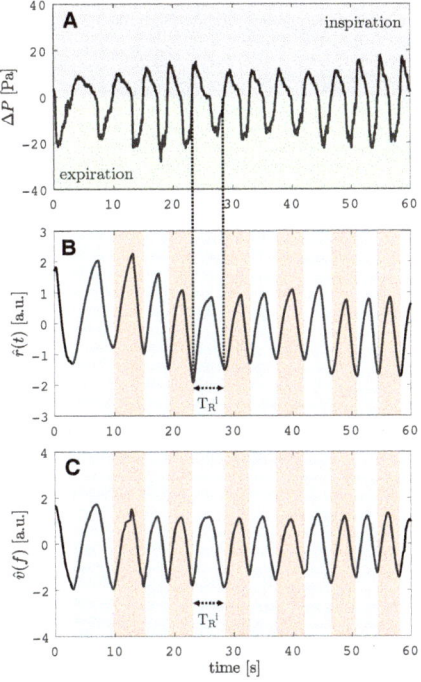

Figure 2. (**A**) ΔP signal recorded by the reference instrument at the level of the nostrils. In grey, the signal collected during the inspiration (positive pressure), while in green, the signal recorded during the expiration (negative pressure). (**B**) Reference respiratory pattern signal ($\hat{r}(t)$) obtained from data processing of ΔP signal. (**C**) Respiratory pattern signal obtained from the proposed measuring system ($\hat{v}(f)$). Figure in (**B**) and (**C**) show similar patterns: during the inspiratory phase the signal increases, while during the expiratory phase they decrease. The duration of one breath ($T_R(i)$) is shown on both the $\hat{r}(t)$ and $\hat{v}(f)$ signals.

3. Tests and Experimental Trials

3.1. Participants and Tests

In this study, we enrolled 12 participants (6 males and 6 females) with a mean age 24 ± 4 years old, mean height of 165 ± 15 cm, mean body mass of 60 ± 10 kg). All the participants provided informed consent. We have created a data set for evaluation of the proposed system. We aim to cover normal breathing (i.e., respiratory frequency in the range 8–25 breaths·min^{-1}), abnormal breathing (i.e., tachypnea) and apnea stages.

Each participant was invited to sit on a chair in front of the web camera at a distance of about 1.2 m. The user adjusted the screen of the laptop in order to record the trunk area (as shown in Figure 1). All the experiments were carried out indoor (in a laboratory room) and with a stable amount of light delivered by neon lights and three windows as sources of illumination. The participants' shoulders were turned towards the furnishings of the room. The windows were lateral to the scene recorded by the camera. Other people were in the room during the data collection but not allowed to pass near the shooting area.

Participants were asked to keep still and seated, and to breathe spontaneously by facing the webcam. Each volunteer was called to breathe quietly for around 5 s, simulate an apnea of duration <10 s, and then to breathe quietly at self-paced f_R for all the duration of the trial (120 s). Each volunteer carried out two trials with the same experimental design: in the first trial, the participant wore a loose-fit t-shirt; in the second trials, a slim-fit t-shirt. Two volunteers were also invited to simulate abnormal breathing (i.e., tachypnea) that is characterized by high f_R values (>35 bpm).

At the same time, respiratory pattern was recorded with a reference instrument described in the following Section 3.2.

3.2. Reference Instrument and Signal

For registering reference pattern, a head-mounted wearable device was used. We already used this system in a similar scenario [31]. This device is based on the recording of the pressure-drop (ΔP) that occurs during the expiratory/inspiratory phases of respiration at the level of nostrils. The device consists of a cannula attached to the jaw with tape: one piece of tape at the end of the nostrils in order to collect part of the nasal flow while the other tap is connected to a static tap of a differential digital pressure sensor (i.e., Sensirion—model SDP610, pressure range up to ±125 Pa). The pressure data were recorded with a dedicated printed circuit board described in [31], at 100 Hz of sample rate. Data were sent to a remote laptop via a wireless connection and archived.

Negative pressure was collected during the expiratory phase and positive pressure during the inspiratory phase, as can be seen in Figure 2A. Then, a temporal standard cumulative trapezoidal numerical integration of the ΔP signal was carried out to obtain a smooth respiratory signal for further analysis ($r(t)$) and to emphasize the maximum and minimum peaks. Afterward, such integrated $r(t)$ has been filtered using a bandpass Butterworth filter in the frequency range 0.05–2 Hz and normalized as in Equation (4) and $\hat{r}(t)$ has been obtained. This $\hat{r}(t)$ is the reference respiratory pattern signal, then used to extract breath-by-breath f_R reference values (i.e., $f_R(i)$).

As shown in Figure 2B, one breath is the portion of the signal between the starting point of the inspiration and the end of the following expiration. During the inspiratory phase, the ΔP signal pass from 0 to positive values (grey area in Figure 2A), and $r(t)$ is an increasing signal. During the expiratory phase, the opposite situation: ΔP signal passes from 0 to negative values (green area in Figure 2A), and $\hat{r}(t)$ is a decreasing signal.

3.3. Respiratory Rate Calculation

The breathing rate can be extracted from both the reference signal $\hat{r}(t)$ and $\hat{v}(f)$ either in the frequency or time domains [21,32]. The analysis in the time domain requires the identification of specific points on the signal. Mainly, two different approaches may be used: (i) based on the identification of the maximum and minimum points; or (ii) the zero-crossing point individuation on the signals. In this work, we used a zero-crossing-based algorithm. We used the same algorithm for the event detection on both the reference signal $\hat{r}(t)$ and $\hat{v}(f)$. The algorithm provides the detection of the zero-crossing points on the signal based on signum function. It allows determining the onset of each respiratory cycle, characterized by a positive going zero-crossing value. The signum function of a real number x is defined as in the following Equation (5):

$$sgn(x): \begin{cases} -1 & \text{if } x_i < 0, \\ 0 & \text{if } x_i = 0, \\ 1 & \text{if } x_i > 0, \end{cases} \quad (5)$$

where x_i is the value x of the signal for frame index i corresponding to the onset of a respiratory cycle. Then, the algorithm provides the location of local minimum points on the signal and their indices between respiratory cycle onsets determined in the first step.

The duration of each i-th breath—$T_R(i)$—is then calculated as the time elapsed between two consecutive minima points (expressed in s). Consequently, the i-th breath-by-breath breathing rate $f_R(i)$, expressed in breaths per minute (bpm), is calculated as in Equation (6):

$$f_R(i) = \frac{60}{T_R(i)}. \quad (6)$$

3.4. Data Analysis

We recorded the breath-by-breath respiratory rate with our system and the reference instrument and evaluated the discrepancies coming from their comparison. Signals obtained from the measuring system have been compared to the reference signals. Firstly the $\hat{r}(t)$ and $\hat{v}(f)$ were synchronized to be directly compared. We used the apnea stage to detect a common event on both signals. All the analysis were carried out on both the $\hat{r}(t)$ and $\hat{v}(f)$ that occur after the first end expiratory point after the apnea stage. The breath-by-breath f_R values have been compared between instruments by extracting such values with the time-domain analysis from $\hat{r}(t)$ (i.e., $f_R(i)$) and $\hat{v}(f)$ (i.e., $\hat{f}_R(i)$).

To compare the values gathered by the reference instrument and computed by the video-based method, we use the mean absolute error (MAE) as in Equation (7):

$$MAE = \frac{1}{n} \cdot \sum_{i=1}^{n} |\hat{f}_R(i) - f_R(i)|, \quad (7)$$

where n is the number of breaths recognized by the algorithm for each subject in the trial.

Then, the standard error of the mean (SE) is calculated as in Equation (8):

$$SE = \frac{SD}{\sqrt{n}}, \quad (8)$$

where SD is the standard deviation of the absolute difference between estimations and reference data $\hat{f}_R(i) - f_R(i)$. Standard error was used to provide a simple estimation of uncertainty.

Lastly, the percentage difference between instruments was calculated as in Equation (9), per each volunteer:

$$\%E = \frac{1}{n} \cdot \sum_n \frac{\hat{f}_R(i) - f_R(i)}{f_R(i)} \cdot 100. \quad (9)$$

Additionally, we used the Bland–Altman analysis to investigate the agreement between the proposed method and the reference, in the whole range of f_R measurement. With this graphical method we investigated if the differences between the two techniques against the averages of the two techniques presented a tendency at the different f_R collected during the trials. The Bland–Altman analysis was used to obtain the mean of the Differences (MOD) and the limits of Agreements (LOAs) values [33] that are typically reported in other studies and extremely useful when comparing our results with the relevant scientific literature [2].

To fulfill the scope of this paper we carried out three separate analyses using these metrics for comparisons. Firstly, we used the data collected with slim-fit and loose-fit clothing to investigate the influence of clothing on the performance of the proposed method, using both male and female data.

Then, we separately use the data collected from male and from female to investigate the influence of sex on performance. Lastly, the overall performance of the proposed measuring system has been tested considering all the breath-by-breath f_R (n = 411). Preliminary tests have been also done using data collected from two volunteers during tachypnea.

4. Experimental Results

The detection of apnea stages used for synchronizing the signals on $\hat{r}(t)$ and $\hat{v}(f)$ was always possible. Therefore, no trials were excluded from the analysis. During the apnea, the signal collected by the reference instrument is a constant and null ΔP; constant signals were also found in $\hat{v}(f)$.

Table 1 summaries the number of breaths, average $\hat{f}_R$ and f_R values, MAE, SE and %E for each subject, at the two t-shirt fittings. MAE value was always lower than 0.78 bpm, while standard error was <0.24 bpm in all the volunteers. %E values were both negative and positive: the maximum value was 0.62%. The performance of the proposed method in the measurement of breath-by-breath respiratory frequencies can be appreciated in Figure 3.

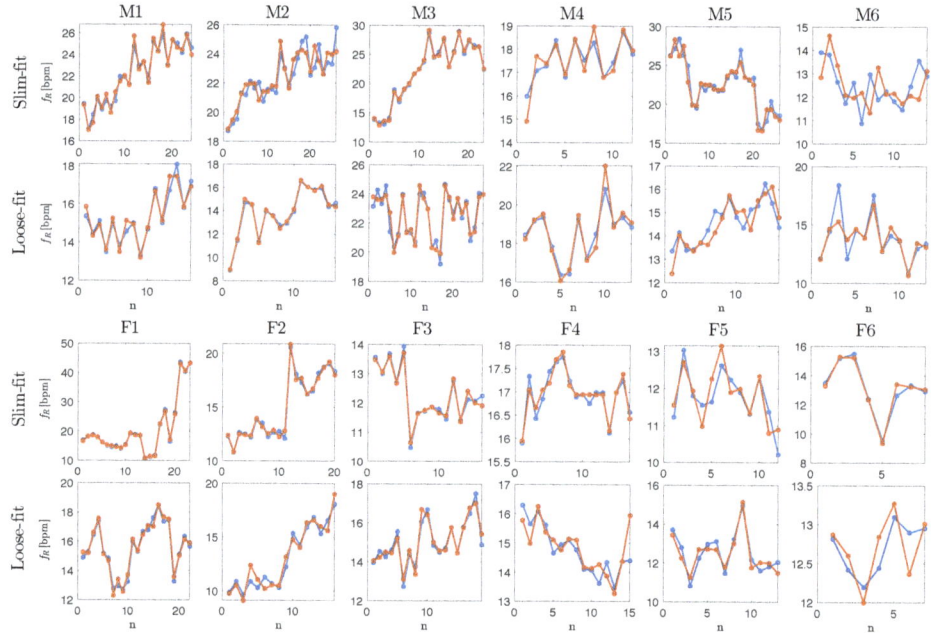

Figure 3. Breath-by-breath values of the respiratory rate collected by the reference system (blue dots and lines) and by the proposed measuring system (orange dots and lines). Data from male (i.e., M1, M2, M3, M4, M5, M6) and female (F1, F2, F3, F4, F5, F6) volunteers wearing slim-fit and loose-fit clothing are reported. Details about MAE, SE and %E values per each volunteer with slim-fit and loose-fit clothing are reported in Table 1.

4.1. Influence of Clothing Type

The influence of clothing was investigated by analyzing the difference (i.e., $\hat{f}_R(i) - f_R(i)$) distribution considering all the data obtained from male and female together. Since the sample size and bin width of the histograms are different between slim-fit (n = 211) and loose-fit (n = 203) data, it is difficult to compare them. So, we normalize the histograms so that all the bar heights add to 1, and we use a uniform bin width (0.1 bpm). With the slim-fit clothing, the 28% of the differences between the two instruments were in the range ±0.1 bpm (94% of data in the range ±1 bpm), while with the loose-fit clothing only 19% of data (94% of data in the range ±1 bpm). For details refers to Figure 4A. The Bland–Altman showed a bias of -0.02 ± 1.07 bpm and 0.01 ± 0.98 bpm in the case of loose-fit and slim-fit clothing, respectively. From the Bland–Altman plot, neither proportional error nor magnitude of measurements dependence were found.

Table 1. Breath-by-breath analysis: average $\hat{f}_R$, average f_R, mae, se and %e values per each volunteer at the different t-shirt fitting. MAE: Mean Absolute Error ; SE: Standard Error of the mean.

Vol.	T-Shirt Fitting	# Breaths	$\hat{f}_R$ [bpm]	f_R [bpm]	MAE [bpm]	SE [bpm]	%E [%]
M1	slim	24	22.29	22.28	0.76	0.18	−0.52
	loose	16	15.33	15.31	0.27	0.05	0.18
M2	slim	17	13.90	13.86	0.58	0.09	0.46
	loose	26	22.48	22.39	0.14	0.02	0.28
M3	slim	23	22.21	22.18	0.27	0.04	0.14
	loose	27	22.55	22.55	0.35	0.0	0.04
M4	slim	12	17.53	17.55	0.32	0.09	0.19
	loose	13	18.57	18.52	0.33	0.09	−0.16
M5	slim	26	22.32	22.46	0.65	0.13	−0.52
	loose	16	14.51	14.60	0.43	0.08	−0.62
M6	slim	14	12.49	12.51	0.78	0.14	0.21
	loose	13	13.82	13.92	0.60	0.24	−0.10
F1	slim	23	20.62	20.67	0.24	0.04	−0.13
	loose	22	15.61	15.57	0.23	0.03	0.26
F2	slim	20	15.08	15.07	0.27	0.04	0.14
	loose	16	13.14	13.07	0.60	0.10	0.55
F3	slim	16	12.27	12.30	0.11	0.02	−0.15
	loose	19	15.08	15.06	0.25	0.04	0.18
F4	slim	17	16.96	16.95	0.11	0.02	0.07
	loose	15	14.85	14.78	0.37	0.10	0.53
F5	slim	12	11.83	11.78	0.35	0.07	0.50
	loose	13	12.50	12.55	0.36	0.04	−0.32
F6	slim	8	13.16	13.14	0.23	0.08	0.17
	loose	7	12.71	12.69	0.23	0.07	0.16
Overall	-	414	-	-	0.39	0.02	0.07

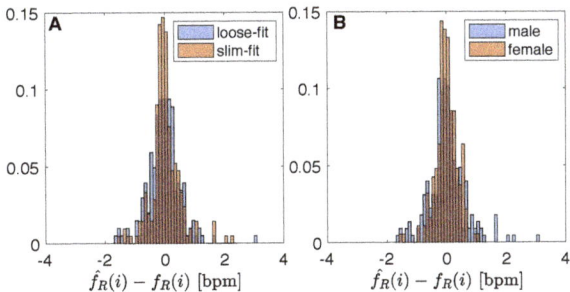

Figure 4. Difference distribution: (**A**) influence of clothing type (i.e., slim-fit vs loose-fit); (**B**) influence of sex (i.e., male vs female).

4.2. Influence of Sex

The influence of sex on the performance of the measuring system was investigated by analyzing the difference ($\hat{f}_R(i) - f_R(i)$) distribution considering all the data obtained from data collection carried out with slim-fit and loose-fit clothing. Normalized histograms with uniform bin widths (0.1 bpm) were used since the difference sample size between male data ($n = 226$) and female data ($n = 188$). In the male group, 21% of data show difference between instrument in the range ±0.1 bpm (90% of data in the range ±1 bpm), while in the female group was 27% of the data (98% of data in the range ±1 bpm). Figure 4B shows the two distributions. The Bland–Altman analysis revealed a bias of 0.01 ± 1.22 bpm (see Figure 5C) and −0.01 ± 0.73 bpm (see Figure 5D) for male and female volunteers, respectively. All the f_R values recorded by the male volunteers are between 10 and 30 bpm (mean 19.14 bpm, SD 4.55 bpm). In female volunteers, five f_R values over 25 bpm can be observed in Figure 5D, while 96% of the data are in the range of 10–20 bpm (mean 14.99 bpm, SD 4.47). Bland–Altman analysis shows the absence of proportional error and magnitude of measurements dependence.

4.3. Overall Performance

All the $f_R(i)$ extracted from $\hat{r}(t)$ and $\hat{v}(f)$ per each subject with slim-fit and loose-fit clothing are presented in Figure 3. Data extracted from signal collected with the proposed measuring system follow the data extracted from reference signal in each subject, both a low f_R and high f_R. Similar variations in f_R estimates can be clearly observed in that figure.

Figure 5A shows the difference distribution of all the 414 breaths collected: the 24% of the differences are in the interval of ±0.1 bpm, and only 6% of data shows differences higher than ±1 bpm. Bland–Altman analysis (Figure 5B) demonstrates a bias with a MOD close to 0 (i.e., −0.01 bpm) and LOAs of 1.02 bpm. Bland–Altman analysis allows us to assess the absence of proportional error and magnitude of measurements dependence.

4.4. Preliminary Results during Tachypnea

The proposed measuring system has also been preliminarily tested on two subjects during tachypnea. Figure 6 reports two examples of 30 s data collection on two volunteers. By applying the algorithm for the f_R calculation, we found a MAE of 1.05 bpm, a SE 0.13 bpm and a %E of −0.24% for the first volunteer; second volunteer data show a MAE of 0.48 bpm, SE of 0.08 bpm and %E of 0.04%. Due to the small sample size, Bland–Altman was not used to summarize bias between methods.

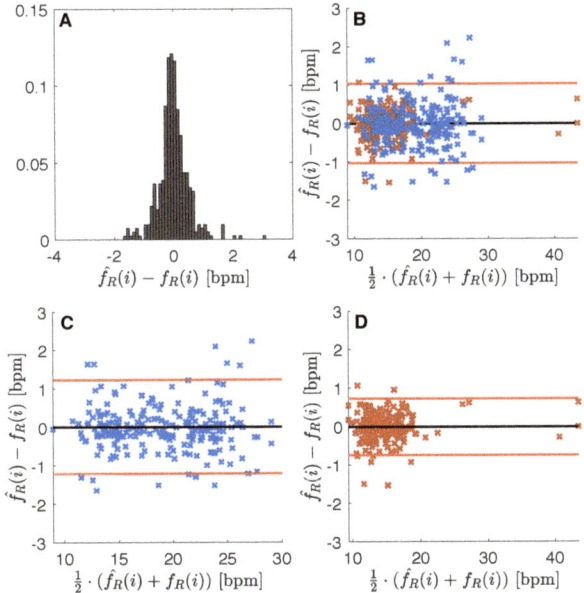

Figure 5. (**A**) Difference distribution between proposed method and reference respiratory rate values; (**B**) Bland–Altman plot obtained considering all the data recorded by male and female volunteers: black line is the MOD, red lines are the LOAs (i.e., ±1.96 times the standard deviation); (**C,B**) Bland–Altman plot obtained considering data recorded by male volunteers; (**D**) Bland–Altman plot obtained considering data recorded by female volunteers.

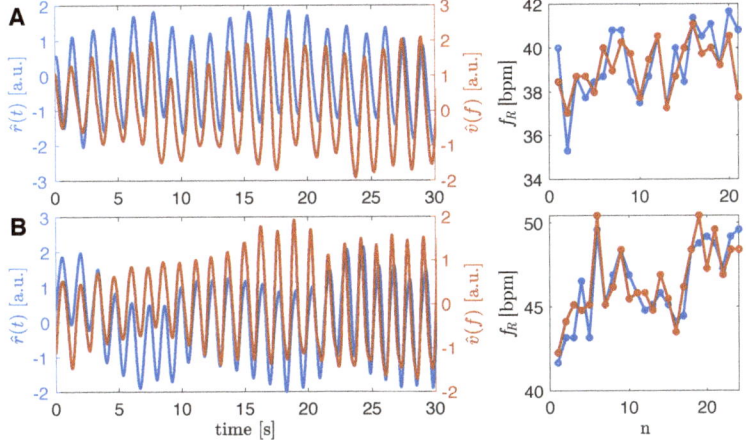

Figure 6. Two patterns collected from two volunteers simulating tachypnea. In blue, the reference signal $\hat{r}(t)$, in orange the $\hat{v}(f)$ signal. In the first volunteer (**graphs A**), the average $\hat{f}_R$ is 39.14 bpm while the average f_R is 39.34 bpm. In the second volunteer (**graphs B**), the average $\hat{f}_R$ is 46.44 bpm while the average f_R is 46.28 bpm.

5. Discussion

In this paper, a single built-in camera system is proposed for the extraction of the respiratory pattern and the estimation of breath-by-breath f_R. The built-in camera of a commercial laptop allows the non-intrusive, ecological, and low-cost recording of chest wall movement. The algorithm for the processing of images allows (i) the chest wall video recording at sufficient frame rate (i.e., 30 Hz), (ii) the selection of a pixel for further semi-automatic selection of a ROI for the measurement of the pixel intensity change, in order to extract video-based respiratory pattern $\hat{v}(f)$, and (iii) the post-processing of the $\hat{v}(f)$ signal to estimate breath-by-breath f_R values. The proposed system has been tested on healthy participants. Tests were carried out on male and female participants wearing both slim-fit and loose-fit t-shirts to simulate real respiratory monitoring conditions (e.g., a subject at home, patient in a medical room, etc.). In the literature, rarely authors take into account the influence of sex and clothing when camera-based methods are used. Additionally, in this paper, we used an unobtrusive head-mounted wearable as reference instrument to not compromise the area recorded by the camera.

Signals obtained with the proposed method allow clear identification of the apnea stages, breathing pattern at quiet pace and during tachypnea in all the trials. Considering the breath-by-breath $f_R(i)$ values, we obtained comparable MAE and SE values in the two groups (slim-fit vs. loose-fit). From the analysis of the bias revealed by the Bland–Altman plots, we found slightly better results with volunteers wearing slim-fit clothing (LOAs of ±0.98 bpm against ±1.07 bpm with loose-fit clothing). These results confirm those obtained in [29]. Considering the sex, results demonstrated good performance with both males and females with slightly lower bias in females (−0.01 ± 0.73 bpm) than in males (0.01 ± 1.22 bpm). By considering all 414 breaths, the Bland–Altman analysis demonstrates a bias of −0.01 ± 1.02 bpm of the proposed method when compared to the f_R values gathered by the reference instrument. The method proposed in [20] achieves bias of −0.32±1.61 bpm when tested in similar setting and participants. Then, the bias we found is comparable with the one reported in [34] (i.e., −0.02 ± 0.83 bpm) where the pseudo-Wigner–Villetime frequency analysis was used (with a f_R resolution of 0.7324 bpm). The performances we obtained are better than those obtained in [35] where the average f_R were considered (bias of 0.37 ± 1.04 bpm), and advanced signal and video processing techniques, including developing video magnification, complete ensemble empirical mode decomposition with adaptive noise, and canonical correlation analysis were used in the post-processing phase. When compared to depth sensors used on participant in supine position [16], our method demonstrates comparable results with simplicity and cost (∼0.01 ± 0.96 bpm in [16]). Despite the absence of contact with the subject, the proposed method shows overall performance similar to those obtained with wearable device for f_R monitoring requiring direct contact with the torso (e.g., garment with optical fibers showed bias of −0.02 ± 2.04 bpm in [36], during quiet breathing). In contrast to other research studies, we did not use a background behind the user to test the system in conditions resembling real application scenarios. Further tests might be focused on extracting respiratory volumes by using a more structured environment during video collection as in [37].

One of the main limitations of this study is the limited number of subjects included in the analysis. For this reason, we did not perform any statistical analysis because population size does not allow any statistically significative conclusions. Additionally, we tested the proposed method at one distance between camera and subject (i.e., 1.2 m).

Further effort will be mainly devoted to addressing these points. Tests will be carried out to investigate the performance of the system in different scenarios at different subject–camera relative distances, and on many subjects. Furthermore, performance of the method will be tested in a wide range of atypical respiratory pattern (i.e., tachypnea, deep breaths, Cheyne-Stokes) and in extracting additional respiratory parameters (e.g., duration of expiratory and inspiratory parameters, inter-breathing variations). We are already testing the validity of additional techniques based on pixel flow analysis to remove unrelated breathing movements. Additionally, we are working on feature selection approaches to use the proposed method for respiratory monitoring when small movements of the user happen. We hope to use the proposed measuring system for respiratory monitoring even with undesired subject' motion, also by implementing a fully automatic process to detect ROI from video frames. These steps will allow automatic and long-term data collection.

Author Contributions: Conceptualization, C.M. and E.S.; Data curation, C.M.; Formal analysis, C.M.; Funding acquisition, C.M.; Investigation, C.M., D.L.P. and D.F.; Methodology, C.M., D.L.P., D.F., S.S. and E.S.; Project administration, C.M.; Resources, C.M. and E.S.; Software, C.M.; Supervision, C.M., D.F., S.S. and E.S.; Validation, C.M.; Visualization, C.M., D.L.P., D.F., S.S. and E.S.; Writing—original draft, C.M.; Writing—review & editing, D.L.P., D.F., S.S. and E.S.

Funding: This research received no external funding.

Conflicts of Interest: The authors declare no conflict of interest.

References

1. Cretikos, M.A.; Bellomo, R.; Hillman, K.; Chen, J.; Finfer, S.; Flabouris, A. Respiratory rate: The neglected vital sign. *Med. J. Aust.* **2008**, *188*, 657–659. [PubMed]
2. Nicolò, A.; Massaroni, C.; Passfield, L. Respiratory frequency during exercise: The neglected physiological measure. *Front. Physiol.* **2017**. [CrossRef] [PubMed]
3. Smith, I.; Mackay, J.; Fahrid, N.; Krucheck, D. Respiratory rate measurement: A comparison of methods. *Br. J. Healthc. Assist.* **2011**, *5*, 18–23. [CrossRef]
4. Barthel, P.; Wensel, R.; Bauer, A.; Müller, A.; Wolf, P.; Ulm, K.; Huster, K.M.; Francis, D.P.; Malik, M.; Schmidt, G. Respiratory rate predicts outcome after acute myocardial infarction: A prospective cohort study. *Eur. Heart J.* **2012**, *34*, 1644–1650. [CrossRef] [PubMed]
5. Younes, M. Role of respiratory control mechanisms in the pathogenesis of obstructive sleep disorders. *J. Appl. Physiol.* **2008**, *105*, 1389–1405. [CrossRef] [PubMed]
6. Rantonen, T.; Jalonen, J.; Grönlund, J.; Antila, K.; Southall, D.; Välimäki, I. Increased amplitude modulation of continuous respiration precedes sudden infant death syndrome: Detection by spectral estimation of respirogram. *Early Hum. Dev.* **1998**, *53*, 53–63. [CrossRef]
7. Schena, E.; Massaroni, C.; Saccomandi, P.; Cecchini, S. Flow measurement in mechanical ventilation: A review. *Med. Eng. Phys.* **2015**, *37*, 257–264. [CrossRef]
8. Brochard, L.; Martin, G.S.; Blanch, L.; Pelosi, P.; Belda, F.J.; Jubran, A.; Gattinoni, L.; Mancebo, J.; Ranieri, V.M.; Richard, J.C.M.; et al. Clinical review: Respiratory monitoring in the ICU-a consensus of 16. *Crit. Care* **2012**, *16*, 219. [CrossRef]
9. Massaroni, C.; Nicolò, A.; Lo Presti, D.; Sacchetti, M.; Silvestri, S.; Schena, E. Contact-based methods for measuring respiratory rate. *Sensors* **2019**, *19*, 908. [CrossRef]
10. Massaroni, C.; Di Tocco, J.; Presti, D.L.; Longo, U.G.; Miccinilli, S.; Sterzi, S.; Formica, D.; Saccomandi, P.; Schena, E. Smart textile based on piezoresistive sensing elements for respiratory monitoring. *IEEE Sens. J.* **2019**. [CrossRef]
11. Dionisi, A.; Marioli, D.; Sardini, E.; Serpelloni, M. Autonomous wearable system for vital signs measurement with energy-harvesting module. *IEEE Trans. Instrum. Meas.* **2016**, *65*, 1423–1434. [CrossRef]
12. Gilbert, R.; Auchincloss, J., Jr.; Brodsky, J.; Boden, W.A. Changes in tidal volume, frequency, and ventilation induced by their measurement. *J. Appl. Physiol.* **1972**, *33*, 252–254. [CrossRef] [PubMed]
13. Al-Naji, A.; Gibson, K.; Lee, S.H.; Chahl, J. Monitoring of cardiorespiratory signal: Principles of remote measurements and review of methods. *IEEE Access* **2017**, *5*, 15776–15790. [CrossRef]
14. Deng, F.; Dong, J.; Wang, X.; Fang, Y.; Liu, Y.; Yu, Z.; Liu, J.; Chen, F. Design and Implementation of a Noncontact Sleep Monitoring System Using Infrared Cameras and Motion Sensor. *IEEE Trans. Instrum. Meas.* **2018**, *67*, 1555–1563. [CrossRef]
15. Lai, J.C.Y.; Xu, Y.; Gunawan, E.; Chua, E.C.; Maskooki, A.; Guan, Y.L.; Low, K.; Soh, C.B.; Poh, C. Wireless Sensing of Human Respiratory Parameters by Low-Power Ultrawideband Impulse Radio Radar. *IEEE Trans. Instrum. Meas.* **2011**, *60*, 928–938. [CrossRef]
16. Bernacchia, N.; Scalise, L.; Casacanditella, L.; Ercoli, I.; Marchionni, P.; Tomasini, E.P. Non contact measurement of heart and respiration rates based on Kinect™. In Proceedings of the 2014 IEEE International Symposium on Medical Measurements and Applications (MeMeA), Lisbon, Portugal, 11–12 June 2014, pp. 1–5.
17. Marchionni, P.; Scalise, L.; Ercoli, I.; Tomasini, E. An optical measurement method for the simultaneous assessment of respiration and heart rates in preterm infants. *Rev. Sci. Instrum.* **2013**, *84*, 121705. [CrossRef] [PubMed]

18. Scalise, L.; Ercoli, I.; Marchionni, P.; Tomasini, E.P. Measurement of respiration rate in preterm infants by laser Doppler vibrometry. In Proceedings of the 2011 IEEE International Workshop on Medical Measurements and Applications Proceedings (MeMeA), Bari, Italy, 30–31 May 2011; pp. 657–661.
19. Sirevaag, E.J.; Casaccia, S.; Richter, E.A.; O'Sullivan, J.A.; Scalise, L.; Rohrbaugh, J.W. Cardiorespiratory interactions: Noncontact assessment using laser Doppler vibrometry. *Psychophysiology* **2016**, *53*, 847–867. [CrossRef] [PubMed]
20. Lin, K.Y.; Chen, D.Y.; Tsai, W.J. Image-Based Motion-Tolerant Remote Respiratory Rate Evaluation. *IEEE Sens. J.* **2016**. [CrossRef]
21. Massaroni, C.; Lopes, D.S.; Lo Presti, D.; Schena, E.; Silvestri, S. Contactless Monitoring of Breathing Patterns and Respiratory Rate at the Pit of the Neck: A Single Camera Approach. *J. Sens.* **2018**, *2018*, 4567213. [CrossRef]
22. Bartula, M.; Tigges, T.; Muehlsteff, J. Camera-based system for contactless monitoring of respiration. In Proceedings of the 2013 35th Annual International Conference of the IEEE Engineering in Medicine and Biology Society (EMBC), Osaka, Japan, 3–7 July 2013; pp. 2672–2675.
23. Koolen, N.; Decroupet, O.; Dereymaeker, A.; Jansen, K.; Vervisch, J.; Matic, V.; Vanrumste, B.; Naulaers, G.; Van Huffel, S.; De Vos, M. Automated Respiration Detection from Neonatal Video Data. In Proceedings of the International Conference on Pattern Recognition Applications and Methods ICPRAM, Lisbon, Portugal, 10–12 January 2015; pp. 164–169.
24. Antognoli, L.; Marchionni, P.; Nobile, S.; Carnielli, V.; Scalise, L. Assessment of cardio-respiratory rates by non-invasive measurement methods in hospitalized preterm neonates. In Proceedings of the 2018 IEEE International Symposium on Medical Measurements and Applications (MeMeA), Rome, Italy, 11–13 June 2018; pp. 1–5.
25. Bernacchia, N.; Marchionni, P.; Ercoli, I.; Scalise, L. Non-contact measurement of the heart rate by a image sensor. In *Sensors*; Springer: Berlin, Germany, 2015; pp. 371–375.
26. Bai, Y.W.; Li, W.T.; Chen, Y.W. Design and implementation of an embedded monitor system for detection of a patient's breath by double Webcams in the dark. In Proceedings of the 12th IEEE International Conference on e-Health Networking Applications and Services (Healthcom), Lyon, France, 1–3 July 2010; pp. 93–98.
27. Janssen, R.; Wang, W.; Moço, A.; De Haan, G. Video-based respiration monitoring with automatic region of interest detection. *Physiol. Meas.* **2015**. [CrossRef]
28. Poh, M.Z.; McDuff, D.J.; Picard, R.W. Advancements in noncontact, multiparameter physiological measurements using a webcam. *IEEE Trans. Biomed. Eng.* **2011**, *58*, 7–11. [CrossRef] [PubMed]
29. Massaroni, C.; Schena, E.; Silvestri, S.; Taffoni, F.; Merone, M. Measurement system based on RBG camera signal for contactless breathing pattern and respiratory rate monitoring. In Proceedings of the 2018 IEEE International Symposium on Medical Measurements and Applications (MeMeA), Rome, Italy, 11–13 June 2018; pp. 1–6.
30. Massaroni, C.; Nicolò, A.; Girardi, M.; La Camera, A.; Schena, E.; Sacchetti, M.; Silvestri, S.; Taffoni, F. Validation of a wearable device and an algorithm for respiratory monitoring during exercise. *IEEE Sens. J.* **2019**. [CrossRef]
31. Taffoni, F.; Rivera, D.; La Camera, A.; Nicolò, A.; Velasco, J.R.; Massaroni, C. A Wearable System for Real-Time Continuous Monitoring of Physical Activity. *J. Healthc. Eng.* **2018**, *2018*, 1878354. [CrossRef]
32. Welch, P. The use of fast Fourier transform for the estimation of power spectra: A method based on time averaging over short, modified periodograms. *IEEE Trans. Audio Electroacoust.* **1967**, *15*, 70–73. [CrossRef]
33. Altman, D.G.; Bland, J.M. Measurement in medicine: The analysis of method comparison studies. *Statistician* **1983**, *32*, 307–317. [CrossRef]
34. Reyes, B.A.; Reljin, N.; Kong, Y.; Nam, Y.; Chon, K.H. Tidal Volume and Instantaneous Respiration Rate Estimation using a Volumetric Surrogate Signal Acquired via a Smartphone Camera. *IEEE J. Biomed. Health Inform.* **2017**, *21*, 764–777. [CrossRef] [PubMed]
35. Al-Naji, A.; Chahl, J. Simultaneous tracking of cardiorespiratory signals for multiple persons using a machine vision system with noise artifact removal. *IEEE J. Translat. Eng. Health Med.* **2017**, *5*, 1–10. [CrossRef] [PubMed]

36. Massaroni, C.; Venanzi, C.; Silvatti, A.P.; Lo Presti, D.; Saccomandi, P.; Formica, D.; Giurazza, F.; Caponero, M.A.; Schena, E. Smart textile for respiratory monitoring and thoraco-abdominal motion pattern evaluation. *J. Biophotonics* **2018**, *11*, e201700263. [CrossRef] [PubMed]
37. Liu, C.; Yang, Y.; Tsow, F.; Shao, D.; Tao, N. Noncontact spirometry with a webcam. *J. Biomed. Opt.* **2017**, *22*, 057002. [CrossRef] [PubMed]

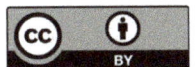

© 2019 by the authors. Licensee MDPI, Basel, Switzerland. This article is an open access article distributed under the terms and conditions of the Creative Commons Attribution (CC BY) license (http://creativecommons.org/licenses/by/4.0/).

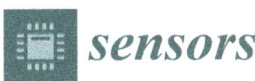

Article

Cardio-Respiratory Monitoring in Archery Using a Smart Textile Based on Flexible Fiber Bragg Grating Sensors

Daniela Lo Presti [1,*], Chiara Romano [1], Carlo Massaroni [1], Jessica D'Abbraccio [2], Luca Massari [2,3], Michele Arturo Caponero [4], Calogero Maria Oddo [2], Domenico Formica [5] and Emiliano Schena [1]

1. Unit of Measurement and Biomedical Instrumentation, Università Campus Bio-Medico di Roma, Via Alvaro del Portillo, 00128 Rome, Italy
2. Neuro-Robotic Touch Laboratory, Biorobotics Institute, Sant'Anna School of Advanced Studies, 56025 Pisa, Italy
3. Department of Linguistics and Comparative Cultural Studies, Ca' Foscari University of Venice, 30123 Venice, Italy
4. Photonics Micro- and Nanostructures Laboratory, ENEA Research Center of Frascati, 00044 Rome, Italy
5. Unit of Neurophysiology and Neuroengineering of Human-Technology Interaction, Università Campus Bio-Medico di Roma, Via Alvaro del Portillo, 00128 Rome, Italy
* Correspondence: d.lopresti@unicampus.it; Tel.: +39-062-2541-9650

Received: 2 August 2019; Accepted: 16 August 2019; Published: 17 August 2019

Abstract: In precision sports, the control of breathing and heart rate is crucial to help the body to remain stable in the shooting position. To improve stability, archers try to adopt similar breathing patterns and to have a low heartbeat during each shot. We proposed an easy-to-use and unobtrusive smart textile (ST) which is able to detect chest wall excursions due to breathing and heart beating. The sensing part is based on two FBGs housed into a soft polymer matrix to optimize the adherence to the chest wall and the system robustness. The ST was assessed on volunteers to figure out its performance in the estimation of respiratory frequency (f_R) and heart rate (HR). Then, the system was tested on two archers during four shooting sessions. This is the first study to monitor cardio-respiratory activity on archers during shooting. The good performance of the ST is supported by the low mean absolute percentage error for f_R and HR estimation (≤1.97% and ≤5.74%, respectively), calculated with respect to reference signals (flow sensor for f_R, photopletismography sensor for HR). Moreover, results showed the capability of the ST to estimate f_R and HR during different phases of shooting action. The promising results motivate future investigations to speculate about the influence of f_R and HR on archers' performance.

Keywords: fiber Bragg gratings; smart textiles; wearable systems; cardiac monitoring; respiratory monitoring; precision sports; archery

---

1. Introduction

Archery is a precision sport which requires consistency and stability of movements [1]. A mismatch of physical, physiological, and psychophysical factors can influence athletic performance and deteriorate archers' accuracy and precision [2–5].

In precision sports, both breathing and heart rate (HR) influence the athlete's performance [5–7]. The control of such physiological activities facilitates the performance of repetitive shots in the same, stable posture [8]. Lakie et al. demonstrated that high values of HR can cause sway movements, tremor, and shaking of the body when aiming at the target [8]. Mohammed et al. showed that HR variations affect breathing capacity, thus inconsistent breathing patterns can also impose a negative effect on the heart rate, and in general on the athlete's performance [9].

In archery, the shooting action can be separated into three main phases: set-up, aiming, and release. During the set-up phase, shoulders are brought in line with the target, hips are rotated forward, and the hand position on the bow grip is set-up. During the aiming phase, the focus is completely diverted to the target and the alignment of bow-sight-target is performed. The shooting of the arrow takes place in the release phase. It is highly recommended that archers start to inhale during the set-up phase of shooting, and to either exhale or hold their breath during the aiming phase. This allows for reducing the level of body rigidity and, simultaneously, preparing the body for the release phase [5,10].

As a result of training, master marksmen know exactly how to time the release of the arrow with the pattern of their breathing and cardiac cycle, thus minimizing the body jerk caused by the breathing process and the heart contraction [11]. Expert athletes experience similar breathing patterns and low HR values during each shot. On the contrary, unskilled archers hold their breath for longer during the aiming phase. The forced breathing process often leads to sway movements due to muscular contraction and an increase of ventricular depolarization, compromising body stability during the aiming phase [12–14]. Thus, comprehensive monitoring of breathing and heart beating during the shooting phases can improve the scheduling of exercises and optimize the training strategies [9].

Breathing and cardiac activities can be monitored by several solutions [15,16]. Among them, smart textiles based on fiber Bragg grating sensors (FBGs) have gained broad interest to monitor the mentioned vital signs in an unobtrusive and comfortable way [17,18]. FBGs can be easily incorporated into textiles thanks to their small size and lightweight. In addition, the high sensitivity and adequate bandwidth make these sensors an optimal solution for such an application. Some potential drawbacks may include the difficulty to handle bare optical fibers, their tiny resistance to mechanical stress, and the requirement to be connected to an optical spectrum interrogator. The encapsulation of FBGs into soft and flexible polymer matrices allows for mitigating the mentioned limits [19–21]. This solution makes easy to handle the fiber and improve the contact compliance with the body, leading to more accurate measurement of parameters from the chest surface movements. At the same time, recent progress towards the development of miniature FBG interrogation systems may broaden the application of FBGs for continuous and remote monitoring [22].

The aim of the present study is the feasibility assessment of a custom ST based on flexible FBG sensors for cardio-respiratory monitoring in archery. The proposed system was assessed on volunteers during quiet breathing and apnea, as well as on archers during shooting sessions.

2. Principle of Work of the Custom Smart Textile

Two flexible sensors were used to develop a ST consisting of two elastic bands (600 mm × 40 mm × 2.1 mm, 10 kgf of maximum load and 100% of polyamide) worn around the thorax and the abdomen, respectively. The fit of each band was adjusted by VELCRO® fastener to put the two FBGs in contact to the chest in correspondence of the xiphoid process and the umbilicus. The use of anatomical landmarks allows the FBGs to be worn on the same measurement points. Each sensor consists of an FBG (Bragg wavelengths λ_B of 1541 nm and 1545 nm for the band around the thorax and the abdomen, grating length of 10 mm and reflectivity of 90%; At Grating Technologies), previously housed in a flexible polymer packaging (90 mm × 24 mm × 1 mm) made of Dragon Skin® 20 (Smooth-On, Inc. USA) as shown in Figure 1. A detailed description of the manufacturing process and of the sensors' metrological properties are reported in [19].

FBGs work as stop band filters of wavelength because they back-reflect a small portion of light traveling along the fiber at a specific wavelength (i.e., λ_B). The FBG working principle is well described by the following equation:

$$\lambda_B = 2 \cdot \eta_{eff} \cdot \Lambda \tag{1}$$

where η_{eff}, is the effective refractive index of the fiber core and Λ, the grating period. The dependence of η_{eff} and Λ from temperature and strain makes FBGs an optimal solution for the development of measurement systems able to sense these two parameters [23].

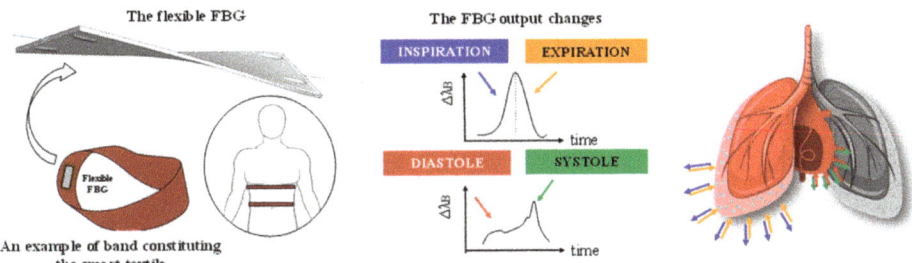

Figure 1. Schematic representation of the sensing element and the smart textile with typical FBG output changes induced by breathing and heart beating.

Regarding the application of interest, breathing and heart beating cause periodic displacements of the chest and, in turn, stretch the flexible sensors embedded in the ST, as schematically reported in Figure 1.

3. Feasibility Assessment of the Smart Textile on Healthy Volunteers

3.1. Population and Experimental Protocol

The ST for cardio-respiratory monitoring was assessed on nine healthy volunteers (four males and five females) whose age and anthropometric characteristics are shown in Table 1.

Table 1. Population.

Volunteer	Age (years)	Height (cm)	Weight (kg)	$C_T{}^1$ (cm)	$C_A{}^1$ (cm)
1	28	182	70	82	74
2	22	168	74	60	80
3	30	163	81	62	84
4	29	180	82	69	91
5	26	153	69	48	71
6	22	166	67	58	76
7	27	173	82	71	90
8	25	160	74	60	78
9	22	172	67	55	72

[1] C_T: thoracic circumference; C_A: abdominal circumference.

Each participant was asked to perform a protocol consisting of three main phases: *i*) a short apnea useful to synchronize the reference instruments (i.e., flowmeter for f_R, photopletismography sensor -PPG- for HR) and the FBG outputs; *ii*) 16 quiet breaths; *iii*) a final apnea as long as each volunteer can. The study was approved by the local ethical committee (protocol number 27/18).

3.2. Experimental Set-Up

The vital signs under investigation were monitored by the ST. The flexible sensors were positioned corresponding to the xiphoid process and the umbilicus (see Figure 2). Each FBG embedded into ST (FBG^T for the band around the thorax and FBG^A for the band around the abdomen, *a* box in Figure 2) was connected to an optical spectrum interrogator (si425, Micro Optics Inc., *b* box) which worked at the sampling frequency of 250 Hz. The reference signal for the respiratory activity was collected by a commercial flow sensor (SpiroQuant P, EnviteC, Alter Holzhafen, Wismar, Germany, *c* box in Figure 2) connected to a differential pressure sensor (163PC01D75, Honeywell, Minneapolis, MN, USA). The output of reference system used for the respiratory monitoring was collected by using a DAQ (NI USB-6009, National Instrument, Rockville, MD, USA, *d* box in Figure 2) and a custom virtual instrument developed in LabVIEW®environment, at the sampling frequency of 250 Hz. The reference system for the cardiac monitoring was a photopletismography sensor (*e* box in Figure 2), placed on the index fingertip of the left hand, as in [24]. The PPG sensor was input into two other analogue ports of the same DAQ used for the respiratory monitoring and collected at the sampling frequency of 250 Hz.

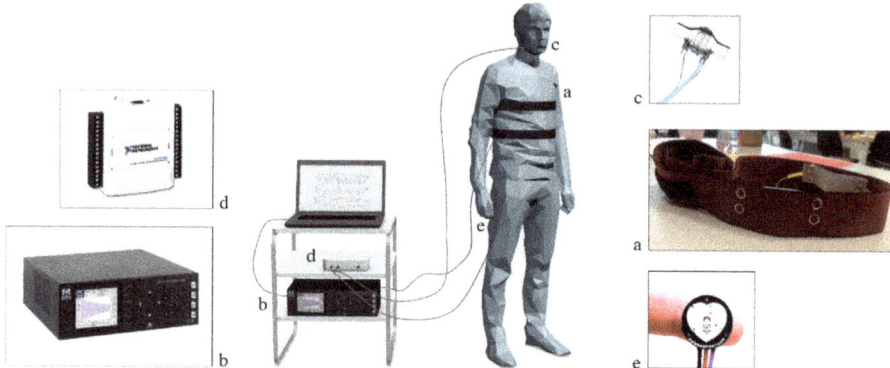

Figure 2. Experimental set-up: (**a**) smart textile consisting of two elastic bands instrumented by flexible FBGs, (**b**) FBG interrogator, (**c**) flow sensor, (**d**) DAQ, and (**e**) PPG sensor.

3.3. Data Analysis and Results

This paragraph will be grouped into two subsections according to the stages of the protocol (i.e., quiet breathing and apnea). Each subsection describes the data analysis performed to estimate f_R (during quiet breathing) and HR (during apnea), and the obtained results.

3.3.1. Respiratory Frequency Estimation During Quiet Breathing

For each volunteer, data were processed following four main steps: *i)* the outputs of the FBGs and the flow sensor were synchronized by selecting the first minimum points (i.e., starting points) after the starting apnea (see Figure 3); *ii)* the quiet breathing stage was selected by cutting all the synchronized signals from the mentioned starting points and considering all the 16 breaths performed during the protocol (see Figure 3); *iii)* a filtering stage consisting of a second order pass-band filter (lower cut-off frequency of 0.05 Hz and higher cut-off frequency of 0.5 Hz) was applied on both FBGs and flow sensor outputs; *iv)* a custom algorithm was used to select the maximum peaks of each signal (see Figure 4).

The respiratory periods (i.e., T_R^A and T_R^T for the band around the abdomen and the thorax, respectively, and T_R^{FLOW} for the flow sensor) were calculated as the time interval between two consecutive maximum peaks. Then, the f_R values estimated by both the FBGs (i.e., f_R^A and f_R^T) and the flow sensor (i.e., f_R^{FLOW}) were calculated as the ratio between 60 and the related respiratory periods in order to express f_R in acts per minute (i.e., apm).

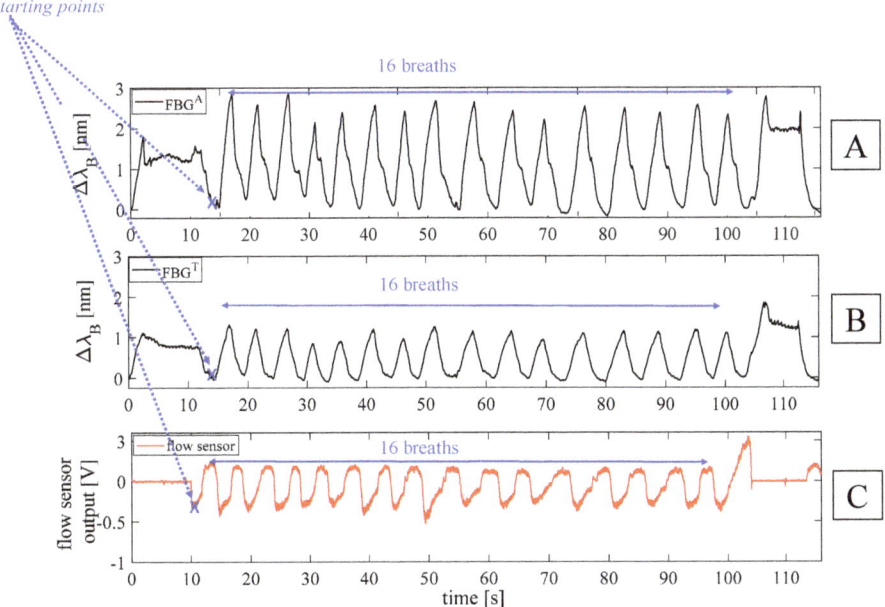

Figure 3. Outputs of the FBGs embedded into the smart textile and of the flow sensor on a whole experiment performed by a volunteer: (**A**) output changes of FBG^A, placed in correspondence of the umbilicus; (**B**) output changes of FBG^T, placed in correspondence of xiphoid process; (**C**) output of the flow sensor.

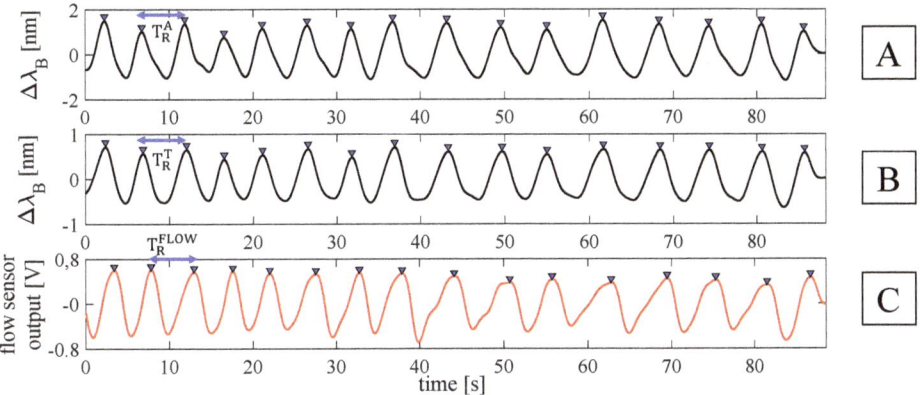

Figure 4. Outputs of the FBGs embedded into the smart textile and of the flow sensor during quiet breathing: (**A**) filtered output changes of FBG^A; (**B**) filtered output changes of FBG^T; (**C**) filtered output changes of the flow sensor. The respiratory periods for the band around the abdomen (i.e., T_R^A), around the thorax (i.e., T_R^T), and for the flow sensor (i.e., T_R^{FLOW}) were also reported.

The ST was assessed in terms of both breath-by-breath and mean f_R values. The Bland-Altman analysis was performed to describe the agreement between f_R values estimated by the proposed system and the reference one [25]. This analysis considered all the f_R values of the enrolled volunteers (i.e., a total of 135 f_R values for each Bland-Altman analyses) for the calculation of the mean of difference (MOD) and the limits of agreement (LOA$^+$ = MOD + 1.96·SD and LOA$^-$ = MOD − 1.96·SD, where SD is the standard deviation of the differences between the data collected by the proposed system and the reference one). The mentioned analysis was performed considering data provided by each flexible sensor. The mean absolute percentage error in the f_R estimation (i.e., MAPE^{fR}) was used to compare mean f_R values and was calculated as:

$$MAPE^{f_R} = \frac{1}{n} \cdot \sum \frac{|f_R^{smart\_textile} - f_R^{reference}|}{f_R^{reference}} \cdot 100 \qquad (2)$$

where $f_R^{smart\_textile}$ and $f_R^{reference}$ denote the values of the f_R obtained by the proposed system and the reference one, respectively.

Results of the breath-by-breath analysis are shown in Figure 5 and in Table 2. The good agreement between the f_R values measured by the proposed system and the reference one is confirmed by the high value of the correlation coefficient (R^2) for both FBG^T and FBG^A and by the low value of both MOD and MAPE^{fR}.

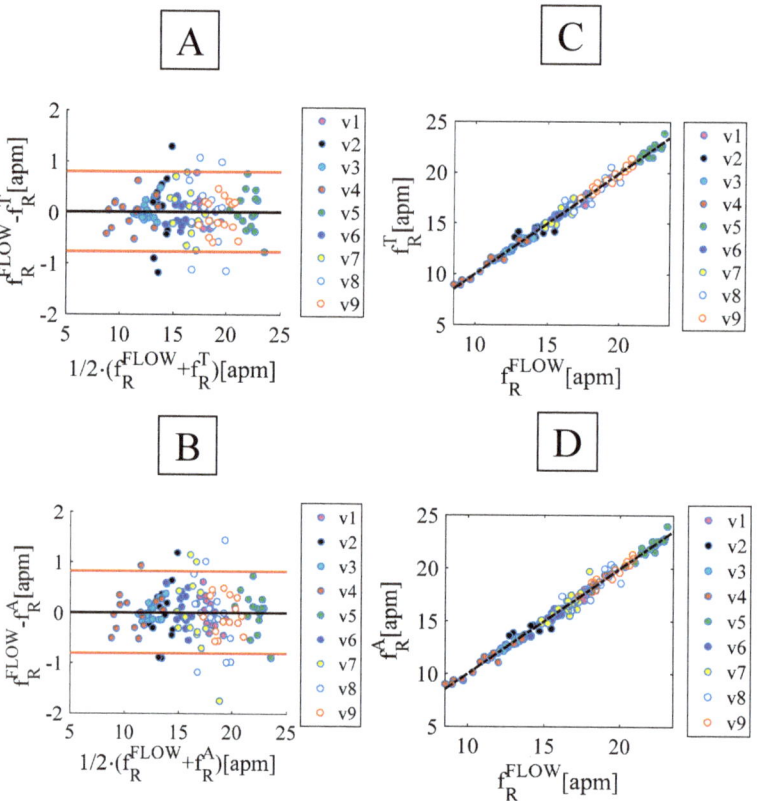

Figure 5. Breath-by-breath analysis: (**A**) and (**B**) Bland-Altman plots using the FBGs placed on the umbilicus, FBG^A and xiphoid process, FBG^T, (**C**) and (**D**) linear regression of the results obtained by the FBGs placed on the umbilicus -FBG^A- and xiphoid process -FBG^T- vs. the reference system.

Table 2. Performance of the smart textile in respiratory monitoring: results of Bland-Altman analysis, linear regression and MAPE^{fR}.

	R^2	MOD (apm)	LOAs (apm)	MAPE^{fR} (%)
$f_R{}^T$	0.99	0.014	−0.804; 0.832	1.92
$f_R{}^A$	0.98	0.004	−0.811; 0.819	1.97

3.3.2. Heart Rate Estimation During the Apnea.

The HR estimation during the apnea was performed according to the following four main phases: *i)* for each trial, the first minimum points after the holding of breath were selected on the FBGs output to define the starting point of the apnea stage for the FBGs and the PPG sensors; *ii)* the same time interval (i.e., 10 s) was chosen to estimate HR of all the volunteers during the apnea (see Figure 6); *iii)* a fourth-order Butterworth pass-band filter with a lower cut-off frequency of 0.6 Hz and a higher cut-off frequency of 20 Hz was applied on the signals. This band of frequency was chosen according to the frequency components of vibrations induced on the chest wall by the blood flow ejection into the vascular bed [26]; *iv)* a custom algorithm was used to select minimum peaks (blue markers in Figure 7) on each filtered FBG signal. The beat-by-beat cardiac period (T_C) from the FBG outputs was calculated considering the minimum peaks, as the time elapsed between two consecutive minimum peaks ($T_C{}^T$ and $T_C{}^A$ from the band around the thorax and the abdomen, respectively). Minimum peaks were chosen because they are easier to detect on the filtered FBG signals, automatically. Beat-by-beat cardiac periods were calculated considering the time interval between two consecutive maximum peaks on the filtered PPG signal ($T_C{}^{PPG}$). The HR values (i.e., HR^A, HR^T, and HR^{PPG}) were calculated as the ratio between 60 and $T_C{}^T$, $T_C{}^A$, and $T_C{}^{PPG}$, in this way HR is expressed in bpm.

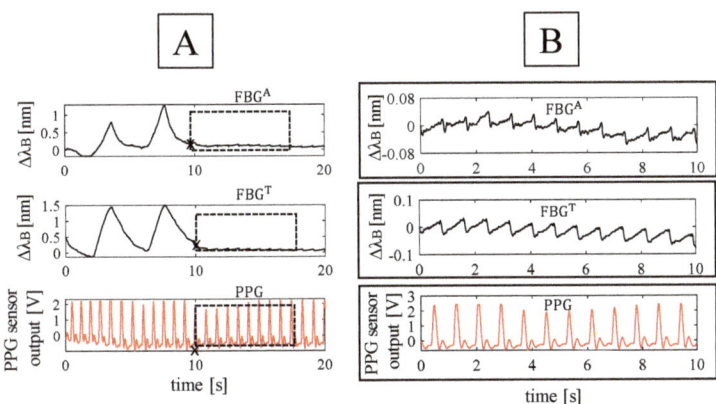

Figure 6. (**A**) Starting points selected on the synchronized signals and (**B**) zoom of the 10 s-window of apnea considering the outputs of FBG^A, FBG^T, and PPG.

The ST capability of monitoring HR was assessed in terms of beat-by-beat and mean HR values. The Bland-Altman analysis was performed by comparing HR values estimated by the proposed system and the reference one, considering all the volunteers for a total number of 149 beats. The mean absolute percentage error (i.e., MAPE^{HR}) was also calculated as follows:

$$MAPE^{HR} = \frac{1}{n} \cdot \sum \frac{|HR^{smart\_textile} - HR^{reference}|}{HR^{reference}} \cdot 100 \qquad (3)$$

where $HR^{smart\_textile}$ and $HR^{reference}$, values estimated by the smart textile and the PPG sensors, respectively. Results of the beat-by-beat analysis are shown in Figure 8 and Table 3. The good agreement between the f_R values measured by the proposed system and the reference one is confirmed by the high value of the R^2 for both FBG^T and FBG^A and by the low value of both MOD and $MAPE^{HR}$.

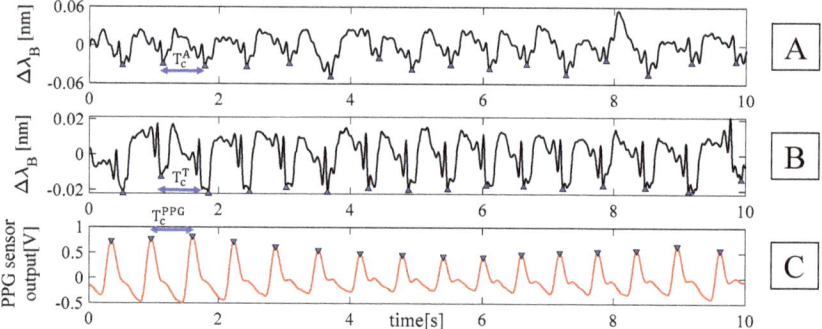

Figure 7. Peaks detection on the filtered signal: (**A**) filtered output changes of FBG^A, (**B**) filtered output changes of FBG^T, and (**C**) filtered output changes of PPG sensor. The cardiac periods for the band around the abdomen (i.e., T_C^A), around the thorax (i.e., T_C^T), and for the flow sensor (i.e., T_C^{PPG}) were also reported.

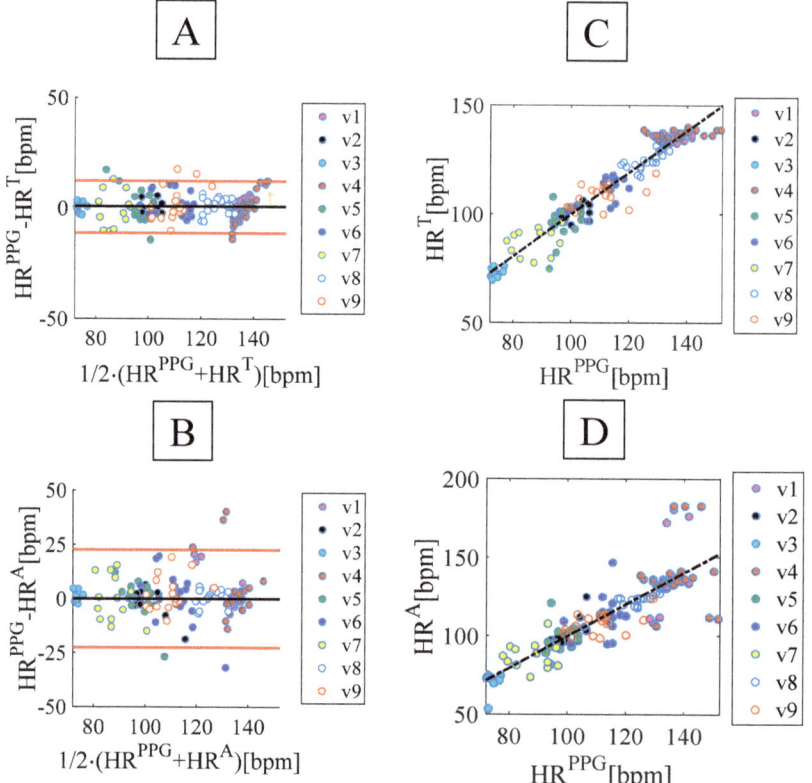

Figure 8. (**A**) and (**B**) Bland-Altman plots using FBG^A and FBG^T, (**C**) and (**D**) linear regression of the results obtained by FBG^A and FBG^T vs. the reference system.

Table 3. Bland-Altman of beat-by-beat analysis.

	R^2	MOD (bpm)	LOAs (bpm)	$MAPE^{HR}$ (%)
HR^A	0.76	0.059	−22.54; +22.65	5.74
HR^T	0.91	0.664	−11.15; +12.48	3.92

4. Tests on Archers During Shooting Sessions

4.1. Population and Experimental Protocol

The ST was tested on two archers (a male and a female). Their characteristics are listed in Table 4.

Table 4. Archers' characteristics.

	Age (years)	Height (cm)	Weight (kg)	C_T (cm)	C_A (cm)	Experience (years)	Training Frequency (days per week)
Archer 1	20	167	65	97	80	3	3
Archer 2	33	165	64	75	60	2	6

[1] C_T: thoracic circumference; C_A: abdominal circumference.

Archers were invited to perform two shooting sessions. Each session consists of six arrows to be shot in five minutes at designed 70 m targets. The first session is a practice round. In this round the arrows are shot at the beginning and do not count as part of the score. Instead, the second one is a scoring round with an awardable maximum score of 60 points (10 points per arrow).

4.2. Experimental Set-Up

During each session of shooting, archers worn the flexible sensors on the same positions investigated during tests on volunteers (see Figure 9). The optical spectrum interrogator (si425, Micro Optics Inc. Hackettstown, NJ, USA) for the acquisition of the FBGs output was placed at 3 m of distance from the archer. The sampling frequency was 250 Hz. Since the assessment of the ST was performed on volunteers (Section 3), no reference instruments were used during the shooting action to not impair the archer movements.

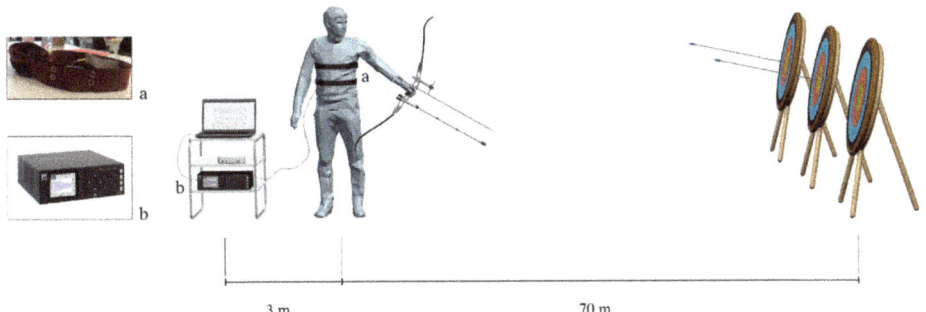

Figure 9. Experimental scenario during shooting session: (**a**) one of the band worn by the archer at designed 70 m targets and (**b**) the FBG interrogator at 3 m of distance from the archer.

4.3. Data Analysis and Results

Changes of FBG^T and FBG^A output of the two practice shooting sessions are plotted in Figure 10.

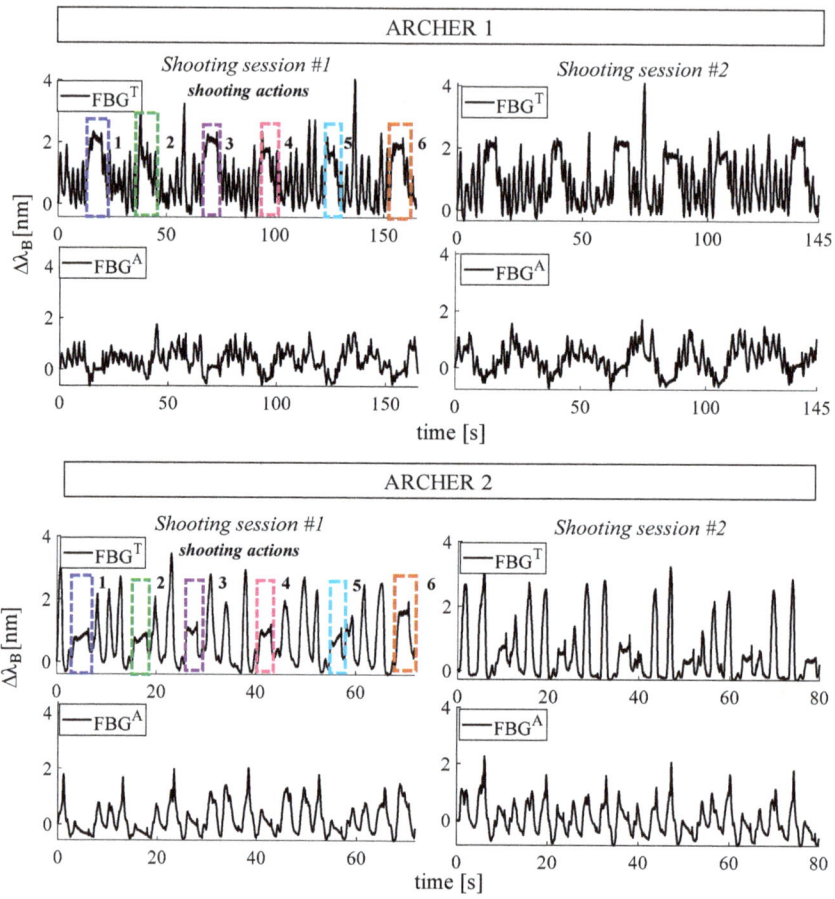

Figure 10. Outputs of the two flexible FBG sensors are shown for the four trials (2 shooting sessions for each archer). By way of example, the shooting actions of the first session are highlighted by dashed rectangular boxes.

The analysis was performed by selecting FBG^T output because the respiratory acts and the shooting phases are clearly discernible while FBG^A output has a more irregular trend (see Figure 10). FBG^T output changes were analyzed following three main phases: *i)* the six shooting actions were selected, as shown in Figure 10; *ii)* for each shooting action, the signal related to the aiming phase was filtered and its minimum peaks were detected to calculate the HR values (Figure 11); *iii)* the signal related to the breathing activity which precedes the shooting actions was filtered and its maximum peaks were detected to estimate the f_R values. Results in terms of f_R and HR for all the four trials are summarized in Table 5.

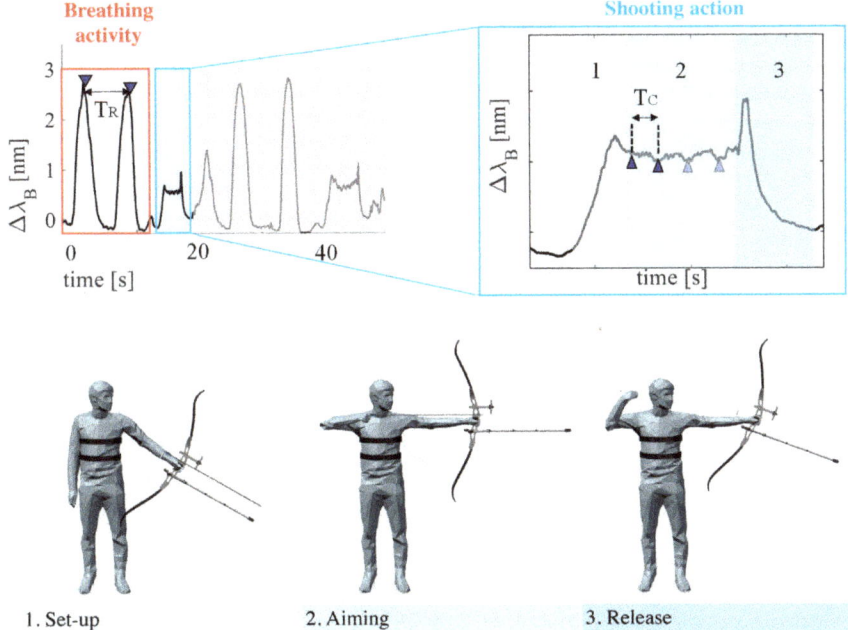

Figure 11. Output of the sensor changes during both breathing activity and shooting action.

Table 5. Values of f_R and HR during the first and the second shooting sessions.

	Shooting Session #1						Shooting Session #2					
Shot	1	2	3	4	5	6	1	2	3	4	5	6
	f_R (apm)						f_R (apm)					
Archer 1	23.9	24.6	20.0	26.5	21.9	20.5	24.1	25.0	20.6	26.5	25.6	23.9
Archer 2	15.2	13.3	9.3	8.6	10.1	8.4	7.4	8.5	7.6	8.8	9.0	7.1
	HR (bpm)						HR (bpm)					
Archer 1	101.8	101.3	97.3	96.7	100.0	94.9	116.4	113.7	108.9	104.7	120.5	115.9
Archer 2	87.6	89.2	94.3	89.3	97.3	94.1	97.2	88.3	92.0	92.3	82.1	90.5

5. Discussion and Conclusions

This work is focused on cardio-respiratory monitoring in archery using a custom ST based on flexible FBGs.

The feasibility of the system was assessed on nine volunteers during both quiet breathing and apnea. The system showed promising results in terms of both f_R and HR estimation, as shown in Tables 2 and 3. The position of FBGs does not influence the system performance in the f_R estimation, while FBG^T allows a more accurate HR monitoring than FBG^A (see Tables 2 and 3).

In a previous work [19], we already characterized the proposed sensing element. The flexible FBG sensors showed sensitivity to strain of 0.125 nm·mε^{-1}, sensitivity to temperature changes of 0.012 nm·°C^{-1} and negligible influence of relative humidity on its response. We were the first group that used Dragon skin®20 as polymer matrix to improve the sensor robustness and skin adherence for the cardio-respiratory monitoring. The main novelties of this work were the assessment of the custom ST on volunteers for the monitoring of both respiratory and cardiac activities and the ST application on archers during shooting sessions.

In the literature, FBGs encapsulated into flexible materials for cardio-respiratory monitoring were mainly proposed for clinical applications (e.g., during magnetic resonance exams). These technological solutions consist of FBG sensors encapsulated into polydimethylsiloxane, PDMS [27], polyvinyl chloride, PVC [28], and fiberglass [21]. In [27], an FBG was encapsulated into PDMS matrix (dimensions: 85 mm × 85 mm × 5 mm). Tests were carried out by positioning the sensing element on the back of two males and two females during MR examination. Results showed maximum relative errors of 4.41% and 5.86% for respiratory and cardiac monitoring, respectively. In [28], PVC was used as flexible matrix to house an FBG for simultaneous respiratory and cardiac monitoring. System showed good performances in the estimation of f_R and HR. In [21], an FBG was housed into fiberglass matrix (dimensions: 30 mm × 10 mm × 0.8 mm). The accuracy of the proposed sensor was characterized by relative error <4.64% for f_R and <4.87% for HR. In the present study, tests performed on volunteers showed promising results in both the estimation of f_R and HR (i.e., $MAPE^{fR} \leq 1.97\%$ and $MAPE^{HR} \leq 5.74\%$).

Focusing on the shooting sessions, results showed that the proposed ST can detect all the six shooting actions and, in turn, monitor f_R during the breathing activity and HR during the aiming phase. In the literature, commercially available devices able to monitor only one of these parameters (f_R and HR) were used on archers. Breathing activity and patterns were studied in [9] by using Zephyr Bio-Harness devices (Model PSM Research version 1.5, single transmitter and receiver, Annapolis, MD, USA). In [2,5,7] HR values were monitored by using Polar FT4, three silver-silver chloride chest electrodes, and Fitbit Charge HR (Fitbit, Inc. Boston, MA, USA), respectively.

These studies showed that both f_R and HR are important since they influence archers' performance. Therefore, the main improvement of the proposed system is the possibility to monitor both f_R and HR with high accuracy during the different phases of the shooting action using the same sensing element. Since the sensing element can be connected to the optical interrogator by means of long, flexible and lightweight fiber optic, the proposed system does not impair the shooting action. This feature encourages further assessment of the proposed system in sports science applications (e.g., during walking running on treadmill and during cycling).

In future works, a high number of archers will be enrolled to investigate how f_R and HR influence the shooting performance, and how HR can be estimated in the presence of breathing. These findings will aid the optimization of training strategies according to the experience of each archer and the maximization of their shooting action and scores.

Author Contributions: Conceptualization, D.L.P., C.R., M.A.C.and E.S.; Data curation, D.L.P. and C.R.; Funding acquisition, C.M., D.F. and E.S.; Investigation, D.L.P., C.R., M.A.C.and E.S.; Methodology, D.L.P., C.M., J.D., L.M., M.A.C., C.M.O., D.F. and E.S.; Supervision, C.M., M.A.C., C.M.O., D.F. and E.S.; Validation, D.L.P.; Writing—original draft, D.L.P., C.R. and E.S.; Writing—review & editing, D.L.P., J.D., L.M., C.M.O. and E.S.

Funding: This research was partially funded by 2018 BRIC INAIL ID10/2018 SENSE-RISC project and partially by MONREAB project financed by Fondazione Baroni.

Acknowledgments: We gratefully acknowledge A.A.; computer graphics artist at the Biorobotics Institute, Sant'Anna School of Advanced Studies for his assistance in designing figures.

Conflicts of Interest: The authors declare no conflict of interest

References

1. Park, J.-M.; Hyun, G.-S.; Jee, Y.-S. Effects of Pilates core stability exercises on the balance abilities of archers. *J. Exerc. Rehabil.* **2016**, *12*, 553–558. [CrossRef] [PubMed]
2. Clemente, F.; Couceiro, M.; Rocha, R.; Mendes, R. Study of the heart rate and accuracy performance of archers. *J. Phys. Educ. Sport* **2011**, *11*, 434–437.
3. Davis, J.R.; Campbell, A.D.; Adkin, A.L.; Carpenter, M.G. The relationship between fear of falling and human postural control. *Gait posture.* **2009**, *29*, 275–279. [CrossRef] [PubMed]
4. Spratford, W.; Campbell, R. Postural stability, clicker reaction time and bow draw force predict performance in elite recurve archery. *Eur. J. Sport Sci.* **2017**, *17*, 539–545. [CrossRef] [PubMed]

5. Keast, D.; Elliott, B. Fine body movements and the cardiac cycle in archery. *J. Sports Sci.* **1990**, *8*, 203–213. [CrossRef]
6. Robazza, C.; Bortoli, L. Nougier V Emotions, heart rate and performance in archery. A case study. *J. Sport. Med. Phys.* **1999**, *39*, 169–176.
7. Mohamed, M.N.; Wan Norman, W.M.N.; Linoby, A.; Sariman, M.H.; Mohd Azam, M.Z. The Importance of Being Calm: The Impact of Heart Rate Towards Performance. In Proceedings of the International Business Management and Computing Research Colloquium (BMCRC), Raub, Malaysia, 25 May 2016.
8. Lakie, M. The influence of muscle tremor on shooting performance. *Exp. Physiol. Issue Rev.* **2010**, *95*, 441–450. [CrossRef]
9. Mohamed, M.N.; Wan Norman, W.M.N.; Linoby, A.; Sariman, M.H.; Mohd Azam, M.Z. Breathing Pattern Influence to the Shooting Performance. In *Proceedings of the International Colloquium on Sports Science, Exercise, Engineering and Technology (ICoSSEET 2014)*; Springer: Singapore, 2014; pp. 321–333.
10. Sorrells, B. *Beginner's Guide to Traditional Archery*; Stackpole Books: Mechanicsburg, PA, USA, 2004; ISBN 0811731332.
11. Konttinen, N.; Mets, T.; Lyytinen, H.; Paananen, M. Timing of triggering in relation to the cardiac cycle in nonelite rifle shooters. *Res. Q. Exerc. Sport* **2003**, *74*, 395–400. [CrossRef]
12. MIYAMOTO, M. Changes of Heart Rate, Somatic Anxiety, and Performance of Japanese Archers during Practices and Matches. *Jpn. J. Exp. Soc. Psychol.* **2012**, *33*, 191–200. [CrossRef]
13. Taylor, A. The contribution of the intercostal muscles to the effort of respiration in man. *J. Physiol.* **1960**, *151*, 390–402. [CrossRef]
14. Lorenzi-Filho, G.; Dajani, H.R.; Leung, R.S.T.; Floras, J.S.; Bradley, T.D. Entrainment of blood pressure and heart rate oscillations by periodic breathing. *Am. J. Respir. Crit. Care Med.* **1999**, *159*, 1147–1154. [CrossRef]
15. Massaroni, C.; Nicolò, A.; Lo Presti, D.; Sacchetti, M.; Silvestri, S.; Schena, E. Contact-Based Methods for Measuring Respiratory Rate. *Sensors* **2019**, *19*, 908. [CrossRef]
16. Ernst, G. *Heart Rate Variability*; Springer: Berlin, Germany, 2014; ISBN 9781447143093.
17. Düking, P.; Hotho, A.; Holmberg, H.C.; Fuss, F.K.; Sperlich, B. Comparison of non-invasive individual monitoring of the training and health of athletes with commercially available wearable technologies. *Front. Physiol.* **2016**, *7*, 71. [CrossRef]
18. Lo Presti, D.; Massaroni, C.; Formica, D.; Giurazza, F.; Schena, E.; Saccomandi, P.; Caponero, M.A.; Muto, M. Respiratory and cardiac rates monitoring during MR examination by a sensorized smart textile. In Proceedings of the I2MTC 2017—2017 IEEE International Instrumentation and Measurement Technology Conference, Torino, Italy, 22–25 May 2017.
19. Lo Presti, D.; Massaroni, C.; D'Abbraccio, J.; Massari, L.; Caponero, M.; Longo, U.G.; Formica, D.; Oddo, C.; Schena, E. Wearable system based on flexible FBG for respiratory and cardiac monitoring. *IEEE Sens. J.* **2019**, 7391–7398. [CrossRef]
20. Ferreira Da Silva, A.; Goncalves, A.F.; De Almeida Ferreira, L.A.; Araujo, F.M.M.; Mendes, P.M.; Correia, J.H.; Correia, J.H. A smart skin PVC foil based on FBG sensors for monitoring strain and temperature. *IEEE Trans. Ind. Electron.* **2011**, *58*, 2728–2735. [CrossRef]
21. Nedoma, J.; Fajkus, M.; Martinek, R.; Nazeran, H. Vital sign monitoring and cardiac triggering at 1.5 tesla: A practical solution by an mr-ballistocardiography fiber-optic sensor. *Sensors* **2019**, *19*, 470. [CrossRef]
22. Mendoza, E.A.; Esterkin, Y.; Kempen, C.; Sun, Z. Multi-channel monolithic integrated optic fiber bragg grating sensor interrogator. *Photonic Sens.* **2011**, *1*, 281–288. [CrossRef]
23. Erdogan, T. Fiber grating spectra. *J. Light. Technol.* **1997**, *15*, 1277–1294. [CrossRef]
24. Lo Presti, D.; Massaroni, C.; Formica, D.; Saccomandi, P.; Giurazza, F.; Caponero, M.A.; Schena, E. Smart Textile Based on 12 Fiber Bragg Gratings Array for Vital Signs Monitoring. *IEEE Sens. J.* **2017**, *17*, 6037–6043. [CrossRef]
25. Martin Bland, J.; Altman, D.G. Statistical Methods For Assessing Agreement Between Two Methods Of Clinical Measurement. *Lancet* **1986**, *327*, 307–310. [CrossRef]
26. Allsop, T.; Lloyd, G.; Bhamber, R.S.; Hadzievski, L.; Halliday, M.; Webb, D.J.; Bennion, I. Cardiac-induced localized thoracic motion detected by a fiber optic sensing scheme. *J. Biomed. Opt.* **2014**, *19*, 117006. [CrossRef]

27. Nedoma, J.; Fajkus, M.; Novak, M.; Strbikova, N.; Vasinek, V.; Nazeran, H.; Vanus, J.; Perecar, F.; Martinek, R. Validation of a novel fiber-optic sensor system for monitoring cardiorespiratory activities during mri examinations. *Adv. Electr. Electron. Eng.* **2017**, *15*, 536–543. [CrossRef]
28. Silva, A.F.; Carmo, J.P.; Mendes, P.M.; Correia, J.H. Simultaneous cardiac and respiratory frequency measurement based on a single fiber Bragg grating sensor. *Meas. Sci. Technol.* **2011**, *22*, 075801. [CrossRef]

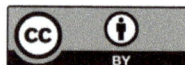

© 2019 by the authors. Licensee MDPI, Basel, Switzerland. This article is an open access article distributed under the terms and conditions of the Creative Commons Attribution (CC BY) license (http://creativecommons.org/licenses/by/4.0/).

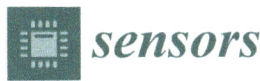

Article

Measurement of Pulse Wave Signals and Blood Pressure by a Plastic Optical Fiber FBG Sensor

Yuki Haseda [1], Julien Bonefacino [2], Hwa-Yaw Tam [2], Shun Chino [3], Shouhei Koyama [4,*] and Hiroaki Ishizawa [5]

1. Gratuate School of Medicine, Science and Technology, Shinshu University, 3-15-1 Tokida, Ueda, Nagano 386-8567, Japan; 19hs115f@shinshu-u.ac.jp
2. Department of Electrical Engineering, Photonics Research Centre, The Hong Kong Polytechnic University, 11 Yuk Choi Road, Hung Hom, Kowloon, Hong Kong, China; jeebonef@polyu.edu.hk (J.B.); Hwa-yaw.tam@polyu.edu.hk (H.-Y.T.)
3. Interdisciplinary Graduate School of Science and Technology, Shinshu University, 3-15-1 Tokida, Ueda, Nagano 386-8567, Japan; 17st108j@shinshu-u.ac.jp
4. Faculty of Textile Science and Technology, Shinshu University, 3-15-1 Tokida, Ueda, Nagano 386-8567, Japan
5. Institute for Fiber Engineering, Shinshu University, 3-15-1 Tokida, Ueda, Nagano 386-8567, Japan; zawa@shinshu-u.ac.jp
* Correspondence: shouhei@shinshu-u.ac.jp; Tel.: +81-268-21-5603

Received: 31 October 2019; Accepted: 18 November 2019; Published: 21 November 2019

Abstract: Fiber Bragg grating (FBG) sensors fabricated in silica optical fiber (Silica-FBG) have been used to measure the strain of human arteries as pulse wave signals. A variety of vital signs including blood pressure can be derived from these signals. However, silica optical fiber presents a safety risk because it is easily fractured. In this research, an FBG sensor fabricated in plastic optical fiber (POF-FBG) was employed to resolve this problem. Pulse wave signals were measured by POF-FBG and silica-FBG sensors for four subjects. After signal processing, a calibration curve was constructed by partial least squares regression, then blood pressure was calculated from the calibration curve. As a result, the POF-FBG sensor could measure the pulse wave signals with an signal to noise (SN) ratio at least eight times higher than the silica-FBG sensor. Further, the measured signals were substantially similar to those of an acceleration plethysmograph (APG). Blood pressure is measured with low error, but the POF-FBG APG correlation is distributed from 0.54 to 0.72, which is not as high as desired. Based on these results, pulse wave signals should be measured under a wide range of reference blood pressures to confirm the reliability of blood pressure measurement uses POF-FBG sensors.

Keywords: fiber Bragg grating; plastic optical fiber; non-invasive measurement; pulse wave signals; blood pressure; partial least squares regression

---

1. Introduction

In recent years, the increase of medical expenses and lack of medical workers have become a social problem due to the aging society [1,2]. Therefore, self-management of health conditions and prevention of sickness by measuring vital signs continuously in daily life has become more important. However, current commercial measurement systems are not suitable for continuous measurement because the majority of them are for stationary use and apply physical constraints. For example, in the blood pressure measurement, a cuff is usually attached on the upper arm of subject. When the measurement begins, the cuff is pressured by injected air and then the arm of subject is also pressured. Thus, the subject feels pain and cannot take any movements during the measurement. To resolve those problems, various wearable vital sign measurement systems have been used globally [3–7]. For example, it was demonstrated that heart rate could be measured by photoplethysmography (PPG) using the Apple Watch™ [3]. Using the PPG method, vital signs such as heart rate or stress can easily be measured by attaching sensors to the fingertip [4]. In addition, only a light emitting diode (LED) as the light source, a photodetector, and microcontroller are required to implement a measurement device. Therefore, it is easy to miniaturize measurement devices. However, there is no report that blood pressure and blood glucose level can be measured using PPG. Moreover, in the situation such as perspiration on the skin surface, the light intensity detected by the photodetector will decrease and measurement becomes difficult.

To resolve those problems, we are developing a non-invasive, wearable, and minimally constraining multi vital sign measurement system using a fiber Bragg grating (FBG) sensor. An FBG sensor is a small and light weight strain sensor fabricated in optical fiber, which has high sensitivity. In previous research, it is demonstrated that vital signs can be determined using pulse wave signals measured by a silica-FBG sensor [8–13]. However, silica optical fiber is easily broken by bending or extension. In addition, silica optical fiber produces sharp edges when break, representing a danger for the user, and prohibiting washing of the fiber and measurements during exercise. Therefore, there is a crucial need for safe FBG sensors for vital sign measurements.

In this report, an FBG sensor fabricated in plastic optical fiber (POF-FBG) sensor was used to resolve those problems. The plastic optical fiber is more flexible, resulting in resistance to bending and extension breaks, and a sharp cross section is not formed when breaks do occur. Furthermore, the plastic optical fiber is biocompatible because it is made from organic compounds like polymethyl methacrylate (PMMA) [14]. These features make it suitable for vital sign measurement. In addition, Bonefacino et al. reported the first demonstration of heartbeats measurements at the brachial artery location using POF-FBG [14]. It is further reported that use of a POF-FBG sensor results in a 20-fold sensitivity improvement over silica-FBG sensors. However, no attempt to calculate blood pressure from wavelength shifts measured by the POF-FBG sensor is made. In this report, we describe the results of measurement of pulse wave signals and the calculation of blood pressure from these signals.

2. Principle of the FBG Sensor

In this report, the FBG sensor system (SM130: Micron Optics, Inc., Atlanta, GA, USA) was used. This system is composed of a laser light source and an interrogator. The FBG sensor has a diffraction grating fabricated in the core of the optical fiber as shown in Figure 1. When broadband light is incident on the diffraction grating, only the specific wavelength corresponding to the Bragg wavelength is reflected, and the remaining light is transmitted. The Bragg wavelength is determined by the period of the diffraction grating and the effective refractive index as described by Equation (1).

$$\lambda_B = 2n_{eff}\Lambda \tag{1}$$

In Equation (1), n_{eff} and Λ are the effective refraction index and the period of the diffraction grating, and λ_B is the corresponding Bragg wavelength. When pressure is applied to the grating, the Bragg wavelength shifts because the period of the diffraction grating changes. The FBG sensor system measures pressure by detecting and calculating the shift of the Bragg wavelength.

Table 1 shows the core diameter, cladding diameter, and Bragg wavelength of the POF-FBG and silica-FBG sensors used in this report. As shown in Table 1, the Bragg wavelength of the POF-FBG sensor is in the near infrared. However, POFs have high attenuation in the IR region [14]. Therefore, a 50 mm POF was used, in which an FBG sensor was fabricated. The POF was attached to an angle-cut silica optical fiber as shown in Figure 2. One end of the silica fiber was cleaved with angle of ≈8° to avoid Fresnel reflection and glued to the POF using UV curable glue (NORLAND 78), ensuring low coupling losses and strong joint. The other end of the silica fiber was spliced to an ferule connector/angled physical contact (FC/APC) connector linked to the interrogator. Near infrared light incident on the silica optical fiber via the FC/APC connector can thus be propagated to the plastic optical fiber with low attenuation. As a result, the POF-FBG reflected Bragg wavelength has sufficient light power to be detected by the interrogator.

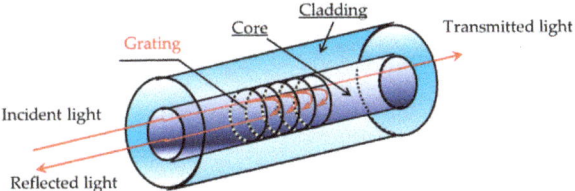

Figure 1. Schematic view of the sensor (fiber Bragg grating).

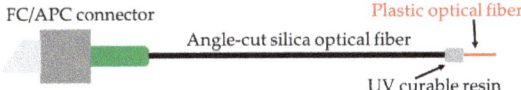

Figure 2. Schematic view of the optical fiber showing the fiber Bragg grating sensor fabricated in plastic optical fiber (POF-FBG) sensor.

Table 1. Fiber characteristics of silica-FBG and POF-FBG sensors.

	Core (µm)	Cladding (µm)	Bragg Wavelength (nm)
Silica-FBG sensor	8.2	125	1543
POF-FBG sensor	5.5	120	1553

3. Experimental Methods

3.1. Measurement of Pusle Wave Signals and Reference Blood Pressure

Figure 3 shows a photograph of experimental measurement. In this report, both the pulse wave signals and reference blood pressure were measured simultaneously 120 times for each of four subjects. Subject A and subject B were healthy males in their 20s, and subject C and subject D were healthy males in their 30s and 40s, respectively. In previous research, it was shown that FBG sensors could measure pulse wave signals at various points of the human body because of its high sensitivity [8]. In addition, when the height of the blood pressure measuring point differs from that of the heart, the blood pressure was measured with a large error because of the effects of gravity. If the measuring point is higher than the heart, the blood pressure increases to supply the blood against gravity. Whereas, if the measuring point is lower than the heart, the blood pressure decreases because the supply of blood is assisted by gravity. To suppress these effects, the POF-FBG sensor was installed on the brachial artery of the left elbow in the seated position. In addition, the silica-FBG sensor was installed in close proximity to the POF-FBG sensor for comparison of the respective SN ratios and waveforms. Both the POF-FBG and silica-FBG sensors were attached to the brachial artery by surgical tape. Pulse wave signals were measured at a sampling frequency of 1 kHz, at which it was previously demonstrated that blood pressure could be measured by an FBG sensor [15].

The FBG sensor cannot measure the blood pressure directly. Therefore, the blood pressure was calculated using a calibration curve constructed for each pulse wave signal from the signal and a reference blood pressure [15]. Both systolic blood pressure (SBP) and diastolic blood pressure (DBP) were measured 120 times as the reference blood pressure at the right upper arm by an electrical sphygmomanometer (HEM-7510C: OMRON Corporation, Kyoto, Japan), which can measure the blood pressure with an accuracy of ±3 mmHg.

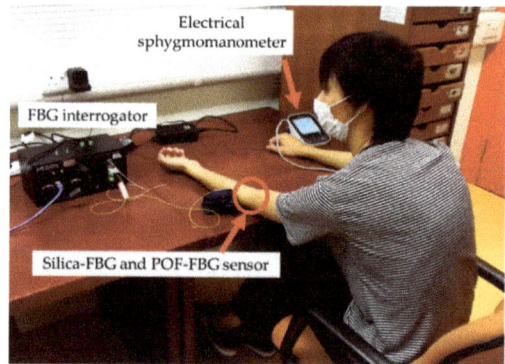

Figure 3. Experimental measurement of a subject.

3.2. Processing and Analysis

In the processing and analysis of pulse wave signals, sixth processing was used for blood pressure prediction. These processing are (1) filtering processing, (2) first differentiation, (3) separation from peak to peak, (4) averaging, (5) normalization, and (6) blood pressure calculation by partial least squares regression (PLSR). These processing were performed from (1) to (6) in order.

Raw pulse wave signals include high frequency noise, which decreases the calculation precision of the blood pressure. Therefore, as in previous research, a band pass filter with a pass band from 0.5 to 5 Hz was used to reduce high frequency noise prior to blood pressure calculation [8–13].

Figure 4 shows the waveform of the acceleration plethysmograph (APG) and the waveform obtained by differentiation after the filtering process of previous research. APG is obtained by differentiating the volume plethysmograph, which shows volume fluctuations of the blood vessel. In addition, it is demonstrated that FBG sensors can measure pulse wave signals, which are similar to those of volume plethysmographs [15]. Extrema A–E are observed in the APG waveform. It is known that the heights of the extrema change when the blood pressure changes. Therefore, it is expected that the blood pressure can be calculated from the changes in height of the extrema. Thus, the first derivative was taken post-filtering.

After the first differentiation process, pulse wave signals were separated to acquire a single pulse wave corresponding to one heartbeat. Single pulse wave signals were acquired by cutting pulse wave signals from peak to the next peak. Next, the averaged pulse wave signals were acquired by averaging assembled single pulse wave signals. Then, normalized pulse wave signals were acquired by normalizing the averaged pulse wave signals along the horizontal axis. Each maximum and minimum value of the vertical axis was normalized to 1 and 0, respectively. The number of sampling points on the horizontal axis was unified in the fewest number of sampling points.

After normalization process, partial least squares regression (PLSR) was used to construct a calibration curve and predict the blood pressure from the processed FBG data. PLSR is a multivariate analysis method, in which the objective variables are regarded as having error. In addition, the reference blood pressure also has error. Furthermore, PLSR can be used to construct a reasonable calibration curve with fewer factors than principal components regression (PCR). Therefore, PLSR is suitable. Firstly, principal components analysis was performed on the pulse wave signals, and the feature vector called the PLS factor was calculated. Objective variables were represented by the linear combination of PLS factors acquired from explanatory variables. The optimal number of PLS factors were statistically tested at the 5% significance level. Finally, the calibration curve represented by the optimal PLS factors was used for calculation of the blood pressure. In this report, the explanatory variable was the normalized pulse wave signal, and the objective variable was the reference blood pressure. Four PLS factors were used to represent the objective variables. In this research, 120 data sets were prepared for PLSR by using raw data measured 120 times, which were composed of the normalized pulse wave signals and reference blood pressure. Eighty data sets were selected randomly and used for the construction of the calibration curve, and the remaining data sets were used for validation. For the evaluation of the error in the calibration curve and blood pressure calculation, the standard error of calibration (SEC) and the standard error of prediction (SEP) were used. SEC can be obtained by calculating the standard deviation of the difference between the reference blood pressure and calculated blood pressure by PLSR. In this calculation method, by using not the calculated blood pressure by PLSR but the calculated blood pressure by the calibration curve, SEP also can be obtained.

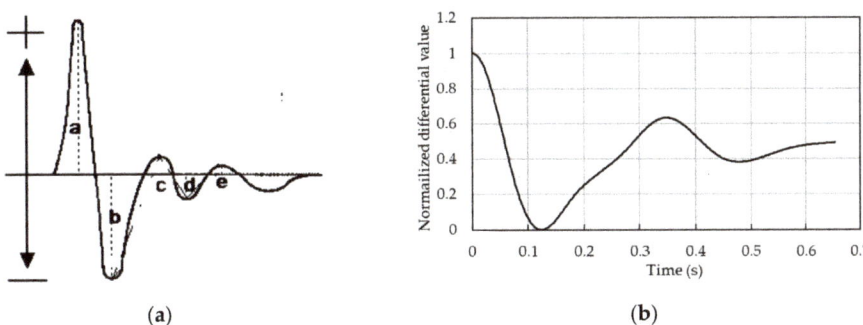

Figure 4. Comparison of acceleration plethysmograph (APG) and silica-FBG waveforms: (**a**) APG waveform and (**b**) silica-FBG sensor waveform.

4. Experimental Results and Discussion

4.1. Pulse Wave Signals Measured by POF-FBG

Figures 5–8 show single pulse wave signals measured by both the POF-FBG and Silica-FBG sensors in one measurement time for each of the four subjects, respectively. These single pulse wave signals were obtained after filtering, first differentiation, averaging, and the normalization process. As shown in the pulse wave signals of the silica-FBG sensor, the detailed waveform could not be determined because of high frequency noise remnants. However, the detailed waveform could be confirmed without the effect of noise in the pulse wave signals of the POF-FBG sensor. Therefore, it was demonstrated that the POF-FBG sensor could measure the pulse wave signals with a higher SN ratio compared to the silica-FBG sensor. In addition, the single pulse wave signals measured by the POF-FBG sensor were similar to the waveform of the APG shown in Figure 4. Thus, it was demonstrated that the POF-FBG sensor could also measure a waveform similar to the APG for an adequate SN ratio.

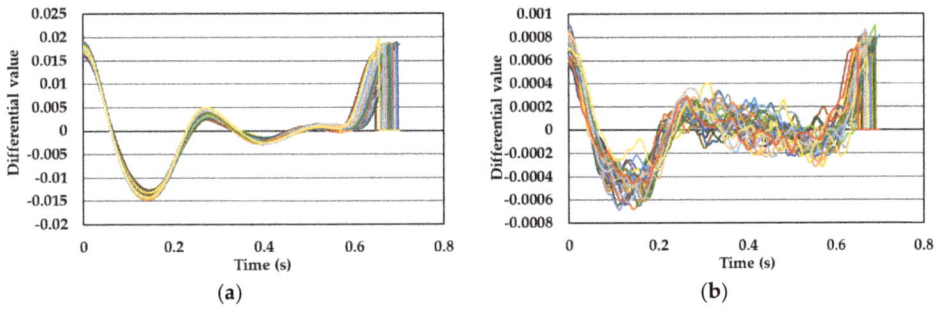

Figure 5. The single pulse wave signals of subject A: (**a**) POF-FBG sensor and (**b**) silica-FBG sensor.

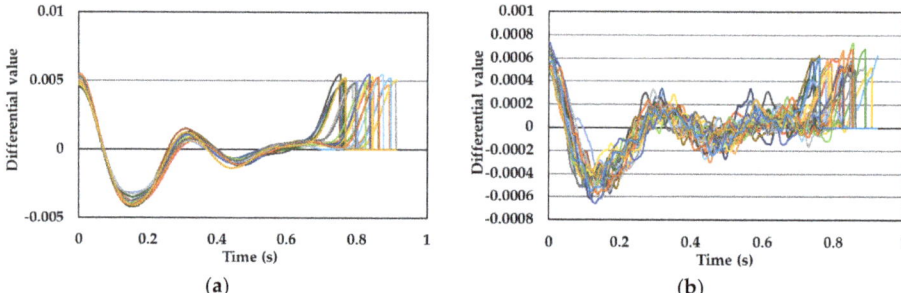

Figure 6. The single pulse wave signals of subject B: (**a**) POF-FBG sensor and (**b**) silica-FBG sensor.

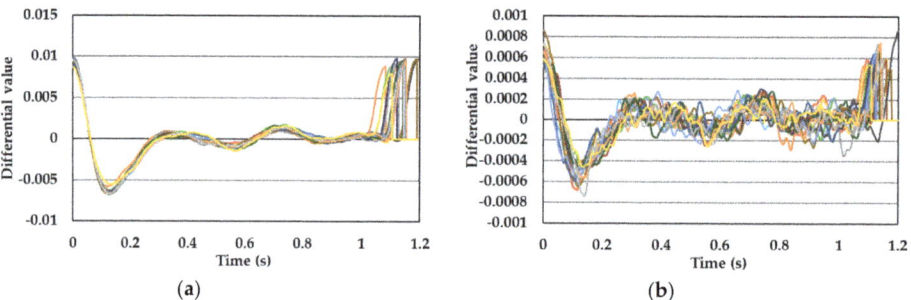

Figure 7. The single pulse wave signals of subject C: (**a**) POF-FBG sensor and (**b**) silica-FBG sensor.

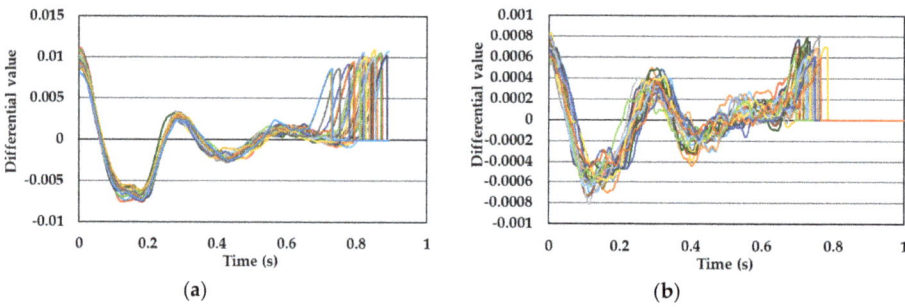

Figure 8. The single pulse wave signals of subject D: (**a**) POF-FBG sensor and (**b**) silica-FBG sensor.

In this research, both the POF-FBG and silica-FBG sensors were attached to the same measuring points using surgical tape. Therefore, as shown in previous research, the SN ratio of the pulse wave signals were improved by at least eight times, due to the difference in sensitivity between the POF-FBG and silica-FBG sensors [14].

4.2. Calculation of Blood Pressure using Pulse Wave Signals

The data from subjects C and D could not be used because the SN ratio of pulse wave signals were poor. Therefore, the data from subjects A and B was used for PLSR. Figures 9–12 show the results of calibration and validation of SBP and DBP. Table 2 shows the detail information of reference blood pressure in calibration and validation. Table 3 shows the correlation coefficient (R), SEC and SEP. In the calibration graph, the vertical axis indicates the calculated blood pressure using PLSR. In the validation graph, vertical axis indicates the blood pressure predicted by the calibration curve. Horizontal axis indicates the reference blood pressure in both calibration and validation graph.

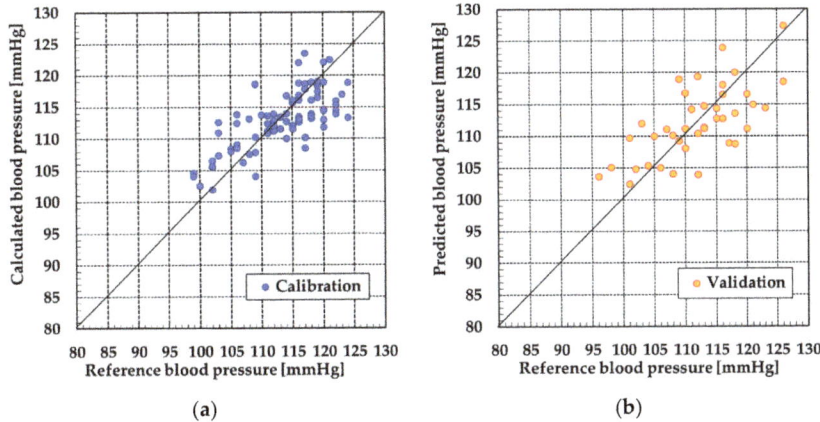

Figure 9. Result at systolic blood pressure (SBP) by partial least squares regression (PLSR) of subject A: (**a**) calibration and (**b**) validation.

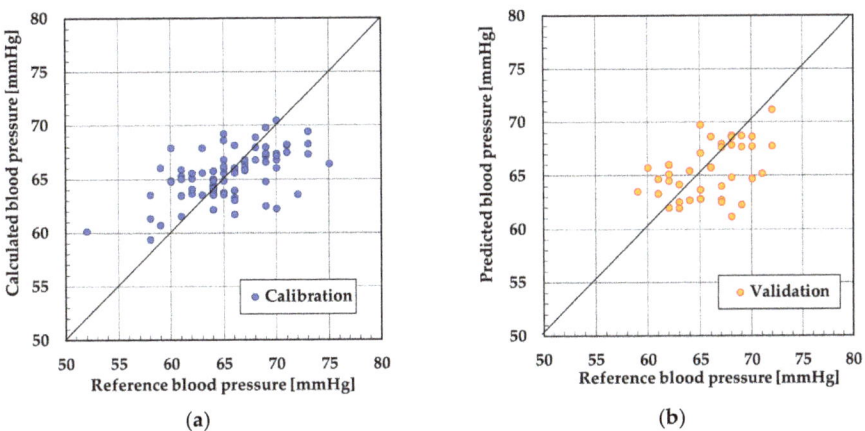

Figure 10. Result at diastolic blood pressure (DBP) by PLSR of subject A: (**a**) calibration and (**b**) validation.

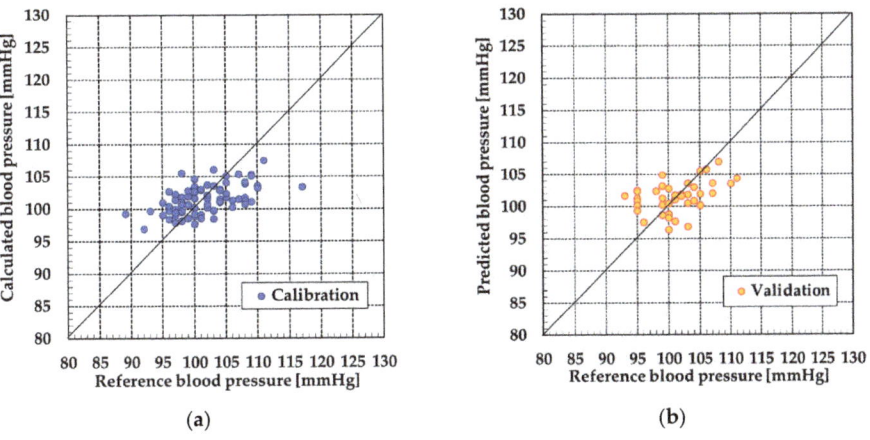

Figure 11. Result at SBP by PLSR of subject B: (**a**) calibration and (**b**) validation.

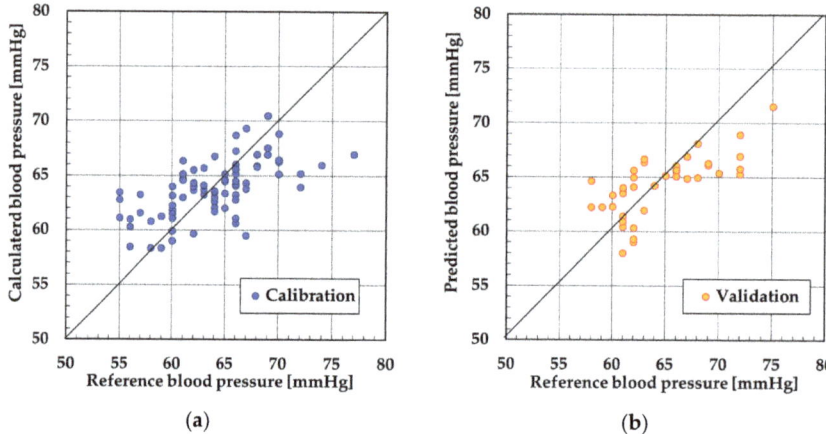

Figure 12. Result at DBP by PLSR for subject B: (**a**) calibration and (**b**) validation.

Table 2. Details of reference blood pressure at calibration and validation.

Subject (Gender)	Cardiac Cycle	Number of Measurements	Value of Blood Pressure (mmHg)		
			Maximum	Minimum	Average
Calibration Data Sets					
A (male)	SBP	80	124	99	113
	DBP	80	75	52	65
B (male)	SBP	80	117	89	102
	DBP	80	77	55	64
Validation Data Sets					
A (male)	SBP	40	126	96	112
	DBP	40	72	59	66
B (male)	SBP	40	111	93	101
	DBP	40	75	58	64

Table 3. Calibration and validation results for each subject.

Subject	Cardiac Cycle	PLS Factor	Calibration		Validation
			R	SEC (mmHg)	SEP (mmHg)
A	SBP	4	0.72	5	6
	DBP	4	0.58	4	3
B	SBP	4	0.54	4	4
	DBP	4	0.63	4	3

For subject A, the correlation coefficient of the calibration curve exceeded 0.7 at SBP. However, the error exceeded 6 mmHg in validation. The SEC and SEP at DBP were smaller than the values at SBP. However, the correlation coefficient was only 0.58. For subject B, the SEC and SEP of both SBP and DBP were almost equal to the error of the electrical sphygmomanometer. However, similarly to the DBP of subject A, the correlation coefficient was not high for SBP or DBP.

4.3. Adequancy of Blood Pressure Measurement Using a POF-FBG Sensor

Judging from Sections 4.1 and 4.2, pulse wave signals were measured at an adequate SN ratio by the POF-FBG sensor. However, although the SEC and SEP were adequately small, the correlation coefficient was poor, with the exception of subject A. For subject A, high correlation was confirmed between the reference blood pressure and blood pressure calculated by the calibration curve at SBP. To discuss these results, we focused on the range of the reference blood pressure and single pulse wave signals.

For subject A at SBP, the calibration and validation plots of Figure 9 were evenly distributed over the range of 25 mmHg. However, in the other calibration and validation results, almost all the plots were distributed over the range of 10 or 15 mmHg. When the range of the reference blood pressure was narrow, the validation of correlation between the reference blood pressure and calculated blood pressure over a wide range was difficult. Therefore, as a future task, it is necessary that the reference blood pressure be measured over a wide range to improve the correlation with the measured blood pressure.

Figure 13 shows all of the normalized pulse wave signals measured with the silica-FBG sensor for one subject from previous research. In this graph, a peak (reflected pulse wave signal) could be observed at approximately 0.22 s as indicated by the circle. Reflected pulse wave signals occur at points where the blood vessel divides into another vessel, or peripheral blood vessels exist. When the blood flow reaches these points, a component of the blood flow is reflected and is propagated to the measuring point, and the strain of blood vessel caused by the reflected pulse wave is detected by the FBG sensor. In addition, it is demonstrated that the reflected pulse wave signal significantly contributes to the calculation of the blood pressure in PLSR [16]. Figure 14 shows all of the normalized pulse wave signals for subjects A and B. As can be seen from these figures, the presence of reflected pulse wave signals between the first minima and second peak was not obvious. Reflected pulse wave signals had the characteristic that they were easily measured at points where peripheral vessels exist. Therefore, as a future task, pulse wave signals should be measured with reflected pulse wave signals so as to improve the accuracy of the calibration curve and calculation of the blood pressure.

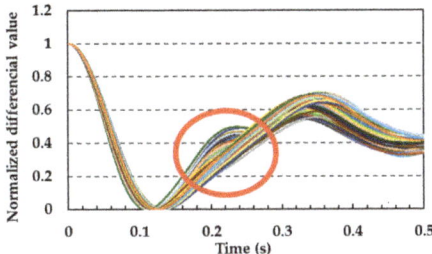

Figure 13. Reflected pulse wave signals (enclosed by circle).

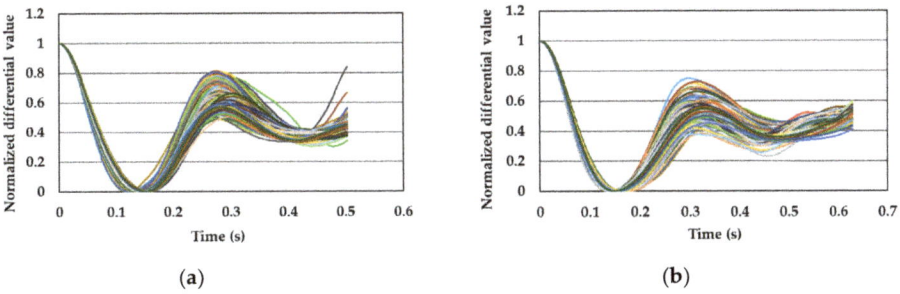

Figure 14. Normalized pulse wave signals: (**a**) subject A and (**b**) subject B.

5. Conclusions

In this paper, we focused on the validity of pulse wave signal measurement and calculation of blood pressure using a POF-FBG sensor. The pulse wave signals were measured by a POF-FBG sensor, and SBP and DBP were calculated by PLSR. In the measurement of pulse wave signals, the POF-FBG sensor was able to measure the pulse wave signals with SN ratio improved by at least eight times compared to the silica-FBG sensor for all subjects. Moreover, the single pulse wave signals measured by the POF-FBG sensor were significantly similar to the waveform of APG. Therefore, it was demonstrated that the POF-FBG sensor could measure pulse wave signals accurately and with very good repeatability.

On calculation of the blood pressure, a high correlation coefficient was confirmed at SBP for subject A. However, the correlation result at SBP for subject B was poor, as were the results at DBP for both subjects A and B. Regarding the accuracy of the calibration curve and the validation of blood pressure, the SEC and SEP at SBP of subject A were high. At SBP for subject B, and DBP for both subjects A and B, the SEC and SEP were almost equal to the accuracy of the electrical sphygmomanometer used in this report. To improve the correlation coefficient of the calibration curve, and accommodate a wide range of blood pressure measurements, it is necessary that the reference blood pressure be measured over a wide range in future experiments. In addition, the measurement of pulse wave signals that take reflected pulse wave signals into account should be performed to improve the accuracy of blood pressure measurement.

It is demonstrated that FBG sensor system can measure the pulse rate, respiratory rate, and blood pressure simultaneously and continuously [8–13]. By applying the flexible POF-FBG sensor to our FBG sensor system, we aimed for real-world implementation of safety FBG sensor system for users.

Author Contributions: Conceptualization, Y.H., S.K. and H.I.; formal analysis, Y.H., S.C. and S.K.; investigation, Y.H., S.C., J.B. and H.-Y.T.; supervision, S.K. and H.I.; writing—original draft preparation, Y.H.

Funding: This work was supported by JSPS KAKNHI, grant Number JP16H01805 and the Wearable Vital Signs Measurement System Development Project at Shinshu University. This work was also supported by a Grant-in-Aid for the Shinshu University Advanced Leading Graduate Program by the Ministry of Education, Culture, Sports, Science and Technology (MEXT), Japan. This research is partially supported by the Creation of a development platform for implantable/wearable medical devices by a novel physiological data integration system of the Program on Open Innovation Platform with Enterprises, Research Institute and Academia (OPERA) from the Japan Science and Technology Agency (JST), grant Number JPMJOP1722. This work was supported by the General Research Fund Project (PolyU 152207/18E) and PolyU Central Grant project 1-ZVGB.

Conflicts of Interest: The authors declare no conflict of interest.

References

1. Ministry of Health, Labour and Welfare. Estimated Number of Patients (per Day), 2014 Summary of Patient Survey. Available online: https://www.mhlw.go.jp/english/database/db-hss/dl/sps_2014_01.pdf (accessed on 10 June 2019).
2. Cabinet Office, Government of Japan. Situation on Aging, Annual Report on the Aging Society 2015. Available online: http://www8.cao.go.jp/kourei/english/annualreport/2015/pdf/c1-1.pdf (accessed on 10 June 2019).
3. Grant, A.; James, B.; Amanda, C.B.; Abbott, D. The validity and inter-device variability of the Apple Watch™ for measuring maximal heart rate. *J. Sports Sci.* **2018**, *36*, 1447–1452.
4. Mallick, B.; Patro, A.K. Heart rate monitoring system using fingertip through arduino and processing software. *Int. J. Sci. Eng. Technol. Res. (IJSETR)* **2016**, *5*, 84–89.
5. Pang, Y.; Tian, H.; Tao, L.; Li, X.; Wang, X.; Deng, N.; Yang, Y.; Ren, T.L. Flexible, Highly Sensitive, and Wearable Pressure and Strain Sensors with Graphene Porous Network Structure. *ACS Appl. Mater. Interfaces* **2016**, *8*, 26458–26462. [CrossRef] [PubMed]
6. Lin, H.; Xu, W.; Guan, N.; Ji, D.; Wei, Y.; Yi, W. Noninvasive and Continuous Blood Pressure Monitoring Using Wearable Body Sensor Networks. *IEEE Intell. Syst.* **2015**, *30*, 38–48. [CrossRef]
7. Yilmaz, T.; Foster, R.; Hao, Y. Detecting Vital Signs with Wearable Wireless Sensors. *Sensors* **2010**, *10*, 10837–10862. [CrossRef] [PubMed]
8. Chino, S.; Ishizawa, H.; Hosoya, S.; Koyama, S.; Fujimoto, K. Non-invasive Blood Pressure Measurement, The Study of Measuring Points. In Proceedings of the SICE Annual Conference 2016, Tsukuba, Japan, 20–23 September 2016; pp. 1706–1709.

9. Miyauchi, Y.; Ishizawa, H.; Koyama, S.; Sato, S.; Hattori, A. Development of the Pulse Rate Measuring System by FBG Sensors. In Proceedings of the 10th JSMBE Symposium Nagano district, Nagano, Japan, 2012; pp. 13–14.
10. Miyauchi, Y.; Ishizawa, Z.; Niimura, M. Measurement of Pulse Rate and Respiration Rate Using Fiber Bragg Grating Sensor. *Trans. Soc. Instrum. Control Eng.* **2013**, *49*, 1101–1105. [CrossRef]
11. Koyama, S.; Ishizawa, H.; Fujimoto, K.; Chino, S.; Kobayashi, Y. Influence of Individual Differences on the Calculation Method for FBG-Type Blood Pressure Sensors. *Sensors* **2017**, *17*, 48. [CrossRef] [PubMed]
12. Sato, S.; Kawamura, M.; Miyauchi, Y.; Koyama, S.; Ishizawa, H. Simultaneous Measurement of the Pulse Rate and Respiratory Rate by Fiber Bragg Gratins Sensors. In Proceedings of the 28th SICE Sensing Forum, Yokohama, Japan, 13–14 October 2011; pp. 97–100.
13. Katsuragawa, Y.; Ishizawa, H. Non-invasive Blood Pressure Measurement by Pulse Wave Analysis Using FBG sensor. In Proceedings of the 2015 IEEE International Instrument and Measurement Technology Conference (I2MTC), Pisa, Italy, 11–14 May 2015; pp. 511–515.
14. Bonefacino, J.; Tam, H.Y.; Glen, T.S.; Cheng, X.; Pun, C.F.J.; Wang, J.; Lee, P.H.; Tse, M.L.V.; Boles, S.T. Ultra-fast polymer optical fiber Bragg grating inscription for medical devices. *Light Sci. Appl.* **2018**, *7*, 1–10. [CrossRef] [PubMed]
15. Haseda, Y.; Ishizawa, H.; Koyama, S.; Ogawa, K.; Fujita, K.; Chino, S.; Fujimoto, K. Fundamental research of pulse wave and blood pressure measurement using passive edged filter integrated in Fiber Bragg Grating measurement system. In Proceedings of the SICE Annual Conference 2018, Nara, Japan, 11–14 September 2018; pp. 1685–1689.
16. Chino, S.; Ishizawa, H.; Koyama, S.; Fujimoto, K. Influence of Installing Method on Pulse Wave Signal in Blood Pressure Prediction by FBG Sensor. In Proceedings of the 2018 IEEE International Symposium on Medical Measurements and Applications, Rome, Italy, 11–13 June 2018; pp. 570–575.

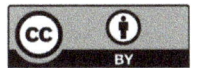

© 2019 by the authors. Licensee MDPI, Basel, Switzerland. This article is an open access article distributed under the terms and conditions of the Creative Commons Attribution (CC BY) license (http://creativecommons.org/licenses/by/4.0/).

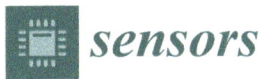

Article

Active Body Pressure Relief System with Time-of-Flight Optical Pressure Sensors for Pressure Ulcer Prevention

Kang-Ho Lee [1,†], Yeong-Eun Kwon [1,2,†], Hyukjin Lee [1], Yongkoo Lee [1], Joonho Seo [1], Ohwon Kwon [1], Shin-Won Kang [2,*] and Dongkyu Lee [1,*]

1. Daegu Research Center for Medical Devices, Korea institute of Machinery and Materials, Daegu 42994, Korea
2. School of Electronics Engineering, College of IT Engineering, Kyungpook National University, Daegu 41566, Korea
* Correspondence: swkang@knu.ac.kr (S.-W.K.); dongkyu@kimm.re.kr (D.L.)
† These authors contributed equally to this work.

Received: 14 August 2019; Accepted: 4 September 2019; Published: 6 September 2019

Abstract: A body pressure relief system was newly developed with optical pressure sensors for pressure ulcer prevention. Unlike a conventional alternating pressure air mattress (APAM), this system automatically regulates air flow into a body supporting mattress with adaptive inflation (or deflation) duration in response to the pressure level in order to reduce skin stress due to prolonged high pressures. The system continuously quantifies the body pressure distribution using time-of-flight (ToF) optical sensors. The proposed pressure sensor, a ToF optical sensor in the air-filled cell, measures changes in surface height of mattress when pressed under body weight, thereby indirectly indicating the interface pressure. Non-contact measurement of optical sensor usually improves the durability and repeatability of the system. The pressure sensor was successfully identified the 4 different-predefined postures, and quantitatively measured the body pressure distribution of them. Duty cycle of switches in solenoid valves was adjusted to 0–50% for pressure relief, which shows that the interface pressure was lower than 32 mmHg for pressure ulcer prevention.

Keywords: body pressure distribution; air-filled cell; alternating pressure air mattress; time of flight; air flow; active control system

---

1. Introduction

Generally, pressure ulcers are caused by a local breakdown of soft tissue due to prolonged high pressures at the interface of body and contact surface [1–3]. In order to relieve the interface pressure, manual repositioning of patients or support surfaces such as cushions has been required [1–3]. Recently, alternating pressure air mattresses (APAMs) have been often used for the prevention and treatment of pressure ulcers [4–8]. Air cells of APAMs sequentially inflate and deflate to relieve pressure for short periods. However, commercial available APAMs have a passive control mechanism that simply repeats inflation and deflation into air cells, which occurs regardless of the pressed regions and pressure level. It is difficult to show even and lower pressure distributions against different stress regions across the body.

To maximize the effect of the pressure relief through APAMs, a robust and reliable measurement of the body pressure is required simultaneously [1,5,8]. Usually, the main types of sensors to measure the interface pressure are based on the measurement of variations in resistance or capacitance from a deformable sensing component [9–13]. The capacitive pressure sensor measures changes in thickness between layers when pressed. Although the sensor has high sensitivity, it is subject to an interference environment due to the external electric field and requires complex readout circuitry such as a charge amplifier, a discharging resistor, and so on [12]. The resistive pressure sensor measures changes in conductivity of sensing material when pressed. This sensor has thin and flexible structures, and the sensor needs simple circuitry. However, its output signal is nonlinear with a slow response, and it shows high power consumption [13,14]. Both capacitive and resistive sensors have been reported that they have hysteresis limitation of the measured value drifts over time [14,15]. In addition, electric pressure sensors are usually weak in durability due to the deformation of a sensing element caused by physical contact force. The transducer placed on the contact surface across the body can also impose artificially high pressures on the tissues and poor resolution due to the thickness of the transducer [15,16]. As an alternative to the electric sensor, the optical sensor has provided good durability and external noise immunity [17–19]. Some device measured the pressure distribution for foot plantar using optic fiber [20]. In this study, a time-of-flight (ToF) optical sensor was used to measure the interface pressure. The ToF optical sensor identifies the distance away to the nearest object by measuring the time that the light takes to travel and reflect [21]. We implemented commercial ToF optical sensors on the bottom surface of air-filled cells in the mattress rather than the contact surface with body skin. The ToF optical sensor measures variations in the surface height of mattress after deformation. For the proof of concept, the optical pressure sensor visualized body pressure distribution and identified the 4 different postures. Here, we developed the APAM with an active control mechanism based on the ToF optical pressure sensor. This system has adaptive inflation (or deflation) duration of air mattress in response to the pressure level for body pressure relief of patient-specific interface regions. To investigate the performance of active body pressure relief system, we confirmed the rapid reduction of lower than 32 mmHg pressure using the system. It is expected that the proposed system can prevent pressure ulcers and improve sleep comfort and quality [22,23].

2. Materials and Methods

2.1. System Structure and Operation Principle

Figure 1 shows a schematic diagram of the proposed active pressure relief system with body pressure sensors. The system includes a mattress with air-filled cells, ToF optical pressure sensors, solenoid valves, a main control unit, and a compressor. The top surface of a mattress has a lot of air-filled cells which directly support the human body. Here, the ToF optical pressure sensors are placed on the internal bottom surface of the air-filled cells, which means that these sensors are physically non-contacted from the interface surface of the body. The signals (P_sig) from the ToF optical sensors are collected together to the main control unit. The main control unit visualizes the body pressure distribution with the corresponding colors.

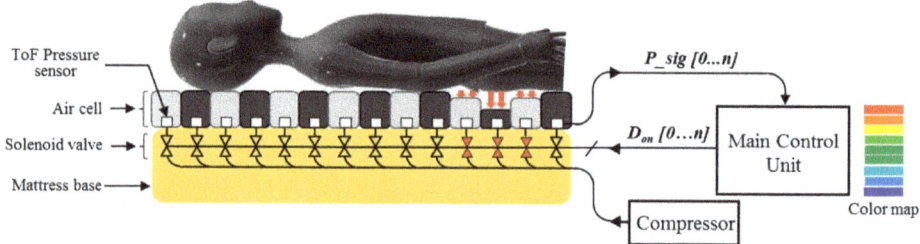

Figure 1. The schematic diagram of the proposed active pressure relief system with body pressure sensors.

In the system, air flow is regulated by a negative feedback control mechanism. In other words, repetitive inflation and deflation duration in air-filled cell are determined by adjusting a duty cycle of solenoid valve switches in response to the magnitude of the measured pressure. As shown in Figure 1, if air-filled cells are strongly pressed (red arrows at the hip area), the corresponding solenoid valves with red color begin to regulate their air flow. Our system updates the pressure data after every cycle when air flow is at a steady-state. Therefore, we consider a simple, single-loop feedback system as shown in Figure 2. The output of the system *P_sig* is fed back with the unity-feedback gain and then, compared with the reference value *Ref_P*. The system periodically calculates error values as the difference between desired and measured pressure levels. The error value is analogue, classified by the predefined thresholds, and then duty cycle D_{on} is changed. The D_{on} describes the proportion of ON time to the regular interval. The D_{on} is a result of pulse-width modulation (PWM) [24]. The output of the PWM is digital, switches the opening of the solenoid valves while regulating air flow applied by the compressor. In the system, the control loop uses a distance value as a feed-back variable. Therefore, the *Ref_P* means an initial distance without deformation and the measured distance is periodically compared with the *Ref_P* to determine the D_{on} of switches in solenoid valves.

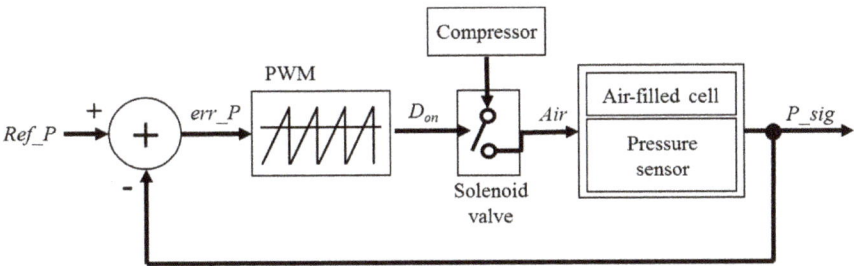

Figure 2. The block diagram of the closed-loop control mechanism in the system.

2.2. Design of the ToF Optical Pressure Sensor

Figure 3a,b show pictures of the developed ToF optical pressure sensor and mounting inside of the air-filled cell, respectively. The ToF optical pressure sensor includes a microcontroller, a ToF unit and a communication component for external interface. As a ToF unit, we used an off-the-shelf component, VL6180X (STMicroelectronics, Plan-les-Ouates, Switzerland). In Figure 3c, air-filled cells on the mattress were closely arranged with a shape of semicircular cover on supporting walls. Therefore, when air-filled cells were pressed by the body, those were mainly deformed in vertical direction while leaning by each other. The ToF optical pressure sensor, which is placed on the bottom surface of air-filled cell, can measure the lowered height by using applied force. Therefore, we used the ToF optical sensor to indirectly measure the interface pressure under body weight. The ToF optical unit transfers its data to the microcontroller unit through the inter-integrated circuit bus (I2C bus). And both ends of the sensor share a common communication line that can be connected to other sensors. Although parallel sensors in other works may require a number of interface wires [9,11,25], our sensors are connected serially, minimizing the number of wires. The RS-485 communication technique needs only differential data lines for external interface [26]. All sensors can be independently separated with the assigned slave addresses. The sensor has a small size of 20(L) × 20(W) mm, which is suitable for using at any location as an independent module. It consumes a current of 30 mA from a 5 V supply.

Figure 4 shows the description of mounting pressure sensors in the air-filled cells of the mattress at a regular distance. The prototype was designed to fit the hip size of body, because the pressure is most focused on the hip of body parts [1,2]. The air-filled cell was fabricated with PVC (polyvinylchloride) film, which has a size of 760(L) × 90(W) × 68(H) mm. Total of 18 sensors in 6 air-filled cells of the prototype system were located. The 6 air-filled cells were arranged longitudinally. The serially connected 18 sensors have individual slave addresses of index numbers of 0–17 as shown in Figure 4. Hose pipe connects the side of the air-filled cells into the solenoid valve, as shown in the left inset of Figure 4.

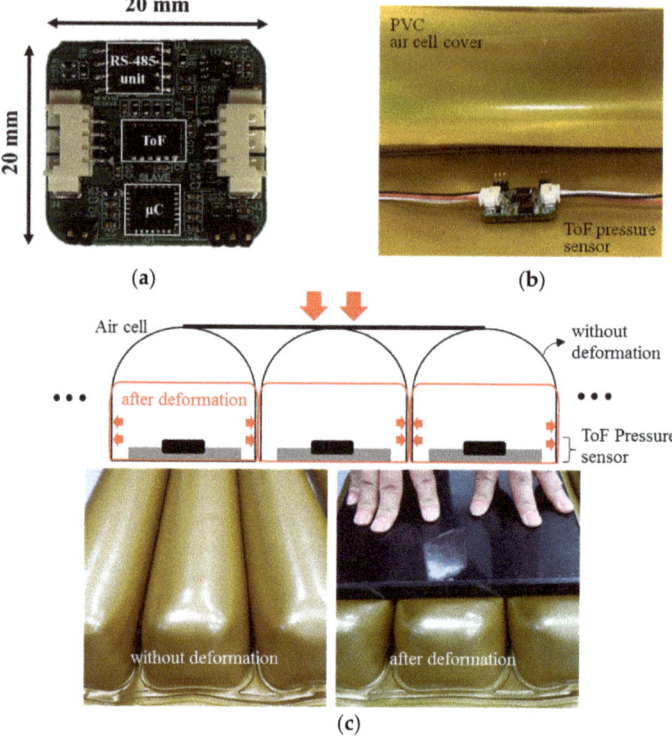

Figure 3. Pictures of (**a**) the developed ToF optical pressure sensor; (**b**) mounting the sensor inside of air-filled cell; (**c**) description of air-filled cell without and with deformation.

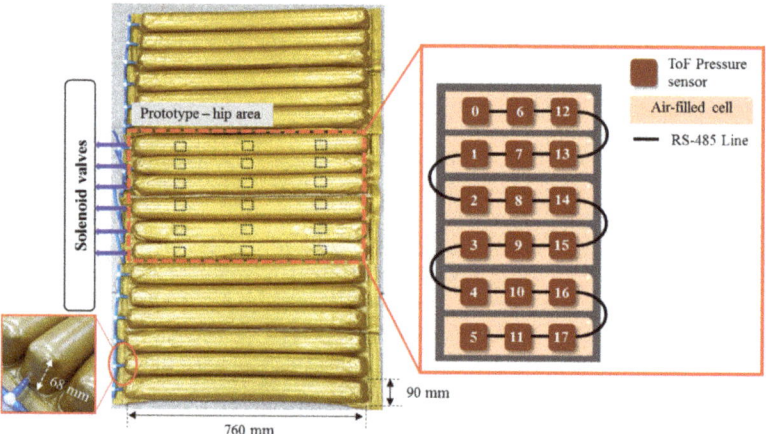

Figure 4. Description of pressure sensor location in air-filled cells of the mattress. The right inset shows the connection diagram of sensors with different addresses from 0 to 17. The left inset shows the hose pipe connected with the side of the air-filled cell.

2.3. Design of the Solenoid Valve System and Its Operation

Figure 5 shows pictures of solenoid valves and their control board. The solenoid valve is an electromechanical device in which the solenoid uses an electric current to generate a magnetic field and thereby operate by a mechanism which regulates the opening of fluid flow in a valve [27]. In our system, each of the air-filled cells is connected to the respective solenoid valve. All solenoid valves were placed together on a common manifold as shown in Figure 5. The valve has the 3-way ports of dose, release, and distribution for air flow. If the valve is open, then an inlet port from compressor is connected to a distribution port to mattress air-filled cell, and air is injected to distribution port. If the valve is closed, then ports are isolated, and air is released through the exhaust port. The valve control board determines whether the electric current is passed through the solenoid, communicating with the main control unit. The solenoid valve consumes a current of 200 mA from a 5 V supply.

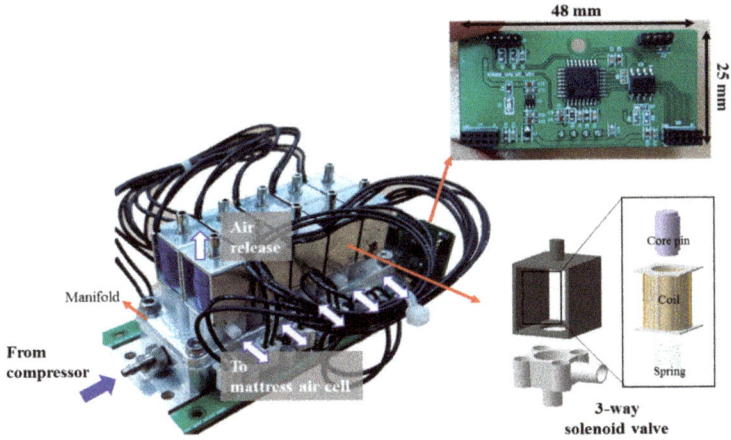

Figure 5. Pictures of the 3-way solenoid valves and a control board.

Figure 6 shows the timing diagram for a solenoid valve control. In the prototype, the 6 air-filled cells were alternately controlled during a cycle period. When the valve switch is ON with logic high, the valve is opened, and then air is injected from the compressor to air-filled cell, thereby inflating the air-filled cell. When the switch is OFF with logic low, the valve is closed, and the air is released from air-filled cell. The system sequentially determines the duration of inflation (or deflation) at the entrance of $t_1 - t_6$. For example, if the pressure level is at its lowest, D_{on} of switches in solenoid valves is 50%, which means that the ON time for inflation is same with the OFF time for deflation, as shown in the air-filled cell #1-5 of Figure 6. If the higher pressure is detected, then the D_{on} begins to decrease while at the same time increasing the deflation rate, as shown in the air-filled cell #6 of Figure 6. Therefore, the system is able to adaptively supply the corresponding air as the interface pressure changes, which results in the reducing effect in the interface pressure.

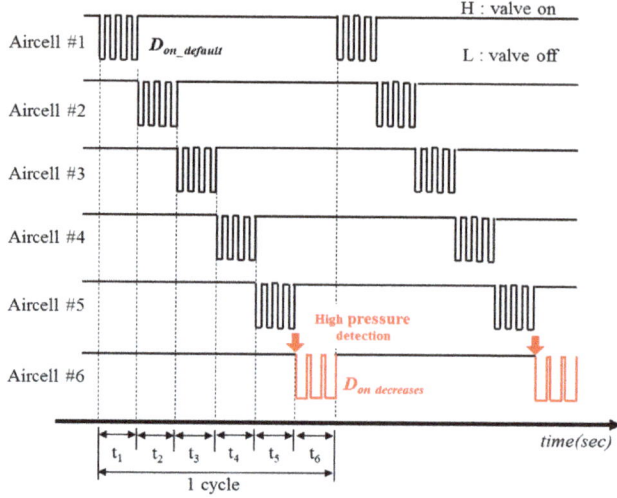

Figure 6. The timing diagram for solenoid valve control.

3. Results and Discussion

3.1. Performance of the TOF Optical Pressure Sensor

The ToF optical pressure sensor is designed by positioning the commercial ToF optical sensor inside of air-filled cell. The ToF optical sensor can measure distance between bottom and top surface of air-filled cell. In Figure 7, the signals of the ToF optical sensor were compared with the height (h) of the air-filled cell after deformation. Figure 7a shows the Z-axis stage equipment that can precisely change the height of the air-filled cell in the vertical direction. Using the Z-axis stage equipment with a ruler, the air-filled cell was manually pressed while recording the actual height of air cell. The height of air cell was compared with the results from the ToF sensor in Figure 7b. The air-filled cell had a maximum height of 68 mm without deformation. The air cell was gradually pressed to reach the height of 10 mm. It is verified that the measured distance by the ToF optical sensor had an accuracy of ±0.57% compared with the actual height of the air-filled cell.

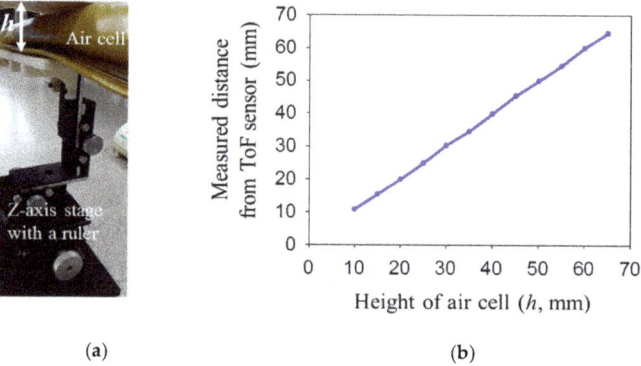

Figure 7. Measuring performance of the ToF optical sensor; (**a**) Setup for pressing the air-filled cell; (**b**) comparison of the measured distance by ToF optical sensor with actual height of air-filled cell by Z-axis stage.

Figure 8 shows the calibration curve of the relative ratio in the measured distance at different pressures. The relative ratio in the measured distance is the ratio of the changed distance after deformation compared with initial distance. This relative value is effective to objectively evaluate the multiple sensors' performance, excluding the common noise. Figure 8a shows the picture for the measurement method to validate the relation between the measured distance and the interface pressure. The commercial equipment X3Pro (XSENSOR, Calgary, AB, Canada) is placed on air-filled cells to investigate the interface pressure. And different forces were manually applied in downward direction using a push-pull gauge (IMADA, Japan). Figure 8b shows the relative ratio of measured distance as different pressures applied by a push-pull gauge. At the same time, the interface pressures were measured by X3Pro as shown in Figure 8c. Our system is capable of measuring the minimum pressure level of 24 mmHg, which is comparable to a commercialized sensor [11]. This system has a linear response under the interface pressure of 35 mmHg. The slope of the interface pressure to the applied pressure is calculated to be 0.3 over 35 mmHg.

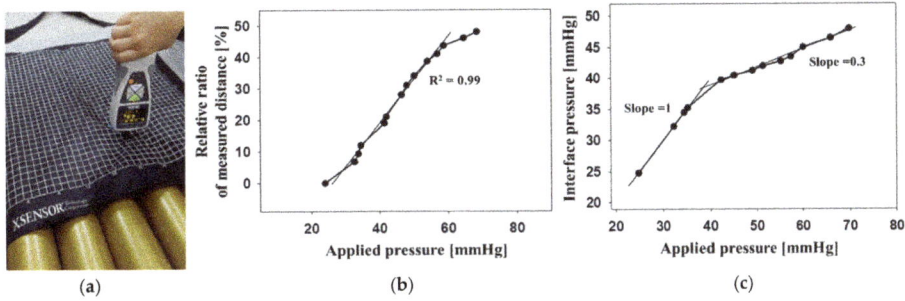

Figure 8. (a) Picture for measurement method, (b) the relative ratio in the measured distance and (c) the interface pressure at pressures applied by manual forces.

3.2. Prototype of Active Body Pressure Relief System with the Optical Pressure Sensor

Figure 9 shows the prototype system including air-filled cells, solenoid valves, a main control unit, and a compressor. As a proof of concept, 6 air-filled cells were tested under the hip placement. The air-filled cells have the ToF optical sensors inside them. The main control unit receives the pressure signal from the ToF optical pressure sensor and regulates air flow by controlling the switches of solenoid valves. In particular, the main control unit has a 7-inch LCD to use for user's interface while visualizing the body pressure distribution in real time. The inset in Figure 9 shows the LCD screen window. The screen shows sections of (a) valve ON and OFF status, (b) color map responding to the pressure level and the measured (c) absolute and (d) relative distance values.

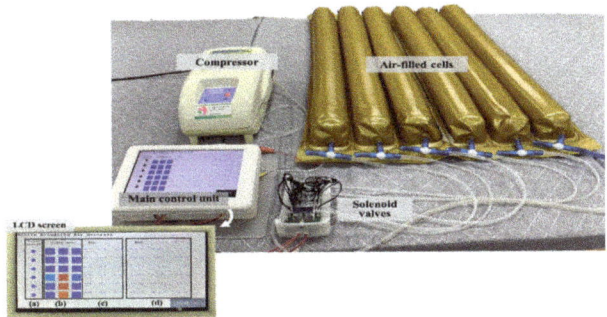

Figure 9. Picture of the prototype system including air-filled cells, solenoid valves, a main control unit and a compressor.

The optical pressure sensor could quantitatively measure the body pressure distribution when a participant was taking different postures on the mattress. Postures are as follows: (a) a supine position, (b) a left lateral position, (c) a right lateral position and (d) a sitting position. Table 1 shows the color visualization and the measured corresponding data at different postures, respectively. The pressure was defined as red color when the relative distance ratio was larger than 45%. The distance ratio of 0% was expressed with the blue color. The distance ratio was classified with a total of 1024 colors between the red and the blue color. In a supine position of posture at Table 1a, the sensors of index of 6 to 11 mainly responded to applied pressure. The sensor of index 9 was matched with the coccyx of the body bones representing the highest pressure with red color. As expected, in the left lateral position of posture at Table 1b, the left-side sensors of index 12 to 17 showed the largest changes in color. We could recognize the left pelvic bone from the colors in the sensors of index 15 and 16. In case of the right lateral position of posture at Table 1c, a participant was lying across the middle and right regions. Therefore, lower and even pressures were visualized due to the pressure redistribution. In (d) of Table 1, a participant was sitting on the mattress. Through the color changes in the sensors of index 3, 9 to 11 and 15, the coccyx and pelvic bones of body could be clearly recognized. In these experiments, the proposed system successfully quantified the body pressure distribution in real time.

Table 1. The color visualization and measured corresponding data when a participant was taking different postures on the mattress; (**a**) a supine position, (**b**) a left lateral position, (**c**) a right lateral position and (**d**) a sitting position.

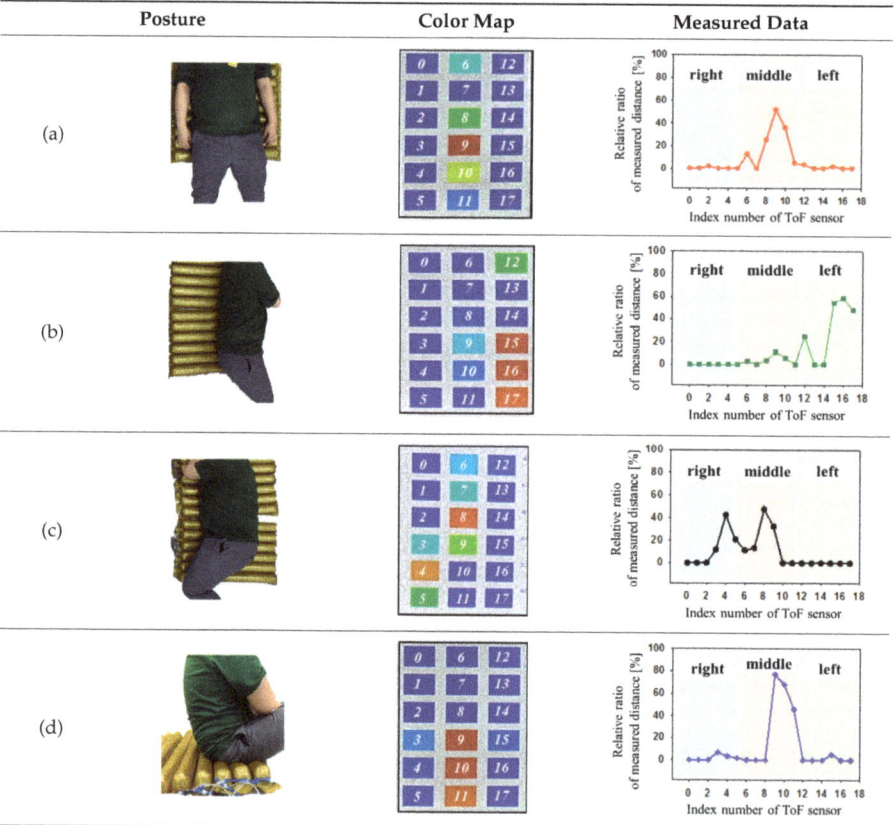

The pressure relieving effect was confirmed by investigating the interface pressure with commercial equipment X3Pro when a participant was taking a supine posture on the air-filled cells. In Figure 10, the changes in interface pressure without any flow control, with a passive air-flow control, and an active control mechanism were investigated, respectively, when the third one of air cells (square dashed line) is inflated and deflated. The pressure distribution was captured in 50 seconds. The red color represents the pressure level over than 32 mmHg. This value is the critical pressure level as a criterion for the occurrence of a pressure ulcer [28,29]. Figure 11a shows the changes of the average pressure in a length of air cell over time at different air-flow controls. In Figure 11b, the peak pressure values at ToF sensor position (circle dashed line) were compared (1) without any flow control, (2) with a passive air-flow control, and (3) an active flow control after 50 seconds. Without any air-flow control in Figure 10a, the surface area in the dashed line had an average pressure of 34.3 mmHg and peak pressure of 45 mmHg, which means that the pressure level may lead to the presence of pressure ulcer. In a passive air-flow control of Figure 10b, which equals to the D_{on} of 50%, the interface pressure decreased to the average of 26.2 mmHg and peak pressure of 32.4 mmHg after 50 seconds. When air flow was actively regulated in response to the pressure level in Figure 10c, the interface pressure was reduced to an average of 20.3 mmHg and peak pressure of 8.4 mmHg. Here, a white spot in the center of Figure 10c means the pressure level of zero. Also, it is showing a rapid decrease of pressure compared with passive air-flow control. Consequently, the ability of the active controlled mattress was to achieve a more even and lower distribution of stress regions across the body. Therefore, the system successfully performed the active pressure relieving mechanism, maintaining the interface pressure at a low enough level to prevent the pressure ulcer.

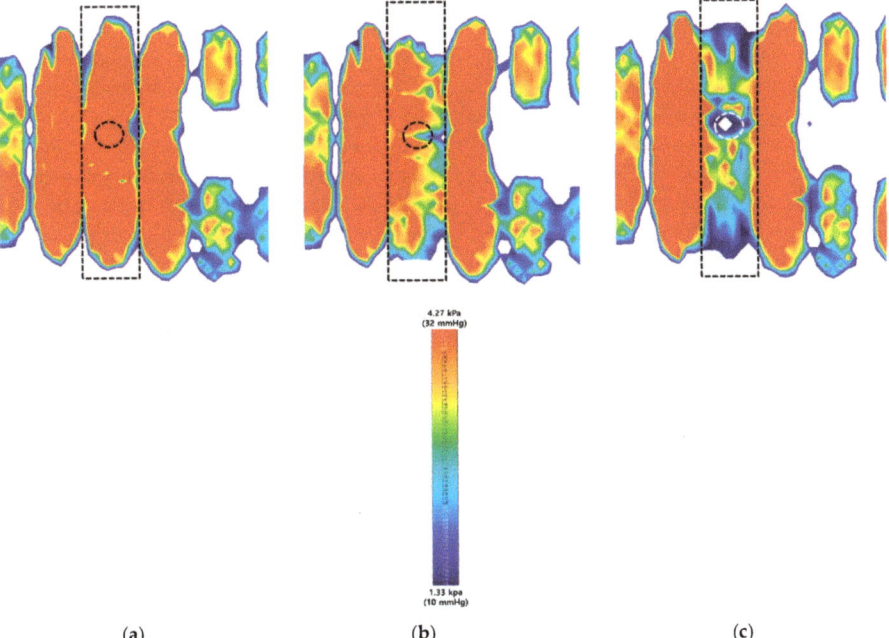

Figure 10. Description of changes in interface pressure, (**a**) without any air-flow control, (**b**) with a passive air-flow control, and (**c**) with an active air-flow control. These colors were visualized by commercial equipment of X3Pro.

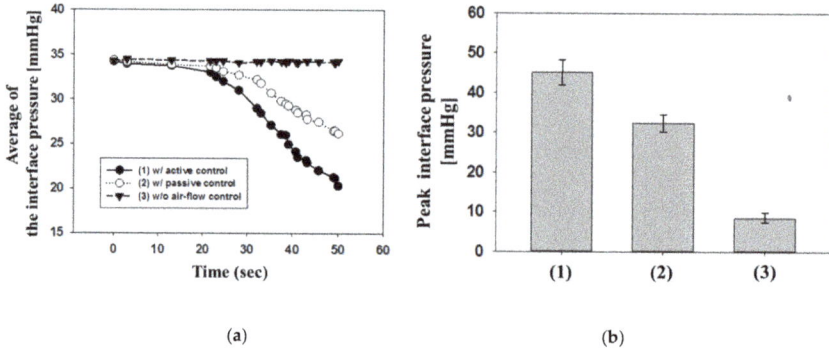

Figure 11. (a) The changes of the average pressure in a length of air cell over time and (b) peak pressure values at ToF sensor position at different air-flow controls of (1) without any air-flow control, (2) with a passive air-flow control, and (3) with an active air-flow control.

4. Conclusions

In this study, an active body pressure relief system was developed to prevent pressure ulcer. The system is an alternating pressure air mattress with adaptive control of air flow in response to the pressure level. The system continuously quantifies the body pressure distribution by indirectly measuring the interface pressure with the ToF optical pressure sensor. This optical sensor is placed on the bottom surface of the air-filled cell. Non-contact characteristic of optical sensor contributes to improved durability and repeatability. Our system can effectively reduce the pressure stress through active control mechanism based on the negative feedback loop. If the interface pressure is higher, the body supporting air-filled cell is more deflated, then the pressure decreases again. It was demonstrated that the system successfully quantified the body pressure distribution at different postures. We could recognize the bones and bump regions of the body, although the prototype measured pressures in discrete regions. It was verified that the pressure relief mechanism performed well keeping the interface pressure low enough to prevent the pressure ulcer. In further work, we will arrange an array of air cells with high resolution expecting a fully relief of high pressure. The system can be potentially used for various bedding applications for measuring the body pressure distribution and relieving the pressure stress.

Author Contributions: K.-H.L. and Y.-E.K. carried out the experiment, analyzed data, validated the concept and wrote the manuscript. S.-W.K. and D.L. conceived the idea, designed the experiment and revised the manuscript. H.L., Y.L., J.S. and O.K. carried out the experiment and analyzed data. All authors provided feedback and discussion of experimental results. Authorship must be limited to those who have contributed substantially to the work reported.

Acknowledgments: This research was partially supported by the Global Excellent Technology Innovation funded by the Ministry of Trade, Industry & Energy(MOTIE, Korea)(10076839) and by a grant(2019-MOIS32-028) of Disaster-Safety Industry Promotion Program funded by Ministry of Interior and Safety(MOIS, Korea). In addition, this research was partially supported by NK217F projects of Korea Institute of Machinery and Materials (KIMM).

Conflicts of Interest: The authors declare no conflict of interest.

References

1. Moysidis, T.; Niebel, W.; Bartsch, K.; Maier, I.; Lehmann, N.; Nonnemacher, M.; Kroeger, K. Prevention of pressure ulcer: Interaction of body characteristics and different mattresses. *Int. Wound J.* **2011**, *8*, 578–584. [CrossRef]
2. Grey, J.E.; Enoch, S.; Harding, K.G. Pressure ulcers. *BMJ* **2006**, *332*, 472–475. [CrossRef]
3. Reddy, M.; Gill, S.S.; Kalkar, S.R.; Wu, W.; Anderson, P.J.; Rochon, P.A. Treatment of pressure ulcers: A systematic review. *JAMA* **2008**, *300*, 2647–2662. [CrossRef]

4. Attard, J.; Rithalia, S.V.S.; Kulkarni, J. Pressure relief characteristics in alternating pressure air cushions. *Prosthet. Orthot. Int.* **1997**, *21*, 229–233.
5. Rithalia, S.V.S.; Gonsalkorale, M. Quantification of pressure relief using interface pressure and tissue perfusion in alternating pressure air mattresses. *Arch. Phys. Med. Rehabil.* **2000**, *81*, 1364–1369. [CrossRef]
6. Vanderwee, K.; Grypdonck, M.H.F.; Defloor, T. Effectiveness of an alternating pressure air mattress for the prevention of pressure ulcers. *Age Ageing* **2005**, *34*, 261–267. [CrossRef]
7. Vanderwee, K.; Grypdonck, M.; Defloor, T. Alternating pressure air mattresses as prevention for pressure ulcers: A literature review. *Int. J. Nurs. Stud.* **2008**, *45*, 784–801. [CrossRef]
8. Goossens, R.H.M.; Rithalia, S.V.S. Physiological response of the heel tissue on pressure relief between three alternating pressure air mattresses. *J. Tissue Viability* **2007**, *17*, 10–14. [CrossRef]
9. X. Technology. Pressure Sensors. Available online: https://xsensor.com/sensors (accessed on 4 August 2019).
10. Higer, S.; James, T. Interface pressure mapping pilot study to select surfaces that effectively redistribute pediatric occipital pressure. *J. Tissue Viability* **2016**, *25*, 41–49. [CrossRef]
11. Tekscan. Body Pressure Measurement System. Available online: http://www.tekscan.com (accessed on 4 August 2019).
12. Chang, W.; Chen, C.; Chang, C.; Yang, C. An enhanced sensing application based on a flexible projected capacitive-sensing mattress. *Sensors* **2014**, *14*, 6922–6937. [CrossRef]
13. Zhao, S.; Wang, W.; Guo, W.; Zhang, C. A human body pressure distribution imaging system based on wavelet analysis and resistance tomography. *Sensors* **2017**, *17*, 2634. [CrossRef]
14. Ashruf, C.M.A. Thin flexible pressure sensors. *Sens. Rev.* **2002**, *22*, 322–327. [CrossRef]
15. Gyi, D.E.; Porter, J.M.; Robertson, N.K. Seat pressure measurement technologies: Considerations for their evaluation. *Appl. Ergon.* **1998**, *27*, 85–91. [CrossRef]
16. Treaster, D.; Marras, W.S. Measurement of seat pressure distributions. *Hum. Factors* **1987**, *29*, 563–575. [CrossRef]
17. Cusano, A.; Cutolo, A.; Albert, J. Polymer Fiber Bragg Gratings. In *Fiber Bragg Grating Sensors: Recent Advancements, Industrial Applications and Market Exploitation*; Bentham Science Publishers: Potomac, MD, USA, 2009.
18. Webb, D.J. Fibre Bragg grating sensors in polymer optical fibres. *Meas. Sci. Technol.* **2015**, *26*, 092004. [CrossRef]
19. Neeharika, V.; Pattnaik, P.K. Optical MEMS pressure sensors incorporating dual waveguide bragg gratings on diaphragms. *IEEE Sens. J.* **2016**, *16*, 681–687. [CrossRef]
20. Vilarinho, D.; Theodosiou, A.; Leitao, C.; Leal, A.G.; Domingues, M.D.F.; Kalli, K.; Andre, P.; Antunes, P.; Marques, C. POFBG-embedded cork insole for plantar pressure monitoring. *Sensors* **2017**, *17*, 2924. [CrossRef]
21. Wiley, W.C.; Mclaren, I.H. Time-of-Flight mass spectrometer with improved resolution. *Rev. Sci. Instrum.* **1955**, *26*, 1150–1157. [CrossRef]
22. Lee, H.; Park, S. Quantitative effects of mattress types (comfortable vs. uncomfortable) on sleep quality through polysomnography and skin temperature. *Int. J. Ind. Ergon.* **2006**, *36*, 943–949. [CrossRef]
23. Wu, J.; Yuan, H.; Li, X. A novel method for comfort assessment in a supine sleep position using three-dimensional scanning technology. *Int. J. Ind. Ergon.* **2018**, *67*, 104–113. [CrossRef]
24. Holtz, J. Pulsewidth modulation for electronic power conversion. *Proc. IEEE* **1994**, *82*, 1194–1214. [CrossRef]
25. Lee, W.; Hong, S.; Oh, H. Characterization of elastic polymer-based smart insole and a simple foot plantar pressure visualization method using 16 electrodes. *Sensors* **2019**, *19*, 44. [CrossRef]
26. Marais, H. RS-485/RS-422 Circuit Implementation Guide. Available online: https://atnel.pl/download/poradniki/rs485/AN-960.pdf (accessed on 4 August 2019).
27. Vaughan, N.D.; Gamble, J.B. The modeling and simulation of a proportional solenoid valve. *J. Dyn. Syst. Meas. Control* **1996**, *118*, 120–125. [CrossRef]
28. Patterson, R.P.; Fisher, S.V. Sitting pressure-time patterns in patients with quadriplegia. *Phys. Med. Rehabil.* **1986**, *67*, 812–814.
29. Wytch, R.; Neil, G.; Kalisse, C. Skin orthosis interface pressure transducers: a review. *Care Sci. Pract.* **1989**, *7*, 100–104.

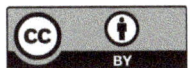

© 2019 by the authors. Licensee MDPI, Basel, Switzerland. This article is an open access article distributed under the terms and conditions of the Creative Commons Attribution (CC BY) license (http://creativecommons.org/licenses/by/4.0/).

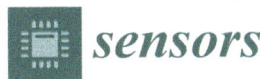

Article

In Vivo Measurement of Cervical Elasticity on Pregnant Women by Torsional Wave Technique: A Preliminary Study

Paloma Massó [1,2]**, Antonio Callejas** [1,3]**, Juan Melchor** [1,3,4,]*****, Francisca S. Molina** [1,2] **and Guillermo Rus** [1,3,4]

1. Instituto de Investigación Biosanitaria, ibs.GRANADA, 18012 Granada, Spain
2. San Cecilio University Hospital, 18016 Granada, Spain
3. Department of Structural Mechanics, University of Granada, 18071 Granada, Spain
4. Excellence Research Unit, "Modelling Nature" (MNat), University of Granada, 18071 Granada, Spain
* Correspondence: jmelchor@ugr.es

Received: 4 June 2019; Accepted: 22 July 2019; Published: 24 July 2019

Abstract: A torsional wave (TW) sensor prototype was employed to quantify stiffness of the cervix in pregnant women. A cross-sectional study in a total of 18 women between 16 weeks and 35 weeks + 5 days of gestation was performed. The potential of TW technique to assess cervical ripening was evaluated by the measurement of stiffness related to gestational age and cervical length. Statistically significant correlations were found between cervical stiffness and gestational age ($R^2 = 0.370$, $p = 0.0074$, using 1 kHz waves and $R^2 = 0.445$, $p = 0.0250$, using 1.5 kHz waves). A uniform decrease in stiffness of the cervical tissue was confirmed to happen during the complete gestation. There was no significant correlation between stiffness and cervical length. A stronger association between gestational age and cervical stiffness was found compared to gestational age and cervical length correlation. As a conclusion, TW technique is a feasible approach to objectively quantify the decrease of cervical stiffness related to gestational age. Further research is required to evaluate the application of TW technique in obstetric evaluations, such as prediction of preterm delivery and labor induction failure.

Keywords: torsional wave; cervix; pregnancy; cervical stiffness

1. Introduction

Approximately, 15 million babies are born preterm (before 37 weeks of gestation) per year, i.e., more than 1 in 10 newborns, and this number is rising in both developing countries and Europe [1,2]. Worldwide, complications of preterm birth are the main cause of child mortality under five years of age [1,3]. Prematurity often leads to long-term disabilities such as learning, visual and hearing problems. Clinical and social risk factors of preterm birth have been identified to develop feasible and cost-effective care measures to save children [1]. Nonetheless, a high proportion of spontaneous preterm birth remains unpredictable.

Current models based on cervical length, obstetric history, digital vaginal examination and echography of the cervix are not able to accurately predict a preterm birth with sufficient anticipation, and there is a lack of evidence on how to prevent preterm delivery [4,5]. Even though there is an agreement that cervical ripening plays a fundamental role during pregnancy, histological changes and biomechanical properties of the cervix are not entirely characterized. The current lack of a clinical tool for the quantitative evaluation of the biomechanic parameters of the cervix is probably a barrier to advance in preventing spontaneous preterm birth [6]. Since 2012, the WHO is encouraging to accelerate research into the causality of preterm birth, and to test effective approaches that would lead to save babies. Recently, elastography techniques are being put forward in the literature to assess quantitatively the stiffness of the cervix as a promising tool to estimate preterm birth risk, as well as to predict the success of labor induction [7–12].

Quasi-static elastography methods have been used to evaluate the cervical stiffness at different gestational ages. The result is a qualitative deformation gradient map, called elastogram. However, all methods have shown unclear results regarding reproducibility and associations between stiffness and gestational age [13–16]. The measurements are also liable to the sensor pressure applied by the clinician, which is not accounted for.

In contrast, dynamic elastography techniques have the strength to provide the absolute quantitative values of stiffness as an objective criterion to evaluate the process of cervical ripening [17,18]. This technology relies on shear ultrasonic waves that travel through the soft tissue. The measurement of the shear wave propagation speed allows characterizing shear stiffness. The commercially available dynamic Supersonic Shear Imaging (SSI) technique employs ultrasonics radiation force to generate shear waves. Shear wave speed in cervix was statistically significant lower in women delivered preterm and inpatients with preterm uterine dynamics compared to women delivered at term [12]. Peralta et al. [19] evaluated SSI elastography to quantify cervical stiffness in real time and its evolution in induced labor in ewes, concluding that stiffness decreases during maturation in induced labor. The Acoustic Radiation Force Imaging (ARFI) is based on displacements generated by an ultrasound beam using the same imaging probe. ARFI has already been proved to evaluate differences in mature versus immature cervical tissue ex vivo [20] and in vivo in pre- and post-labor induction [21]. Both studies agree that shear waves speeds are statistically significantly different in mature versus immature cervical tissue. Viscoelasticity maps of uterine corpus and cervix were assessed thought magnetic resonance elatography in nonpregnant women [22]. Results show a higher elasticity in uterine corpus, and similar viscosity compared with cervix.

The presented measurements data are taken using an alternative dynamic technique: torsional wave (TW) technique [23]. This is based on the propagation of shear waves through the tissue not only in depth but also radially, which makes the technique suitable for applications such as cervical tissue. Axis-symmetric waves allows the precise interrogation of soft tissue mechanical functionality in cylindrical geometries, which are challenged by current elastography approaches in small organs.

This work was aimed at evaluating the reliability and feasibility of TW technique to provide consistent data on the changes of the cervical stiffness during pregnancy. Eighteen singleton-pregnant women were recruited. The hypothesis were: (1) torsional wave technique has the capacity to quantify cervical stiffness defined by its elastic modulus; and (2) stiffness decreases along pregnancy. The second hypothesis stems from the fact that the cervical tissue behavior depends on changes in its multi-scale structure from a mechanical point of view. The cervical stroma microstructure is formed of cross-linked mesh of collagen immersed into viscous proteoglycan [24]. These biochemical compounds exist on different scales whose length is variable by several orders of magnitude. They provide a tractive and compressive strength to the cervical tissue. Despite the fact that cervical architecture changes during ripening [25], these modifications along pregnancy are still not well studied.

2. Materials and Methods

2.1. Design of the Study

A cross-sectional study in healthy pregnant women was performed to assess stiffness modifications in cervix.

2.2. Healthcare Settings

The pre-pilot test study was carried out at San Cecilio University Hospital in Granada. The data were analyzed in the Ultrasonics Laboratory in the University of Granada.

2.3. Ethical Issues

The study met the principles of the Declaration of Helsinki. Approvals of the Ethical Committee in Human Research of University of Granada and Ethical Commission and Health Research of San Cecilio University Hospital in Granada were achieved.

2.4. Subjects

Eighteen healthy women were recruited from their routine medical visits during pregnancy, and TW technique explorations were performed in the Fetal Medicine Unit. The entire population of women in the study had pregnancies without any complication with a median of 26.4 (16 weeks to 35 weeks + 5 days) gestation weeks, and there was no twin pregnancy. A statistical power analysis was designed to estimate the size of the population. A multivariate continuous regression with a power of 80%, estimated significance in a two-tail distribution, and a recommended effect size ES = 0.30, yielded a sample size of 17 subjects. Exclusion criteria were multiple pregnancies, previous cervical surgeries and patients with information relative to malignant changes in the cervical tissue. All women enrolled in the evaluation provided agreement by signing a written consent and reading the information of the patient report.

For the exploration with TW technique, the participants emptied their bladder before the exploration and then were placed in the dorsal lithotomy position. The intravaginal device was allocated in contact with the cervical internal OS (see Figure 1). The measurements of cervical length were obtained by a transvaginal sonography probe, which was directed in the anterior fornix. A sagital view was obtained. Three TW technique and cervical length measurements per women were performed.

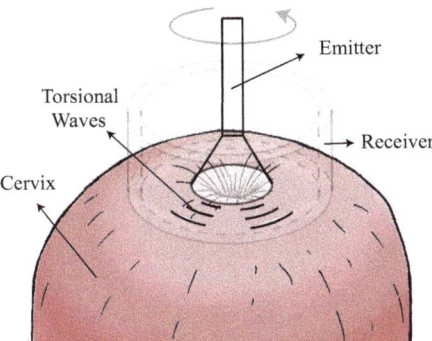

Figure 1. Schematic diagram for the exploration with TW technique.

2.5. Torsional Wave Technique

Elastography quantification was achieved by the TW probe [26–28], which generated waves under safe threshold of energies. The device consisted in three parts: a torsional wave sensor (probe), an electronic system for generating and receiving the signal, and an interface software (Figure 2).

The probe was manufactured in 2017 and was composed of: (1) an electromechanical actuator which deleted electronic cross-talk [23]; (2) a receiver based on two polylactic acid rings where the piezoelectric elements were fitted; and (3) a case to contain the emitter and the receiver. The shear modulus was obtained assuming an elastic and incompressible medium by the following equation,

$$\mu = \rho c_s^2 \qquad (1)$$

where ρ is the density of the medium and c_s is the torsional wave velocity, which is based on shear wave group velocity.

The excitation signal was a burst composed of a one-cycle frequency f ranging from 0.5 to 1.5 kHz with 10× averaging. The frequencies were chosen according to the results obtained in the work carried out by Callejas et al. [23].

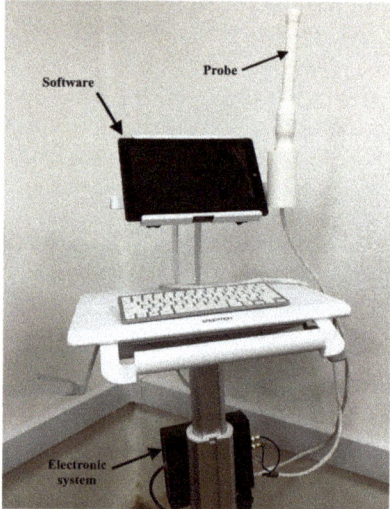

Figure 2. The prototyped TW probe.

An example of three different emitted and received signals is shown in Figure 3. The shear wave group velocity calculation algorithm was based on dividing the distance by the torsional wave time-of-flight. The signals were preprocessed by a low-pass filter close to the central frequency of the received signal. The time of flight was computed using three procedures: (1) searching the first time the signal raises 30% above zero; (2) subtracting a quarter of the period (inverse of the received signal central frequency) from the first peak; and (3) subtracting three quarters of the period (inverse of the received signal central frequency) from the second peak. All three methods provided similar estimates of the velocity, as shown in the results.

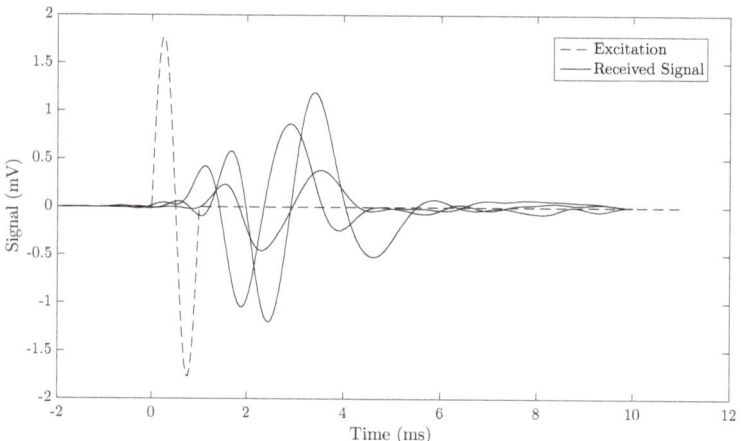

Figure 3. Example of three emitted and received 1 kHz signals.

Safety Considerations

A new medical diagnostic equipment needs to follow the specifications described in the Food and Drug Administration (FDA) guidelines [29] for the application in clinical practice. It is necessary that the Torsional Wave technique be safe for humans. There are three parameters that should be evaluated according to the acoustic output in the use of Fetal Imaging and Other (FDA): the mechanical index ($MI < 1.9$), the spatial peak pulse average intensity ($ISPPA < 190$ W/cm^2), and the spatial peak temporal average intensity ($ISPTA < 94$ mW/cm^2). The calculation of these parameters was made as follows:

$$MI = PRP/\sqrt{F_c} \quad (2)$$

where PRP is the peak rarefractional pressure of the torsional wave in (MPa) and Fc is the center frequency (MHz).

$$ISPPA = P_0^2/(2 * \rho * c) \quad (3)$$

where P_0 is the maximal acoustic pressure generated by the electromechanical actuator, ρ is the density of the medium, and c is the sound speed in the medium.

$$ISPTA = ISPPA * \Delta t/1 \quad (4)$$

where Δt is the excitation pulse duration.

The three parameters were experimentally estimated. The excitation signal used was a low-frequency ultrasonic sine-burst at a central frequency of 1 kHz, consisting of one cycle of 1 ms and 16 Vpp amplitude. This excitation signal was generated by a wave generator (Agilent 33220A, Santa Clara, CA, USA). The response signal was registered using a decibel sensor (YH-610 Environment Multimeter). The signal traveled through a water layer before arriving to the decibel sensor and different distances from 5 cm to 0 cm. To convert the pressure recorded by the decibel sensor into water acoustic pressure, the equation that relates the impedances of the two media (air–water) was used:

$$T = \frac{2 * Z_{air}}{(Z_{air} + Z_{water})^2} \quad (5)$$

where T is the transmission coefficient and Z_{air} and Z_{water} are the acoustic impedance of the air and water, respectively.

2.6. Statistic Analysis

The evolution of cervical stiffness tissue during pregnancy was quantified. Normal distribution of the data was checked for each velocity calculation algorithm by the normal quantile–quantile plot (Q–Q plot) and the Shapiro–Wilk test. The mean values for each velocity calculation procedure were compared to the normal distribution of these values. The coefficient of determination (R^2) for linear regression analysis was calculated to provide the correlations: (a) between gestational age and cervical velocity (c_s) using 0.5, 1 and 1.5 kHz torsional waves, for the three velocity calculation algorithms; (b) between gestational age and cervical length; and (c) between stiffness and cervical length. Data were analyzed using the MATLAB (Release 2014b Mathworks, Natick, MA, USA). T-test was calculated to estimate p-values. A statistically significance for $p < 0.05$ was assumed.

3. Results

The experimental results obtained to evaluate the three security parameters according to the Food and Drug Administration guidelines were as follows.

The maximum pressure registered after converting the pressure recorded by the decibel sensor into water acoustic pressure was 3.99×10^{-5} MPa. The maximal acoustic pressure and the peak rarefractional pressure of the torsional wave in water was $P_0 = 3.99 \times 10^{-4}$ bars. The three previous parameters were obtained with the cited experimental conditions:

$$MI = 0.0013 < 1.9 \tag{6}$$

$$ISPPA = P_0^2/(2*\rho*c) = 5.3 \text{ W/cm}^2 < 190 \text{ W/cm}^2 \tag{7}$$

considering the density of the medium $\rho = 1000 \text{ kg/m}^3$, and the sound speed in the medium 1500 m/s.

$$ISPTA = ISPPA * \Delta t/1 = 5.3 \text{ mW/cm}^2 < 94 \text{ mW/cm}^2 \tag{8}$$

A normal distribution for the three velocity calculation procedures was found through Q–Q test (Figure 4) and Shapiro–Wilk test. The obstetric characteristics of the population in the study are shown in Table 1.

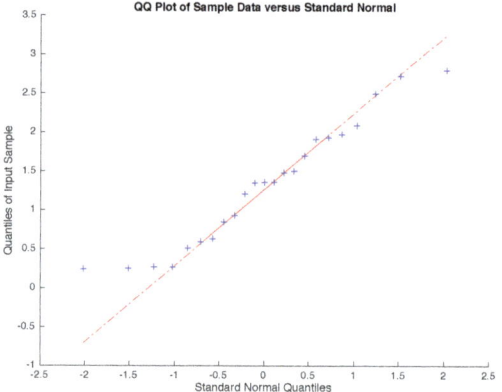

(a) The first velocity calculation procedure

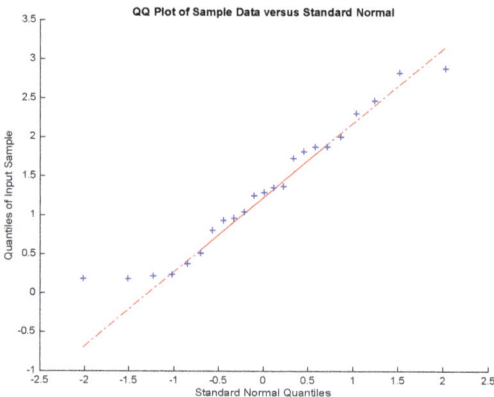

(b) The second velocity calculation procedure

Figure 4. Cont.

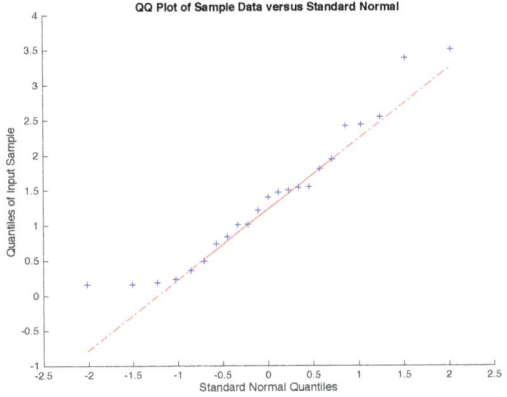

(c) The third velocity calculation procedure

Figure 4. Normal quantile–quantile plots for the three velocity calculation procedures.

Table 1. Features of the population in the study.

Characteristics	Value
Total population (N)	18
Gestational age at test (weeks)	26.4 (16 weeks to 35 weeks + 5 days)
Nulliparous (N)	2 (11 %)
Cervical length (mm)	33 (10–49)

Three measurements of TW stiffness and cervical length per subject were determined from all women. Box plots of these data observed in each patient were calculated and a linear regression was fitted with 80% confidence intervals (see Figure 5). In this work, the three frequencies were used to study the effect of attenuation on the cervical tissue. The selected frequency configuration was 1 kHz, which was the optimal measure to yield the highest amplitude signals, the best shear wave speed reconstructions and a significant correlation with gestational age. In some measurements, frequencies ≥ 1.5 kHz, yielded amplitudes of signal similar to the amplitude of noise probably due to attenuation, and consequently anomalous values of the cervical stiffness were obtained. In contrast, the noise masked the amplitude of the signal in some data with frequencies ≤ 0.5 kHz. All missing data were due to signal noise.

The decrease of the stiffness was computed from the data in Figure 5 using Equation (1). The error bars are estimated from the three velocity estimation algorithms described in the methods. The three overlapping regressions (continuous and dashed lines in Figures 5–7) correspond to each velocity estimation algorithms.

Similar correlations are shown in Figures 6 and 7 for 1.5 kHz and 0.5 kHz, respectively, where some of the measurements were rejected due to noise in the signal. A stronger association between gestational age and cervical stiffness was found ($R^2 = 0.370$, $p = 0.0074$, Figure 5) compared to gestational age and cervical length correlation ($R^2 = 0.025$, $p = 0.6043$, Figure 8).

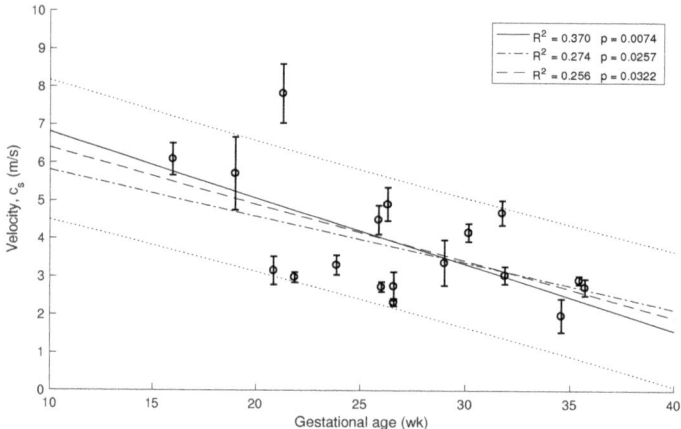

Figure 5. Relationship between cervical stiffness assessed by shear wave speed using 1 kHz waves and gestational age at time of examination.

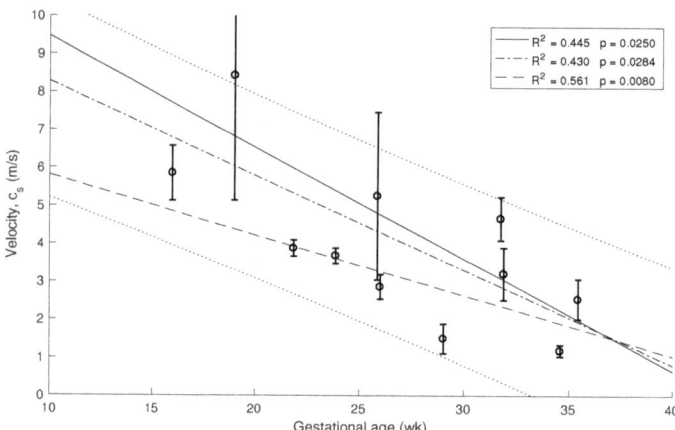

Figure 6. Relationship between cervical stiffness assessed by shear wave speed using 1.5 kHz waves and gestational age at time of examination.

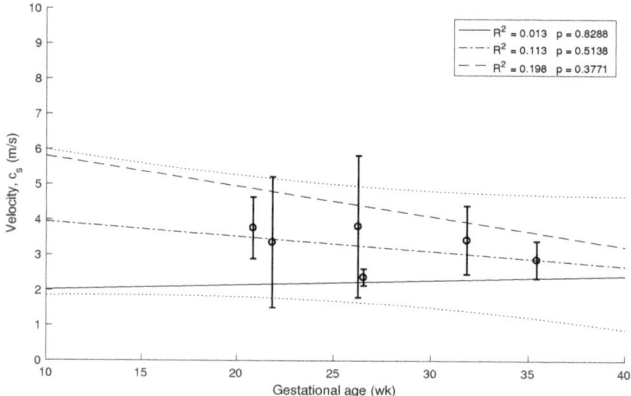

Figure 7. Relationship between cervical stiffness assessed by shear wave speed using 0.5 kHz waves and gestational age at time of examination.

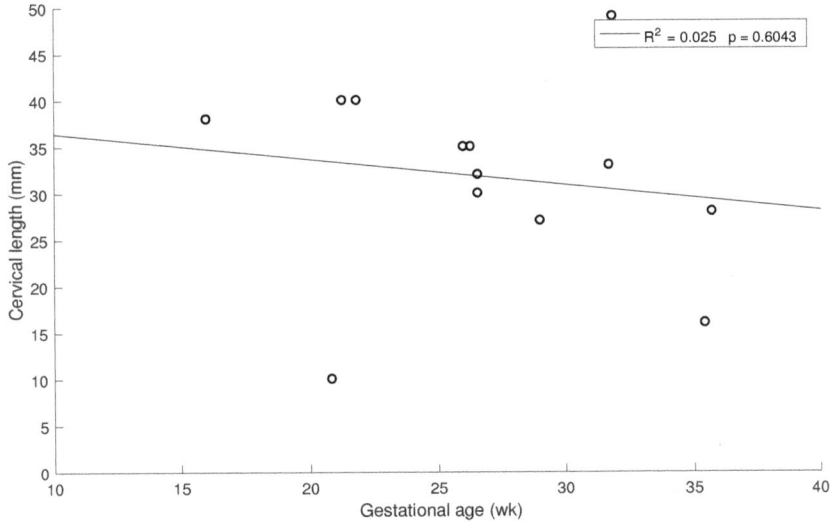

Figure 8. Relationship between cervical length and gestational age at time of examination.

No high associations ($R^2 < 0.5$ for all cases) and no significant correlation ($p > 0.05$) were obtained between stiffness and cervical length (Figure 9).

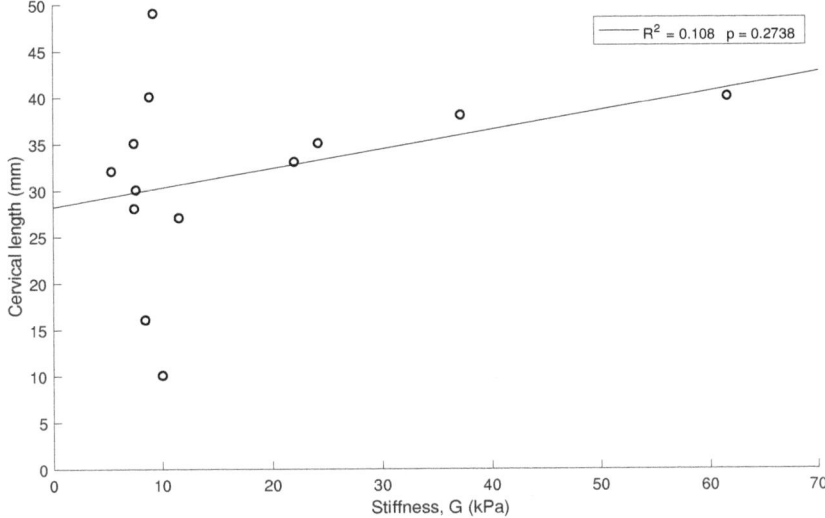

Figure 9. Relationship between cervical stiffness and cervical length.

4. Discussion

This study focused on assessing the feasibility of torsional wave technique to quantify the changes in cervical stiffness during pregnancy, which were measured by shear wave speed. The presented results show, for the first time in vivo, the viability of torsional waves to objectively measure cervical elasticity in pregnant women. The observed data therefore support Hypothesis 1 that torsional wave technique has the capacity to quantify cervical stiffness defined by its elastic modulus.

The presented observations also support Hypothesis 2 that shear stiffness decreases during pregnancy. Cervical stiffness was shown to significantly decrease with gestational age, which is compatible with observations by former researchers that assessed cervical ripening by different techniques [8,30–32]. A gradual reduction from about 40 kPa at the beginning of pregnancy to close to zero at delivery was obtained in the study carried out by Peralta et al. [30]. A correction due to the difference of range of shear wave frequencies of ARFI was considered, about a higher order of magnitude, which affect the apparent stiffness given the viscoelastic behaviour of cervical tissue. Thus, cervical ripening is directly related to the time to delivery. Correlation between cervical stiffness and gestational age assessed by TW technique showed a higher correlation to gestational aged compared to quantification through shear wave speed (SSI) ($R^2 = 0.37$ vs. $R^2 = 0.29$) [12].

A weaker correlation was found between cervical stiffness and cervical length than with gestational age, which is compatible with previous studies [11,30], using dynamic and quasi-static elastography, respectively, but contrary to observations by Hernandez-Andrade et al. [16], who found that associations between cervical tissue strain and cervical length was higher than with gestational age. This inconsistency feeds a debate, which could be at least partially explained by the inherent limitations of the commercially available quasi-static elastography technologies [14–17], as this technique provides a qualitative estimation of the cervical stiffness through an indirect measurement.

The experiment results support that TW technique is safe to be used in pregnant women. All the values obtained were far below the thresholds according to the Food and Drug Administration (FDA) guidelines reference parameters in Fetal Imaging and Other. The mechanical index (MI) was 0.0013 (<1.9), the spatial peak pulse average intensity ($ISPPA$) was 5.3 W/cm^2 (<190 W/cm^2), and the spatial peak temporal average intensity ($ISPTA$) was 5.3 mW/cm^2 (<94 mW/cm^2).

The limitations of this research are linked to the nature of propagation of torsional wave in cervical tissue as well as its complex microarchitecture. Some mechanical hypotheses have been raised in the literature about the hystologic features of the cervix to estimate the shear stiffness elasticity, assuming homogeneous, non viscous, isotropic and semi-infinite medium [20,33–36]. The equation employed in this study to estimate the cervix stiffness is only based on shear wave group velocity. However, the behavior of cervical tissue is dispersive, that is, the higher are the shear wave frequencies, the higher are the shear waves speeds and, therefore, phase–velocity-based techniques would lead to a direct calculation of shear modulus. The time-of-tflight technique measured the shear wave group velocity, which is dependent on the envelope of the propagating elastic wave.

Finally, due to the exploratory nature of this study about the feasibility of torsional wave technique to assess cervical maturation, a small population of patients was recruited. To extend the validity and reliability of the proposed technology, larger complementary studies are needed. The protocol of measurements by TW technique will be enhanced by applying the optimal contact conditions between the probe and the cervix [37]. We are positive that torsional waves are a tool with potential to objectively diagnose early cervical ripening disorders and preterm birth.

5. Conclusions

The presented experimental observations prove that, firstly, cervical stiffness was a valuable predictor variable of gestational age at the moment of evaluation. Secondly, TW technique is a tool that allows quantifying cervical shear stiffness during pregnancy. Finally, this technique is safe to be used in pregnant women.

TW technique might provide clinically relevant data on the cervical ripening in addition to that obtained from digital exploration and standard sonography. Further research is required to assess the TW technique feasibility in obstetric evaluations, such as probabilistic inverse problems based on viscoelastic models for the prediction of preterm delivery and labor induction failure.

Author Contributions: P.M., A.C., J.M. and G.R. conceived and designed the study. P.M., F.S.M. and G.R. performed the measurements. P.M., A.C., J.M. and G.R. analyzed the data and wrote the paper.

Funding: This research was funded by the Ministry of Education grant numbers DPI2017-83859-R, DPI2014-51870-R and UNGR15-CE-3664, Ministry of Health grant numbers DTS15/00093 and PI16/00339, and Junta de Andalucía grant numbers, PI-0107-2017 and PIN-0030-2017.

Acknowledgments: We thank the Department of Electronics and Computer Technology for assistance with the electronic system of the torsional wave sensor.

Conflicts of Interest: Massó has nothing to disclose. Molina, Rus, Melchor and Callejas are partners of INNITIUS, a company to develop ultrasonic sensors; they have not receive funding from the company for the submitted work.

Abbreviations

The following abbreviations are used in this manuscript:

TW	Torsional Wave
WHO	World Health Organization
ARFI	Acoustic Radiation Force Imaging
SSI	Supersonic Shear Imaging
PLA	Polylactic Acid
Internal OS	Internal Orifice of the Cervix
ES	Effect size

References

1. WHO. *March of Dimes, The Partnership for Maternal, Newborn & Child Health, and Save the Children 2012*; Born too Soon: The global Action Report on Preterm Birth; *Magn. Reson. Med.*; Howson, C.P., Kinney, M.V., Lawn, J.E., Eds.; WHO: Geneva, Switzerland, 2012.
2. Zeitlin, J.; Szamotulska, K.; Drewniak, N.; Mohangoo, A.D.; Chalmers, J.; Sakkeus, L.; Irgens, L.; Gatt, M.; Gissler, M.; Blondel, B.; et al. Wideband MR elastography for viscoelasticity model identification. *BJOG Int. J. Obstet. Gynecol.* **2013**, *120*, 1356–1365. [CrossRef] [PubMed]
3. WHO. *Fact Sheet—Preterm Birth*; *Magn. Reson. Med.*; WHO: Geneva, Switzerland, 2016.
4. Sananes, N.; Langer, B.; Gaudineau, A.; Kutnahorsky, R.; Aissi, G.; Fritz, G.; Boudier, E.; Viville, B.; Nisand, I.; Favre, R. Prediction of spontaneous preterm delivery in singleton pregnancies: where are we and where are we going? A review of literature. *J. Obstet. Gynaecol.* **2014**, *34*, 457–461. [CrossRef] [PubMed]
5. Ross, M.G.; Beall, M.H. Prediction of preterm birth: Nonsonographic cervical methods. *Semin. Perinatol.* **2009**, *33*, 312–316. [CrossRef] [PubMed]
6. Feltovich, H.; Hall, T.J.; Berghella, V. Beyond cervical length: Emerging technologies for assessing the pregnant cervix. *Am. J. Obstet. Gynecol.* **2012**, *207*, 345–354. [CrossRef]
7. Khalil, M.R.; Thorsen, P.; Uldbjerg, N. Cervical ultrasound elastography may hold potential to predict risk of preterm birth. *Ultrasound Obstet. Gynecol.* **2013**, *60*, A4570.
8. K'obbing, K.; Fruscalzo, A.; Hammer, K.; M'ollers, M.; Falkenberg, M.; Kwiecien, R.; Klockenbusch, W.; Schmitz, R. Quantitative elastography of the uterine cervix as a predictor of preterm delivery. *J. Perinatol.* **2014**, *34*, 774. [CrossRef]
9. Swiatkowska-Freund, M.; Preis, K. Elastography of the uterine cervix: Implications for success of induction of labor. *Ultrasound Obstet. Gynecol.* **2011**, *38*, 52–56. [CrossRef]
10. Pereira, S.; Frick, A.P.; Poon, L.C.; Zamprakou, A.; Nicolaides, K.H. Successful induction of labor: Prediction by pre-induction cervical length, angle of progression and cervical elastography. *Ultrasound Obstet. Gynecol.* **2014**, *44*, 468–475. [CrossRef]
11. Wozniak, S.; Czuczwar, P.; Szkodziak, P.; Milart, P.; Wozniakowska, E.; Paszkowski, T. Elastography in predicting preterm delivery in asymptomatic, low-risk women: A prospective observational study. *BMC Pregnancy Childbirth* **2014**, *14*, 238. [CrossRef]
12. Muller, M.; Aït-Belkacem, D.; Hessabi, M.; Gennisson, J.L.; Grangé, G.; Goffinet, F.; Lecarpentier, E.; Cabrol, D.; Tanter, M.; Tsatsaris, V. Assessment of the cervix in pregnant women using shear wave elastography: A feasibility study. *Ultrasound Med. Biol.* **2015**, *41*, 2789–2797. [CrossRef]

13. Thomas, A.; Kummel, S.; Gemeinhardt, O.; Fischer, T. Real-time sonoelastography of the cervix: Tissue elasticity of the normal and abnormal cervix. *Acad. Radiol.* **2007**, *14*, 193–200. [CrossRef] [PubMed]
14. Molina, F.S.; Gómez, L.F.; Florido, J.; Padilla, M.C.; Nicolaides, K.H. Quantification of cervical elastography: A reproducibility study. *Ultrasound Obstet. Gynecol.* **2012**, *39*, 685–689. [CrossRef] [PubMed]
15. Fruscalzo, A.; Schmitz, R.; Klockenbusch, W.; Steinhard, J. Reliability of cervix elastography in the late first and second trimester of pregnancy. *Ultraschall Med. Eur. J. Ultrasound* **2012**, *33*, E101–E107. [CrossRef] [PubMed]
16. Hernandez-Andrade, E.; Hassan, S.S.; Ahn, H.; Korzeniewski, S.J.; Yeo, L.; Chaiworapongsa, T.; Romero, R. Evaluation of cervical stiffness during pregnancy using semiquantitative ultrasound elastography. *Ultrasound Obstet. Gynecol.* **2013**, *41*, 152–161. [CrossRef]
17. Feltovich, H.; Hall, T.J. Quantitative imaging of the cervix: Setting the bar. *Ultrasound Obstet. Gynecol.* **2013**, *41*, 121–128. [CrossRef] [PubMed]
18. Bamber, J.; Cosgrove, D.; Dietrich, C.F.; Fromageau, J.; Bojunga, J.; Calliada, F. EFSUMB guidelines and recommendations on the clinical use of ultrasound elastography. Part I: Basic principles and technology. *Ultraschall Med.* **2013**, *34*, 169–184. [CrossRef] [PubMed]
19. Peralta, L.; Mourier, E.; Richard, C.; Chavette-Palmer, P.; Muller, M.; Tanter, M.; Rus, G. 117 in vivo evaluation of the cervical stiffness evolution during indiced labor in ewes using elastohraphy. *Reprod. Fertil. Dev.* **2015**, *27*, 150–151. [CrossRef]
20. Carlson, L.C.; Feltovich, H.; Palmeri, M.L.; Dahl, J.J. Muñoz del Rio, A.; Hall, T.J. Estimation of shear wave speed in the human uterine cervix. *Ultrasound Obstet. Gynecol.* **2014**, *43*, 452–458. [CrossRef]
21. Carlson, L.C.; Romero, S.T.; Palmeri, M.L.; Muñoz del Rio, A.; Esplin, S.M.; Rotemberg, V.M.; Feltovich, H. Changes in shear wave speed pre and post induction of labor: A feasibility study. *Ultrasound Obstet. Gynecol.* **2014**. [CrossRef]
22. Jiang, X.; Asbach, P.; Streitberger, K.J.; Thomas, A.; Hamm, B.; Braun, J.; Sack, I.; Guo, J. In vivo high-resolution magnetic resonance elastography of the uterine corpus and cervix. *Eur. Radiol.* **2014**, *24*, 3025–3033. [CrossRef]
23. Callejas, A.; Gomez, A.; Melchor, J.; Riveiro, M.; Massó, P.; Torres, J.; López-López, M.; Rus, G. Performance study of a torsional wave sensor and cervical tissue characterization. *Sensors* **2017**, *17*, 2078. [CrossRef] [PubMed]
24. House, M.; Kaplan, D.L.; Socrate, S. Relationships between mechanical properties and extracellular matrix constituents of the cervical stroma during pregnancy. *Semin. Perinatol.* **2009**, *33*, 300–307. [CrossRef] [PubMed]
25. Timmons, B.; Akins, M.; Mahendroo, M. Cervical remodeling during pregnancy and parturition. *Trends Endocrinol. Metab.* **2010**, *21*, 353–361. [CrossRef] [PubMed]
26. Melchor, J.; Rus, G. Torsional ultrasonic transducer computational design optimization. *Ultrasonics* **2014**, *54*, 1950–1962. [CrossRef] [PubMed]
27. Melchor, J.; Muñoz, R.; Rus, G. Torsional ultrasound sensor optimization for soft tissue characterization. *Sensors* **2017**, *17*, 1402. [CrossRef] [PubMed]
28. Rus, G.; Muñoz, R.; Melchor, J.; Molina, R.; Callejas, A.; Riveiro, M.; Massó, P.; Torres, J.; Moreu, G.; Molina, F.; et al. Torsion ultrasonic sensor for tissue mechanical characterization. In Proceedings of the 2016 IEEE International Ultrasonics Symposium (IUS), Tours, France, 18–21 September 2016; pp. 1–4.
29. Food and Drug Administration. *Information for Manufacturers Seeking Marketing Clearance of Diagnostic Ultrasound Systems and Transducer*; U. S. Department Health and Human Services, Food and Drug Administration, Center for Devices and Radiological Health: Washington, DC, USA, 1997.
30. Peralta, L.; Molina, F.; Melchor, J.; Gómez, L.; Massó, P.; Florido, J.; Rus, G. Transient elastography to assess the cervical ripening during pregnancy: A preliminary study. *Ultraschall Med. Eur. J. Ultrasound* **2015**. [CrossRef] [PubMed]
31. Badir, S.; Mazza, E.; Zimmermann, R.; Bajka, M. Cervical softening occurs early in pregnancy: Characterization of cervical stiffness in 100 healthy women using the aspiration technique. *Prenat. Diagn.* **2013**, *33*, 737–741. [CrossRef]
32. Parra-Saavedra, M.; Gomez, L.; Barrero, A.; Parra, G.; Vergara, F.; Navarro, E. Prediction of preterm birth using the cervical consistency index. *Ultrasound Obstet. Gynecol.* **2011**, *38*, 44–51. [CrossRef]
33. Gennisson, J.L.; Deffieux, T.; Fink, M.; M, T. Ultrasound elastography: Principles and techniques. *Diagn. Interv. Imaging* **2013**, *94*, 487–495. [CrossRef]

34. Peralta, L.; Rus, G.; Bochud, N.; Molina, F.S. Mechanical assessment of cervical remodelling in pregnancy: Insight from a synthetic model. *J. Biomech.* **2015**, *144*, 1557–1565. [CrossRef]
35. Peralta, L.; Rus, G.; Bochud, N.; Molina, F.S. Assessing viscoelasticity of shear wave propagation in cervical tissue by multiscale computational simulation. *J. Biomech.* **2015**, *48*, 1549–1556. [CrossRef] [PubMed]
36. Yasar, T.K.; Royston, T.J.; Magin, R.L. Wideband mr elastography for viscoelasticity model identification. *Magn. Reson. Med.* **2013**, *70*, 479–489. [CrossRef] [PubMed]
37. Rus, G.; Riveiro, M.; Molina, F. Effect of Contact Conditions of Torsional Wave Elastographic Probe on Human Cervix. *Math. Probl. Eng.* **2018**, *2018*, 6494758. [CrossRef]

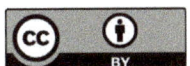 © 2019 by the authors. Licensee MDPI, Basel, Switzerland. This article is an open access article distributed under the terms and conditions of the Creative Commons Attribution (CC BY) license (http://creativecommons.org/licenses/by/4.0/).

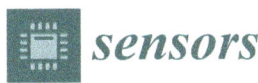

Article

An fMRI Compatible Smart Device for Measuring Palmar Grasping Actions in Newborns

Daniela Lo Presti [1], Sofia Dall'Orso [2,3], Silvia Muceli [2,3], Tomoki Arichi [3,4], Sara Neumane [3,5,6], Anna Lukens [4], Riccardo Sabbadini [1], Carlo Massaroni [1], Michele Arturo Caponero [7], Domenico Formica [8], Etienne Burdet [9] and Emiliano Schena [1,*]

1. Unit of Measurements and Biomedical Instrumentation, Università Campus Bio-Medico di Roma, Via Alvaro del Portillo, 00128 Rome, Italy; d.lopresti@unicampus.it (D.L.P.); r.sabbadini@unicampus.it (R.S.); c.massaroni@unicampus.it (C.M.)
2. Division of Signal Processing and Biomedical Engineering, Department of Electrical Engineering, Chalmers University of Technology, SE-412 96 Gothenburg, Sweden; dallorso@chalmers.se (S.D.); muceli@chalmers.se (S.M.)
3. Centre for the Developing Brain, School of Biomedical Engineering and Imaging Sciences, King's College London, London WC2R 2LS, UK; tomoki.arichi@kcl.ac.uk (T.A.); sara.neumane@kcl.ac.uk (S.N.)
4. Paediatric Neurosciences, Evelina London Children's Hospital, Guy's and St Thomas' NHS Foundation Trust, London SE1 7EH, UK; anna.lukens@gstt.nhs.uk
5. NeuroDiderot Unit UMR1141, Université de Paris, INSERM, F-75019 Paris, France
6. UNIACT, Université Paris-Saclay, CEA, NeuroSpin, F-91191 Gif-sur-Yvette, France
7. Photonics Micro- and Nanostructures Laboratory, ENEA Research Center of Frascati, 00044 Frascati (RM), Italy; michele.caponero@enea.it
8. Unit of Neurophysiology and Neuroengineering of Human-Technology Interaction (NeXt Lab), Università Campus Bio-Medico di Roma, Via Alvaro del Portillo, 00128 Rome, Italy; d.formica@unicampus.it
9. Department of Bioengineering, Imperial College London, London SW7 2AZ, UK; e.burdet@imperial.ac.uk
* Correspondence: e.schena@unicampus.it; Tel.: +39-062-2541-9650

Received: 25 September 2020; Accepted: 21 October 2020; Published: 23 October 2020

Abstract: Grasping is one of the first dominant motor behaviors that enable interaction of a newborn infant with its surroundings. Although atypical grasping patterns are considered predictive of neuromotor disorders and injuries, their clinical assessment suffers from examiner subjectivity, and the neuropathophysiology is poorly understood. Therefore, the combination of technology with functional magnetic resonance imaging (fMRI) may help to precisely map the brain activity associated with grasping and thus provide important insights into how functional outcomes can be improved following cerebral injury. This work introduces an MR-compatible device (i.e., smart graspable device (SGD)) for detecting grasping actions in newborn infants. Electromagnetic interference immunity (EMI) is achieved using a fiber Bragg grating sensor. Its biocompatibility and absence of electrical signals propagating through the fiber make the safety profile of the SGD particularly favorable for use with fragile infants. Firstly, the SGD design, fabrication, and metrological characterization are described, followed by preliminary assessments on a preterm newborn infant and an adult during an fMRI experiment. The results demonstrate that the combination of the SGD and fMRI can safely and precisely identify the brain activity associated with grasping behavior, which may enable early diagnosis of motor impairment and help guide tailored rehabilitation programs.

Keywords: fiber Bragg grating sensors (FBGs); functional magnetic resonance imaging (fMRI); grasping actions detection; motor assessment; MR-compatible measuring systems

1. Introduction

Human infants exhibit a range of spontaneous movements and primitive reflexes as they develop across the first few months following birth. Among these, the grasping reflex is considered a key behavior that enables their first interactions with their surroundings [1]. The absence of such a reflex during the first days after birth or its long-lasting persistence after sixth months of age is associated with underlying brain injury and considered to be predictive of later neuromotor impairment, e.g., cerebral palsy (CP) [2]. For this reason, clinical assessment tools for neurodevelopment disorders and brain abnormalities in the infant period (particularly for those born preterm or at high risk of developing later CP) usually incorporate a component that involves eliciting the grasp reflex [3,4].

Clinical assessment of palmar grasp is currently performed by applying light pressure on the infant's palm with an object or the examiner's finger to induce hand closure. This approach is entirely qualitative and based on the use of functional scales and the examiner's expertise [5] and is therefore potentially affected by inter-rater variability [6]. Furthermore, whilst clinicians and physiotherapists may develop discriminative experience about the quality of this reflex, they will still lack the sensitivity to identify subtle features not perceivable by a human observer (e.g., the discrimination of active/passive touch or the quantitative measurement of grasping strength and holding time). Therefore, a quantitative measure of grasping actions may provide new and valuable information about infant motor behavior. Consequently, there is a pressing need for new technologies that could enable the accurate measurement of grasping behavior and thus objectively evaluate sensorimotor function in the newborn. The use of such a technology could provide further insights into the relationship between motor behavior and underlying patterns of brain activity when combined with neuroimaging techniques [7]. This knowledge may be crucial in the context of early brain injury at a time when there is a high capacity for compensatory neural plasticity and thus the potential to improve functional outcome through patient-specific tailored therapies [8,9].

Functional magnetic resonance imaging (fMRI) allows for the non-invasive study of human brain function and has been successfully applied even with very young subjects [10–13]. In a typical fMRI experiment, brain responses when performing a task (which can be either an active action or passive stimulation) are identified by measuring temporal changes in the blood oxygen level dependent (BOLD) signal. However, a large challenge in performing fMRI studies with newborn infants is designing and effectively providing a task to this inherently uncooperative population. Technology can potentially resolve this difficulty and enable fMRI studies by allowing precise patterns of safe stimulation or accurate measures of spontaneous behavior while the subject is inside the scanner [6,8].

With the advance of sensor technology, several solutions have been proposed to quantitatively assess grasping behavior in infants and thus remove subjectivity. The majority of these studies have utilized technologies to assess grasping behavior in terms of strength and holding time, as well as to investigate the relationship between grasping pattern and intrinsic (e.g., infant gender, weight, premature births) and extrinsic factors (e.g., object shape and texture) [14,15]. The aforementioned measuring systems have used pressure transducers based on electrical components which are unusable inside the MRI scanner [6,16–19]. MR-compatible technology requires unconventional solutions to ensure safety due to the strong static magnetic field and avoid electromagnetic interference (EMI), with further attention required for successfully imaging infant subjects. Fiber Bragg gratings (FBGs) may be a solution to overcome this issue [20]. They are highly sensitive, small-sized, light, non-toxic, and immune to EMI [21]. Therefore, these features meet the technical and clinical requirements (e.g., MR-compatibility and safety) of devices for detecting and measuring grasping in preterm and term neonates both inside and outside the MRI scanner [6].

To date, only a few studies have systematically investigated functional brain activity in newborn infants using assistive technologies [8,9]. In [16], a customized robotic interface was used to passively move the limbs of preterm infants and identify the corresponding brain responses within the sensorimotor cortex. This study showed that the human brain is already functionally organized even at a very young age and paved the path for future investigations of task-related functional responses in preterm infants. Whilst the authors investigated the somatosensory response related to passive movements, they were unable to detect grasping actions.

The present study aims to develop an FBG-based measuring system (hereinafter called the smart graspable device (SGD)) to detect grasping actions in newborns. The SGD consists of an FBG sensor encapsulated into a soft silicone matrix. The FBG ensures that the device has EMI and the ideal safety profile for working with infants and inside the MRI environment. The device softness and cylindrical shape mimicking the ones of a finger additionally provides easy affordance and usability. Assessing grasp with the proposed device is based around the principle of the transduction of external forces (F_{ext}) applied by an infant's hand on the device into grating strain (ε) via squeezing and releasing of the silicone. In this paper we firstly described the design and fabrication of the proposed device so as to fulfill all technical and clinical requirements according to the target population (i.e., preterm and term newborns). Then, the sensitivity of the SGD to F_{ext} was estimated. Finally, two preliminary trials were carried out to investigate the performances of the proposed device when used by a preterm infant in the neonatal intensive care unit and an adult during an fMRI experiment.

2. Basic Requirements and Components of the Smart Graspable Device

2.1. Technological and Clinical Requirements

Designing a sensing device able to detect natural grasping actions and work simultaneously within an fMRI experiment is very challenging. Furthermore, there are additional constraints set by the target population (i.e., preterm and term newborn infants), which are not fulfilled by the majority of devices currently proposed in the literature [6,22]. In addition, the electromagnetic field inside the MRI environment can affect the working capability of most electronic devices proposed for grasp measurements and can induce currents in metal loops leading to infant contact burns [23,24]. In the same way, ferromagnetic elements widely used as components of electronic graspable devices may cause artefacts on the MRI images themselves, affecting diagnostic image quality [25].

As newborn infants are inherently uncooperative subjects, a further requirement of the device is that their natural movements can be safely measured under natural conditions [6,19]. To allow for handling by a newborn infant, the proposed tool should be small and lightweight, and its shape should be appropriate to improve engagement and encourage palmar grasping [26]. Moreover, high sensitivity to a low range of loads is necessary to detect the hand closure of a newborn infant, as well as being biocompatible and easily cleaned to reduce the risk of cross-infection between subjects [15,27].

To meet all of these technical and clinical requirements, an FBG sensor was chosen as the sensing element. A flexible and non-toxic silicone rubber (i.e., Dragon Skin™ 10) was used as a squeezable matrix to encapsulate the FBG sensor [28]. Lastly, a polylactic acid (PLA) structure characterized by a linkage mechanism filled with the soft silicone was designed according to the index finger dimensions of an adult human, as this is typically used to insert into the infant's palm to elicit the grasping reflex. The proposed solution is highly sensitive, robust, safe, affordable, and infant-friendly.

2.2. Fiber Bragg Gratings Working Principles

An FBG sensor is a distributed Bragg grating inscribed into a short segment of an optical fiber produced by creating a perturbation of the effective refractive index (η_{eff}) of the fiber core. In its simplest form, this periodic perturbation is sinusoidal with Λ, the constant grating pitch.

Generally, an FBG works in reflection as a notch filter; when a broadband spectrum of light is guided within the core and hits on the grating segment, a smooth Gaussian-shaped narrow spectrum is reflected and represents the output of the FBG. The center of the reflected Gaussian peak is known as the Bragg wavelength (λ_B) and satisfies the Bragg condition [29].

$$\lambda_B = 2\,\eta_{eff}\Lambda \tag{1}$$

Strain along the fiber longitudinal axis (ε) and temperature changes (ΔT) induce variations of Λ and η_{eff}, which result in a λ_B shift ($\Delta\lambda_B$) as in

$$\Delta\lambda_B = \lambda_B \left[(1 - P_e)\,\varepsilon + (\alpha_\Lambda + \xi)\,\Delta T\right] \tag{2}$$

The first term of Equation (2) represents the ε effect on the grating, with P_e the effective strain-optic constant; the second term represents the ΔT effect, with α_Λ and ξ denoting the thermal expansion and the thermo-optic coefficients of the fiber, respectively. When the effects of ΔT are negligible, Equation (2) in [29] can be rewritten as

$$\Delta\lambda_B = \lambda_B\,(1 - P_e)\,\varepsilon \tag{3}$$

In this work, the SGD is able to detect grasping forces applied by a newborn infant through the compression of the silicone encapsulation that allows transducing loads applied on the device into longitudinal ε experienced by the FBG.

Based on the need for a physical connection to a dedicated device (i.e., the FBG interrogator) for enlightening the gratings and reading their outputs, a patch cord can be used to connect the FBG-based device inside the MRI scanner to the interrogator placed in the control room. This connection allows separation of the SGD inside the MRI scanner room from the measuring circuitry located in the control room.

2.3. Dragon Skin™ Silicones

Dragon Skin™ materials (commercialized by Smooth On Inc., Macungie, PA, USA) are platinum care bicomponent silicone rubbers used in a variety of scenarios, including medical fields (e.g., in prosthetics as cushioning materials and in physiological monitoring for flexible sensor development [30,31]). They are highly compliant and highly flexible. Moreover, they are skin safe in compliance with ISO 10993-10 (Biological evaluation of medical devices—Part 10: Tests for irritation and skin sensitization) [28,32].

Dragon Skin™ silicones are commercialized as liquid silicone rubbers in the form of an elastomer kit containing two components (A and B). Part A contains the platinum catalyst, part B the crosslinker [33]. The manufacturer recommends mixing Dragon Skin™ silicones in the proportion of 1A:1B by weight and thinning the liquid formulation with Silicon Thinner™ to lower the viscosity of the mix for easier pouring and vacuum degassing [34]. Curing temperature and time are also defined in the technical bulletin. Dragon Skin™ silicones are commercialized in different hardnesses expressed in terms of Shore A Scale: 10 (Very Fast, Fast, Medium, Slow), 20, and 30, with curing time ranging from 4 min to 45 min according to the silicone hardness.

In this work, the mechanical properties of Dragon Skin™ 10 Medium, 20, and 30 were investigated in terms of stress–strain properties. To better quantify the compression behavior of Dragon Skin™ silicones, the Young modulus E (expressed in MPa) was calculated to facilitate the selection of the material that best satisfies all the requirements mentioned above. Considering the scenario of interest and target population, the application of low squeezing forces will induce a compression on the silicone rubber with ε values lower than 10% of the rubber sample (l_0). Thus, the stress–strain relationship can be described by Hooke's law [33]:

$$\sigma = E\,\varepsilon \tag{4}$$

where σ is the stress (i.e., the external force applied to the sample per its cross-sectional area) and ε is calculated as $(l - l_0)/l_0$.

The standard ISO 7743:2017 (Rubber, vulcanized or thermoplastic—Determination of compression stress–strain properties) was used for defining the dimensions of the cylindrical pieces used for the compression tests. The test piece B (method C) with a diameter of 17.8 ± 0.2 mm and a height of 25.0 ± 0.2 mm was chosen [35]. Dragon Skin™ 10 Medium, 20, and 30 were poured into a cylindrical mold designed in Solidworks (Dassault Systemes, Waltham, MA, USA) and 3D printed using PLA. As suggested by the technical bulletin, the curing process was carried out at room temperature for 5 h, 4 h, and 16 h for Dragon Skin™ 10, 20, and 30, respectively. A total of fifteen specimens were fabricated, five pieces for each hardness level.

Compression tests were carried out using a testing machine (Instron®, Norwood, MA, USA, model 3365, load cell with a range of measurement of ±10 N, an accuracy of 0.02 N, and a resolution of 10^{-5} N) to apply controlled ε values (from 0% to 25% of l_0 as suggested by the standard ISO 7743:2017) in a quasi-static condition (at a low displacement rate of 2 mm·min^{-1}). The static assessment of each specimen was executed by positioning the cylinder-shaped sample between the lower and the upper plates of the machine, as shown in Figure 1. A total of five repetitive compression tests were carried out at room temperature for a total of twenty tests per sample. The loads and the displacements applied by the compression machine to the specimen were recorded at a sampling frequency of 100 Hz using Instron® Bluehill Universal software.

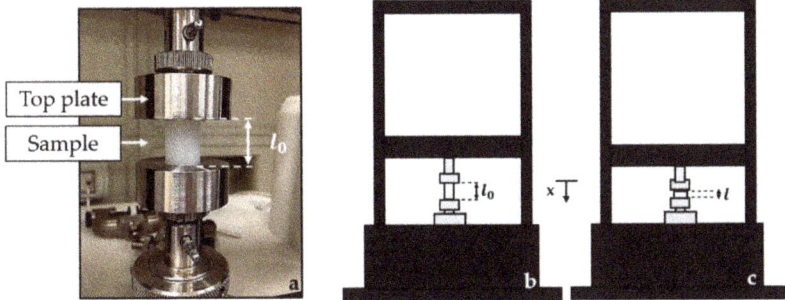

Figure 1. Set-up of the compression tests (**a**): the cylinder-shaped sample between the lower and the upper plates of the Instron machine and the initial sample length before (l_0) and during the compression (l) are illustrated ((**b**,**c**), respectively). The top plate moves at constant speed parallel to the *x*-axis (**c**).

The stress–strain relationships (σ vs. ε) of each Dragon Skin™ material were obtained by processing the collected data through a custom algorithm. The mean value of experimental σ (σ_{exp}) and the repeatability of the system response were determined by calculating the related uncertainty across the twenty tests by considering a t-Student reference distribution with 19 degrees of freedom and a level of confidence of 95% [36]. The best fitting line of the calibration curve was obtained, and its angular coefficient was calculated to estimate E. Lastly, the linearity error was calculated by using Equation (5) in terms of the maximum linearity error (% u_L^{max}).

$$\% u_L^{max} = \{\max [\sigma_{exp}(\varepsilon) - \sigma_{th}(\varepsilon)] \cdot \sigma^{fs}_{exp}{}^{-1}\} \cdot 100 \tag{5}$$

where σ^{fs}_{exp} is the full-scale output range, $\sigma_{exp}(\varepsilon)$ the experimental stress experienced by the sample at a specific ε, and $\sigma_{th}(\varepsilon)$ is the theoretical stress obtained by the linear model at the same ε value.

Results showed E values of 0.24 MPa, 0.47 MPa, and 0.74 MPa for Dragon Skin™ 10, 20, and 30, respectively (see Figure 2). R-square (R^2) values higher than 0.98 were found for all the responses, and linearity errors of 5.7%, 7.8%, and 8.9% were obtained for Dragon Skin™ 10, 20, and 30, respectively.

Our results quantified the mechanical properties of Dragon Skin™ in terms of compression behavior. As expected, Dragon Skin™ 10 was found to be more flexible than Dragon Skin™ 20 and Dragon Skin™ 30. In particular, the E value of Dragon Skin™ 10 was approximately half that of Dragon Skin™ 20 (i.e., 0.24 MPa vs. 0.47 MPa) and one-third that of Dragon Skin™ 30 (i.e., 0.24 MPa vs. 0.74 MPa). The high R^2 values (for all tests $R^2 > 0.98$) indicated good agreement between the experimental data and the linear model. Moreover, the Dragon Skin™ 10 response showed the best linear behavior as testified by the % u_L^{max} value (i.e., 5.7%), which was lower than those of Dragon Skin™ 20 (i.e., 7.8%) and Dragon Skin™ 30 (i.e., 8.9%), as shown in the respective plots in Figure 2.

Finally, Dragon Skin™ 10 showed the best results in terms of uncertainty (maximum uncertainty of 0.004 MPa) when compared to Dragon Skin™ 20 (i.e., 0.01 MPa) and Dragon Skin™ 30 (i.e., 0.007 MPa).

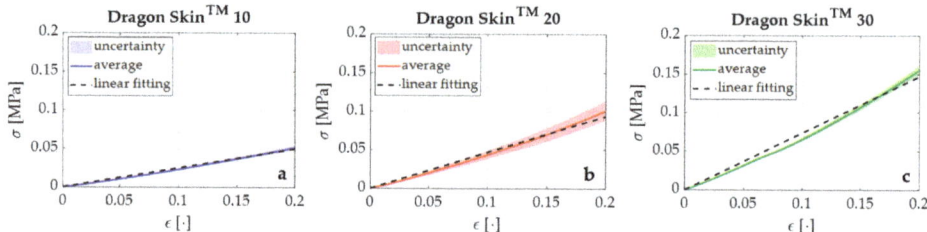

Figure 2. The σ–ε relationships for Dragon Skin™ 10, 20, and 30 are shown in blue (**a**), red (**b**), and green (**c**), respectively. In particular, the continuous lines represent the average σ_{exp} values, the shaded areas the related uncertainties, and the black dotted lines the σ_{th} values obtained by the best linear fitting model.

These findings demonstrated that Dragon Skin™ 10 is best suited to meet the technical requirements of the SGD, particularly given the expected low ranges of F_{ext} applied by newborn infants, which would likely require high flexibility; Dragon Skin™ 10 allows the SGD to be easily squeezed by a newborn for the F_{ext} transduction into grating ε.

3. The Smart Graspable Device

3.1. Design and Manufacturing of the Smart Graspable Device

The idea behind the system design and manufacturing was based on the need for it to be sensitive enough to detect F_{ext} applied by the infant and able to transduce F_{ext} into grating ε measured by the FBG sensor. At the same time, the device should be robust and safe enough to be handled and grasped by a newborn infant in a variety of settings.

The medium consists of a PLA-based structure characterized by a linkage mechanism and filled by flexible silicone (i.e., Dragon Skin™ 10). The transduction mechanism exploits four-bar linkages hinged to the PLA structure ends to convert the applied F_{ext} into ε via the silicone squeezing and releasing. When the newborn infant grasps the device, the silicone is squeezed and the FBG is strained; it is then unstrained once the SGD is released again (see Figure 3).

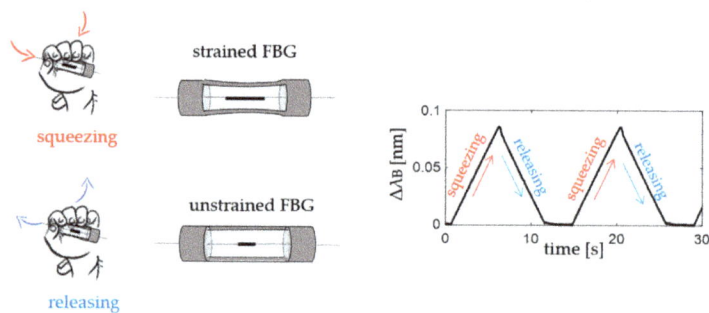

Figure 3. The smart graspable device (SGD) principle of working during grasping: squeezing (in red) and releasing (in blue) phases.

The PLA structure is a hollow cylinder made up of two semi-cylindrical pieces (see Figure 4A,B). Each piece is constituted of two end parts perpendicularly spaced by two bar linkages (40 mm of length, 4.2 mm of width, and 1 mm of depth). The bar linkages are hinged along the ends with a uniform interval of 60° to form a symmetrical structure (Figure 4A, top and front views). One semi-cylinder has a 10-mm long conduit to accommodate the jacket (yellow cable in Figure 4B). The jacket is the last layer of protection of the optical fiber from the end of the PLA structure to the interrogation unit.

The outer diameter of the PLA structure is 12 mm, and its overall length is 50 mm, which corresponds roughly to the dimensions of a human finger. The sensing element embedded into the PLA structure consists of an FBG sensor (λ_B of 1547 nm and grating length of 10 mm, commercialized by AtGrating Technologies, Shenzhen, China) configured with the middle part of the optical fiber encapsulated into a Dragon Skin™ 10 silicone matrix.

The encapsulation was fabricated as follows:

1. the optical fiber was tightly suspended inside the PLA structure by firmly gluing its two ends inside the small grooves fabricated at the center of the structure ends. This configuration utilized pre-tension to keep the FBG in a stretched state in order to improve its resolution and sensitivity (stage 1 in Figure 4B);
2. the PLA structure was placed inside a mold to allow cavity filling without any silicone spilling. The silicone rubber was synthesized by mixing A and B liquid components of Dragon Skin™ polymer at a ratio of 1:1; the mix was degassed and poured into the cavity (stage 2 in Figure 4B);
3. a curing process of 5 h was carried out at room temperature, as suggested in the technical bulletin [28], to allow the silicone rubber vulcanization before extracting the SGD from the mold (stage 3 in Figure 4B).

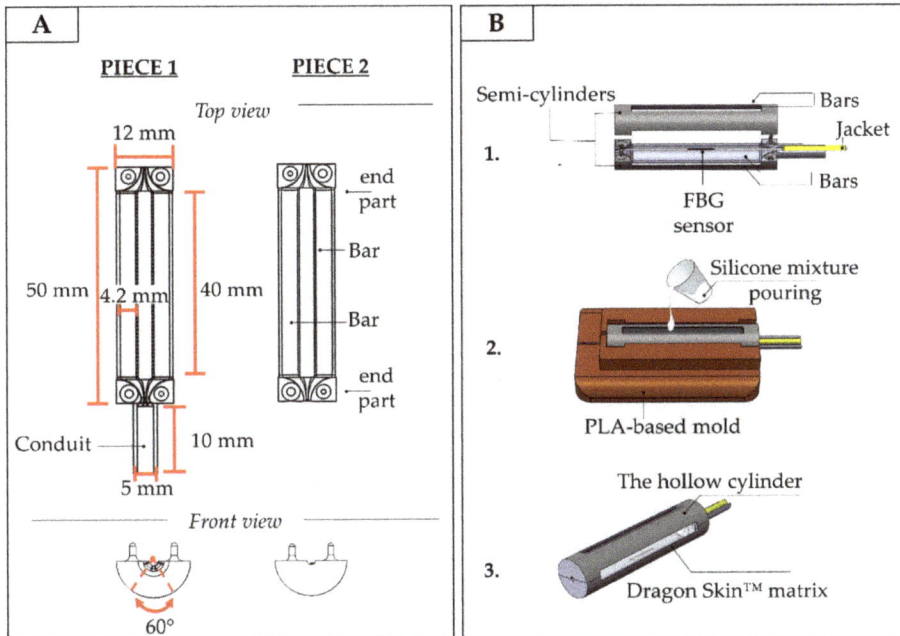

Figure 4. (**A**) The geometrical features of an SGD; (**B**) The main manufacturing steps: the FBG sensor positioning (step 1), the silicone mixture pouring (step 2), and the SGD removed from the mold after the rubber vulcanization (step 3).

Two nominally identical SGDs (from now on referred to as SGD^1 and SGD^2) were developed following the same manufacturing stages previously described.

To improve the SGDs usability during fMRI, both the devices were designed to also be able to instrument an already existing fMRI-compatible robotic interface for conducting experiments with newborn infants described in [8,9]. This interface was designed to accommodate the infant's forearm on a central non-sensitive platform and to passively guide the flexion and extension of the infant wrist while the hand was wrapped around a bar. The instrumentation of the robotic interface with the proposed SGD was performed by switching the non-sensorized handlebar with the SGD, thus allowing the investigation of brain activity related to grasping and spontaneous movements (Figure 5A,B). To fit the SGD to the robotic interface, two temporary PLA-based anchoring systems were fabricated (see Figure 5A). The anchoring mechanism was designed to allow quick and easy fitting of the SGD according to the fMRI investigation being performed.

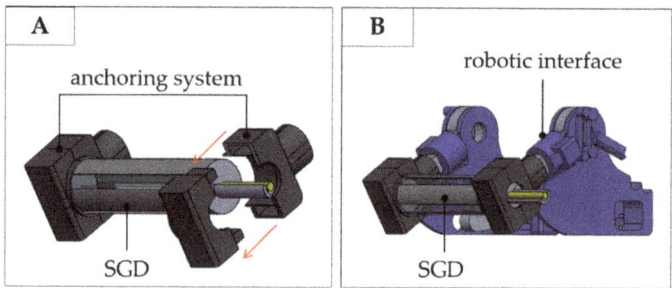

Figure 5. (**A**) A detail of the anchoring system elements designed to allow fitting of the SGD within an already existing robotic interface; (**B**) the SGD together with the robotic interface.

3.2. Metrological Characterization of the Smart Graspable Device

To estimate SGD sensitivity to F_{ext} (S_F), compression tests were performed by using a tensile testing machine (Instron, model 3365, load cell with a range of measurement of ±10 N, an accuracy of 0.02 N, and a resolution of 10^{-5} N). The blocking system shown in Figure 6 was designed to avoid any axial rotation of SGD during the application of loads on the SGD bars. This system consisted of a support plate with two clamps to securely lock the SGD through M4 fixings.

Each sensor (i.e., SGD^1 and SGD^2) was placed on the lower base of the machine blocked to the support place by using the 3D-printed clamps. External loads in the range 0 N–2 N were applied on each bar of the SGD at a low compression rate of 2 mm·min^{-1} to simulate quasi-static conditions (see Figure 6).

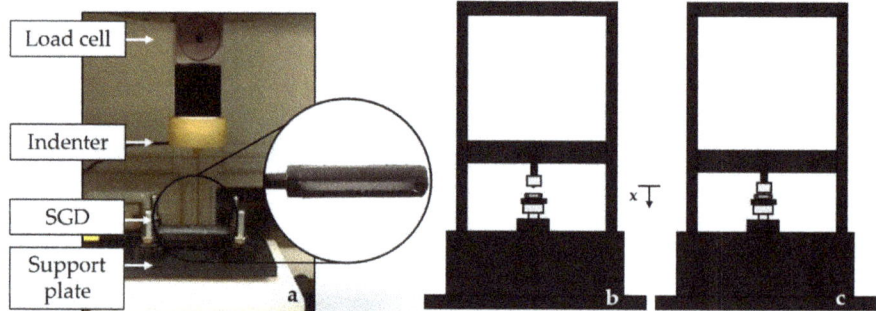

Figure 6. The SGD in the blocking system, the load cell, and the mechanical indenter are shown (**a**). A schematic representation of the SGD between the lower and the upper plates of the Instron machine is illustrated (**b**). The top plate moves at constant speed parallel to the *x*-axis (**c**).

The load was applied to the center of each bar by using a mechanical indenter (5 mm diameter). A total of five compression tests were performed on each of the four bars for a total of 20 tests. Once the five tests related to a single bar ended, the SGD was rotated 90° along its longitudinal axis, re-blocked to the support, and the second bar was loaded. The same procedure was repeated for the remaining two bars. The S_F value of each SGD was found averaging the twenty responses of all the bars to the applied loads.

During each test, the output from the tensile machine was collected at a sampling frequency of 100 Hz. The $\Delta\lambda_B$ values were simultaneously recorded using the optical spectrum interrogator (si255, Hyperion Platform, Micro Optics Inc., Atlanta, GA, USA) at the same sampling frequency.

The calibration curve ($\Delta\lambda_B$ vs. F_{ext}) was obtained by processing the collected data through a custom algorithm to evaluate the average value of $\Delta\lambda_B$ vs. F_{ext}. The first step was the synchronization of the experimental values of $\Delta\lambda_B$ and F_{ext}. Then, both the average value and the expanded uncertainty of $\Delta\lambda_B$ were calculated across the twenty tests. The expanded uncertainty was calculated by using a t-Student reference distribution (with 19 degrees of freedom and a level of confidence of 95%). Finally, a linear regression to find the equation of the line which best fits the experimental data (i.e., $\Delta\lambda_B$ vs. F_{ext}) was performed. Its slope represents the S_F value for SGD^1. The same procedure was followed for SGD^2 (see Figure 7).

Results showed a S_F value of ~0.23 nm·N^{-1} for both devices, suggesting a good reproducibility of the fabrication process. Moreover, an $R^2 > 0.99$ indicated excellent agreement between the experimental data and the linear fitting model.

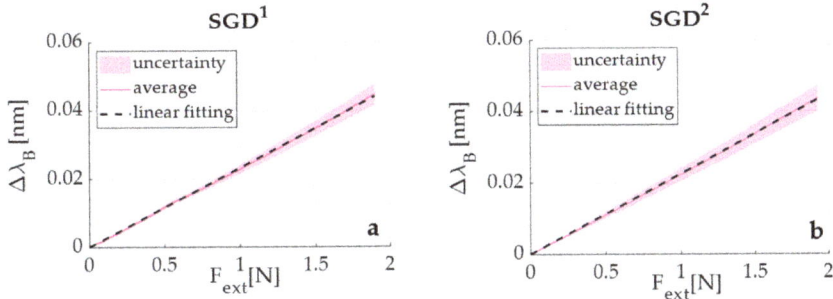

Figure 7. The $\Delta\lambda_B$ vs. F_{ext} of SGD^1 (**a**) and SGD^2 (**b**): in continuous magenta lines the average $\Delta\lambda_B$ vs. F_{ext} responses, in shaded magenta areas the related uncertainties, and in dotted black lines the best linear fitting.

4. Experimental Validation of the Smart Graspable Device

To assess the proposed SGDs performance in a real scenario, two explorative tests were performed with a newborn infant and an adult subject. Given the high agreement in S_F values between SGD^1 and SGD^2, SGD^1 was used for the following tests and for simplicity is now referred to as SGD. First, an explorative test was performed on a healthy newborn infant in the neonatal intensive care unit of St. Thomas Hospital (London, UK) to test compatibility of the SGD and assess its ability to detect a newborn infant's grasp. A further explorative trial within an fMRI experiment was then carried out to validate the device performances inside the MRI scanner and to confirm that activation within the brain areas associated with the grasping action detected by SGD could be identified with fMRI.

4.1. Experimental Trial on a Newborn: Protocol and Results

To assess the capability of SGD to detect grasping behavior in newborn infants, three healthy infants were recruited at St Thomas' Hospital (London, UK). Of them, only one infant (gestational age at birth: 36 weeks + 6 days, postmenstrual age at the time of recording: 37 weeks + 2 days) was in a suitable awake state at the time of the recording. The study was approved by the NHS research ethics committee (REC code: 12/LO/1247), and informed written consent was obtained from parents prior to participation. A neonatal physiotherapist under the supervision of a physician handled the SGD and applied light pressure on the infant's palm to induce hand closure around the device and elicit grasping behavior. Data from the SGD were collected using the FBG interrogator (si425, Micron Optics Inc., Atlanta, GA, USA) at a sampling frequency of 250 Hz, and a video used as reference was simultaneously recorded using a camera (Handycam, Sony, Minato-ku, Tokyo, Japan).

After data acquisition, the physiotherapist and the physician checked the recorded video to identify the time windows corresponding to the grasping action performed by the newborn infant. A total of five grasping events were identified (see Figure 8A).

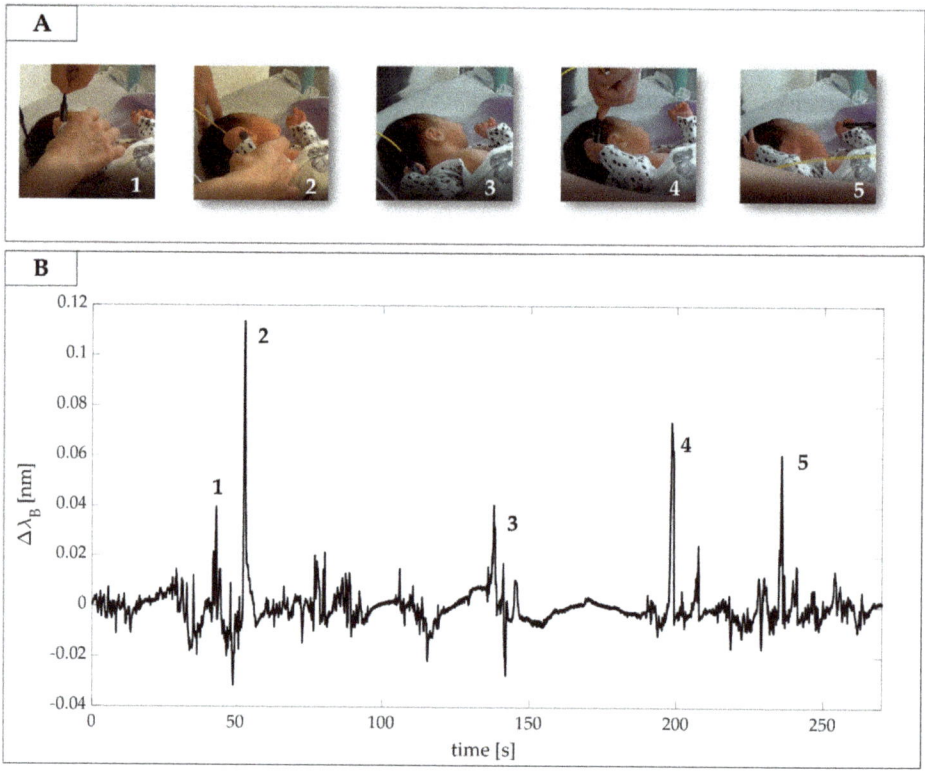

Figure 8. (**A**) Video frames of grasping actions identified by the clinicians; (**B**) the related signals collected by the SGD. Grasps actions are enumerated from 1 to 5.

Those time windows were then used to highlight changes in the SGD output associated with grasping actions. The signal showed evident peaks during the specific time windows related to presumed SGD squeezing and releasing actions (see Figure 8B). Results showed $\Delta\lambda_B$ values ranging from 0.04 nm to 0.11 nm that corresponded to forces ranging from ~0.17 N to ~0.48 N.

4.2. Experimental Trial on an Adult during fMRI: Protocol and Results

The second trial was performed on a healthy volunteer (32 years old, adult female volunteer) inside a 3 Tesla MRI scanner (Philips Achieva, Best, The Netherlands) located at St Thomas Hospital with a 32-channel receive head coil. High resolution structural T1-weighted and T2-weighted images were acquired for image registration purposes. BOLD contrast fMRI data with an EPI GRE sequence with parameters: x/y/z resolution: 3.5 mm × 3.5 mm × 6 mm; TR: 1500 ms; TE: 45 ms; FA 90°.

The subject was studied with her right hand fitted inside the instrumented robotic interface described in [8,9] with the right index and middle fingers strapped to the SGD on the handle bar.

The subject was then asked to use their two fingers to apply a brief force on the SGD at spontaneous and random times during an acquisition session lasting 225 s (corresponding to 150 images). The SGD signal was collected using the FBG interrogator (si425, Micron Optics Inc., Atlanta, GA, USA) at a sampling frequency of 250 Hz, and the recording started synchronously with the fMRI image acquisition so that the timing of task could be related to the fMRI timeseries. The task was designed to simulate a situation in which the experimenter is unaware of the timing of the task inside the scanner, as would be the case when studying spontaneous motor behavior in infants but can obtain this information from the output of the SGD. The experimental set-up and data flow are shown in Figure 9.

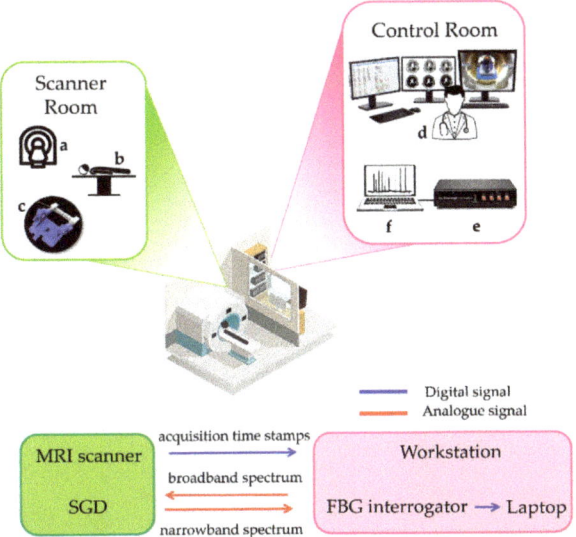

Figure 9. Experimental set-up of fMRI trial with the data flow: the MRI scanner (**a**), the patient (**b**), and the robotic interface instrumented by the SGD (**c**) in the scanner room, and the workstation (**d**), the FBG interrogator (**e**), and the laptop (**f**) in the control room. Digital and analogue data flows between the scanner and control rooms are shown using blue and red arrows, respectively.

The acquisition volume trigger markers (via a TTL pulse) were transmitted to the scanner workstation and used offline to synchronize the fMRI data with the signal recorded by the SGD. Data from the SGD were analyzed in the MATLAB R2019b environment (Mathworks, Natick, MA, USA). As shown in Figure 10A, the device was able to detect the force applied by the subject without prior knowledge of its timing (i.e., 26 actions in the SGD output across the period of acquisition) from which the event-related occurrence of the task could be defined for the fMRI data analysis.

In order to identify which voxels of the brain images were active during the task, it is possible to use a simple general linear model (GLM) to fit the BOLD time series within each voxel with a temporal model of the predicted activation, and the strength of each fit is used to generate a z-statistics map across the whole brain (z-score map in Figure 10). The predicted activation used as a model is built as the convolution of the experimental design (a vector that represents the timing of action vs. rest) and the hemodynamic response function (HRF) that act as a temporal smoothing kernel. The SGD-derived task pattern was then expressed in a binary vector form (with 1's representing action and 0's representing rest) where the events were identified using the *findpeaks* function on the normalized SGD signal in the MATLAB environment (see Figure 10A). Each event was represented by 8 ms centered at the peak of the action, and the binary vector was then convolved with the canonical hemodynamic response function (HRF) to generate the design model for the general linear model fMRI analysis (see Figure 10A). MRI data were processed using tools implemented in the FMRIB software library (FSL) in [37] following a standard pipeline which included high pass temporal filtering (with 0.02 Hz cut-off frequency), MCFLIRT rigid body motion correction, slice timing correction, brain extraction using BET, spatial smoothing (Gaussian of FWHM 5 mm), univariate general linear model (GLM) with additional 6 motion parameters derived from the rigid body motion correction as confound regressors, and cluster correction (p threshold 0.05). As predicted, significant clusters of positive BOLD activity were located in the primary contralateral (left) somatosensory and motor cortices and supplementary motor area correlating to the task performed by the subject, and the main cluster of activation was located at the hand knob on the precentral gyrus (see left (L) and right (R) lateral and top view on the 3D rendered brain images in Figure 10B).

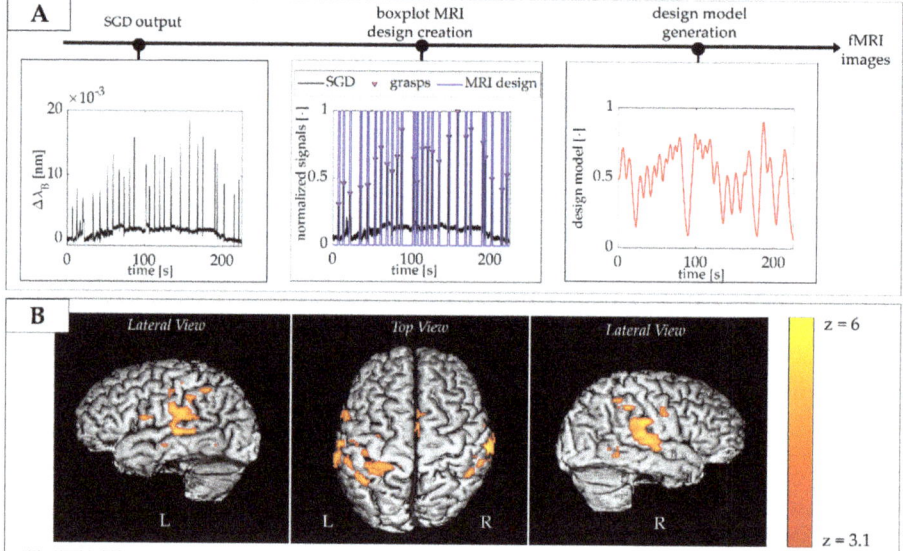

Figure 10. (**A**) Flow of data analysis. The peak in $\Delta\lambda_B$ coming from the SGD were used to infer the timing of the action and create a boxplot MRI design. This was convolved with the hemodynamic response function (HRF) to generate the design model for the general linear model (GLM); (**B**) Significant cluster of functional response to the task (in red and yellow) overlaid onto the subject's T1-weighted brain image with the z-score map.

5. Discussion

The key elements of the present study are the development of a novel smart device (i.e., the SGD), which can quantitatively measure the grasping behavior of newborn infants even within the MRI scanner environment. The design of the proposed device was guided by technical and clinical requirements predicated by the target population and with the intended use including small size, lightweight, high sensitivity, biocompatibility, and safety. In addition, the SGD was also designed to easily instrument an existing robotic interface used for fMRI studies of newborn infants.

To the best of our knowledge, the proposed SGD is the first fMRI-compatible device based on FBG able to detect and measure palmar grasp in preterm and term infants. The SGD is shaped and sized appropriately to be handled by a newborn infant's hand, easily squeezed, and able to detect low grasping F_{ext}. Furthermore, the FBGs' EMI compatibility ensures safety and working capability both outside and inside the MRI environment.

Two identical devices were fabricated (i.e., SGD[1] and SGD[2]). Both the responses of SGD[1] and SGD[2] to F_{ext} showed a linear behavior, which reached an average S_F value of ~0.23 nm·N^{-1}. This finding confirmed the high reproducibility of the manufacturing process as well as the capability of the SGD to detect the low ranges of F_{ext} applied by the target infant population. Two pilot tests were carried out to investigate the performance of the proposed SGD on a newborn infant in the neonatal intensive care unit and on an adult during an fMRI experiment. These preliminary validation experiments revealed that the SGD was capable of working in both cases, namely on a non-collaborative subject (i.e., the newborn infant) and within the MRI environment.

In the literature, pioneering work describing grasping behavior in infants began in the 1930s [38–40]. These first studies were based on functional scales or on the direct observation of infant responses to the application of light pressure on the palm [41]. These methods suffer from several limitations, including examiner subjectivity and incapability of quantifying grasping actions in terms of strength and duration. With the advancement of technological devices, novel methods emerged for assessing motor function in early infancy [7,14–16,18,19,42,43]. In particular, grasping behavior was studied in infants in terms of strength and holding time, with some studies proposing novel systems to investigate the relationship of these variables with intrinsic (e.g., infant sex [15], weight [27], preterm birth [1]) and extrinsic factors (e.g., object shape and texture [7]). Moreover, systems for objective assessment of grasping actions were developed to detect early abnormal neuromotor development and based on the premise that this could guide prompt intervention to improve functional outcome [43,44]. The main findings of the state-of-the-art showed a higher grasping strength and pronounced handedness symmetry in males more than females [15]; a decrease in holding time when the same object was repetitively put in the newborn infant's hand and an increase when its shape and smoothness changed [7]; and longer holding times in preterm in comparison to term neonates with significant differences related to sex [15].

Existing technological tools developed for measuring grasping in newborn infants can be grouped into devices worn on the examiner's finger [18] or those that are directly handled by an infant [16,18,19,43]. Very few of these systems were also specifically designed to be used by newborn infants in the first days following birth. All of these systems are based on pressure transducers with electrical components (i.e., piezoresistive sensors [16], force sensing resistors (FSR) [19], capacitive sensors [18], and conductive polymer layers [43]). These features do not allow their employment inside the MRI scanner. In contrast, our device is designed to be directly handled by a newborn infant and can be used in fMRI owing to the FBG sensor EMI immunity and the SGD's affordable shape.

In [16], as in our study, the device was designed to be directly grasped by a newborn infant without active involvement from the examiner during the experimental trial. An electrical sensing element (i.e., a piezoresistive pressure transducer) was used to develop a ring-shaped device consisting of a silicone-filled chamber hung within a rigid case and connected to the transducer (total diameter of 93 mm). This allowed for the measuring of infant grasping activity generated by chamber internal pressure changes due to the silicon squeezing. Our device is different, as the proposed SGD is based on optical technology instead of electrical components, is softer (10 A vs. 50 A), and is considerably lighter (8 g vs. 115 g). All of these features make our system more suitable for studying a wider range of infant populations including preterm and term infants.

Future studies will aim to investigate the feasibility of SGD assessment on a wider range of newborn infants both inside and outside the MRI scanner. Moreover, two SGDs can be used together in longitudinal studies to study the emergence of hand dominance and (bi)manual grasping to investigate developmental motor disorders resulting from localized brain injury. Further investigation may also be focused on optimizing the SGD for use with older infants, for instance across their first year as the transition to volitional prehension occurs. These studies will require a remodulation of system requirements (e.g., change in dimensions, FBG numbers, and silicone hardness) to optimize the SGD measuring properties for a different target population. Lastly, changes in grasping variables according to age, sex, and object texture could be performed to provide new insights into behavioral neurophysiology and neuropathology.

6. Conclusions

This paper described the first fMRI-compatible technological solution (SGD) based on FBG for detecting grasping actions in newborn infants. The use of such a device in conjunction with fMRI can shed new light on associated cerebral processes and may provide novel insight into the neuromotor impairments that result from neonatal brain injury. This knowledge may be crucial in the context of prompt diagnoses of atypical task-related brain activations and early brain injuries such as CP, at a time when there is a high capacity for compensatory neural plasticity. Furthermore, the technology-aided assessment of neurodevelopmental deviation from normal physiological development can provide useful biomarkers for establishing patient-tailored therapies and optimizing the rehabilitation outcomes.

Author Contributions: Conceptualization, D.L.P., S.D., S.M., R.S., T.A., D.F., E.B., E.S.; methodology, M.A.C., C.M., D.F., E.B., E.S.; software, D.L.P., S.D., R.S.; validation, D.L.P., S.D., T.A., S.N., A.L., E.S.; formal analysis, D.L.P., S.M., T.A., C.M., M.A.C., D.F., E.B., E.S.; investigation, D.L.P., S.D., T.A., S.N., A.L., E.S.; resources, T.A., M.A.C., C.M., E.B., E.S.; data curation, D.L.P., S.D., R.S.; writing—original draft preparation, D.L.P., S.D.; writing—review and editing, S.M., T.A., S.N., A.L., R.S., C.M., M.A.C., D.F., E.B., E.S.; visualization, D.L.P., S.D., S.M.; supervision, D.F., E.B., E.S.; project administration, D.L.P., D.F., B.E., E.S.; funding acquisition, D.L.P., S.M., T.A., D.F. All authors have read and agreed to the published version of the manuscript.

Funding: This article was supported by ReSTART (Sistema indossabile per il Recupero poST-ictAle sensoRiale e moTorio) project (funded by Fondazione G.B. Baroni), by the European Union's Horizon 2020 research and innovation programme under the Marie Sklodowska-Curie grant agreement No 846679 (INFANTPATTERNS), by CONBOTS (H2020-ICT-871803), by the Life Science Engineering Area of Advance at Chalmers University of Technology, and by MRC Clinician Scientist Fellowship (MR/P008712/1).

Conflicts of Interest: The authors declare no conflict of interest. The funders had no role in the design of the study; in the collection, analyses, or interpretation of data; in the writing of the manuscript; or in the decision to publish the results.

Ethical Statement: All subjects gave their informed consent for inclusion before they participated in the study. The study was conducted in accordance with the Declaration of Helsinki, and the protocol was approved by the UK NHS research Ethics Committee (12/LO/1247).

References

1. Lejeune, F.; Audeoud, F.; Marcus, L.; Streri, A.; Debillon, T.; Gentaz, E. The manual habituation and discrimination of shapes in preterm human infants from 33 to 34+6 post-conceptional age. *PLoS ONE* **2010**, *5*, e9108. [CrossRef] [PubMed]
2. Nelson, K.B.; Lynch, J.K. Stroke in newborn infants. *Lancet Neurol.* **2004**, *3*, 150–158. [CrossRef]
3. Mercuri, E.; Ricci, D.; Pane, M.; Baranello, G. The neurological examination of the newborn baby. *Early Hum. Dev.* **2005**, *81*, 947–956. [CrossRef] [PubMed]
4. Glick, T.H. Toward a more efficient and effective neurologic examination for the 21st century. *Eur. J. Neurol.* **2005**, *12*, 994–997. [CrossRef] [PubMed]
5. Moraes, M.V.M.; Tudella, E.; Ribeiro, J.; Beltrame, T.S.; Krebs, R.J. Reliability of the M-FLEX^{TM}: Equipment to measure palmar grasp strength in infants. *Infant Behav. Dev.* **2011**, *34*, 226–234. [CrossRef] [PubMed]
6. Allievi, A.G.; Arichi, T.; Gordon, A.L.; Burdet, E. Technology-aided assessment of sensorimotor function in early infancy. *Front. Neurol.* **2014**, *5*, 197. [CrossRef] [PubMed]
7. Molina, M.; Sann, C.; David, M.; Touré, Y.; Guillois, B.; Jouen, F. Active touch in late-preterm and early-term neonates. *Dev. Psychobiol.* **2015**, *57*, 322–335. [CrossRef] [PubMed]
8. Allievi, A.G.; Melendez-Calderon, A.; Arichi, T.; Edwards, A.D.; Burdet, E. An fMRI compatible wrist robotic interface to study brain development in neonates. *Ann. Biomed. Eng.* **2013**, *41*, 1181–1192. [CrossRef]
9. Dall'Orso, S.; Steinweg, J.; Allievi, A.G.; Edwards, A.D.; Burdet, E.; Arichi, T. Somatotopic mapping of the developing sensorimotor cortex in the preterm human brain. *Cereb. Cortex* **2018**, *28*, 2507–2515. [CrossRef]
10. Stippich, C.; Freitag, P.; Kassubek, J.; Sörös, P.; Kamada, K.; Kober, H.; Scheffler, K.; Hopfengärtner, R.; Bilecen, D.; Radü, E.; et al. Motor, somatosensory and auditory cortex localization by fMRI and MEG. *NeuroReport* **1998**, *9*, 1953–1957. [CrossRef]
11. Stippich, C.; Hofmann, R.; Kapfer, D.; Hempel, E.; Heiland, S.; Jansen, O.; Sartor, K. Somatotopic mapping of the human primary somatosensory cortex by fully automated tactile stimulation using functional magnetic resonance imaging. *Neurosci. Lett.* **1999**, *277*, 25–28. [CrossRef]

12. Moore, C.I.; Stern, C.E.; Corkin, S.; Fischl, B.; Gray, A.C.; Rosen, B.R.; Dale, A.M. Segregation of somatosensory activation in the human rolandic cortex using fMRI. *J. Neurophysiol.* **2000**, *84*, 558–569. [CrossRef] [PubMed]
13. Blatow, M.; Nennig, E.; Durst, A.; Sartor, K.; Stippich, C. fMRI reflects functional connectivity of human somatosensory cortex. *Neuroimage* **2007**, *37*, 927–936. [CrossRef] [PubMed]
14. Molina, M.; Jouen, F. Weight perception in 12-month-old infants. *Infant Behav. Dev.* **2003**, *26*, 49–63. [CrossRef]
15. Molina, M.; Jouen, F. Modulation of the palmar grasp behavior in neonates according to texture property. *Infant Behav. Dev.* **1998**, *21*, 659–666. [CrossRef]
16. Del Maestro, M.; Cecchi, F.; Serio, S.M.; Laschi, C.; Dario, P. Sensing device for measuring infants' grasping actions. *Sens. Actuators A Phys.* **2011**, *165*, 155–163. [CrossRef]
17. Baldoli, I.; Cecchi, F.; Guzzetta, A.; Laschi, C. Sensorized graspable devices for the study of motor imitation in infants. In Proceedings of the Annual International Conference of the IEEE Engineering in Medicine and Biology Society, EMBS, Milan, Italy, 25–29 August 2015; pp. 7394–7397.
18. Muhammad, T.; Lee, J.S.; Shin, Y.B.; Kim, S. A wearable device to measure the palmar grasp reflex of neonates in neonatal intensive care unit. *Sens. Actuators A Phys.* **2020**, *304*, 111905. [CrossRef]
19. Cecchi, F.; Serio, S.M.; Del Maestro, M.; Laschi, C.; Sgandurra, G.; Cioni, G.; Dario, P. Design and development of "biomechatronic gym" for early detection of neurological disorders in infants. In Proceedings of the 2010 Annual International Conference of the IEEE Engineering in Medicine and Biology Society, EMBC'10, Buenos Aires, Argentina, 31 August–4 September 2010; pp. 3414–3417.
20. Lo Presti, D.; Massaroni, C.; Leitao, C.S.J.; Domingues, M.F.; Sypabekova, M.; Barrera, D.; Floris, I.; Massari, L.; Oddo, C.M.; Sales, S.; et al. Fiber Bragg Gratings for medical applications and future challenges: A review. *IEEE Access* **2020**, *8*, 156863–156888. [CrossRef]
21. Othonos, A. Fiber Bragg gratings. *Rev. Sci. Instrum.* **1997**, *68*, 4309–4341. [CrossRef]
22. Gassert, R.; Burdet, E.; Chinzei, K. MRI-compatible robotics. *IEEE Eng. Med. Biol. Mag.* **2008**, *27*, 12–14. [CrossRef] [PubMed]
23. Dempsey, M.F.; Condon, B.; Hadley, D.M. MRI safety review. *Semin. Ultrasound CT MRI* **2002**, *23*, 392–401. [CrossRef]
24. Dempsey, M.F.; Condon, B. Thermal injuries associated with MRI. *Clin. Radiol.* **2001**, *56*, 457–465. [CrossRef] [PubMed]
25. Krupa, K.; Bekiesińska-Figatowska, M. Artifacts in magnetic resonance imaging. *Pol. J. Radiol.* **2015**, *80*, 93–106. [PubMed]
26. Hall, J.G.; Ursula, G.F.I.; Allanson, J.E. *Oxford Medical Publications: Handbook of Normal Physical*; Cambridge University Press: Cambridge, UK, 1989.
27. Molina, M.; Jouen, F. Manual cyclical activity as an explanatory tool in neonates. *Infant Behav. Dev.* **2004**, *27*, 42–53. [CrossRef]
28. Smooth-On Dragon Skin® High Performance Silicone Rubber. Available online: https://www.smooth-on.com/product-line/dragon-skin/ (accessed on 23 July 2020).
29. Erdogan, T. Fiber grating spectra. *J. Light. Technol.* **1997**, *15*, 1277–1294. [CrossRef]
30. Massaroni, C.; Zaltieri, M.; Lo Presti, D.; Tosi, D.; Schena, E. Fiber Bragg Grating Sensors for Cardiorespiratory Monitoring: A Review. *IEEE Sens. J.* **2020**. [CrossRef]
31. Lo Presti, D.; Carnevale, A.; D'Abbraccio, J.; Massari, L.; Massaroni, C.; Sabbadini, R.; Zaltieri, M.; Di Tocco, J.; Bravi, M.; Miccinilli, S.; et al. A multi-parametric wearable system to monitor neck movements and respiratory frequency of computer workers. *Sensors* **2020**, *20*, 536. [CrossRef]
32. BSI Biological Evaluation of Medical Devices Part 10: Tests for Irritation and Skin Sensitization. Available online: https://www.iso.org/standard/40884.html (accessed on 25 August 2020).
33. Mazurek, P.; Vudayagiri, S.; Skov, A.L. How to tailor flexible silicone elastomers with mechanical integrity: A tutorial review. *Chem. Soc. Rev.* **2019**, *48*, 1448–1464. [CrossRef]
34. Silicone Thinner® Product Information | Smooth-On, Inc. Available online: https://www.smooth-on.com/products/silicone-thinner/ (accessed on 25 August 2020).
35. ISO 7743:2011 Rubber, Vulcanized or Thermoplastic—Determination of Compression Stress-Strain Properties. Available online: https://www.iso.org/standard/72784.html (accessed on 25 August 2020).
36. Willink, R.; Willink, R. Guide to the Expression of Uncertainty in Measurement. In *Measurement Uncertainty and Probability*; Cambridge University Press: Cambridge, UK, 2013; pp. 237–244, ISBN 9267101889.

37. Jenkinson, M.; Beckmann, C.F.; Behrens, T.E.J.; Woolrich, M.W.; Smith, S.M. Review FSL. *Neuroimage* **2012**, *62*, 782–790. [CrossRef]
38. Halverson, H.M. An experimental study of prehension in infants by means of systematic cinema records. *Genet. Psychol. Monogr.* **1931**, *10*, 107–286.
39. Halverson, H.M. A further study of grasping. *J. Gen. Psychol.* **1932**, *7*, 34–64. [CrossRef]
40. Halverson, H.M. Studies of the grasping responses of early infancy: I. *Pedagog. Semin. J. Genet. Psychol.* **1937**, *51*, 371–392. [CrossRef]
41. Amiel-Tison, C.; Barrier, G.; Shnider, S.M.; Hughes, S.C.; Stefani, S.J. A new neurologic and adaptive capacity scoring system for evaluating obstetric medications in full-term newborns. *Anesthesiol. J. Am. Soc. Anesthesiol.* **1980**, *53*, S322. [CrossRef]
42. Forssberg, H.; Kinoshita, H.; Eliasson, A.C.; Johansson, R.S.; Westling, G.; Gordon, A.M. Development of human precision grip—II. Anticipatory control of isometric forces targeted for object's weight. *Exp. Brain Res.* **1992**, *90*, 393–398. [PubMed]
43. Cecchi, F.; Serio, S.M.; Perego, P.; Mattoli, V.; Damiani, F.; Laschi, C.; Dario, P. A mechatronic toy for measuring infants' grasping development. In Proceedings of the 2nd Biennial IEEE/RAS-EMBS International Conference on Biomedical Robotics and Biomechatronics, BioRob 2008, Scottsdale, AZ, USA, 19–22 October 2008; pp. 397–401.
44. Cioni, G.; Bos, A.F.; Einspieler, C.; Ferrari, F.; Martijn, A.; Paolicelli, P.B.; Rapisardi, G.; Roversi, M.F.; Prechtl, H.F.R. Early neurological signs in preterm infants with unilateral intraparenchymal echodensity. *Neuropediatrics* **2000**, *31*, 240–251. [CrossRef]

Publisher's Note: MDPI stays neutral with regard to jurisdictional claims in published maps and institutional affiliations.

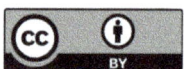

© 2020 by the authors. Licensee MDPI, Basel, Switzerland. This article is an open access article distributed under the terms and conditions of the Creative Commons Attribution (CC BY) license (http://creativecommons.org/licenses/by/4.0/).

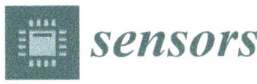

Article

EEG-Brain Activity Monitoring and Predictive Analysis of Signals Using Artificial Neural Networks

Raluca Maria Aileni *, Sever Pasca and Adriana Florescu

Department of Applied Electronics and Information Engineering, Faculty of Electronics, Telecommunications and Information Technology, Politehnica University of Bucharest, 060042 Bucharest, Romania; pasca@colel.pub.ro (S.P.); adriana.florescu@upb.ro (A.F.)
* Correspondence: raluca.maria.aileni@gmail.com

Received: 19 April 2020; Accepted: 8 June 2020; Published: 12 June 2020

Abstract: Predictive observation and real-time analysis of the values of biomedical signals and automatic detection of epileptic seizures before onset are beneficial for the development of warning systems for patients because the patient, once informed that an epilepsy seizure is about to start, can take safety measures in useful time. In this article, Daubechies discrete wavelet transform (DWT) was used, coupled with analysis of the correlations between biomedical signals that measure the electrical activity in the brain by electroencephalogram (EEG), electrical currents generated in muscles by electromyogram (EMG), and heart rate monitoring by photoplethysmography (PPG). In addition, we used artificial neural networks (ANN) for automatic detection of epileptic seizures before onset. We analyzed 30 EEG recordings 10 min before a seizure and during the seizure for 30 patients with epilepsy. In this work, we investigated the ANN dimensions of 10, 50, 100, and 150 neurons, and we found that using an ANN with 150 neurons generates an excellent performance in comparison to a 10-neuron-based ANN. However, this analyzes requests in an increased amount of time in comparison with an ANN with a lower neuron number. For real-time monitoring, the neurons number should be correlated with the response time and power consumption used in wearable devices.

Keywords: EEG; PPG; EMG; epilepsy; signal processing; brain monitoring; artificial neural network; predictive analysis

1. Introduction

1.1. Aim of the Work

Epilepsy is a disease that affects about 1% of the world's population. Crisis identification involves multi-channel EEG monitoring for 24–72 h. Crisis detection (grand mal) is essential for the diagnosis of epilepsy, the control of the crisis, and warning the patients in sufficient time before the seizure. Moreover, the observation and investigation of the biomedical signals values before an epileptic seizure are beneficial for developing prevention and support systems for patients because by informing the patient that an epilepsy seizure is about to occur, he or she can take his or her safety measures promptly. The correlations and covariance between the biomedical signals that EEG, PPG, and EMG collect from sensors are essential because, in the case of the patients with epilepsy, the heart rate increases, and uncontrolled tremors of the muscles or their stiffening may occur.

In the case of the patients with epilepsy, the real-time monitoring based on wearable devices with EEG, PPG, EMG integrated, and biomedical signals predictive analysis based on neural network systems with reduced processing time and low power computing is essential for warning before a seizure, and patients fall prevention.

1.2. State-of-the-Art

There are scientific studies that specify the use of artificial intelligence, using methods such as deep neural networks for patients' ECG-based authentication [1], ResNet-based signal recognition [2], arrhythmia detection [3,4], or learning feed-forward and recurrent neural networks [5]. The automatic signal detection was used in studies based on the discrete wavelet transform (DWT) for automated detection [4] or automated heartbeat classification [6].

The electrical activity of the brain monitoring by EEG (electroencephalogram) is useful to study the disease pathologies by analyzing the numerical distribution of data and correlating the brain signals (EEG) with other types of biomedical signals such as electrical activity of the heart obtained by electrocardiogram (ECG), heart rate monitoring by photoplethysmograph (PPG), and electrical activity produced by muscles by electromyography (EMG) [7–9].

To analyze the pathology of chronic diseases, the researchers also used the multivariate analysis of EEG, ECG, and PPG signals [10,11].

Mainly for predictive analysis of influence factors that generate a pathology or of the biomedical signal changes that could anticipate the existence of pathology are software applications for signal acquisition from sensors (EEG, ECG, PPG, or EMG), correlations [12], univariate, bivariate [13–15] or multivariate analyzes [16,17] of numerical data used, but computational methods [18] based on mathematical models are also used. Thus, computational models use studies on large populations (e.g., 274 patients [19]) and a large volume of data (e.g., 183 seizures recorded in 3565 h [20]). These analyses aim to find valid patterns [21] for a large population with similar independent variables (age, gender).

For the prediction of epileptic seizures, researchers used technologies such as machine learning, data mining, artificial neural networks [22] (backpropagation algorithm-for recognition and classification of EEG signals [23,24]), fuzzy systems [25], and predictive analysis statistics (multivariate [26], bivariate or univariate).

The study of the correlations between various electrical signals captured (e.g., EEG, ECG, PPG, and EMG) from the human body is essential because, in the case of patients with neurological disorders, the phenomenon of comorbidity exists and consists of overlapping of several diseases.

The electroencephalogram (EEG) represents a set of fluctuating field potentials produced by the simultaneous activity of a large number of neurons [27] and captured by electrodes located on the scalp. The EEG system consists of 10–20 metal electrodes distributed on the skin surface of the head and connected by 36 wires to the recording device. It measures the electrical potential detected by each electrode. EEG can be used in monitoring the brain during anesthesia [28], surgical procedures [29], and investigations of brain disorders (psychoses [30], meningoencephalitis [31], Parkinson [9], Alzheimer [32–37], dementia [38], epilepsy [39–42], central motor neuron syndrome [43], cerebral palsy [44–46], and muscular dystrophy [47]). Mainly, EEG systems are used to diagnose and monitor patients with neuropathology, especially in diagnosis of epilepsy and in studying the seizures, as well as the monitoring of treatment and evolution.

Electroencephalographic reactivity is evaluated using simple tests: eye-opening, hyperpnea (slow and full breathing), and intermittent light stimulation obtained with short and intense light discharges with gradually increasing frequency. The EEG assessment takes approximately 20 min and does not require hospitalization [48].

In the case of an electroencephalogram, the risks are minimal. Still, intermittent light stimulation or hyperventilation can produce epileptic seizures. Therefore, the examination is performed under the supervision of a physician who can recognize the crisis and immediately establish appropriate safety and therapeutic measures.

Epilepsy is a chronic disease of the brain that manifests through partial (focal) or generalized seizures due to spontaneous electrical discharges that occur in the brain.

Manifestations consist of involuntary movements of different body segments and abnormal neuro-vegetative sensations in the body. EEG analysis can be used to diagnose and monitor the patient in various stages of the disease (focal or generalized seizures, sleep) [38–41].

1.3. Contribution

In this paper, we present an efficient method for the detection of seizures based on artificial neural networks and correlations between biomedical signals.

Our study included 30 subjects from the CAP Sleep Database [49,50]. Our selected records were sampled at 160 Hz. The records consisted of both normal EEG and EEG spikes specific to epileptic seizures. The signals captured were from 13 EEG channels, submentalis and bilateral anterior tibialis EMG, and an earlobe PPG sensor. We used the artificial neural network and the Levenberg–Marquardt backpropagation optimization algorithm in MATLAB for implementing the classification and 3D plots. Data pre-processing and feature extraction were implemented using MATLAB 2019a (Mathworks, Santa Clara, CA, USA). All the experiments were carried out in Windows 8.1, 8 GB RAM, and 64-bit operating system.

The rest of the paper is structured as follows: the methods for signals decomposition, filtering, EEG biomedical signals, and theoretical methodology are presented in Section 2. Section 3 presents the predictive analysis of the signals using artificial neural networks. Aspects concerning the biomedical signals covariance are discussed in Section 4. The conclusions of the work are presented in Section 5.

2. Materials and Methods

The proposed method was tested using the CAP Sleep Database. The CAP Sleep Database comprises 40 recordings of patients (male and female) diagnosed with nocturnal frontal lobe epilepsy. The record duration is 8 h, approximately.

Our study included 30 subjects from the CAP Sleep Database. Our selected records were sampled at 160 Hz. The records consist of both normal EEG and EEG spikes specific to epileptic seizures. We analyzed 30 EEG recordings 10 min before a seizure and during the seizure in 30 patients with epilepsy. The signals analyzed are from 13 EEG channels, submentalis and bilateral anterior tibialis EMG, and an earlobe PPG sensor.

Within this research, the topic has used the detection of electrical signals from the brain using the EEG head with non-invasive electrodes (for the available biomedical signals in the PhysioNet databases).

In the discrete-time domain, digital filters (low-pass filter for signals with a frequency lower than a selected cutoff frequency and a high-pass filter that passes signals with a frequency higher than a cutoff frequency chosen) have been used for signal analysis.

Discrete wavelet transformation (DWT) [48] is calculated by additional high-pass and successive low-pass filters and sub-sampling using the Mallat algorithm [51]. Additional filtering applied to a real EEG signal leads to double the number of data from the original one being requested after each filtration to reduce the number of samples by sub-sampling of the EEG signal. DWT uses the dyadic variant. In the wavelet analysis, approximations (a (n)) and details (d (n)) are used (Figures 1 and 2):

1. Approximations (a (n)) are the components at high scales and low frequencies;
2. Details (d (n)) are components at low levels and high rates.

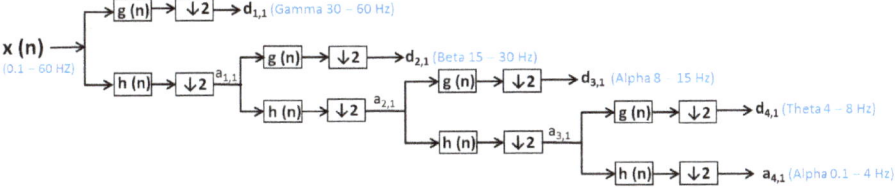

Figure 1. Electroencephalogram (EEG) from a patient with no seizure-signal filtering and decomposition using the discrete wavelet transform (DWT) method.

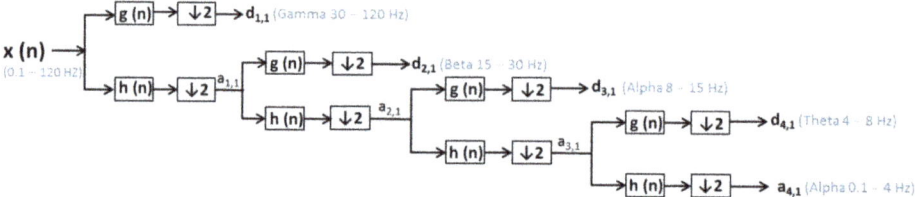

Figure 2. EEG from a patient with epileptic seizure-signal filtering and decomposition using the DWT method.

To reduce the continuous-time signal to a discrete-time signal, the EEG signals were sampled with a sampling frequency (fs = 160 Hz). EEG signals were filtered by a low-pass filter (60 Hz) and a high-pass filter (0.1 Hz) and decomposed using the discrete wavelet transform [52,53] for patients without epilepsy (Figure 1).

In the case of epilepsy, seizures detection consists of finding EEG segments with seizures and onset and offset points [53]. For pattern profiling, it is necessary to monitor a large population of patients with epilepsy for 24–48 h. Because gamma frequency oscillations (30–120 Hz) often precede interictal epileptiform spike discharges (IEDs) [54], we used DWT with Daubechies function, and we considered the low-pass filter 120 Hz to observe the gamma wave specific to an epileptic seizure. Some scientific papers report the values around 100–600 Hz for gamma waves—that is, not associated with IEDs, but occurring during epileptic seizures [54,55]. However, other researchers [54,56] reported the fluctuation of gamma wave values.

EEG signals were filtered by a low-pass filter (120 Hz) and a high-pass filter (0.1 Hz) and decomposed using the discrete wavelet transform for patients with epileptic seizures (Figure 2).

x (n)—signal (0.1–60 Hz), respective for patient with seizure x (n)—signal (0.1–120 Hz);
h(n)—low-pass filter (LPF);
g (n)—high-pass filter (HPF);
d (n)—the signal of the detail produced by HPF, e.g., d1, 1, d2, 1, d3, 1, d4, 1;
a (n)—the signal produced by LPF, is a rough approximation, e.g., a1, 1, a2, 1, a3, 1, a4, 1;
↓2—down sampling by two.

The wavelet transform is a way to implement a particular type of signal representation called multi-resolution analysis [57,58]. The analyzed signal is described by a succession of details and approximations that contain more information. Each level of approximation (Figures 1 and 2) contains information available at the previous level, which is an added component of detail. In Figure 3, the signal processed by discrete wavelet transform and Daubechies method using four decomposition levels for a patient before and after a short seizure is presented. In Figure 3, detail d1 represents gamma waves, detail d2 represents beta waves, detail d3 represents alpha waves, detail d4 represents theta waves, and the approximation a4 represents delta waves.

In Figure 4, the signal processed by discrete wavelet transform and Daubechies method using four decomposition levels for a patient with epileptic seizures is presented. In Figure 4, the detail d1 represents gamma waves, detail d2 represents beta waves, detail d3 represents alpha waves, detail d4 represents theta waves, and the approximation a4 represents delta waves. From Figure 4, it is evident that the presence of the gamma waves with values equal to or greater than 120 shows that a seizure phase is present. Moreover, the epileptic spikes are very evident in Figure 4.

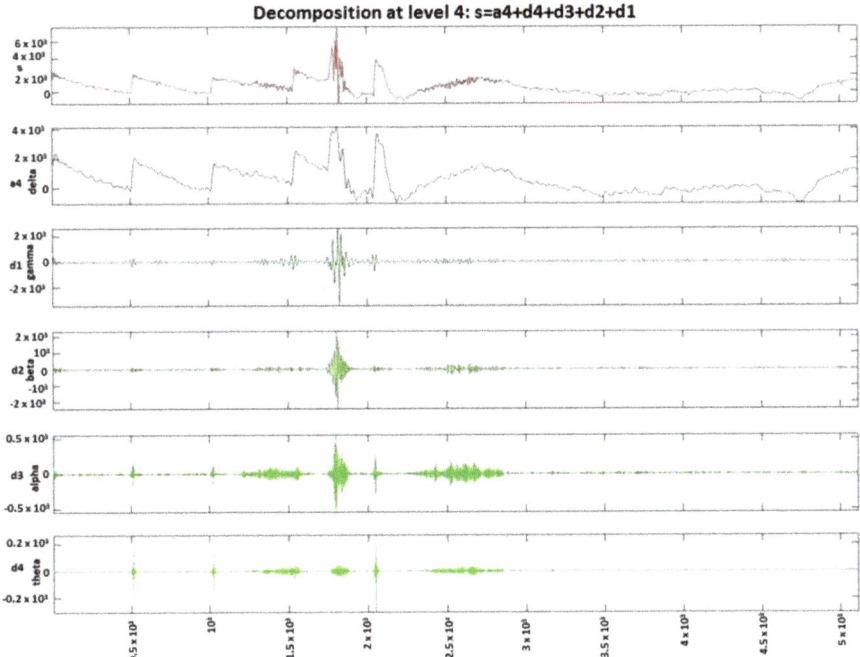

Figure 3. Patient before and after the seizure, signal decomposition on four levels using DWT.

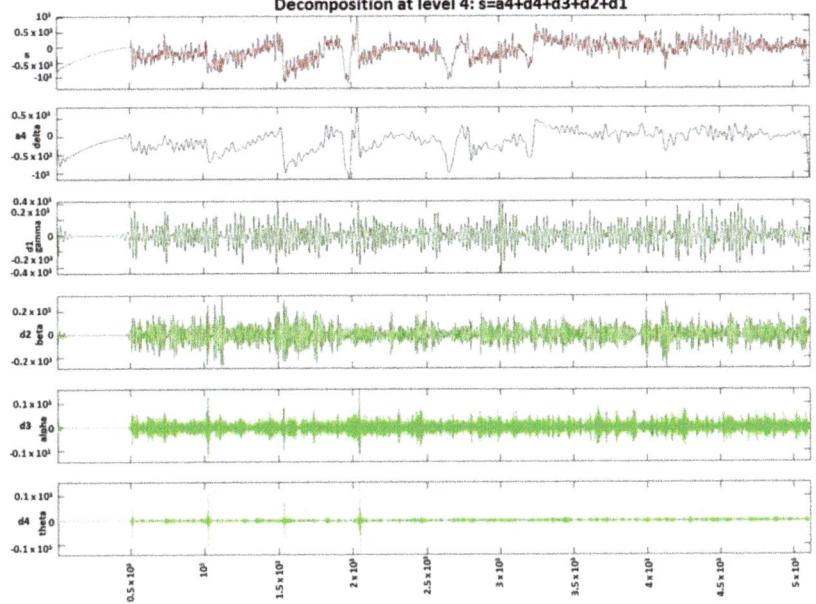

Figure 4. Patient with epileptic seizure, signal decomposition on four levels using DWT.

In Figure 5, the 3D spectrogram of the signals from all 13 channels of electro-cap used for monitoring a patient with an epileptic seizure is presented. The epileptic gamma waves spikes (with the yellow-red color market on the graphic) that are over 200 or 400, indicating abnormal frequencies for gamma waves that occur on seizures, are also evident from Figure 5.

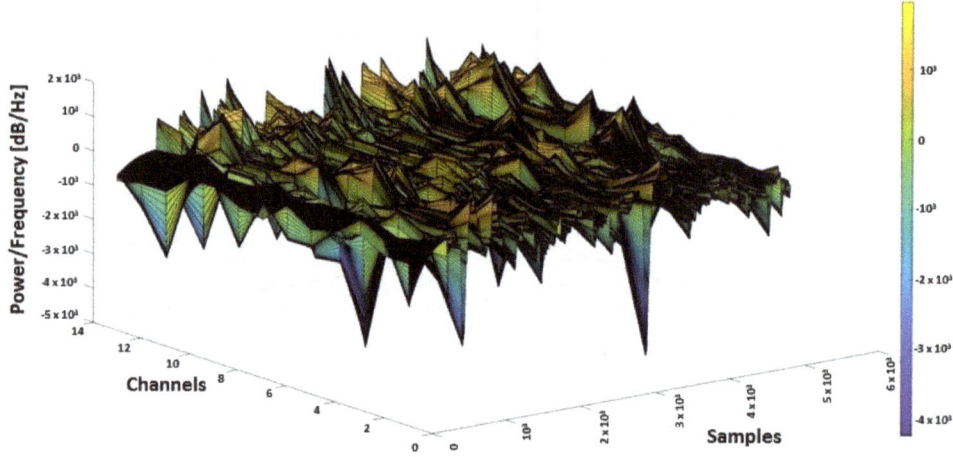

Figure 5. 3D spectrogram of EEG signals from 13 channels.

3. Biomedical Signal Selection

To analyze the correlation and covariance between signals, signals such as EEG (related to the frontal lobes FP1-F3, FP2-F4), EMG, and PPG from a patient n1 with no epileptic seizures and a patient n2 with epileptic seizures were selected.

The purpose of using PPG and EMG signals in correlation with EEG was to find a modification of the biomedical signals collected from wearable devices that could anticipate an epilepsy seizure and to use a software system to send medical alerts in advance [59–65]. From the CAP Sleep Database, the biomedical signals taken from 2 patients (n1 and n2) were used for the actual study. In Figures 6 and 7, the 3D spectrograms for the EEG signals (Fp2-F4, F4-C4, C4-P4, P4-O2, F8-T4, T4-T6, FP1-F3, F3-C3, C3-P3, P3-O1, F7-T3, T3-T5, C4-A1) taken from patients n1 and n2 are presented. In the case of patient n1, the epileptic spikes for gamma waves cannot be observed (Figure 6), but in the case of patient n2, these spikes are evident, marked with yellow-orange in the 3D spectrogram (Figure 7) and being above the 120 Hz threshold.

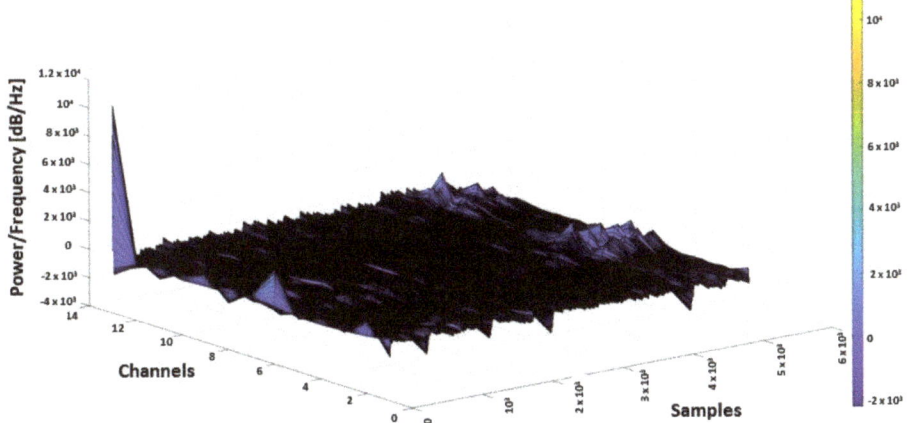

Figure 6. 3D spectrogram of signals EEG from 13 channels for patient n1 with no epileptic seizures.

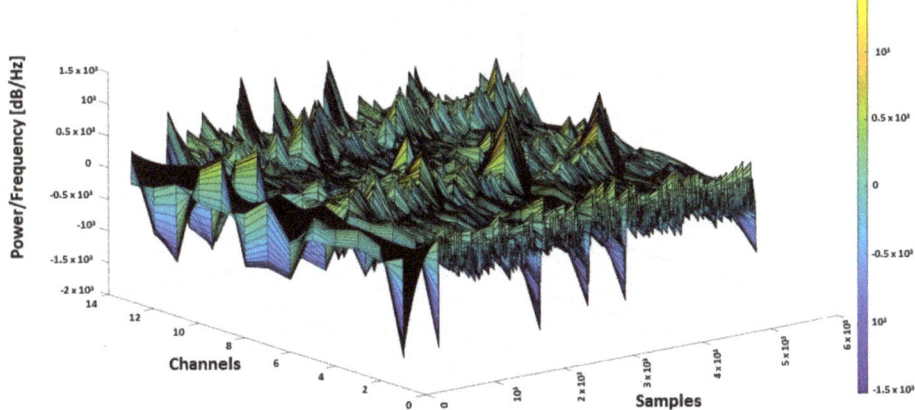

Figure 7. 3D spectrogram signals EEG from 13 channels for patient n2 with epileptic seizures.

4. Results Based on Predictive Analysis of the Signals Using Artificial Neural Networks

For predictive analysis of EEG signals, artificial feed-forward neural networks are used based on the Levenberg–Marquardt backpropagation optimization algorithm.

The functional units within the neural networks consisted of:

- Input units represented by the values of the EEG matrix for patients with epilepsy seizures.

  Hidden groups (data) given by the number of neurons (10, 50, 100, and 150 neurons, respectively).

- Outputs are represented by the values of the EEG matrix for patients who do not have seizures.

For optimization, the Levenberg–Marquardt algorithm was used, which approximates the Hessian matrix (H) as follows (1):

$$H = J^T J \qquad (1)$$

where:

- J is the Jacobian matrix containing the derivatives of the error function concerning weights (w) and biases (b);
- J^T is the transposed Jacobian matrix;
- e is the vector of errors.

The Levenberg–Marquardt algorithm uses the following parameter updating rule (Equation (2)):

$$x_{k+1} = x_k - \left[J^T J + \mu I\right]^{-1} J^T e \qquad (2)$$

For this purpose, four neural networks were designed with n hidden neurons (Figure 8), where $n \in \{10, 50, 100, 150\}$, to estimate the occurrence of epilepsy seizures, compared with EEG signals taken from a healthy patient, respectively, with EEG signals received from the patient with no seizures. The artificial neural network (ANN) architecture models (with 10, 50, 100, and 150 respective hidden neurons) used for the prediction of the epileptic seizures have a two-layer feed-forward network with hidden sigmoid neurons and linear output neurons, and allow the training and evaluation of the performance using mean square error (MSE) and regression analysis (R). The proposed ANNs structures are based on the principal elements:

- input data (matrix 13 × 5120 samples);
- hidden layer with n neurons, $n \in \{10, 50, 100, 150\}$;
- output (target) data (matrix 13 × 5120 samples);
- train set (70% of samples) that is used to provide an independent measure of network performance during and after training;
- test set (15% of samples) that is used during training, and the network is adjusted according to its error;
- validation set (15% of samples) is used to measure network generalization, and to halt training when generalization stops improving.

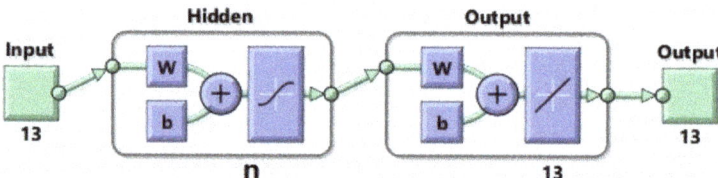

Figure 8. Artificial neural network (ANN) with n neurons, $n \in \{10, 50, 100, 150\}$.

In Table 1, the principal parameters for ANNs with 10, 50, 100, and 150 neurons are presented.

Table 1. ANN parameters.

Neurons No.	Input Data [Samples EEG3]	Output (Target) Data [Samples EEG1]	Train Set [Samples]	Test Set [Samples]	Validation Set [Samples]
10	Matrix 13 × 5120	Matrix 13 × 5120	3584	768	768
50	Matrix 13 × 5120	Matrix 13 × 5120	3584	768	768
100	Matrix 13 × 5120	Matrix 13 × 5120	3584	768	768
150	Matrix 13 × 5120	Matrix 13 × 5120	3584	768	768

Prediction and optimization were made with a feed-forward backpropagation multi-layer neural network.

The input data-independent variables (matrix input) X_1 = EEG signal (EEG3) taken when the patient does not have seizures.

The target data-dependent variables (matrix target) Y_1 = EEG signal (EEG1) taken from a patient with epilepsy. The target (Y_1) represents the desired output for the given input, X_1. We consider the real output matrix (D).

The continuous training of neural networks is based on extensive datasets; 70% (3584 samples) of the total data generated by the ANNs were used to train the model, while 15% (768 samples) of the data was used for testing and 15% (768 samples) for validation (Figures 9–12). Regression analysis of the ANN model showed the R^2 (regression) values for training between 0.57316 for the ANN with ten neurons, 0.65267 for the ANN with 50 neurons, 0.85089 for the ANN with 100 neurons, and 0.81819 for the ANN with 150 neurons, showing the higher accuracy and significance of the ANN model for the ANN with 100 neurons, respective to the ANN with 150 neurons.

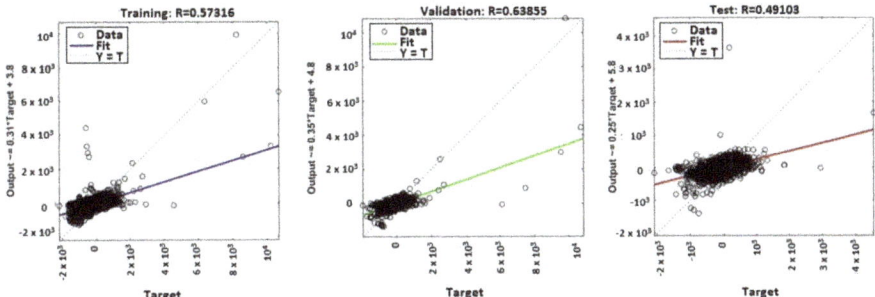

Figure 9. Regression (R^2) for validation, test, and training—ANN with ten neurons.

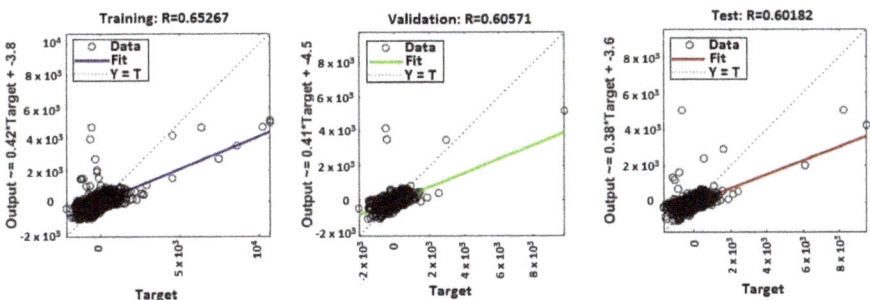

Figure 10. Regression (R^2) for validation, test, and training—ANN with 50 neurons.

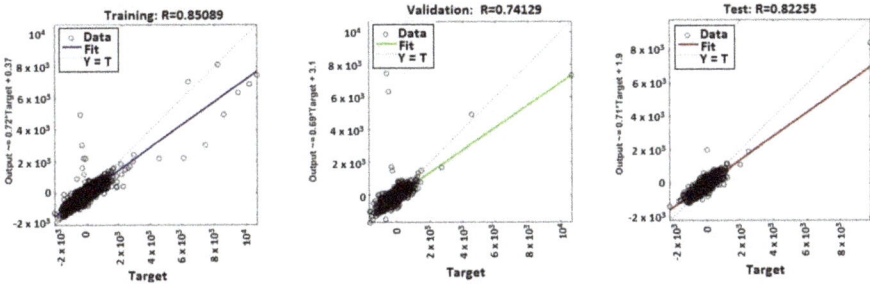

Figure 11. Regression (R^2) for validation, test, and training—ANN with 100 neurons.

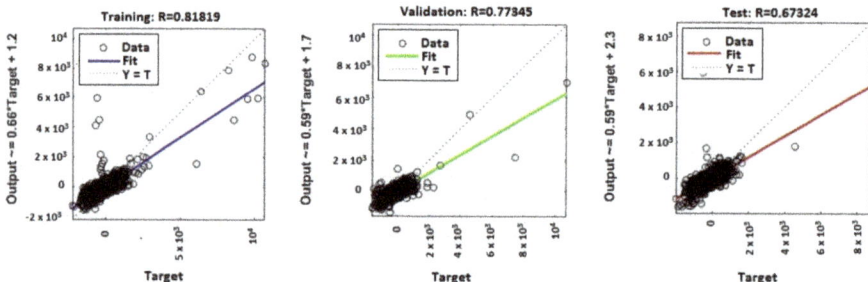

Figure 12. Regression (R^2) for validation, test, and training—ANN with 150 neurons.

MATLAB libraries were used to perform the functions and the code sequences within the neural networks. The regression plots (9–12) show a regression between network outputs and network targets. The parameterized linear regression model is given by mathematical relation (3). The R (Equation (3)) value indicates the relationship between the outputs (y) and targets. If $R = 1$, this indicates that there is an exact linear relationship between outputs and targets. If the R-value is close to zero, then there is no linear relationship between the outputs and targets.

$$R = D = \sum_{j=1}^{M} w_j x_j + \varepsilon \Leftrightarrow R = w^T x + \varepsilon \quad (3)$$

where:

- ε is the error;
- w_j is synaptic weight;
- x is the input matrix;
- M is the model order;
- T denotes matrix transposition (Equations (4) and (5)).

$$w = [w_1, w_2, \ldots, w_M]^T \quad (4)$$

$$x = [x_1, x_2, \ldots, x_M]^T \quad (5)$$

From the regression graphs for testing, training, and validation for neural networks with 10, 50, 100, and 150 neurons (Figures 9–12), and from values presented on Table 1, it is evident that the value of the R regression for training, validation, and testing is in a direct relationship with the number of neurons of the network. The regression value R close to zero indicates that is no linear relationship between outputs and targets. Moreover, if R is very close to 1, it shows a good match and an exact linear relationship between the outputs and targets. From the regression graphs, it is observed that the value of the regression for test, training, and validation is close to the value 1, which indicates a good match between inputs, outputs, and objectives. From Figure 9, it can be observed that, in the case of the neural network with ten hidden neurons, the values of the regression for test, validation, and training are in the inequality report $R_{Test} < R_{Training} < R_{Validation}$, the regression is lower than 1, and the higher one is the regression for validation ($R_{Validation} = 0.63855$). From Figure 10, we observed that, in the case of the neural network with 50 hidden neurons, the values of the regression for test, validation, and training are in the inequality report $R_{Test} < R_{Validation} < R_{Training}$, the regression is lower than 1, and the higher one is the regression for training ($R_{Training} = 0.65267$). In Figure 11, it can be observed that, in the case of the neural network with 100 hidden neurons, the values of the regression for test, validation, and training are in the inequality report $R_{Validation} < R_{Test} < R_{Training}$, the regression is lower than 1, and the higher one is the regression for training ($R_{Training}$ = 0.85089). From Figure 12, it is evident that, in the case of the neural network with 150 hidden neurons, the values of the regression for test, validation, and training are in the inequality report $R_{Test} < R_{Validation} < R_{Training}$, the regression is lower than 1, and the higher one is the regression for training ($R_{Training}$ = 0.81819).

From the histograms of errors (Figures 13 and 14), it can be observed that the increase in the number of neurons in the network leads to a decrease in the percentage of errors generated. The error histograms (Figures 13 and 14) show normal distributions with residuals (errors), indicating that many of the residuals fall on or near zero in the case of the ANN with 150 neurons. Analyzing Figures 13 and 14, we can conclude that the ANN model with 150 neurons used for the prediction can generate an excellent prediction of epileptic seizures.

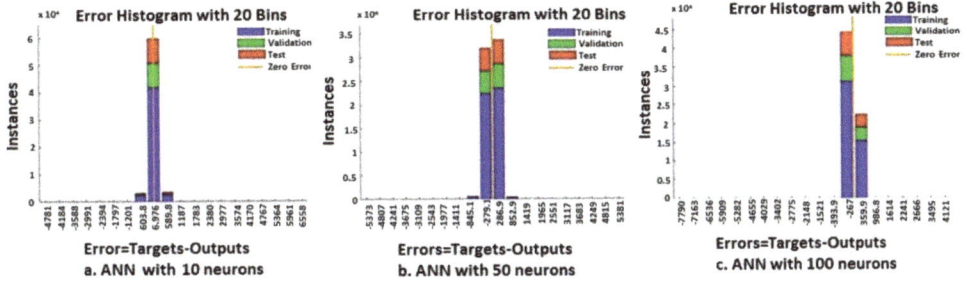

Figure 13. Error histograms—ANN with 10, 50, and 100 neurons.

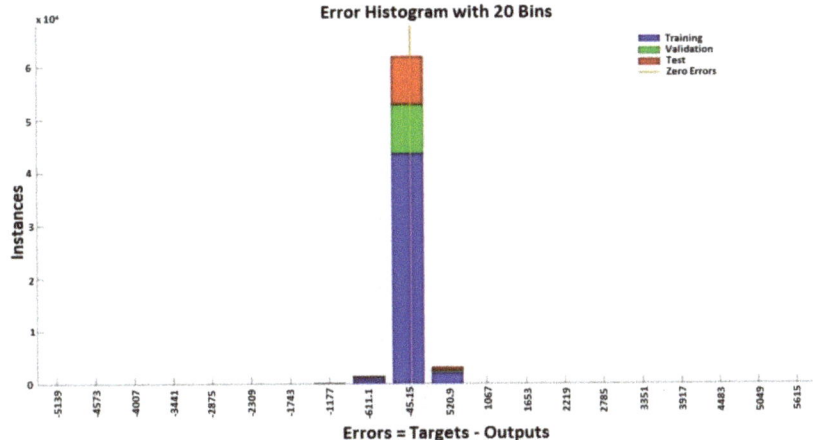

Figure 14. Error histogram—ANN with 150 neurons.

In Table 2 are presented for each neural network developed, the number of hidden neurons allocated, the processing time [seconds] of the neural network, and the values of the regression for training ($R_{Training}$), test (R_{Test}), and validation ($R_{Validation}$). In Table 2, the processing time represents the total time allocated for training, test, and validation.

In the proposed ANN with n (10, 50, 100, and 150) neurons, we defined the training set, test set, and validation set to check over-optimization. The validation set was used to measure network generalization, and to halt training when generalization stopped improving. The evaluation of the performance was done using mean square error (MSE) and regression analysis (R).

Table 2. Value $R = f$ (neural network neurons).

Neurons No.	R Training	R Validation	R Test	Processing Time [s]
10	0.57316	0.63855	0.49103	42
50	0.65267	0.60571	0.60182	745
100	0.85089	0.74129	0.82255	913
150	0.81819	0.77345	0.67324	2784

In Figures 15 and 16, the performances of the neural networks with 10 and 150 neurons, respectively, are presented. In Figures 15 and 16, error vs. epoch is plotted for the validation. The best validation is taken from the epoch with the lowest validation error. On the y axis of the charts, the mean squared error (MSE) (Equation (6)) is presented. The best validation is taken from the epoch with the lowest validation error. Mainly, the error reduces after more epochs of training.

$$MSESE = \frac{1}{n} \sum_{i=1}^{n} (y_i - \hat{y}_i)^2 \tag{6}$$

where:

y_i is the vector of observed values;
$\hat{y}_i$ is the vector of predicted values.

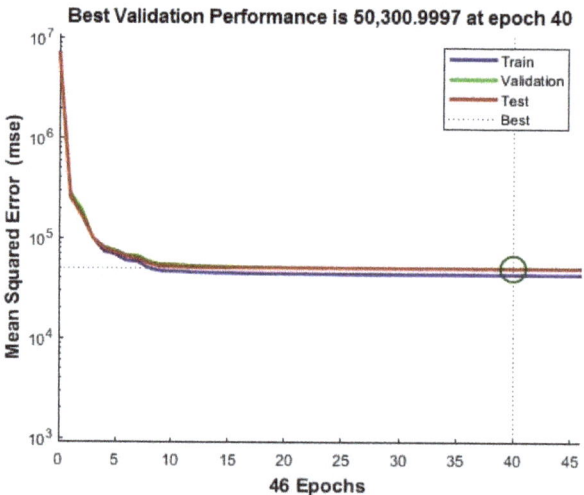

Figure 15. Neural network (10 neurons) best validation performance.

However, the best validation performance was generated in 40 epochs, whereas 47 epochs were run to confirm the model accuracy for the ANN with ten neurons (Figure 15). The best validation performance was generated in 9 epochs, whereas 15 epochs were run to confirm the model accuracy for the ANN with 150 neurons (Figure 16). In comparison with the ANN with ten neurons, the ANN with 150 neurons shows higher performance.

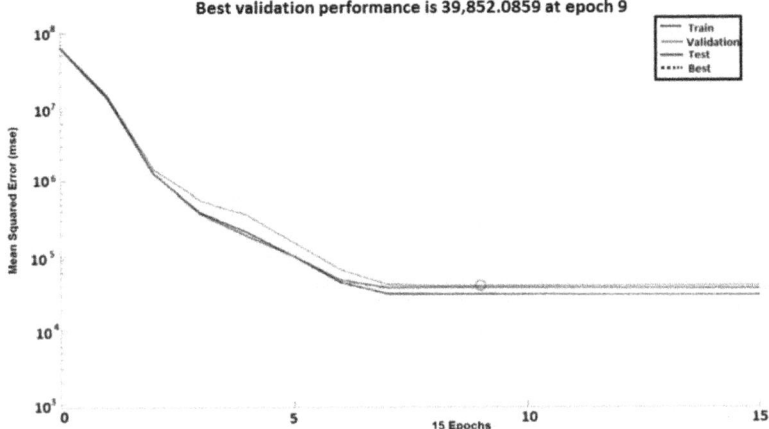

Figure 16. Neural network (150 neurons) best validation performance.

5. Discussion

5.1. Biomedical Signals Covariance Analysis

In order to evaluate if the previously presented biomedical signals (EMG, PPG, and EEG) can be used to predict epileptic seizures, it is necessary to investigate the covariance between all the analyzed signals. Mainly, for two discrete signals, $x(k)$ and $y(k)$, correlation is a discrete function in time (Equation (7)), defined by:

$$r_{xy}(k) = \sum_{n=-\infty}^{+\infty} x(n)y(n-k) \qquad (7)$$

where $k = 0, 1, 2, \ldots$.

Using the correlation function of two signals, the similarity between the signals can be appreciated. The autocorrelation function has a maximum in origin when $k = 0$ and can be used to determine the periodicity of real signals. The autocorrelation function (Equation (8)) is defined by:

$$r_{xx}(k) = \sum_{n=-\infty}^{+\infty} x(n)y(n-k) \qquad (8)$$

where: $k = 0, 1, 2, \ldots$.

The signals EEG1 (no seizure) and EEG3 (with seizure) collected from patient n1, respective to the signals EEG2 (with seizure) and EEG4 (no seizure) collected from patient n2, were sampled at a rate of 160 Hz and filtered using high-pass (0.1 Hz) and low-pass filters (60 Hz for EEG with no seizure activity, respective to 120 Hz for EEG with seizure).

By analyzing the covariance matrix for EEG_i, EEG_j (Equations (9), (11), (13), (15), (17) and (19)), and correlation coefficients (Equations (10), (12), (14), (16), (18) and (20)), we found that:

- between EEG1 and EEG3 is a negative covariance; this means that they are not in a linear dependence (Equation (9)). Because the correlation coefficient is negative (Equation (10)), it follows that EEG1 and EEG3 are in an inverse proportionality relationship.
- between EEG2 and EEG4 is a negative covariance, which means that EEG2 and EEG4 are not in a linear dependence (Equation (11)). Because the correlation coefficient is negative (Equation (12)), it follows that EEG1 and EEG3 are in an inverse proportionality relationship.

- between EEG1 and EEG4 is a positive covariance, which means that EEG1 and EEG4 are in a linear dependence (Equation (13)), and because the correlation coefficient is positive (Equation (14)), it follows that EEG1 and EEG4 are in a direct proportionality relationship.
- between EEG1 and EEG2 is a negative covariance (Equation (15)), which means that EEG1 and EEG2 are not in a linear dependence, and because the correlation coefficient is negative (Equation (16)), it follows that EEG1 and EEG2 are in an inverse proportionality relationship.
- between EEG2 and EEG3 is a positive covariance, which means that EEG2 and EEG3 are in a linear dependence (Equation (17)), and because the correlation coefficient is positive (Equation (18)), it follows that EEG1 and EEG4 are in a direct proportionality relationship.
- between EEG3 and EEG4 is a negative covariance (Equation (19)), which means that EEG3 and EEG4 are not in a linear dependence, and because the correlation coefficient is negative (Equation (20)), it follows that EEG3 and EEG4 are in an inverse proportionality relationship.

$$cov(EEG1, EEG3) = 1.0e+05 * \begin{vmatrix} 0.7206 & -0.0369 \\ -0.0369 & 0.7206 \end{vmatrix} \tag{9}$$

$$R_{EEG1,\ EEG3} = \begin{vmatrix} 1.0000 & -0.0272 \\ -0.0272 & 1.0000 \end{vmatrix} \Leftrightarrow r_{1,2} = r_{2,1} = -0.0272 \tag{10}$$

$$cov(EEG2, EEG4) = 1.0e+05 * \begin{vmatrix} 0.5555 & -0.0900 \\ -0.0900 & 5.7909 \end{vmatrix}, \tag{11}$$

$$R_{EEG2,EEG4} = \begin{vmatrix} 1.0000 & -0.0502 \\ -0.0502 & 1.0000 \end{vmatrix} \Leftrightarrow r_{1,2} = r_{2,1} = -0.0502, \tag{12}$$

$$cov(EEG1, EEG4) = 1.0e+05 * \begin{vmatrix} 0.7206 & 0.0196 \\ 0.0196 & 5.7909 \end{vmatrix}, \tag{13}$$

$$R_{EEG1,\ EEG4} = \begin{vmatrix} 1.0000 & 0.0096 \\ 0.0096 & 1.0000 \end{vmatrix} \Leftrightarrow r_{1,2} = r_{2,1} = 0.0096, \tag{14}$$

$$cov(EEG1, EEG2) = 1.0e+04 * \begin{vmatrix} 7.2061 & -0.5302 \\ -0.5302 & 5.5551 \end{vmatrix}, \tag{15}$$

$$R_{EEG1,\ EEG2} = \begin{vmatrix} 1.0000 & -0.0838 \\ -0.0838 & 1.0000 \end{vmatrix} \Leftrightarrow r_{1,2} = r_{2,1} = -0.0838, \tag{16}$$

$$cov(EEG2, EEG3) = 1.0e+05 * \begin{vmatrix} 0.5555 & 0.3163 \\ 0.3163 & 2.5545 \end{vmatrix}, \tag{17}$$

$$R_{EEG2,EEG3} = \begin{vmatrix} 1.0000 & 0.2655 \\ 0.2655 & 1.0000 \end{vmatrix} \Leftrightarrow r_{1,2} = r_{2,1} = 0.2655, \tag{18}$$

$$cov(EEG3, EEG4) = 1.0e+05 * \begin{vmatrix} 2.5545 & -0.2580 \\ -0.2580 & 5.7909 \end{vmatrix}, \tag{19}$$

$$R_{EEG3,\ EEG4} = \begin{vmatrix} 1.0000 & -0.0671 \\ -0.0671 & 1.0000 \end{vmatrix} \Leftrightarrow r_{1,2} = r_{2,1} = -0.0671 \tag{20}$$

Using the Shapiro–Wilk test (Figure 17) to evaluate the distribution of EEG1, EEG2, EEG3, and EEG4 signals in the Brainstorm application, it can be seen that the values for $W_{EEG1} = 0.9378$, $W_{EEG2} = 0.9236$, $W_{EEG3} = 0.9133$, and $W_{EEG4} = 0.8299$, are very close to 1, which means that the signals have a distribution close to the normal distribution.

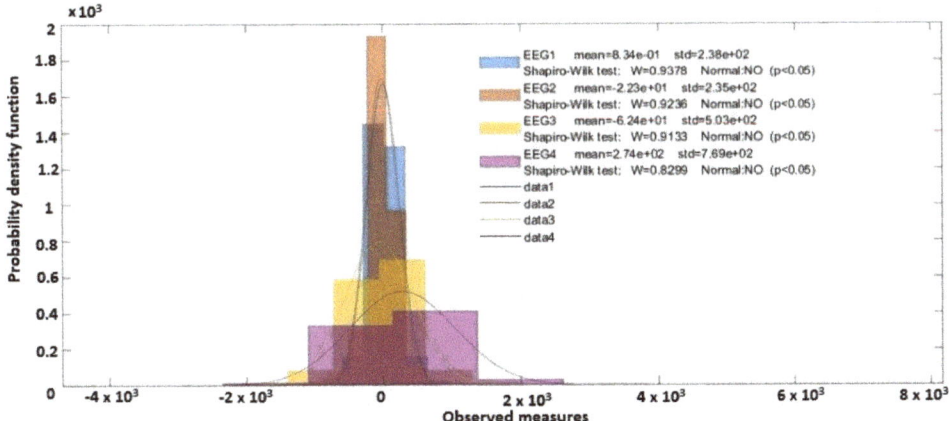

Figure 17. Distribution probabilities (Shapiro–Wilk test, Brainstorm).

The analysis of the covariances and correlations between EMG2 and EEG2 (Equations (21) and (22)) and PPG3 and EEG3 (Equations (23) and (24)), respective of those between EMG3 and EEG3 (Equations (25) and (26)), shows that there is a positive correlation and a direct covariance between signal pairs ((PPG3, EEG3) and (EMG3, EEG3)), respective of those between signal pairs (EMG2, EEG2), which could be exploited in anticipation of epilepsy seizures by predictive analysis using an ANN and a support decision system.

$$cov(EMG2, EEG2) = 1.0e + 04 * \begin{vmatrix} 0.6864 & 0.0422 \\ 0.0422 & 9.2137 \end{vmatrix}, \quad (21)$$

$$R_{EMG2,EEG2} = \begin{vmatrix} 1.0000 & 0.0168 \\ 0.0168 & 1.0000 \end{vmatrix} \Leftrightarrow r_{1,2} = r_{2,1} = 0.0168, \quad (22)$$

$$cov(PPG3, EEG3) = 1.0e + 05 * \begin{vmatrix} 0.2690 & 0.0909 \\ 0.0909 & 4.9304 \end{vmatrix}, \quad (23)$$

$$R_{PPG3, EEG3} = \begin{vmatrix} 1.0000 & 0.0789 \\ 0.0789 & 1.0000 \end{vmatrix} \Leftrightarrow r_{1,2} = r_{2,1} = 0.0789 \quad (24)$$

$$cov(EMG3, EEG3) = 1.0e + 05 * \begin{vmatrix} 2.1729 & 0.0122 \\ 0.0122 & 4.9304 \end{vmatrix}, \quad (25)$$

$$R_{EMG3,EEG3} = \begin{vmatrix} 1.0000 & 0.0037 \\ 0.0037 & 1.0000 \end{vmatrix} \Leftrightarrow r_{1,2} = r_{2,1} = 0.0037, \quad (26)$$

In conclusion, the correlations and covariances between the biomedical signals (EEG, PPG, and EMG) collected from sensors are significant because, in the case of the patients with epilepsy, the heart rate increases and may generate uncontrolled tremors of the muscles or their stiffening. Furthermore, to patients having epilepsy, the comorbidity phenomena are present [66–68] and consist of overlapping of several diseases (diabetes, cardiovascular diseases, etc.).

5.2. Comparative Analysis

To observe the performance of our proposed methodology, we compared our methods (DWT and ANN), validation, and accuracy of the results with the existing methods based on machine learning from the literature. Comparison is presented in Table 3, which contains the feature extraction methods, the machine learning methods, the validation methods, and also the classification accuracy.

Table 3. Methodology description of recent state-of-the-art compared with our results.

Literature	Features Extraction Method	Learning Machine Method	Validation	Classification Accuracy
Method 1	-	[69] Convolutional neural network (CNN) with 3 layers	6-fold cross validation	83.8–95%
Method 2	spectral and spatial features	[70] SVM	-	96%
Method 3	wavelet transform for decomposition	[71] ANN and genetic algorithm	-	-
Method 4	wavelet transform for decomposition	[72] negative correlation learning (NCL) and a mixture of experts (ME)	25% of the train set was randomly selected for the validation set	96.92%
Method 5	Multi-wavelet Transform	[73] ANN	-	90%
Method 6	-	[74] pyramidal one-dimensional CNN (P-1D-CNN)	10-fold cross validation	99.1%
Method 7	-	[75] 13-layer CNN	10-fold cross-validation	88.67%
Method 8	DWT	[76] SVM	-	96%
Method 9	Minimum redundancy maximum relevance (mRMR), Principal component analysis (PCA)	[77] SVM, k-nearest neighbors (k-NN), and discriminant analysis	Leave-one-out cross-validation	51% (SVM) 80% (k-nn with mRMR)
Method 10	-	[78] CNN	20-fold and 10-fold cross-validation	84.26%
Method 11	-	[79] U-Time—convolutional encoder-decoder network	5-fold cross-validation	-
Our work	DWT	ANN	15% of the samples were selected for the validation set	91.1%

5.3. Limitation and Future Scope

The proposed methods give significant results, but the ratio between best validation performance and processing time exhibits an inverse relationship and generates the limitation in real-time data processing because the neural network with 150 neurons has the best validation performance, but the increasing the number of neurons in the ANN generates an increase in the time required for data processing.

The other state-of-the-art methods do not analyze the problem of real-time processing through the perspective of the ratio between best performance validation and time.

However, an investigation for a new set of parameters and to learn algorithms to improve this is needed. Moreover, analyzing other physiological signals such as the heart's electrical activity (ECG) along with EMG, PPG, and EEG may improve the investigations to detect biomedical parameters changes before or during the seizures.

6. Conclusions

In this work, we used artificial neural networks (ANN) for automatic detection of epileptic seizures before onset. We used DWT with Daubechies function for decomposing the signals and analyzing EEG recordings before onset and during the seizure for patients with epileptic seizures and with no epileptic seizures. To design the model, we used the predictive analysis of EEG signals, artificial feed-forward neural networks based on the Levenberg–Marquardt backpropagation optimization algorithm. In addition, we analyzed the covariance between biomedical signals (EEG, PPG, and EMG) to select the signals that can be used on predicting epileptic seizures.

We can conclude that using the ANN with 150 neurons has an excellent performance in comparison with the ANN with ten neurons. However, this ANN analyzes requests an increased time in comparison with an ANN with a lower neuron number (e.g., ten neurons). Even if the use of an ANN with a large number of neurons gives more precision, it requires a very long time for data processing, and it is preferable to choose neural networks that provide an adequate solution about the issues regarding the accuracy of the outputs and the time allocated for processing [80].

The analysis of the covariance and correlation between signals allows the identification of biomedical signals that can be used in the predictive ANN applications for medical alert systems to send alerts if the regression at time *t* has a different value from the regression recorded in the analysis of signals taken from patients with no seizures activity [80].

The proposed methods showed promising results compared to other state-of-the-art methods. Our method opens new perspectives to the successful automatic detection of epileptic seizures before onset, enabling a real-time brain monitoring wearable system.

In the future, we plan to apply this method to epileptic signal detection on wearable devices. Our next research object is to develop a successful seizure forecasting model by analyzing, in addition, heart electrical activity (ECG).

Author Contributions: Conceptualization, R.M.A.; methodology, R.M.A.; software, R.M.A.; validation, R.M.A.; formal analysis, R.M.A., S.P., and A.F.; investigation, R.M.A.; writing—original draft preparation, R.M.A.; writing—review and editing, R.M.A. and A.F.; visualization, R.M.A.; supervision, S.P. and A.F.; project administration, R.M.A., A.F., and S.P.; and funding acquisition, A.F. All authors have read and agreed to the published version of the manuscript.

Funding: This research received no external funding.

Conflicts of Interest: The authors declare no conflict of interest.

References

1. Hammad, M.; Pławiak, P.; Wang, K.; Acharya, U.R. ResNet-Attention model for human authentication using ECG signals. *Expert Syst.* **2020**, e12547. [CrossRef]
2. Tuncer, T.; Ertam, F.; Dogan, S.; Aydemir, E.; Pławiak, P. Ensemble residual network-based gender and activity recognition method with signals. *J. Supercomput.* **2020**, *76*, 2119–2138. [CrossRef]
3. Pławiak, P.; Acharya, U.R. Novel deep genetic ensemble of classifiers for arrhythmia detection using ECG signals. *Neural Comput. Appl.* **2019**, 1–25. [CrossRef]
4. Tuncer, T.; Dogan, S.; Pławiak, P.; Acharya, U.R. Automated arrhythmia detection using novel hexadecimal local pattern and multilevel wavelet transform with ECG signals. *Knowl. Based Syst.* **2019**, *186*, 104923. [CrossRef]
5. Pławiak, P.; Tadeusiewicz, R. Approximation of phenol concentration using novel hybrid computational intelligence methods. *Int. J. Appl. Math. Comput. Sci.* **2014**, *24*, 165–181. [CrossRef]
6. Kandala, R.N.; Dhuli, R.; Pławiak, P.; Naik, G.R.; Moeinzadeh, H.; Gargiulo, G.D.; Gunnam, S. Towards Real-Time Heartbeat Classification: Evaluation of Nonlinear Morphological Features and Voting Method. *Sensors* **2019**, *19*, 5079. [CrossRef] [PubMed]
7. Alqatawneh, A.; Alhalaseh, R.; Hassanat, A.; Abbadi, M. Statistical-Hypothesis-Aided Tests for Epilepsy Classification. *Computers* **2019**, *8*, 84. [CrossRef]
8. Chenane, K.; Touati, Y.; Boubchir, L.; Daachi, B. Neural Net-Based Approach to EEG Signal Acquisition and Classification. *BCI Appl. Comput.* **2019**, *8*, 87.
9. Borghini, G.; Aricò, P.; Di Flumeri, G.; Sciaraffa, N.; Babiloni, F. Correlation and similarity between cerebral and non-cerebral electrical activity for user's states assessment. *Sensors* **2019**, *19*, 704. [CrossRef] [PubMed]
10. Usami, K.; Matsumoto, R.; Sawamoto, N.; Murakami, H.; Inouchi, M.; Fumuro, T.; Shimotake, A.; Kato, T.; Mima, T.; Shirozu, H.; et al. Epileptic network of hypothalamic hamartoma: An EEG-fMRI study. *Epilepsy Res.* **2016**, *125*, 1–9. [CrossRef] [PubMed]

11. Übeyli, E.D.; Cvetkovic, D.; Cosic, I. AR spectral analysis technique for human PPG, ECG and EEG signals. *J. Med. Syst.* **2008**, *32*, 201–206. [CrossRef] [PubMed]
12. Bonita, J.D.; Ambolode, L.C.C.; Rosenberg, B.M.; Cellucci, C.J.; Watanabe, T.A.A.; Rapp, P.; Albano, A.M. Time domain measures of inter-channel EEG correlations: A comparison of linear, nonparametric and nonlinear measures. *Cogn. Neurodyn.* **2013**, *8*, 1–15. [CrossRef] [PubMed]
13. Mirowski, P.; Madhavan, D.; LeCun, Y.; Kuzniecky, R. Classification of patterns of EEG synchronization for seizure prediction. *Clin. Neurophysiol.* **2009**, *120*, 1927–1940. [CrossRef]
14. Kuhlmann, L.; Freestone, D.R.; Lai, A.; Burkitt, A.N.; Fuller, K.; Grayden, D.B.; Seiderer, L.; Vogrin, S.; Mareels, I.; Cook, M.J. Patient-specific bivariate-synchrony-based seizure prediction for short prediction horizons. *Epilepsy Res.* **2010**, *91*, 214–231. [CrossRef] [PubMed]
15. Shibasaki, H.; Rothwell, J.C.; Deuschl, G.; Eisen, A.; EMG-EEG Correlation. Recommendations for the practice of Clinical Neurophysiology: Guidelines of the International Federation of Clinical Neurophysiology. Electroenceph Clin Neurophysiol. Electroenceph. *Clin. Neurophysiol. Suppl.* **1999**, *52*, 269–274.
16. Williamson, J.R.; Bliss, D.W.; Browne, D.W.; Narayanan, J.T. Seizure prediction using EEG spatiotemporal correlation structure. *Epilepsy Behav.* **2012**, *25*, 230–238. [CrossRef]
17. Sharma, A.; Rai, J.K.; Tewari, R.P. Multivariate EEG signal analysis for early prediction of epileptic seizure. In Proceedings of the 2015 2nd International Conference on Recent Advances in Engineering & Computational Sciences (RAECS), Chandigarh, India, 21–22 December 2015.
18. Teixeira, C.; Direito, B.; Bandarabadi, M.; Le Van Quyen, M.; Valderrama, M.; Schelter, B.; Schulze-Bonhage, A.; Navarro, V.; Sales, F.; Dourado, A. Epileptic seizure predictors based on computational intelligence techniques: A comparative study with 278 patients. *Comput. Methods Programs Biomed.* **2014**, *114*, 324–336. [CrossRef] [PubMed]
19. Buchbinder, M. Neural imaginaries and clinical epistemology: Rhetorically mapping the adolescent brain in the clinical encounter. *Soc. Sci. Med.* **2014**, *143*, 304–310. [CrossRef] [PubMed]
20. Bandarabadi, M.; Teixeira, C.; Rasekhi, J.; Dourado, A. Epileptic seizure prediction using relative spectral power features. *Clin. Neurophysiol.* **2015**, *126*, 237–248. [CrossRef]
21. Smith, S.J.M. EEG in the diagnosis, classification, and management of patients with epilepsy. *J. Neurol. Neurosurg. Psychiatry* **2005**, *76*, ii2–ii7. [CrossRef]
22. Costa, R.P.; Oliveira, P.; Rodrigues, G.; Leitao, B.; Dourado, A. Epileptic seizure classification using neural networks with 14 features. In Proceedings of the International Conference on Knowledge-Based and Intelligent Information and Engineering Systems, Budapest, Hungary, 3–5 September 2008; Springer: Berlin, Germany.
23. Damayanti, A.; Pratiwi, A.B. Epilepsy detection on EEG data using backpropagation, firefly algorithm, and simulated annealing. In Proceedings of the 2nd International Conference on Science and Technology-Computer (ICST), Yogyakarta, Indonesia, 27–28 October 2016.
24. Aldabbagh, A.M.; Alshebeili, S.A.; Alotaiby, T.N.; Abd-Elsamie, F.E. Low computational complexity EEG epilepsy data classification algorithm for patients with intractable seizures. In Proceedings of the 2015 2nd International Conference on Biomedical Engineering (ICoBE), Penang, Malaysia, 30–31 March 2015.
25. Harikumar, R.; Shanmugam, A.; Rajan, P. VLSI Synthesis of Heterogeneous and SIRM Fuzzy System for Classification of Diabetic Epilepsy Risk Levels. In Proceedings of the 2008 Cairo International Biomedical Engineering Conference, Cairo, Egypt, 18–20 December 2008.
26. Quintero-Rincón, A.; Prendes, J.; Pereyra, M.; Batatia, H.; Risk, M. Multivariate Bayesian classification of epilepsy EEG signals. In Proceedings of the IEEE 12th Image, Video, and Multidimensional Signal Processing Workshop (IVMSP), Bordeaux, France, 11–12 July 2016.
27. Despre Electroencefalografie. Ce Diagnostice Poate Descoperi? Available online: http://www.unicare.ro/blog/despre-electroencefalografie-ce-diagnostice-poate-descoperi.htm (accessed on 15 December 2017).
28. Kreuzer, M. EEG based monitoring of general anesthesia: Taking the next steps. *Front. Comput. Neurosci.* **2017**, *11*, 56. [CrossRef]
29. Jameson, L.C.; Sloan, T.B. Using EEG to monitor anesthesia drug effects during surgery. *J. Clin. Monit.* **2006**, *20*, 445–472. [CrossRef]
30. Takeda, Y.; Inoue, Y.; Tottori, T.; Mihara, T. Acute psychosis during intracranial EEG monitoring: Close relationship between psychotic symptoms and discharges in amygdala. *Epilepsia* **2001**, *42*, 719–724. [CrossRef]

31. Gandelman-Marton, R.; Kimiagar, I.; Itzhaki, A.; Klein, C.; Theitler, J.; Rabey, J.M. Electroencephalography findings in adult patients with West Nile virus—associated meningitis and meningoencephalitis. *Clin. Infect. Dis.* **2003**, *37*, 1573–1578. [CrossRef]
32. Yi, G.-S.; Jiang, W.; Bin, D.; Xi-Le, W. Complexity of resting-state EEG activity in the patients with early-stage Parkinson's disease. *Cogn. Neurodyn.* **2017**, *2*, 147–160. [CrossRef] [PubMed]
33. Dauwels, J.; Francois, V.; Andrzej, C. Diagnosis of Alzheimer's disease from EEG signals: Where are we standing? *Curr. Alzheimer Res.* **2010**, *7*, 487–505. [CrossRef]
34. Melissant, C.; Alexander, Y.; Edward, E.F.; Cornelis, J.S. A method for detection of Alzheimer's disease using ICA-enhanced EEG measurements. *Artif. Intell. Med.* **2005**, *33*, 209–222. [CrossRef] [PubMed]
35. Jeong, J. EEG dynamics in patients with Alzheimer's disease. *Clin. Neurophysiol.* **2004**, *115*, 1490–1505. [CrossRef]
36. Deng, B.; Li, L.; Shunan, L.; Ruofan, W.; Haitao, Y.; Jiang, W.; Xile, W. Complexity extraction of electroencephalograms in Alzheimer's disease with weighted-permutation entropy. *Chaos Interdiscip. J. Nonlinear Sci.* **2015**, *25*, 043105. [CrossRef]
37. Bonanni, L.; Astrid, T.; Pietro, T.; Bernardo, P.; Sara, V.; Marco, O. EEG comparisons in early Alzheimer's disease, dementia with Lewy bodies and Parkinson's disease with dementia patients with a 2-year follow-up. *Brain* **2008**, *131*, 690–705. [CrossRef]
38. Kumar, S.S.P.; Ajitha, L. Early detection of epilepsy using EEG signals. In Proceedings of the International Conference on Control, Instrumentation, Communication, and Computational Technologies (ICCICCT), Kanyakumari, India, 10–11 July 2014; pp. 1509–1514.
39. Ahmad, M.Z.; Saeed, M.; Saleem, S.; Kamboh, A.M. Seizure detection using EEG: A survey of different techniques. In Proceedings of the International Conference on Emerging Technologies (ICET), Islamabad, Pakistan, 18–19 October 2016; pp. 1–6.
40. Al-Omar, S.; Kamali, W.; Khalil, M.; Daher, A. Classification of EEG signals to detect epilepsy problems. In Proceedings of the 2nd International Conference on Advances in Biomedical Engineering, Tripoli, Lebanon, 11–13 September 2013; pp. 5–8.
41. Sun, Z.; Wang, G.; Li, K.; Zhang, Z.; Bao, G. Cerebral functional connectivity analysis based on scalp EEG in epilepsy patients. In Proceedings of the 7th International Conference on Biomedical Engineering and Informatics, Dalian, China, 14–16 October 2014; pp. 283–287.
42. David, A.S.; Ruth, A.G. Neuropsychological study of motor neuron disease. *Psychosomatics* **1986**, *27*, 441–445. [CrossRef]
43. Lesný, I. Study in Different Forms of Cerebral Palsy. *Dev. Med. Child Neurol.* **2008**, *5*, 593–602. [CrossRef]
44. Screens, Tests and Evaluations. Available online: http://www.cerebralpalsy.org/about-cerebral-palsy/diagnosis/evaluations (accessed on 15 December 2017).
45. Şenbil, N.; Birkan, S.; Ömer, F.A.; Yahya, K.Y.G. Epileptic and non-epileptic cerebral palsy: EEG and cranial imaging findings. *Brain Dev.* **2002**, *24*, 166–169. [CrossRef]
46. Anderson, J.L.; Stewart, I.H.; Rae, C.; Morley, J.W. Brain function in Duchenne muscular dystrophy. *Brain* **2002**, *125*, 4–13. [CrossRef]
47. Electroencephalogram (EEG). Available online: https://www.nhs.uk/conditions/electroencephalogram (accessed on 12 February 2020).
48. Chen, D.; Wan, S.; Xiang, J.; Bao, F.S. A high-performance seizure detection algorithm based on Discrete Wavelet Transform (DWT) and EEG. *PLoS ONE* **2017**, *12*, e0173138. [CrossRef]
49. Terzano, M.G.; Parrino, L.; Smerieri, A.; Chervin, R.; Chokroverty, S.; Guilleminault, C.; Hirshkowitz, M.; Mahowald, M.; Moldofsky, H.; Rosa, A.; et al. Atlas, rules, and recording techniques for the scoring of cyclic alternating pattern (CAP) in human sleep. *Sleep Med.* **2002**, *3*, 187–199. [CrossRef]
50. Goldberger, A.L.; Amaral, L.; Glass, L.; Hausdorff, J.M.; Ivanov, P.C.; Mark, R.G.; Mietus, J.; Moody, G.B.; Peng, C.K.; Stanley, H. PhysioBank, PhysioToolkit, and PhysioNet: Components of a new research resource for complex physiologic signals. *Circulations* **2000**, *101*, e215–e220. [CrossRef]
51. Mingai, L.; Shuoda, G.; Guoyu, Z.; Yanjun, S.; Jinfu, Y. Removing ocular artifacts from mixed EEG signals with FastKICA and DWT. *J. Intell. Fuzzy Syst.* **2015**, *28*, 2851–2861. [CrossRef]
52. Real-Time Meditation Feedback. Available online: http://www.choosemuse.com (accessed on 20 April 2018).
53. Faust, O.; Acharya, R.U.; Adeli, H.; Adeli, A. Wavelet-based EEG processing for computer-aided seizure detection and epilepsy diagnosis. *Seizure* **2015**, *26*, 56–64. [CrossRef]

54. Ren, L.; Kucewicz, M.T.; Cimbalnik, J.; Matsumoto, J.Y.; Brinkmann, B.H.; Hu, W.; Worrell, G.A. Gamma oscillations precede interictal epileptiform spikes in the seizure onset zone. *Neurology* **2015**, *84*, 602–608. [CrossRef]
55. Al-Qazzaz, N.K.; Hamid Bin Mohd Ali, S.; Ahmad, S.A.; Islam, M.S.; Escudero, J. Selection of mother wavelet functions for multi-channel EEG signal analysis during a working memory task. *Sensors* **2015**, *15*, 29015–29035. [CrossRef] [PubMed]
56. Haddad, T.; Ben-Hamida, N.; Talbi, L.; Lakhssassi, A.; Aouini, S. Temporal epilepsy seizures monitoring and prediction using cross-correlation and chaos theory. *Healthc. Technol. Lett.* **2014**, *1*, 45–50. [CrossRef] [PubMed]
57. Orosco, L.; Correa, A.G.; Diez, P.F.; Laciar, E. Patient non-specific algorithm for seizures detection in scalp EEG. *Comput. Boil. Med.* **2016**, *71*, 128–134. [CrossRef]
58. Graps, A. An introduction to wavelets. *IEEE Comput. Sci. Eng.* **1995**, *2*, 50–61. [CrossRef]
59. Fergus, P.; Hussain, A.; Hignett, D.; Al-Jumeily, D.; Abdel-Aziz, K.; Hamdan, H. A machine learning system for automated whole-brain seizure detection. *Appl. Comput. Inform.* **2016**, *12*, 70–89. [CrossRef]
60. Subasi, A.; Ercelebi, E. Classification of EEG signals using neural network and logistic regression. *Comput. Methods Programs Biomed.* **2005**, *78*, 87–99. [CrossRef]
61. Ramgopal, S.; Thomé-Souza, S.; Jackson, M.; Kadish, N.E.; Fernández, I.S.; Klehm, J.; Bosl, W.; Reinsberger, C.; Schachter, S.; Loddenkemper, T. Seizure detection, seizure prediction, and closed-loop warning systems in epilepsy. *Epilepsy Behav.* **2014**, *37*, 291–307. [CrossRef]
62. Jeppesen, J.; Beniczky, S.; Johansen, P.; Sidenius, P.; Fuglsang-Frederiksen, A. Detection of epileptic seizures with a modified heart rate variability algorithm based on Lorenz plot. *Seizure* **2015**, *24*, 1–7. [CrossRef]
63. Osorio, I.; Manly, B.F.J. Probability of detection of clinical seizures using heart rate changes. *Seizure* **2015**, *30*, 120–123. [CrossRef]
64. Stefanidou, M.; Carlson, C.; Friedman, D. The relationship between seizure onset zone and ictal tachycardia: An intracranial EEG study. *Clin. Neurophysiol.* **2015**, *126*, 2255–2260. [CrossRef]
65. Vandecasteele, K.; De Cooman, T.; Gu, Y.; Cleeren, E.; Claes, K.; Van Paesschen, W.; Van Huffel, S.; Hunyadi, B. Automated Epileptic Seizure Detection Based on Wearable ECG and PPG in a Hospital Environment. *Sensors* **2017**, *17*, 2338. [CrossRef]
66. Seidenberg, M.; Pulsipher, D.; Hermann, B. Association of epilepsy and comorbid conditions. *Future Neurol.* **2009**, *4*, 663–668. [CrossRef]
67. Pellock, J.M. Understanding co-morbidities affecting children with epilepsy. *Neurology* **2004**, *62*, S17–S23. [CrossRef]
68. Zaccara, G. Neurological comorbidity and epilepsy: Implications for treatment. *Acta Neurol. Scand.* **2009**, *120*, 1–15. [CrossRef]
69. Zhou, M.; Tian, C.; Cao, R.; Wang, B.; Niu, Y.; Hu, T.; Guo, H.; Xiang, J. Epileptic Seizure Detection Based on EEG Signals and CNN. *Front. Aging Neurosci.* **2018**, *12*, 95. [CrossRef]
70. Shoeb, A.H.; Guttag, J.V. Application of machine learning to epileptic seizure detection. In Proceedings of the International Conference on Machine Learning (Haifa), Haifa, Israel, 21–24 June 2010; pp. 975–982.
71. Patnaik, L.; Manyam, O.K. Epileptic EEG detection using neural networks and post-classification. *Comput. Methods Programs Biomed.* **2008**, *91*, 100–109. [CrossRef]
72. Ebrahimpour, R.; Babakhan, K.; Arani, S.A.A.A.; Masoudnia, S. Epileptic seizure detection using a neural network ensemble method and wavelet transform. *Neural Netw. World* **2012**, *22*, 291. [CrossRef]
73. Akareddy, S.M.; Kulkarni, P. EEG signal classification for Epilepsy Seizure Detection using Improved Approximate Entropy. *Int. J. Public Health Sci. (IJPHS)* **2013**, *2*. [CrossRef]
74. Ullah, I.; Hussain, M.; Qazi, E.-U.-H.; Abualsamh, H.A. An automated system for epilepsy detection using EEG brain signals based on deep learning approach. *Expert Syst. Appl.* **2018**, *107*, 61–71. [CrossRef]
75. Acharya, U.R.; Oh, S.L.; Hagiwara, Y.; Tan, J.H.; Adeli, H. Deep convolutional neural network for the automated detection and diagnosis of seizure using EEG signals. *Comput. Boil. Med.* **2018**, *100*, 270–278. [CrossRef]
76. Acharya, U.R.; Yanti, R.; Swapna, G.; Sree, V.S.; Martis, R.J.; Suri, J.S. Automated diagnosis of epileptic electroencephalogram using independent component analysis and discrete wavelet transform for different electroencephalogram durations. *Proc. Inst. Mech. Eng. Part H J. Eng. Med.* **2012**, *227*, 234–244. [CrossRef]

77. Machado, F.; Sales, F.; Santos, C.; Dourado, A.; Teixeira, C. A knowledge discovery methodology from EEG data for cyclic alternating pattern detection. *Biomed. Eng. Online* **2018**, *17*, 185. [CrossRef] [PubMed]
78. Mousavi, S.; Afghah, F.; Acharya, U.R. SleepEEGNet: Automated sleep stage scoring with sequence to sequence deep learning approach. *PLoS ONE* **2019**, *14*, e0216456. [CrossRef] [PubMed]
79. Perslev, M.; Jensen, M.; Darkner, S.; Jennum, P.; Igel, C. U-time: A fully convolutional network for time series segmentation applied to sleep staging. In Proceedings of the Advances in Neural Information Processing Systems (NeurIPS 2019), Vancouve, BC, Canada, 8–14 December 2019.
80. Maria, A.R. Correlation Analysis of Biomedical Signals for Predictive Modeling. Master's Thesis, Politehnica University of Bucharest, București, Romania, 2019.

© 2020 by the authors. Licensee MDPI, Basel, Switzerland. This article is an open access article distributed under the terms and conditions of the Creative Commons Attribution (CC BY) license (http://creativecommons.org/licenses/by/4.0/).

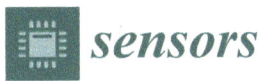

Article

Cost-efficient and Custom Electrode-holder Assembly Infrastructure for EEG Recordings

Yuan-Pin Lin [1,*], Ting-Yu Chen [1,†] and Wei-Jen Chen [1,2,†]

1 Laboratory for Neuroergonomics, Institute of Medical Science and Technology, National Sun Yat-sen University, Kaohsiung 80424, Taiwan; tychen@imst.nsysu.edu.tw (T.-Y.C.); wjc@imst.nsysu.edu.tw (W.-J.C.)
2 Department of Computer Science and Engineering, National Sun Yat-sen University, Kaohsiung 80424, Taiwan
* Correspondence: yplin@mail.nsysu.edu.tw; Tel.: +886-7-5252-000 (ext. 5795)
† These authors contributed equally to this work.

Received: 3 August 2019; Accepted: 1 October 2019; Published: 2 October 2019

Abstract: Mobile electroencephalogram (EEG)-sensing technologies have rapidly progressed and made the access of neuroelectrical brain activity outside the laboratory in everyday life more realistic. However, most existing EEG headsets exhibit a fixed design, whereby its immobile montage in terms of electrode density and coverage inevitably poses a great challenge with applicability and generalizability to the fundamental study and application of the brain-computer interface (BCI). In this study, a cost-efficient, custom EEG-electrode holder infrastructure was designed through the assembly of primary components, including the sensor-positioning ring, inter-ring bridge, and bridge shield. It allows a user to (re)assemble a compact holder grid to accommodate a desired number of electrodes only to the regions of interest of the brain and iteratively adapt it to a given head size for optimal electrode-scalp contact and signal quality. This study empirically demonstrated its easy-to-fabricate nature by a low-end fused deposition modeling (FDM) 3D printer and proved its practicability of capturing event-related potential (ERP) and steady-state visual-evoked potential (SSVEP) signatures over 15 subjects. This paper highlights the possibilities for a cost-efficient electrode-holder assembly infrastructure with replaceable montage, flexibly retrofitted in an unlimited fashion, for an individual for distinctive fundamental EEG studies and BCI applications.

Keywords: mobile EEG recordings; montage-replaceable headsets; BCI

1. Introduction

Mobile electroencephalogram (EEG)-sensing technologies has rapidly progressed and made the access of neuroelectrical brain activity outside the laboratory in everyday life more realistic. The integrity of mobile systems by various manufacturers has been thoroughly validated and reported [1–3]. Owing to its interesting advantages of price, usability, and mobility, a considerable number of recent studies has emerged highlighting the aforementioned advantages to encourage the study of EEG correlates of brain states and functions in multidisciplinary domains, such as preliminary perception (e.g., visual/auditory responses [4–6]), cognition capacity (e.g., attention relocation [7,8], face recognition [1], and memory processing [9,10]), and psychological reaction (e.g., affective response [11,12], mental fatigue [13], and working stress [14]). The exploited state-/task-related EEG associations can be further leveraged with machine learning to underpin a mobile brain-computer interface (BCI) for a vast range of applications, such as rehabilitative exoskeleton control [15], visual function loss [16], attentional responses [17], lapse mitigation [18], quadcopter control [19], and visual-search games [20]. To this end, a mobile EEG device that enables a valid and reliable measurement of EEG signals over the brain is highly demanded and can play a vital role toward mobile BCI applications in real-world scenarios.

Several research-grade and consumer-oriented mobile EEG devices are available in the market, such as Quick/Mobile series (Cognionics, Inc., San Diego, CA, USA), ENOBIO series (Neuroelectrics, Barcelona, Spain), Smarting (mBrainTrain, Inc., Belgrade, Serbia), Ultracortex (OpenBCI, Inc., Brooklyn, New York, USA), EPOC (Emotiv, Inc., San Francisco, California, USA), and MindWare (NeuroSky, Inc., San Jose, CA, USA). Their general technical specifications or other devices can be referred to [2,8,21]. As compared to conventional bulk, tethered systems in laboratory, the mobile system shares common features with miniaturized light-weight amplifier, wireless telemetry, and/or dry/gel/saline electrodes, facilitating the applicability of EEG recording with more naturalistic settings (e.g., non-stationary subjects [5,17]). Aside from commercial products, continuous research effort has been invested in hardware innovation from the aspects of enhancing signal quality, device usability and mobility, cost efficiency, and practical applicability. Most endeavors have been directed to the counterparts of dry electrode [6,22–28], signal amplifier [4,8,22,29–31], and standalone computing [30]. Many commercial or customized mobile devices can be useful and provide acceptable/promising signal quality for specific circumstances. Along with signal validity and reliability, the selection of a mobile device should also consider the electrode montage in terms of the number of electrodes and their positions on the scalp [21]. It is essential to confirm whether its headset coverage offers signal accessibility to the brain regions of interest in an EEG study as well as a BCI task that is to be performed. Given the diversity of manufacturers, electrode density and coverage vary widely, from one single electrode over a single brain region (e.g., NeuroSky MindWare) to high-density electrodes with a whole-brain coverage (e.g., Cognionics Mobile-64/-128). A low-density example may constrain usability because of the sparseness or absence of electrodes over certain brain regions (e.g., Emotiv EPOC does not contain midline electrodes), whereas a high-density example can provide an ideal setting but inevitably poses a financial barrier and time-consuming preparation. The most critical issue is that a whole-brain coverage is plausibly with the presence of a large number of redundant electrodes as long as a specific BCI task is concerned, such as non-posterior electrodes for steady-state visual-evoke potential (SSVEP) [32] and non-sensorimotor electrodes for motor imagery (MI) [33]. The electrode placements for both the low- and high-density headsets are typically designed in an immobile manner. As such, customized headsets made of auxiliary cables, rack/stripe, headband, or soft/elastic cap have been used to secure electrodes for a specific application [8,18,20,26,33,34]. Up until recently, OpenBCI Ultracortex Mark series has gained much attention in the community and can be considered as the state-of-the-art headset frame. It enables to change the montage to a certain extent by voluntarily placing a desired number of electrodes on to a fixed, 3D-printed 35-location frame. Yet, the headset may have redundant electrode holders in use. Moreover, the design of a rigid frame or soft cap in commercial products does not ideally fit well to distinctive head sizes and shapes of individuals in different age groups. A feasible remedy is to offer a headset with different sizes, suitable for a desired range of head circumference (e.g., OpenBCI Ultracortex Mark series and Neuroelectrics ENOBIO series). It is reasonably expected that an inappropriate headset size may compromise the sensor locations and their contact to the scalp, thereby downgrading signal quality to a certain extent. Taken together, a headset with an immobile sensor-holder structure of electrode density and coverage may pose a great challenge with applicability and generalizability to both commercial and custom mobile EEG devices. To date, headsets in the market do not offer a flexible headset frame with a customable montage design.

Therefore, in this study, an electrode-holder assembly infrastructure for EEG recordings was developed, which allows a user to (re)assemble a compact holder grid to accommodate a desired number of electrodes to the brain regions of interest in an unlimited fashion, in accordance to the EEG and BCI study of interest to be performed. During the assembly, the formed headset can iteratively adapt to a given head size and shape, practically ensuring electrode-scalp contact and signal quality. All the conceived assembly elements (e.g., sensor-positioning ring, inter-ring bridge, and bridge shield) were manufactured via a low-end consumer 3D printer and the practicability of the assembled headset was validated through the study of event-related potentials (ERP) and steady-state visual evoked potential (SSVEP) tasks. This study demonstrated exceptional possibilities for a cost-efficient electrode-holder assembly infrastructure with replaceable montage retrofitted for an individual in unlimited manner, for distinctive fundamental EEG investigations and BCI applications.

2. Materials and Methods

2.1. Design and Practice of Sensor-holder Assembly Infrastructure

The assembly infrastructure developed in this study has the following practical benefits for EEG recording as well as BCI deployment. First, the infrastructure allows (re)assembling without limit to accommodate a desired number of electrodes over brain regions of interest, leading to a compact headset without the need for redundant electrodes attached to the head (i.e., saving cost, weight, and calibration time, and improving wearability and comfort). In addition, the infrastructure is capable of optimally retrofitting the headset to a certain head size/circumference for each individual during assembly. This provides the advantage of not only positioning the sensors over the target brain regions as consistently as possible for different age groups in the same study or task but also ensuring the attached electrodes to be in good contact with the scalp for better signal quality. As such, the proposed infrastructure can be considered a design of multi-purpose, with a montage-replaceable headset to record EEG signals from only the brain regions of interest.

The assembled infrastructure was conceived to compose of three primary components including sensor positioning ring, inter-ring bridge, and bridge shield (as shown in Figure 1A). The positioning ring is used to place an EEG electrode, whereas the inter-ring bridge is utilized to assemble a plurality of the rings in a desired montage. The bridge shield covers an assembled junction of the ring and bridge, thereby fastening the connection (i.e., prevent them from falling apart in use). The positioning ring can be fabricated to the required shape and size to comply with the specifications of different EEG sensors. The present form was designed to better accommodate the adopted dry flex electrodes (Cognionics, Inc., San Diego, CA, USA). Analogously, the inter-ring bridge can work in different lengths and curvatures, such that the assembly holders naturally form a desired 3D grid to fit the head size. The bridge and shield were designed empirically to be able to quickly assemble positioning rings to be connected or disassemble them. By leveraging supplementary counterparts of ear and chin strips and holders, a user can easily wear an assembled headset on his/her head or disassemble it. Figure 1B illustrates four plausible embodiments of the proposed holder assembly (simulated by 3D design software) to measure the EEG signals from the entire scalp or individual brain regions of interest, e.g., frontal, sensorimotor, and occipital parts.

To demonstrate the practicality, an 8-electrode holder grid was implemented to accommodate EEG electrodes over the fronto-central midline and parieto-occipital regions (four for each region, as shown in Figure 2A), in accordance with the signal amplifier and experimental tasks employed in this study (described in the later subsections). Note that a supplementary component of tiny bridge extender (blue) was also implemented for the assembly demonstration. The extender shows the capability to prolong a bridge by concatenating multiples bridges if the bridge in a desired length is unavailable. All the assembled components were fabricated by a low-end fused deposition modeling (FDM) 3D printer (layer resolution of 0.3–0.4 mm applied with 100% infill) using polylactide (PLA) or ethylene vinyl acetate (EVA) filaments. The PLA was used to print the stiff positioning ring, whereas the EVA was used to print the bridge and shield in a bendable/flexible manner. The printed components could work supposedly as long as possible in normal use. The Cognionics dry flex electrodes, which were made by Ag/AgCl-covered elastomer, were adopted for EEG measurement. Referring to Figure 2B, the midline locations include Fz, FCz, Cz, and CPz (orange rings), whereas the posterior counterparts include Pz, O1, Oz, and O2 (blue rings). A few auxiliary rings (black), embedding non-conductive comfort pads, were also assembled to further improve wearability. Figure 2C demonstrates the practice of the assembled 8-ch EEG headset wore on an adult head at different view angles. In the present demonstration, the positioning ring inserted a supplementary component of electrode adapter to snap the dry electrode via snap fastener. That is, the adaptor can be made in various forms to accommodate desired electrodes in the market. In detail, the 8-electrode grid was assembled within around 15 minutes by 16 rings (electrode: 8, comfort pad: 8), 27 bridges (11 mm: 14, 13 mm: 9, 40 mm: 2, 50 mm: 2), and 54 shields, which cost less than 5 USD for the filaments.

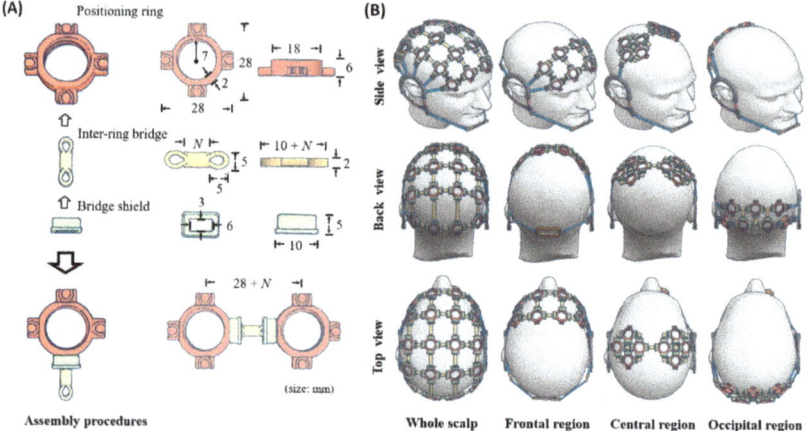

Figure 1. Illustration of the developed electrode-holder assembly infrastructure. (**A**) Three primary components and their assembly procedures. The sizes are in millimeter (N = 11, 13, 40, and 50 used in this work); (**B**) four assembly embodiments with coverages of the entire scalp and individual regions of interest (simulated by 3D design software).

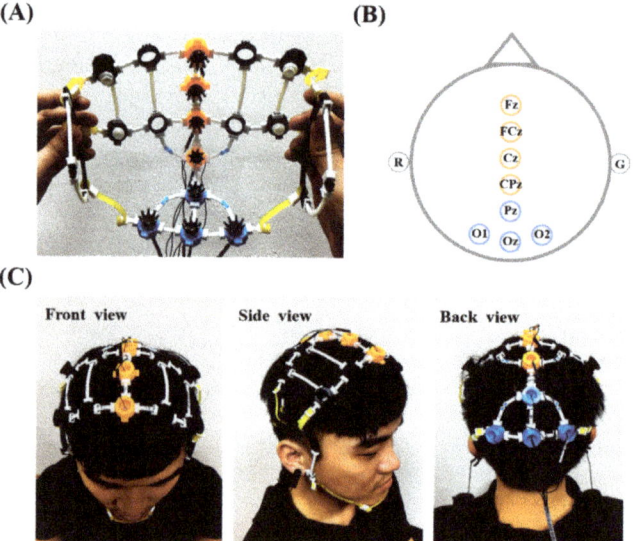

Figure 2. Implementation of an 8-electrode holder assembly grid. (**A**) Assembled headset embedded with Cognionics dry electrodes; (**B**) 8-channel montage; (**C**) headset wore on the head at different view angles.

2.2. EEG Recording

In this study, a portable, custom 8-ch EEG-sensing device [8] was employed to wire the assembled headset to measure the EEG signals. This device had been systematically validated by conducting a simultaneous EEG recording of three subjects in 10 day sessions. Successful measurement of weak, time-locked, and phase-locked ERP signals demonstrated its proficiency in terms of signal quality, reliability, and data-event synchronization. Briefly, its major technical specifications are as follows. This device was designed to measure up to eight channels of analog signal input, filter the signals in a bandwidth of 0.6–56.5 Hz, sample and quantize the signals at 250 Hz with a resolution of 10 bits, and wirelessly transmit the digitized streams (synchronized with events if any) via a typical Bluetooth communication protocol. More details can be found in [8] regarding hardware implementation and verification. The left and right earlobes were set to reference and ground sites, respectively, during recording.

2.3. Participants and Experimental Paradigms

Fifteen healthy participants (six males and nine females; age 22.4 ± 1.4 years.) were recruited to validate the practicability of the assembled electrode-holder grid. They were all students from the Colleges of Science and of Engineering and had normal hearing and normal or corrected-to-normal vision. Participants gave their written informed consent approved by Human Research Protections Program of the local ethics committee and received monetary compensation.

In this study, two stereotypical paradigms were conducted underpinning different modalities of visual perception and cognitive processing through SSVEP and oddball ERP protocols, respectively. These two tasks allowed us to assess the signal quality in terms of time- and phase-locked temporal (i.e., ERP amplitude) and spectral (i.e., SSVEP amplitude) context while wearing the assembled headset. The four central midline electrodes were intended to capture not only the N100 ERP (i.e., negative deflection in the voltage around 100–170 ms after stimulation onset) of early sensory perception but also the P300 ERP (i.e., positive deflection peak by 300–500 ms) for the endogenous process of attentional relocation, engaging in an oddball paradigm [8,35,36]. On the other hand, the four parieto-occipital electrodes attempted to capture frequency-coded responses of SSVEPs originating from the visual cortex that are synchronized to continuous, repetitive visual stimulation [32]. The rationale for performing both tasks was that if the assembled electrode-holder grid cannot integrate its numerous components of the positioning rings, inter-ring bridge, and bridge shields in a proficient structure and position the desired electrodes in a non-uniform curved surface across the head (e.g., fronto-central midline and posterior parts), poor contact for the attached electrodes will result, barely returning the prominent ERP and SSVEP characteristics from the group of 15 participants. The detailed parameters and procedures for the ERP and SSVEP task are depicted as follows.

2.3.1. Auditory Oddball ERP Paradigm

The oddball paradigm consisted of two pure tones in different occurrences. A high-pitched tone (1000 Hz) was infrequently formed (30%, called target tone) as compared to the frequently presented low-pitched tone (500 Hz, called standard tone). Both these tones lasted for 500 ms and were played through the speakers. Each participant was instructed to focus their gaze at the fixation cross located at the center on a 27" LCD monitor, attentively responding to the target tone by pressing a handheld button as fast as possible, while ignoring the frequent standard tone. The paradigm was composed of four blocks; each contained 100 trials with both tones in random order and with an inter-trial jitter of 0.5–1.5 s. The oddball paradigm for each participant corresponded to a total of 120 target trials versus 280 standard trials for sequential ERP analysis.

2.3.2. SSVEP Paradigm

Three repetitive black/white visual flickers (frequency: 10, 12, and 14 Hz; size 5.5 cm × 5.5 cm) located at the vertices of a triangle were presented on a 27-inch LCD monitor. A fixation cross at the triangle center (no flickering) was also presented as control. The participant was instructed to attentively gaze at the fixation cross or at one of the three flickers for four seconds in turn. The paradigm contained four 20-trial blocks; each block presented one of four visual targets five times in a random order. An auditory cure guided the participant to shift their gaze to the next target within an inter-trial duration of 2.5 s. The SSVEP task collected 80 trials (20 per target) from each participant.

During the recording, each participant sat comfortably on a chair in a dimly lit room. They underwent both the aforementioned tasks on different days in a random order. Each task lasted approximately 30 min, which comprised experiment briefing, headset capping, and data recording. The assembled headset was cleaned simply by a wet wipe with a bit of sanitizer before the capping. During the capping, the initial inter-ring bridges with respect to certain positioning rings could be replaced by different lengths for certain individuals because of a distinctive head size. In the meanwhile, the participant was informed about mild to moderate pressure needed for attaching dry electrodes well to the scalp. This procedure typically took 5–10 min to confirm the comfort and ensure the contact between the fronto-central midline and/or parieto-occipital electrodes and the scalp.

2.4. EEG Analysis

This study employed the following procedures to pre-process and analyze the collected ERP and SSVEP sessions, including (1) bandpass filtering (ERP: 1–30 Hz, SSVEP: 7–17 Hz), (2) trial segmentation (ERP: −0.2 to 1 s, SSVEP: 0 to 4 s), (3) trial analysis (ERP: synchronized averaging calculation, SSVEP: power spectral density (PSD) estimation, and (4) signal-to-noise (SNR) calculation on the peaks of interest (ERP: P300 amplitude, SSVEP: 10-, 12-, and 14-Hz amplitude). Other signal modality-specific parameters or steps are depicted below. Data preprocessing, analysis, and visualization were performed using the open source EEGLab toolbox/scripts [37] and self-custom scripts in MATLAB (The Mathworks, Inc., MA, USA).

2.4.1. ERP Analysis

Following trial segmentation, the trials containing extreme amplitudes (>±100 μV) or corresponding to erroneous behavioral responses were removed from further analysis (6.5 ± 0.1% trials discarded on average). In addition, the z-score standardization was applied to the averaged ERP profile of each individual prior to calculate the grand average ERP. The P300 SNR was derived by dividing the P300 peak amplitude (300–500 ms) by the standard deviation of the prestimulus baseline (−200 to 0 ms) as the procedure in [8,38]. Finally, a paired t-test was applied to assess the statistical difference in P300 SNR between the target versus non-target events.

2.4.2. SSVEP Analysis

Synchronized averaging calculation was also applied to the 4-s SSVEP trials corresponding to each of the visual targets after trial segmentation. The short-time Fourier transform (STFT) with 1-s Hamming window (with 80% overlap) was subsequently employed to estimate the EEG spectrogram with a frequency resolution of 1 Hz and yield the averaged PSDs across all time windows. Lastly, SSVEP SNR was defined by the ratio of spectral amplitude in the target frequency (10, 12, or 14 Hz) versus the mean amplitude of its six neighboring frequencies (i.e., three frequencies to each side), as referred to [39].

3. Results

Figure 3 presents the ERP outcome in terms of its temporal profile and P300 SNR for the auditory oddball paradigm. Figure 3A shows the ERP image from the representative subject, whereas Figure 3B,C summarize the ERP profile and P300 SNR of the 15 participants. Note that the ERP image visualizes single ERP trials and sorts them by button-press response time (RT) in ascending order. From the representative target ERP image (see Figure 3A), the salient P300 peak closely followed the RT (black trace) with a distinct amplitude. A longer RT tended to accompany a weaker amplitude and prolonged latency. On the contrary, the non-target ERP image did not exhibit the P300 peak. For the group analysis (see Figure 3B), the target event (red profile) exclusively and reliably elicited the P300 peak (at ~400 ms) against the non-target event (blue profile) for 15 participants, leading to a statistical significance in P300 SNR ($p < 0.01$). The N100 peak (at ~170 ms) time-locked to the stimulus onset was also seen for both events. The topographic mapping of P300 SNR further showed that the highest value was located at Pz as compared to other electrodes for the target event only (see Figure 3C).

Figure 4 shows the measured SSVEP signatures as exposed to frequency-coded visual flickers. Figure 4A,B present the temporal and spectral profiles from the representative subject, where Figure 4C presents the topographic mapping of SNR values over the 15 participants. The single-subject temporal profile was clearly associated with neural activity synchronized to the onset of the visual flickers at 10, 12, and 14 Hz (see Figure 4A). Their spectral profiles also exhibited salient peaks dominated at the corresponding frequencies (see Figure 4B). Furthermore, the topographic SNR mapping in Figure 4C showed that the occipital electrodes accompanied higher SNR values reactive to each of the visual flickers as compared to other electrodes, especially at Oz. Unlike the frequency-modulated flickers, the eye-gaze at the fixation cross barely led to frequency-synchronized neural modulation.

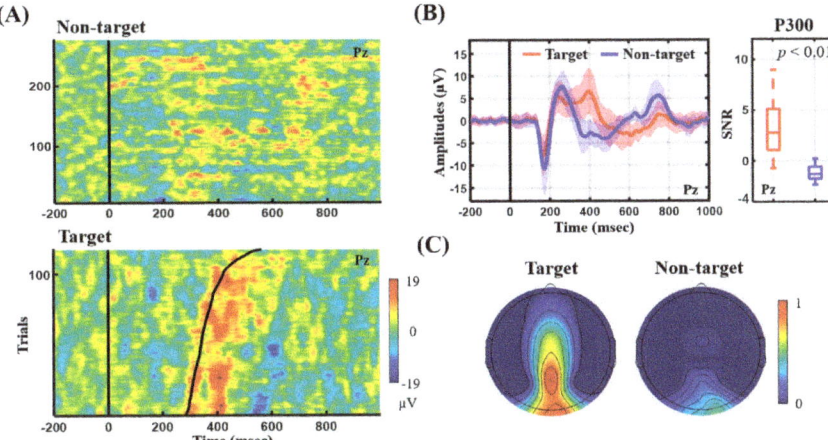

Figure 3. The ERP outcomes recorded in an auditory oddball ERP paradigm. (**A**) ERP images of Pz from a representative subject; (**B**) ERP profiles and P300 SNR (i.e., 300–500 ms) of Pz summarized by 15 participants; (**C**) averaged topographic mapping of P300 SNR using the adopted eight electrodes.

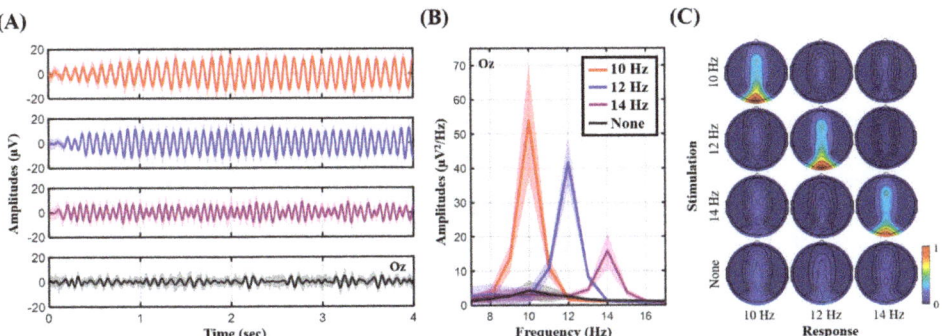

Figure 4. The SSVEP outcomes corresponding to frequency-coded visual flickers against fixation cross. (**A**) Temporal profiles of Oz from a representative subject; (**B**) spectral profiles of Oz from the same representative subject; (**C**) averaged 8-ch topographic mapping of SSVEP SNR using 4-s trials by 15 participants.

4. Discussion

In this study, an electrode-holder infrastructure was developed for EEG recordings through the assembly of three primary components, including sensor positioning ring, inter-ring bridge, and bridge shield. Given one assembly set, a user is able to self-assemble a headset with a desired montage to position electrodes at the brain regions of interest in unlimited manner for fundamental research as well as BCI applications. Whereas most existing headsets exhibit an immobile design, the proposed headset assembly accommodates the use of a compact set of electrodes placed over certain regions but removes other redundant electrodes or counterparts that are used for different purposes. During assembly, the formed 3D structure grid can be retrofitted iteratively to a given head size or shape of individuals in different age groups. In this way, the electrode-scalp contact can be optimized to ensure the signal quality accordingly as compared to that of an immobile headset with an unsuitable size. Most practically, this study demonstrated that the fabrication of the assembly structures can be accomplished using a low-cost FDM 3D printer, which is cheaper to custom manufacture than injection molding. Although the state-of-the-art OpenBCI Ultracortex Mark series is also a 3D-printed design and allows voluntarily placing the electrodes over default 35 locations, its headset frame is fixed (i.e., having redundant electrode holders in use) and only available in three head circumference sizes. Our assembly holder departed from the Ultracortex frame substantially with respect to unlimitedly (re)assembling of a compact holder grid for different purposes or even head sizes given one assembly set of the primary components (i.e., a LEGO-like headset) without additional cost. In addition, as assembling an Ultracortex-like headset frame, our design will cost only about 10 USD (using 35 rings, 58 bridges, and 116 shields) by PLA and EVA filaments. Aside from continuous innovation for electrode and amplifier technologies [4,6,8,22–31], this study contributed to a cost-efficient, montage-customable headset assembly infrastructure for a range of applications. It is worth noting that the proposed assembly grid has the capability of inserting a variety of commercial electrodes (i.e., electrode adaptor required) and wiring them to a commercial amplifier if a direct connection is feasible (e.g., OpenBCI Ganglion/Cyton biosensing board).

To validate the practicability of the conceived electrode-holder assembly, this study implemented an 8-ch electrode-holder grid embedded with Cognionics dry electrodes for incorporation with a portable, custom EEG amplifier [8] for EEG recordings. Its electrode coverage over the fronto-central midline and parieto-occipital regions was intended to capture the prominent ERP P300 and frequency-modulated signal peaks while engaging in the auditory oddball and SSVEP tasks, respectively. Given the EEG recordings of the 15 participants, the resultant ERP and SSVEP outcomes were in line with those found in the literature. From the ERP perspective (c.f., Figure 3), the target tones predominantly aroused the attention-related P300 amplitude, with the highest SNR over the parietal region at Pz [8,35,36]. The single-subject example further demonstrated a clear RT-modulated P300 profile consistently in [8]. In addition, both auditory tones corresponded to the N100 component, early component of exogenous stimulus detection [8,36]. From the SSVEP perspective (c.f., Figure 4), the occipital electrodes exclusively recorded strong SSVEP amplitudes corresponding to the targeted frequencies (Oz with the highest SNR), as SSVEP responses originate from the visual cortex and are synchronized to frequency-coded visual stimulation [5,13]. Taken together, the replication of the time-locked and phase-locked ERP and SSVEP signatures empirically demonstrated the satisfactory electrode-scalp contact and signal quality while wearing the proposed headset assembly for EEG recordings.

There are several possibilities or advantages far beyond the current demonstration of EEG recording. First, the sensor-holder ring can be fabricated with different specifications to organize either homogeneous/heterogeneous sensors or sensors and stimulators on the same headset, e.g., comparing EEG electrodes made by different materials at very adjacent sites [1,5,35,40], facilitating a simultaneous EEG and functional near-infrared spectroscopy (fNIR) recording over the brain regions of interest [31], and monitoring EEG activity while applying transcranial alternating current (TAC) stimulation [41]. In addition, the assembly structure is surely capable of being retrofitted to a head-mounted display system (e.g., AR/VR goggle), worn on the head for stand-alone application [16,19,42]. In contrast, a headset with an immobile design to an end user may make the above applications difficult to implement.

Although this study presented a promising start to a cost-efficient, montage-replaceable headset assembly in mobile EEG technologies, future effort should be devoted to further demonstrating and improving its robustness and generalizability. First, EEG recordings can be replicated on non-stationary subjects (e.g., walking on treadmill [5]). This will be a rigorous yet realistic setting to evaluate the behavior of the electrode-scalp contact under head movement conditions (e.g., bobbing or swaying) in walking. Furthermore, in constructing a truly multi-purpose assembly set with considerable wearability and comfort, it is essential to pay more attention to the mechanical properties of each of the assembled components, such as size, length, curvature, shape, material, and weight, and what should be included, at least for the capacity of retrofitting a desired montage from sparse to high-dense settings over distinct brain regions of interest. It is also helpful to have a guideline following the international 10–20 system of electrode placement. A holder grid can then be customized by selecting suitable components efficiently (e.g., inter-ring bridge noted with length) for distinctive brain regions of interest during assembly.

5. Conclusions

In this study, a cost-efficient, custom EEG-electrode holder infrastructure was developed through the assembly of primary components, including sensor positioning ring, inter-ring bridge, and bridge shield. For different studies or BCI tasks, the user can (re)assemble a compact holder grid in an unlimited fashion to accommodate a desired number of electrodes only to the brain regions of interest and iteratively adapt it to a given head size for optimal electrode-scalp contact and signal quality. This study empirically demonstrated the easy-to-fabricate nature of the infrastructure through a low-cost 3D printer and its practicability in measuring ERP and SSVEP signals was proven over studies with 15 participants. Through this study, a montage-replaceable headset tailored to be applicable for a variety of purposes was explored.

Author Contributions: Y.-P.L. developed the assembly infrastructure, conceived the EEG experiment and analysis, and wrote and revised the paper. T.-Y.C. conducted SSVEP experiment and analysis. W.-J.C. conducted ERP experiment and analysis.

Funding: This work was supported in part by the Collaborative Research of National Sun Yat-sen University and Kaohsiung Chang Gung Memorial Hospital, Taiwan, under Grant CMRPG8I0371.

Conflicts of Interest: The authors declare no conflict of interest.

References

1. Melnik, A.; Legkov, P.; Izdebski, K.; Karcher, S.M.; Hairston, W.D.; Ferris, D.P.; Konig, P. Systems, Subjects, Sessions: To What Extent Do These Factors Influence EEG Data? *Front. Hum. Neurosci.* **2017**, *11*, 150. [CrossRef] [PubMed]
2. Cruz-Garza, J.G.; Brantley, J.A.; Nakagome, S.; Kontson, K.; Megjhani, M.; Robleto, D.; Contreras-Vidal, J.L. Deployment of Mobile EEG Technology in an Art Museum Setting: Evaluation of Signal Quality and Usability. *Front. Hum. Neurosci.* **2017**, *11*, 527. [CrossRef] [PubMed]
3. Oliveira, A.S.; Schlink, B.R.; Hairston, W.D.; König, P.; Ferris, D.P. Proposing Metrics for Benchmarking Novel EEG Technologies Towards Real-World Measurements. *Front. Hum. Neurosci.* **2016**, *10*, 188. [CrossRef] [PubMed]
4. Valentin, O.; Ducharme, M.; Cretot-Richert, G.; Monsarrat-Chanon, H.; Viallet, G.; Delnavaz, A.; Voix, J. Validation and Benchmarking of a Wearable EEG Acquisition Platform for Real-World Applications. *IEEE Trans. Biomed. Circuits Syst.* **2019**, *13*, 103–111. [CrossRef] [PubMed]
5. Lin, Y.P.; Wang, Y.J.; Wei, C.S.; Jung, T.P. Assessing the quality of steady-state visual-evoked potentials for moving humans using a mobile electroencephalogram headset. *Front. Hum. Neurosci.* **2014**, *8*, 182. [CrossRef] [PubMed]

6. Kappel, S.L.; Rank, M.L.; Toft, H.O.; Andersen, M.; Kidmose, P. Dry-Contact Electrode Ear-EEG. *IEEE Trans. Biomed. Eng.* **2019**, *66*, 150–158. [CrossRef]
7. Krigolson, O.E.; Williams, C.C.; Norton, A.; Hassall, C.D.; Colino, F.L. Choosing MUSE: Validation of a Low-Cost, Portable EEG System for ERP Research. *Front. Neurosci.* **2017**, *11*, 109. [CrossRef]
8. Chuang, K.C.; Lin, Y.P. Cost-Efficient, Portable, and Custom Multi-Subject Electroencephalogram Recording System. *IEEE Access* **2019**, *7*, 56760–56769. [CrossRef]
9. Wang, S.Y.; Gwizdka, J.; Chaovalitwongse, W.A. Using Wireless EEG Signals to Assess Memory Workload in the n-Back Task. *IEEE Trans. Hum. Mach. Syst.* **2016**, *46*, 424–435. [CrossRef]
10. Park, J.L.; Donaldson, D.I. Detecting the neural correlates of episodic memory with mobile EEG: Recollecting objects in the real world. *Neuroimage* **2019**, *193*, 1–9. [CrossRef]
11. Katsigiannis, S.; Ramzan, N. DREAMER: A Database for Emotion Recognition Through EEG and ECG Signals from Wireless Low-cost Off-the-Shelf Devices. *IEEE J. Biomed. Health Inform.* **2018**, *22*, 98–107. [CrossRef] [PubMed]
12. Lin, Y.P.; Hsu, S.H.; Jung, T.P. Exploring Day-to-Day Variability in the Relations Between Emotion and EEG Signals. In Proceedings of the Foundations of Augmented Cognition: 9th International Conference, AC 2015, Held as Part of HCI International 2015, Los Angeles, CA, USA, 2–7 August 2015; Schmorrow, D.D., Fidopiastis, C.M., Eds.; Springer International Publishing: Cham, Switzerland, 2015; pp. 461–469.
13. Ruyi, F.; Kai Keng, A.; Zhuo, Z.; Chai, Q. An iterative cross-subject negative-unlabeled learning algorithm for quantifying passive fatigue. *J. Neural Eng.* **2019**, *16*, 056013.
14. Betti, S.; Lova, R.M.; Rovini, E.; Acerbi, G.; Santarelli, L.; Cabiati, M.; Ry, S.D.; Cavallo, F. Evaluation of an Integrated System of Wearable Physiological Sensors for Stress Monitoring in Working Environments by Using Biological Markers. *IEEE Trans. Biomed. Eng.* **2018**, *65*, 1748–1758. [PubMed]
15. Vinoj, P.G.; Jacob, S.; Menon, V.G.; Rajesh, S.; Khosravi, M.R. Brain-Controlled Adaptive Lower Limb Exoskeleton for Rehabilitation of Post-Stroke Paralyzed. *IEEE Access* **2019**, *7*, 1–22. [CrossRef]
16. Nakanishi, M.; Wang, Y.T.; Jung, T.P.; Zao, J.K.; Chien, Y.Y.; Diniz, A.; Daga, F.B.; Lin, Y.P.; Wang, Y.J.; Medeiros, F.A. Detecting Glaucoma with a Portable Brain-Computer Interface for Objective Assessment of Visual Function Loss. *Jama Ophthalmol.* **2017**, *135*, 550–557. [CrossRef]
17. De Vos, M.; Gandras, K.; Debener, S. Towards a truly mobile auditory brain–computer interface: Exploring the P300 to take away. *Int. J. Psychophysiol.* **2014**, *91*, 46–53. [CrossRef] [PubMed]
18. Wang, Y.T.; Huang, K.C.; Wei, C.S.; Huang, T.Y.; Ke, L.W.; Lin, C.T.; Cheng, C.K.; Jung, T.P. Developing an EEG-based on-line closed-loop lapse detection and mitigation system. *Front. Neurosci.* **2014**, *8*, 321. [CrossRef]
19. Wang, M.; Li, R.J.; Zhang, R.F.; Li, G.Y.; Zhang, D.G. A Wearable SSVEP-Based BCI System for Quadcopter Control Using Head-Mounted Device. *IEEE Access* **2018**, *6*, 26789–26798. [CrossRef]
20. Siddharth, S.; Patel, A.; Jung, T.; Sejnowski, T. A Wearable Multi-modal Bio-sensing System Towards Real-world Applications. *IEEE Trans. Biomed. Eng.* **2018**, *66*, 1137–1147. [CrossRef]
21. Lau-Zhu, A.; Lau, M.P.H.; McLoughlin, G. Mobile EEG in research on neurodevelopmental disorders: Opportunities and challenges. *Dev. Cogn. Neurosci.* **2019**, *36*, 100635. [CrossRef]
22. Zhang, Y.; Zhang, X.; Sun, H.; Fan, Z.W.; Zhong, X.F. Portable brain-computer interface based on novel convolutional neural network. *Comput. Biol. Med.* **2019**, *107*, 248–256. [CrossRef] [PubMed]
23. Debener, S.; Emkes, R.; De Vos, M.; Bleichner, M. Unobtrusive ambulatory EEG using a smartphone and flexible printed electrodes around the ear. *Sci. Rep.* **2015**, *5*, 16743. [CrossRef] [PubMed]
24. Chen, Y.H.; Op de Beeck, M.; Vanderheyden, L.; Carrette, E.; Mihajlovic, V.; Vanstreels, K.; Grundlehner, B.; Gadeyne, S.; Boon, P.; Van Hoof, C. Soft, Comfortable Polymer Dry Electrodes for High Quality ECG and EEG Recording. *Sensors* **2014**, *14*, 23758–23780. [CrossRef] [PubMed]
25. Fiedler, P.; Muhle, R.; Griebel, S.; Pedrosa, P.; Fonseca, C.; Vaz, F.; Zanow, F.; Haueisen, J. Contact Pressure and Flexibility of Multipin Dry EEG Electrodes. *IEEE Trans. Neural Syst. Rehabil. Eng.* **2018**, *26*, 750–757. [CrossRef] [PubMed]
26. Huang, Y.J.; Wu, C.Y.; Wong, A.M.K.; Lin, B.S. Novel Active Comb-Shaped Dry Electrode for EEG Measurement in Hairy Site. *IEEE Trans. Biomed. Eng.* **2015**, *62*, 256–263. [CrossRef] [PubMed]
27. Krachunov, S.; Casson, A.J. 3D Printed Dry EEG Electrodes. *Sensors* **2016**, *16*, 1635. [CrossRef] [PubMed]
28. Lee, J.S.; Han, C.M.; Kim, J.H.; Park, K.S. Reverse-curve-arch-shaped dry EEG electrode for increased skin-electrode contact area on hairy scalps. *Electron. Lett.* **2015**, *51*, 1643–1644. [CrossRef]

29. Chiesi, M.; Guermandi, M.; Placati, S.; Scarselli, E.F.; Guerrieri, R. Creamino: A Cost-Effective, Open-Source EEG-based BCI System. *IEEE Trans. Biomed. Eng.* **2018**, *66*, 900–909. [CrossRef]
30. McCrimmon, C.M.; Fu, J.L.; Wang, M.; Lopes, L.S.; Wang, P.T.; Karimi-Bidhendi, A.; Liu, C.Y.; Heydari, P.; Nenadic, Z.; Do, A.H. Performance Assessment of a Custom, Portable, and Low-Cost Brain-Computer Interface Platform. *IEEE Trans. Biomed. Eng.* **2017**, *64*, 2313–2320. [CrossRef]
31. Von Luhmann, A.; Wabnitz, H.; Sander, T.; Muller, K.R. M3BA: A Mobile, Modular, Multimodal Biosignal Acquisition Architecture for Miniaturized EEG-NIRS-Based Hybrid BCI and Monitoring. *IEEE Trans. Biomed. Eng.* **2017**, *64*, 1199–1210. [CrossRef]
32. Wang, Y.; Wang, R.P.; Gao, X.R.; Hong, B.; Gao, S.K. A practical VEP-based brain-computer interface. *IEEE Trans. Neural Syst. Rehabil. Eng.* **2006**, *14*, 234–239. [CrossRef] [PubMed]
33. Lu, N.; Li, T.F.; Ren, X.D.; Miao, H.Y. A Deep Learning Scheme for Motor Imagery Classification based on Restricted Boltzmann Machines. *IEEE Trans. Neural Syst. Rehabil. Eng.* **2017**, *25*, 566–576. [CrossRef] [PubMed]
34. Xing, X.; Wang, Y.J.; Pei, W.H.; Guo, X.H.; Liu, Z.D.; Wang, F.; Ming, G.; Zhao, H.Z.; Gui, Q.; Chen, H.D. A High-Speed SSVEP-Based BCI Using Dry EEG Electrodes. *Sci. Rep.* **2018**, *8*, 14708. [CrossRef] [PubMed]
35. Mathewson, K.E.; Harrison, T.J.L.; Kizuk, S.A.D. High and dry? Comparing active dry EEG electrodes to active and passive wet electrodes. *Psychophysiology* **2017**, *54*, 74–82. [CrossRef] [PubMed]
36. Kerick, S.E.; Oie, K.S.; McDowell, K. Assessment of EEG Signal Quality in Motion Environments. *Army Res. Lab. Rep. ARL-TR-4866* **2009**.
37. Delorme, A.; Makeig, S. EEGLAB: An open source toolbox for analysis of single-trial EEG dynamics including independent component analysis. *J. Neurosci. Methods* **2004**, *134*, 9–21. [CrossRef]
38. Debener, S.; Strobel, A.; Sorger, B.; Peters, J.; Kranczioch, C.; Engel, A.K.; Goebel, R. Improved quality of auditory event-related potentials recorded simultaneously with 3-T fMRI: Removal of the ballistocardiogram artefact. *Neuroimage* **2007**, *34*, 587–597. [CrossRef]
39. Wang, Y.T.; Nakanishi, M.; Wang, Y.J.; Wei, C.S.; Cheng, C.K.; Jung, T.P. An Online Brain-Computer Interface Based on SSVEPs Measured from Non-Hair-Bearing Areas. *IEEE Trans. Neural Syst. Rehabil. Eng.* **2017**, *25*, 11–18. [CrossRef]
40. Di Flumeri, G.; Arico, P.; Borghini, G.; Sciaraffa, N.; Di Florio, A.; Babiloni, F. The Dry Revolution: Evaluation of Three Different EEG Dry Electrode Types in Terms of Signal Spectral Features, Mental States Classification and Usability. *Sensors* **2019**, *19*, 1365. [CrossRef]
41. Kohli, S.; Casson, A.J. Removal of Gross Artifacts of Transcranial Alternating Current Stimulation in Simultaneous EEG Monitoring. *Sensors* **2019**, *19*, 190. [CrossRef]
42. Si-Mohammed, H.; Petit, J.; Jeunet, C.; Argelaguet, F.; Spindler, F.; Évain, A.; Roussel, N.; Casiez, G.; Lécuyer, A. Towards BCI-based Interfaces for Augmented Reality: Feasibility, Design and Evaluation. *IEEE Trans. Vis. Comput. Graph.* **2019**. [CrossRef] [PubMed]

© 2019 by the authors. Licensee MDPI, Basel, Switzerland. This article is an open access article distributed under the terms and conditions of the Creative Commons Attribution (CC BY) license (http://creativecommons.org/licenses/by/4.0/).

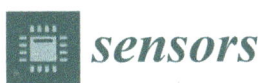

Article

Application of an Improved Correlation Method in Electrostatic Gait Recognition of Hemiparetic Patients

Shanshan Tian, Mengxuan Li, Yifei Wang and Xi Chen *

State Key Laboratory of Mechatronics Engineering and Control, Beijing Institute of Technology, Beijing 100081, China; shanshanbit@126.com (S.T.); formlmx@126.com (M.L.); wangyifeibit@163.com (Y.W.)
* Correspondence: chenxi@bit.edu.cn; Tel.: +86-010-6891-8017

Received: 2 April 2019; Accepted: 30 May 2019; Published: 3 June 2019

Abstract: Hemiparesis is one of the common sequelae of neurological diseases such as strokes, which can significantly change the gait behavior of patients and restrict their activities in daily life. The results of gait characteristic analysis can provide a reference for disease diagnosis and rehabilitation; however, gait correlation as a gait characteristic is less utilized currently. In this study, a new non-contact electrostatic field sensing method was used to obtain the electrostatic gait signals of hemiplegic patients and healthy control subjects, and an improved Detrended Cross-Correlation Analysis cross-correlation coefficient method was proposed to analyze the obtained electrostatic gait signals. The results show that the improved method can better obtain the dynamic changes of the scaling index under the multi-scale structure, which makes up for the shortcomings of the traditional Detrended Cross-Correlation Analysis cross-correlation coefficient method when calculating the electrostatic gait signal of the same kind of subjects, such as random and incomplete similarity in the trend of the scaling index spectrum change. At the same time, it can effectively quantify the correlation of electrostatic gait signals in subjects. The proposed method has the potential to be a powerful tool for extracting the gait correlation features and identifying the electrostatic gait of hemiplegic patients.

Keywords: gait analysis; gait correction; electrostatic gait signal; improved Detrended Cross-Correlation Analysis cross-correlation coefficient

1. Introduction

With the aging of the global population, strokes and other neurological diseases are occurring more frequently. Hemiparesis is one of the common sequelae of these diseases. Hemiplegic patients with body motor dysfunction often show a hemiplegic gait, among other symptoms. Assessing and restoring the walking ability of patients is the main objective of rehabilitation treatment for hemiplegic patients. The literature shows that the use of a variety of sensing methods to obtain hemiplegic gait information in clinical manifestations of hemiparesis [1,2], in order to study the kinematics and mechanics of gait signals and to objectively and quantitatively evaluate the pathological gait characteristics of hemiplegic patients, can provide effective support for the diagnosis and rehabilitation of hemiplegic patients [3,4].

At present, there are two main methods of gait measurement; one is the contact measurement method, which is usually obtained through the subject wearing an inertial unit sensor [5,6] or photoelectric sensor [7,8]; the other is the non-contact method, in which a video analysis system is used [9]. However, these common methods have some limitations. For example, wearing a sensor will affect the natural gait of the subject, while a video system compromises the privacy of the subject and is associated with data processing difficulties. Because of its non-contact, non-intrusive, and long-term continuous monitoring of gait signals, electrostatic detection has gradually become a research focus in the field of gait measurement [10,11]. In Chen's work [12], the equivalent capacitance model of the human body was established by theoretical deduction, and the correctness of the model was verified by simulations and measured signals. In the paper by Li [13], the gait parameters of the "gold standard" plantar pressure system were compared with the electrostatic measurement system, and this proved that the gait time parameters can be effectively measured by the electrostatic field sensing method. The electrostatic gait signal is a non-stationary time series, which contains various motion parameters of the human body, including time, frequency and nonlinear parameters, among others. The related research on feature extraction of the gait signal not only helps explain gait signal fluctuations, obtaining more gait parameters, but also helps to analyze the physiological health status of the human body.

Correlation is an important feature of the non-stationary time series. Correlation analysis of the electrostatic gait signal can demonstrate the inherent characteristics of the signal, and the implicit correlation between the signals. Detrended fluctuation analysis (DFA), first proposed by Peng, is used to study the long-range fluctuation of DNA sequences [14]. After that, DFA was widely used in financial time series [15], meteorological time series [16], and physiological signal series [17,18]. However, the traditional DFA cannot describe a complex biological signal sequence accurately because of its single scale index. In order to better describe the correlation of non-stationary time series, the bi-index analysis method and local index derivation method are studied in the works by Peng and Castiglioni [19,20]; however, there is a limitation in that they cannot describe in detail the dynamic correlation of the signal. Xia Jianan et al. [21] proposed a local moving window combined multiscale detrended fluctuation analysis (MSDFA) method in order to study the dynamics of the correlation of signals, wherein the scale index spectrum is obtained by fitting $logF(n)$ and $log(n)$ in a local moving window to distinguish the ECG signals of healthy and pathological groups, and effectively avoid the influence of extreme values with this method. The correlation expansion of a non-stationary time series can obtain the cross-correlation between two non-stationary time series. The Detrended Cross-Correlation Analysis (DCCA) method proposed by Podobnik and Stanley [22] was first used to calculate the cross-correlation between two non-stationary time series. It has been widely used in financial [23,24], atmospheric [25], physiological, and other fields [26]. However, the single scaling index in the DCCA results still has similar inadequacies to DFA; that is, only a single parameter is used to describe the sequence characteristics. In order to solve this problem, Yin Yi et al. [27] applied the improved multiscale detrended cross-correlation analysis (MSDCCA) method in order to obtain the scaling index spectrum. This method can better show the dynamic changes of the scaling index in different scaling windows, and effectively avoid the influence of outliers, so it has good robustness.

In order to quantitatively analyze the correlation of non-stationary signals, Zebende proposed a DCCA cross-correlation coefficient method based on DFA and DCCA [28]. However, we found that when this method was used to calculate electrostatic gait signals, the results would fluctuate abnormally near the crossover point [29,30]. Further, the traditional DCCA cross-correlation coefficient spectrum of electrostatic gait signals of the same type of subjects has random and incomplete similarity, so it was difficult to distinguish hemiplegic patients from healthy control subjects by the DCCA cross-correlation coefficient. In order to solve this problem, an improved DCCA cross-correlation coefficient method is proposed in this paper. Local moving windows are used instead of the fixed scales in the original algorithm. The results of the improved algorithm show a uniform and regular single peak structure at the crossover points, and have a stable curve structure; moreover, the results of different electrostatic gait signals for hemiplegic patients showed a relatively consistent trend. This method can effectively improve the stability of the DCCA cross-correlation coefficient, and quantify the correlation level of electrostatic gait signals under different scales.

The rest of this paper is arranged as follows: The second part will introduce the principle of electrostatic sensing method and the experimental process of electrostatic gait signal acquisition, as well as how to obtain electrostatic gait signals of hemiplegic patients and healthy control subjects; the third part will introduce in detail the improvement of the traditional DCCA cross-correlation coefficient method; and the fourth part uses the traditional method to analyze the electrostatic gait signals of subjects, from which we find that the traditional method has some shortcomings in the analysis of electrostatic gait signals. Then, we use the improved method to analyze the electrostatic gait signals. Through a comparison between the traditional method and the improved method, it can be concluded that the improved method is more suitable for the correlation analysis of electrostatic gait signals. This method can be better applied to the correlation analysis of human electrostatic gait signals.

2. Methods

2.1. Principle of Electrostatic Field Induction in the Human Foot

The electrostatic phenomenon is a ubiquitous physical phenomenon. The human body is charged with electrostatic energy during movement due to friction between the body and the clothes, as well as friction between the sole and the ground [31,32]. Therefore, with the movement of the foot during walking, the electric field around the human body will change [33]. In Chen's research [12], based on the principle of the electrostatic field, the equivalent model of the human body was established. Because the human body has a certain charge, it will produce equivalent capacitance with the surrounding environment, including the direct coupling capacitance C_f generated by human feet contacting the ground through the sole, and other capacitance C_r (i = 1, 2 ...). The two capacitors are connected in parallel to form the total capacitance of the human body (Formula (1)). The equivalent capacitance model of the human body is shown in Figure 1.

$$C_h = C_f + \sum_{i=1}^{\infty} C_{ri} \tag{1}$$

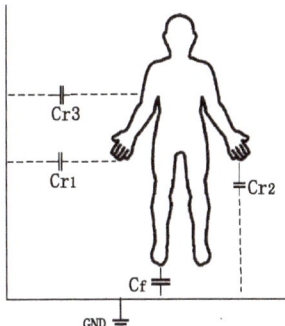

Figure 1. Sketch of the human body equivalent capacitance model.

The left and right feet alternately leave the ground when walking. The capacitance between the foot and the ground is equivalent to a variable capacitance which connected to the height of the foot from the ground in series with C_f. The capacitance value becomes C, resulting in dynamic changes of electrostatic field around the human body. As in the literature [12], assuming that the charge of the human body is Q_B, the induced current I placed on the sensing electrode at a certain distance from the subject is shown in Formula (2).

$$I = \frac{dQ_B}{dt} = C\frac{dU_B}{dt} \propto \frac{1}{S_s}\frac{d}{dt}(h(t)) - \frac{h(t)}{S_s^2}\frac{dS_s}{dt} \tag{2}$$

U_B is the induced potential generated during human walking, $h(t)$ is the height function of human feet leaving the ground when walking, and S_s is the effective bottom area of $h(t)$ from the ground height. The first item in Formula (2) represents the current generated by the foot movement before the foot leaves the ground, and the second item in Formula (2) represents the current caused by the foot and leg movement after the foot leaves the ground completely. Therefore, when the tester moves near the electrodes, we can obtain the electrostatic induction current caused by human motion under non-contact conditions, and then obtain the relevant parameters of the gait by analyzing the current waveform obtained.

2.2. Human Electrostatic Gait Measurement System

The electrostatic signal sensing system includes the induction electrode, electrostatic sensing circuit, signal acquisition and processing circuit. The system schematic diagram is shown in Figure 2. In this system, a copper foil planar electrode is used as the electrode material. The shape of the electrode is a circle with a diameter of 90 mm. The electrostatic sensing circuit allows the amplification and filtering of the electrostatic signal, and realizes the conversion and amplification from the induced charge to the current to the voltage, thereby converting the weak induced charge amount into a voltage signal that can be processed. A low-pass filter with a cut-off frequency of 20 Hz was added before A/D conversion in order to prevent the measured signal from being disturbed by the power frequency signal of the power grid. The signal acquisition and processing circuit converts the amplified and filtered analog signals into digital signals using an A/D conversion with high precision and a wide voltage input, and then processes the collected signals using a microcontroller unit. The sampling frequency of the system is 1 kHz, and the sampled data is sent to a personal computer for storage and processing. According to [13], the current intensity of the induced current is inversely proportional to the distance between the human body and the induction electrode, and the maximum induced current can be generated when the human body directly faces the induction electrode. Therefore, in order to obtain a better gait electrostatic signal, the subject is required to tread 1 m in front of the electrostatic induction electrode.

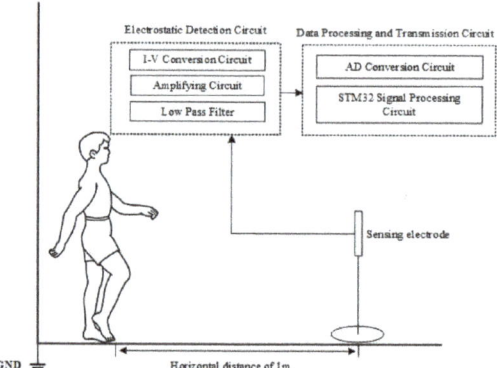

Figure 2. Schematic of the electrostatic sensing system.

2.3. Gait Measurement Experiment

In this experiment, 10 hemiparetic patients and 10 healthy control subjects participated in data collection. The experiment recruited 10 hemiparetic patients (six males and four females) from the Zhongshan People's Hospital of Guangdong Province, China, as the pathological group. Their average height was 1.68 m (height range: 1.58~1.76 m), the average weight was 68.7 kg (56~78 kg), and the average age was 46 years (age range: 31~60 years old). The selection criteria for the hemiparetic patients was: (1) Unilateral hemiparesis after their first stroke, and the condition has been confirmed by computed tomography (CT) or nuclear magnetic resonance (MRI) imaging; (2) able to continuously step or walk for at least three minutes without any help or auxiliary equipment; (3) understands the external orders and follows the experimental procedures; (4) suffers no other diseases known to affect the gait [34]. This research was approved by the Ethics Committee of Zhongshan People's Hospital, and an informed consent form was signed by each subject.

The healthy control group had no neurological damage (six males and four females). Their average height was 1.73 m (height range: 1.58~1.81 m) and the average weight was 61.7 kg (45~78 kg). The average age was 28 years (age range: 24–33 years old).

All subjects gave their informed consent for inclusion before they participated in the study. The study was conducted in accordance with the Declaration of Helsinki, and the protocol was approved by the Ethics Committee of Zhongshan People's Hospital.

In the experiment, the electrostatic testing equipment was placed on a triangle stand at a height of 1 m from the ground. The healthy control group and the hemiplegic patients wore ordinary rubber sole shoes, and they were required to tread at a distance of 1 m in front of the electrostatic induction electrode. The subjects were required to tread in situ at a normal pace. Two groups of signals from the hemiplegic patients and healthy controls were obtained; that is, a total of 40 groups of electrostatic gait signals were collected, each of which was about 60 s in length. The ambient temperature and humidity ranged from 20 to 25 °C, and from 50% to 60%, respectively.

2.4. Preprocessing of the Experimental Data

Figure 3a,b shows the original gait signals of a healthy control person and a hemiplegic patient. The signals are digitally filtered and normalized to intercept 50 s of data from the complete signals. From the figure, we can see that the amplitude of the healthy control is more stable than that of the hemiplegic patient, and the gait cycle of the healthy control is shorter than that of the hemiplegic patient.

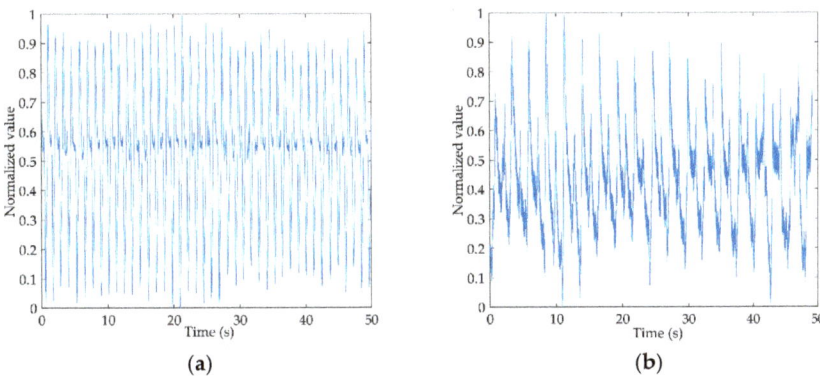

Figure 3. Schematic diagram of the original electrostatic gait signal. (**a**) Preprocessed electrostatic gait signals of a healthy control; (**b**) Preprocessed electrostatic gait signals of a hemiplegic patient.

2.5. Improved DCCA Cross-Correlation Coefficient Method

The DCCA cross-correlation coefficient method has the characteristic of quantifying the cross-correlation level between two non-stationary time series. The DCCA cross-correlation coefficients of two non-stationary time series $x(i)$ and $y(i)$ are defined as:

$$\rho_{DCCA}(n) = \frac{f^2_{DCCA}(n)}{f_{DFAx}(n) \cdot f_{DFAy}(n)} \qquad (3)$$

The DCCA cross-correlation coefficient is calculated from the DFA and DCCA of the sequence. When dealing with electrostatic gait signals, this method is sensitive to the fluctuations of f_{DFA} and f_{DCCA}; it cannot accurately and quantitatively reflect the correlation level. The local moving window can display the details of physiological signal dynamic change and has good robustness. This paper proposes an improved DCCA cross-correlation coefficient algorithm based on the local moving window.

The improved DCCA cross-correlation coefficient method is described as follows: calculate the sample sequence to get the detrended variance function $f_{DFAx}(n)$ and $f_{DFAy}(n)$, and detrended covariance function $f_{DCCA}(n)$, where n is the scale. The fluctuation function curves are divided by the local moving window, then the data in each window is fitted. The expression of the fitted line can be expressed as $(a \cdot n + b)$, where a is the slope of the line, which can also be regarded as the scale index in each local window, while b is the only parameter of the currently fitted straight line in the correlation analysis [21,27]. We are only focused on using the scale index to quantify the correlation, so parameter b is not discussed. Therefore, every window DCCA cross-correlation coefficient can be represented as:

$$\rho_{DCCA}(n) = \frac{(a_{DCCA} \cdot n)^2}{(a_{DFAx} \cdot n) \cdot (a_{DFAy} \cdot n)}, (n \in w_i = [c,d], i = 1, 2, \ldots, m) \quad (4)$$

The method for dividing the local moving window is described as follows: For the sample data with the data length N, set the range of n as ($5 < n < N/10$), then the partial moving window is divided. $w_i = [c, d]$ ($i = 1, 2, \ldots, m$) is expressed as each local moving window, c is the starting value, d is the ending value, the starting value interval is 5, and the ending value is five times the starting value, m is the number of local moving window. s_{wi} indicates the scaled median value of each window, a_{wi} indicates the scale index in the corresponding window, and $a_w = \{a_{w1}, a_{w2}, \ldots, a_{wm}\}$ is the scale index spectrum.

After calculating all the window data, the above formula can be improved to Formula (5):

$$\rho_{MSDCCA}(s_{wi}) = \frac{(a_{wi,DCCA})^2}{(a_{wi,DFA}) \cdot (a_{wi,DFA})}, (i = 1, 2, \ldots, m) \quad (5)$$

We call ρ_{MSDCCA} the multi-scale detrended cross-correlation coefficient. In the results, $\rho_{MSDCCA} > 0$ indicates that there is positive cross-correlation between sequences, while $\rho_{MSDCCA} < 0$ indicates that there is an anti-cross-correlation between sequences. The dynamics of the sequence and the inherent complex structure of the sequence can be observed from the curve of ρ_{MSDCCA} changing with s_{wi}.

3. Results

In this part, we analyzed the electrostatic gait signal of the hemiplegic patients and the healthy control subjects with the traditional method. We found that the traditional method had some deficiencies in the analysis of the electrostatic gait signal correlation. Then, the electrostatic gait signal was analyzed by the improved method proposed in this paper. The results showed that the improved method improved the stability and accuracy of the data results compared with the traditional method, and helped to better identify the electrostatic gait signal of hemiparesis.

3.1. Analysis of the Electrostatic Gait Signal with the Traditional Method

DCCA is used to analyze the correlation between two non-stationary time series, and has been widely used in finance, atmosphere, physiology, and other fields [23–26]. In this paper, the electrostatic gait signals of hemiplegic patients and healthy control subjects are analyzed with the DCCA method, and the logarithmic curve of the cross-correlation fluctuation function and the scale of the electrostatic gait signals are obtained, as shown in Figure 4. From graph (a), we can see that all the cross-correlation wave functions of healthy controls have good consistency, and the curves have a crossover point ($n = 500$). The cross-correlation index spectrum of the electrostatic gait signals of the healthy controls is obviously divided into two sections, with a single index ($a_{DCCA} = 1.84$). From graph (b), we can see that the cross-correlation wave function curves of all hemiplegic patients are scattered. There are two crossover points ($n_1 = 60$, $n_2 = 1200$). The cross-correlation index spectrum of the electrostatic gait signals of hemiplegic patients is obviously divided into three segments. There are two indices for the electrostatic gait signals of hemiplegic patients ($\alpha_{DCCA1} = 1.22$, $\alpha_{DCCA2} = 1.54$). In Figure 4b, the waveform functions of different samples of hemiplegic patients show chaotic waveform characteristics after the first crossover point. This phenomenon is related to the difference of walking ability between hemiplegic patients, but the waveform characteristics cannot be explained by a single index.

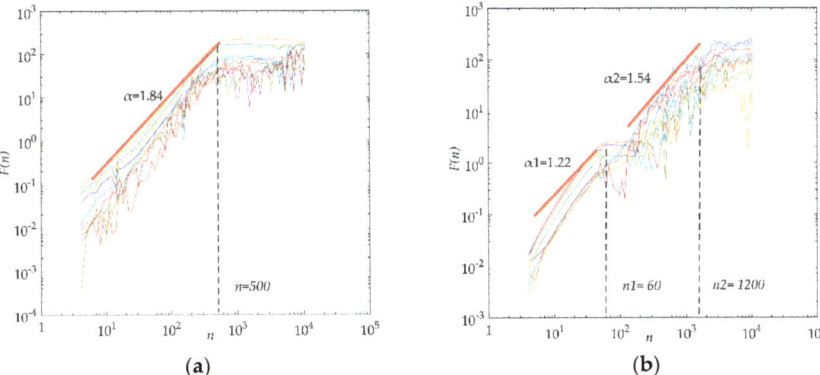

Figure 4. DCCA analysis of healthy controls (a) and hemiplegia patients (b).

Although the cross-correlation wave function spectrogram of the electrostatic gait signals of subjects calculated by the DCCA method can show the difference between them, the long-range cross-correlation of the electrostatic gait signals of hemiplegic patients can be seen from a single index that is weaker than that of the healthy controls. However, this difference is small, and the cross-correlation index cannot quantify the strength of cross-correlation between signals.

DCCA cannot quantify the correlation of electrostatic gait signals. In this paper, the DCCA cross-correlation coefficient method is used to analyze the electrostatic gait signals quantitatively. This method is also widely used in physiological signals [35]. The DCCA cross-correlation coefficient method is defined by DFA and DCCA to quantitatively study the cross-correlation between non-stationary time series. The electrostatic gait signals of hemiplegic patients and healthy controls were calculated and analyzed by the DCCA cross-correlation coefficient method. Figure 5 shows the analyzed electrostatic gait signals of hemiplegic patient 5 (hemi 5) and healthy control 1 (control 1). We can see from the graph that the spectrum of ρ_{DCCA} in hemiplegic patient 5 fluctuates greatly. The first peak ($\rho_{DCCA} = 0.69$) appears at the scale $n_1 = 54$, and then the curve shows a downward trend and a disorderly fluctuation trend. The second peak ($\rho_{DCCA} = 0.68$) appears at the scale $n_2 = 967$, and then the curve decreases and produces two small peaks. The scales corresponding to wave peaks are similar to those of crossover points in DCCA, and on all scales, $\rho_{DCCA} = 0.54 \pm 0.06$. For healthy control 1, the fluctuation of the spectrogram of ρ_{DCCA} was relatively stable, but there was a peak fluctuation on scale $n = 540$ ($\rho_{DCCA} = 0.83$) and $\rho_{DCCA} = 0.69 \pm 0.06$ on all scales.

The DCCA cross-correlation coefficient can quantify the correlation of the electrostatic gait signals in hemiplegic patients and healthy controls. After DCCA cross-correlation coefficient analysis of data from all hemiplegic patients and healthy controls, we found that the fluctuation of ρ_{DCCA} near the crossover point was a common phenomenon, showing a chaotic fluctuation of one main peak and several sub-peaks. The trend of the DCCA cross-correlation coefficient spectrum of electrostatic gait signals of the same type of test population was random and similar.

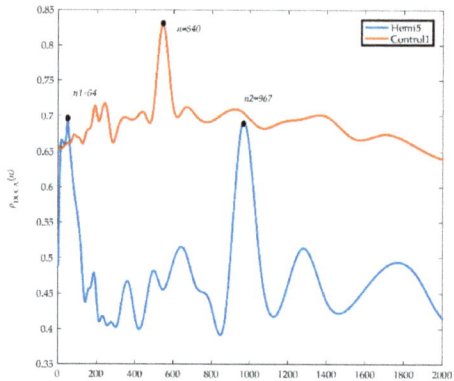

Figure 5. Spectrum of ρ_{DCCA} in healthy control 1 and hemiplegic patient 5.

Due to the different fluctuation characteristics of time series on different time scales, the crossover point phenomenon appears in the DFA and DCCA results, and the complex fluctuation phenomenon appears near the crossover point of the cross-correlation index spectrum, which will affect the quantitative judgment of the cross-correlation. The traditional method has some limitations in the analysis of electrostatic gait signals, so we need to improve the traditional method for better analysis of electrostatic gait signals.

3.2. Improved DCCA Cross-Correlation Coefficient Method for Electrostatic Gait Signal Analysis

Because the traditional DCCA cross-correlation coefficient method has some limitations, the improved method is used to analyze hemiplegic patient 5 and healthy control 1. As shown in Figure 6, we can see from the graph that the spectrum of ρ_{MSDCCA} in hemiplegic patient 5 first decreases, then rises, and finally tends to be stable. The scale window $s_{w1} = 160$ has a trough, the correlation coefficient spectrum in the $160 < s_w < 589$ interval shows an increasing trend, the scale window $s_{w2} = 589$ has a peak, and the correlation coefficient of $s_w > 589$ first decreases to a stable trend. The correlation coefficients near the peak and trough did not fluctuate significantly in the results of ρ_{MSDCCA}. In contrast, the spectral line of healthy control 1 was relatively stable and showed no obvious fluctuation in the whole scale window, and the range of healthy control 1 was $\rho_{MSDCCA} = [1.4, 1.6]$.

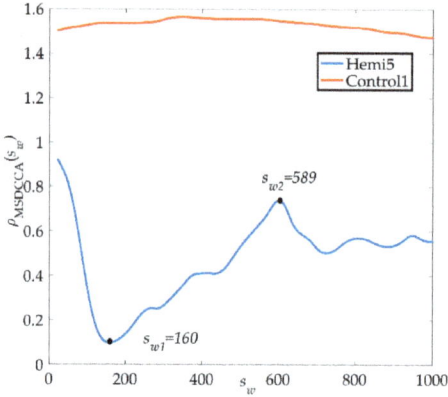

Figure 6. ρ_{MSDCCA} spectrograms of healthy control 1 and hemiplegic patient 5.

Finally, the improved method was used to analyze the electrostatic gait signals of all subjects, and the correlation coefficient spectra of ρ_{MSDCCA} of hemiplegic patients and healthy controls were obtained, as shown in Figure 7. The red bold line in the figure represents the average of all data changes. Figure 7a is a spectrogram of the coefficients of ρ_{MSDCCA} of the healthy control group. The curve tends to be stable in the window scale range. The range of ρ_{MSDCCA} is [1.3, 1.8], and the mean and standard deviation are 1.45 ± 0.12. The gait signals of the healthy control group have a better correlation. The coefficient curve of ρ_{MSDCCA} in the hemiplegic patient group is shown in Figure 7b. From the graph, we can see that the curve first has a downward trend and then an upward trend, and tends to be stable. The fluctuation of the ρ_{MSDCCA} curve in the hemiplegic patients is closely related to the crossing point. The stability range of ρ_{MSDCCA} is [0.6, 1.6], and the mean and standard deviation are 0.93 ± 0.26.

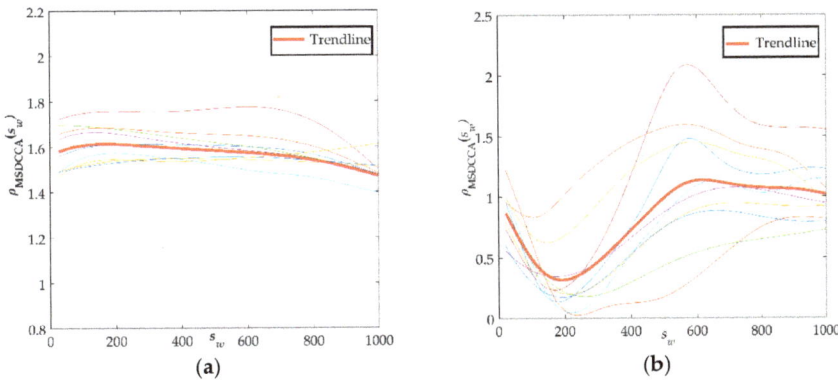

Figure 7. Result curve of ρ_{MSDCCA}. (**a**) Analytical curves of ρ_{MSDCCA} of all healthy controls with respect to the change of moving windows; (**b**) Analytical curves of ρ_{MSDCCA} with the moving window in all hemiplegic patients.

From the spectrum of hemiplegic patients and healthy controls calculated by the improved method, we can clearly see the difference between them, meaning it is possible to effectively distinguish the hemiplegic patient from the healthy control easily. In addition, it can be seen from the spectrum of ρ_{MSDCCA} that the local variation trend of correlation coefficients near the crossover point is identical, with many similarities and good stability. Moreover, the improved method can quantitatively show the difference between the correlation of the gait signals of two groups of subjects, and it can also reflect the differences of walking ability between individual hemiplegic patients.

4. Conclusions

This study analyzes the correlation between the electrostatic gait signals of hemiparetic patients and healthy controls by using an improved method which combines the local moving window method and traditional DCCA cross-correlation coefficient method. Using the improved method to analyze the electrostatic gait signal can mitigate the weaknesses of the traditional method, such as the random trend changes and incomplete similarity. In this paper, the electrostatic gait signals of hemiparetic patients and healthy controls were collected, and the improved method was used for gait analysis. Compared with the ρ_{MSDCCA} coefficient of the healthy control group, the mean value of the ρ_{MSDCCA} coefficient of the hemiparetic patients was smaller, and the trend of change was more complicated, reflecting that the gait stability of the hemiparetic patients was weaker than that of the healthy controls, additionally, a poor correlation was obtained. The improved method can obtain the dynamic changes of the scale index under the multi-scale structure, and quantify the gait difference between the hemiparetic patients and the healthy controls.

We only collected one minute of the patients' gait signal data due to their weakened mobility. This paper does not consider the difference in the gait signal between individual patients due to different rehabilitation stages, which can be considered a limitation. In future research, we will obtain more abundant experimental data, and conduct more in-depth research based on the different rehabilitation stages of hemiparetic patients, and then obtain more accurate and effective characteristic parameters. In the future, multiple characteristic parameters could be used to analyze various abnormal gaits, such as the hemiparesis and Parkinson gaits.

Author Contributions: Conceptualization, S.T. and X.C.; Data curation, M.L. and Y.W.; Formal analysis, M.L. and Y.W.; Funding acquisition, X.C.; Investigation, S.T. and M.L.; Methodology, S.T.; validation, S.T., M.L. and Y.W.; Resources, X.C.; Software, Y.W.; Writing—original draft, S.T.; Writing—review & editing, all authors.

Funding: This work was financially supported by grants from National Natural Science Foundation of China (#51407009, #51777010, #51707008, #U1630130).

Acknowledgments: The authors would like to thank all the participants for their contributions to the study. The authors are particularly grateful to Zhonghua Liu and Liyi Chen for assisting in the completion of the patient's gait data collection experiments.

Conflicts of Interest: The authors declare no conflict of interest.

References

1. Galli, M.; Cimolin, V.; Rigoldi, C.; Tenore, N.; Albertini, G. Gait patterns in hemiplegic children with Cerebral Palsy: Comparison of right and left hemiparetic. *Res. Dev. Disabil.* **2010**, *31*, 1340–1345. [CrossRef] [PubMed]
2. Nasciutti-Prudente, C.; Oliveira, F.G.; Houri, S.F.; de Paula Goulart, F.R.; Neto, M.H.; Teixeira-Salmela, L.F. Relationships between muscular torque and gait speed in chronic hemiparetic subjects. *Disabil. Rehabil.* **2009**, *31*, 103–108. [CrossRef] [PubMed]
3. Jaffe, D.L.; Brown, D.A.; Pierson-Carey, C.D.; Buckley, E.L.; Lew, H.L. Stepping over obstacles to improve walking in individuals with poststroke hemiplegia. *J. Rehabil. Res. Dev.* **2004**, *41*, 283. [CrossRef] [PubMed]
4. Patten, C.; Lexell, J.; Brown, H.E. Weakness and strength training in persons with poststroke hemiplegia: Rationale, method, and efficacy. *J. Rehabil. Res. Dev.* **2004**, *41*, 293. [CrossRef]
5. Device, I.S. Detection of Hemiplegic Walking Using a Wearable Inertia Sensing Device. *Sensors* **2018**, *18*, 1736. [CrossRef]
6. Allseits, E.; Lučarević, J.; Gailey, R.; Agrawal, V.; Gaunaurd, I.; Bennett, C. The development and concurrent validity of a real-time algorithm for temporal gait analysis using inertial measurement units. *J. Biomech.* **2017**, *55*, 27–33. [CrossRef] [PubMed]
7. Carcreff, L.; Gerber, C.N.; Paraschiv-Ionescu, A.; De Coulon, G.; Newman, C.J.; Armand, S.; Aminian, K. What is the best configuration of wearable sensors to measure spatiotemporal gait parameters in children with cerebral palsy? *Sensors* **2018**, *18*, 394. [CrossRef] [PubMed]
8. Bertoli, M.; Cereatti, A.; Trojaniello, D.; Avanzino, L.; Pelosin, E.; Din, D.S. Estimation of spatio-temporal parameters of gait from magneto-inertial measurement units: Multicenter validation among Parkinson, mildly cognitively impaired and healthy older adults. *Biomed. Eng. Online* **2018**, *17*, 58. [CrossRef]
9. Lee, L. *Gait Analysis for Classification*; AI Technical Report AITR-2003-014; Artificial Intelligence Laboratory of Massachusetts Institute of Technology: Cambridge, MA, USA, 2003.
10. Takiguchi, K.; Wada, T.T.S. Human Body Detection that Uses Electric Field by Walking. *J. Adv. Mech. Des. Syst. Manuf.* **2007**, *1*, 294–305. [CrossRef]
11. Fujiwara, O.; Okazaki, M.A.T. Electrification Properties of Human Body by Walking. *IEICE Trans.* **1990**, *73*, 99–107. [CrossRef]
12. Chen, X.; Zheng, Z.; Cui, Z.; Zheng, W. A novel remote sensing technique for recognizing human gait based on the measurement of induced electrostatic current. *J. Electrost.* **2012**, *70*, 105–110. [CrossRef]
13. Li, M.; Li, P.; Tian, S.; Tang, K.; Chen, X. Estimation of temporal gait parameters using a human body electrostatic sensing-based method. *Sensors* **2018**, *18*, 1737. [CrossRef] [PubMed]

14. Peng, C.; Israel, B.; Medical, D.; Buldyrev, S.V.; Havlin, S.; Stanley, H.E. Mosaic organization of DNA nucleotides. *Phys. Rev. E* **1994**, *42*, 1685. [CrossRef]
15. Li, W.; Wang, F.; Havlin, S.; Stanley, H.E. Financial factor influence on scaling and memory of trading volume in stock market Financial factor influence on scaling and memory of trading volume in stock market. *Phys. Rev. E* **2011**, *84*, 046112. [CrossRef] [PubMed]
16. Telesca, L.; Pierini, J.O.; Scian, B. Investigating the temporal variation of the scaling behavior in rainfall data measured in central Argentina by means of detrended fluctuation analysis. *Physica A* **2012**, *391*, 1553–1562. [CrossRef]
17. Goldberger, A.L.; Amaral, L.A.N.; Hausdorff, J.M.; Ivanov, P.C.; Peng, C.-K.; Stanley, H.E. Fractal dynamics in physiology: Alterations with disease and aging. *Proc. Natl. Acad. Sci. USA* **2002**, *99*, 2466–2472. [CrossRef] [PubMed]
18. Dingwell, J.B.; Cusumano, J.P. Re-interpreting detrended fluctuation analyses of stride-to-stride variability in human walking. *Gait Posture* **2010**, *32*, 348–353. [CrossRef]
19. Peng, C.K.; Havlin, S.; Stanley, H.E.; Goldberger, A.L. Quantification of scaling exponents and crossover phenomena in nonstationary heartbeat time series. *Chaos* **1995**, *5*, 82–87. [CrossRef] [PubMed]
20. Castiglioni, P.; Bernard, C.; Castiglioni, P.; Parati, G.; Civijian, A.; Quintin, L.; Rienzo, M.D. Local Scale Exponents of Blood Pressure and Heart Rate Variability by Detrended Fluctuation Analysis: Effects of Posture, Exercise, and Local Scale Exponents of Blood Pressure and Heart Rate Variability by Detrended Fluctuation Analysis: Effects of posture, exercise, and aging. *IEEE Trans. Biomed. Eng.* **2009**, *56*, 675–684. [CrossRef]
21. Xia, J.; Shang, P.; Wang, J. Estimation of local scale exponents for heartbeat time series based on DFA. *Nonlinear Dyn.* **2013**, *74*, 1183–1190. [CrossRef]
22. Podobnik, B.; Stanley, H.E. Detrended Cross-Correlation Analysis: A New Method for Analyzing Two Nonstationary Time Series. *Phys. Rev. Lett.* **2007**, *100*, 084102. [CrossRef]
23. Sukpitak, J.; Hengpunya, V. The influence of trading volume on market efficiency: The DCCA approach. *Phys. A Stat. Mech. Its Appl.* **2016**, *458*, 259–265. [CrossRef]
24. Ikeda, T. A detrended cross correlation analysis for stock markets of the United States, Japan, and the Europe. *Phys. A Stat. Mech. Appl.* **2017**, *484*, 194–198. [CrossRef]
25. Shi, K.; Di, B.; Zhang, K.; Feng, C.; Svirchev, L. Detrended cross-correlation analysis of urban traffic congestion and NO 2 concentrations in Chengdu. *Transp. Res. Part D* **2018**, *61*, 165–173. [CrossRef]
26. Wang, J.; Zhao, D.Q. Detrended cross-correlation analysis of electroencephalogram. *Chin. Phys. B* **2012**, *21*, 028703. [CrossRef]
27. Yin, Y.; Shang, P. Modified DFA and DCCA approach for quantifying the multiscale correlation structure of financial markets. *Physica A* **2013**, *392*, 6442–6457. [CrossRef]
28. Zebende, G.F. DCCA cross-correlation coefficient: Quantifying level of cross-correlation. *Phys. A Stat. Mech. Appl.* **2011**, *390*, 614–618. [CrossRef]
29. Ogata, H.; Tokuyama, K.; Nagasaka, S.; Ando, A.; Kusaka, I.; Sato, N.; Goto, A.; Ishibashi, S.; Kiyono, K.; Struzik, Z.R.; et al. Long-range negative correlation of glucose dynamics in humans and its breakdown in diabetes mellitus. *Am. J. Phys.-Regul. Integr. Comp. Physiol.* **2019**, *291*, 1638–1643. [CrossRef]
30. Varela, M.; Vigil, L.; Rodriguez, C.; Vargas, B.; García-carretero, R. Delay in the Detrended Fluctuation Analysis Crossover Point as a Risk Factor for Type 2 Diabetes Mellitus. *J. Diabetes Res.* **2016**, *2016*, 9–12. [CrossRef]
31. Chubb, J.N.Ã. A Standard proposed for assessing the electrostatic suitability of materials. *J. Electrost.* **2007**, *65*, 607–610. [CrossRef]
32. Gady, B. Identification of electrostatic and van der Waals interaction forces between a micrometer-size sphere and a flat substrate. *Phys. Rev. B* **1996**, *53*, 8065. [CrossRef]
33. Okazaki, M.; Fujiwara, O.; Azakami, T. Characteristic Meas-urement of Human Body Potential due to Stepping on Metal Plate. *J. IEICE* **1991**, *2*, 184.

34. Li, M.; Tian, S.; Sun, L.; Chen, X. Gait Analysis for Post-Stroke Hemiparetic Patient by Multi-Features Fusion Method. *Sensors* **2019**, *19*, 1737. [CrossRef] [PubMed]
35. Chen, Y.; Cai, L.; Wang, R.; Song, Z.; Deng, B.; Wang, J.; Yu, H. DCCA cross-correlation coefficients reveals the change of both synchronization and oscillation in EEG of Alzheimer disease patients. *Phys. A Stat. Mech. Appl.* **2018**, *490*, 171–184. [CrossRef]

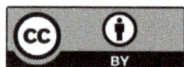

© 2019 by the authors. Licensee MDPI, Basel, Switzerland. This article is an open access article distributed under the terms and conditions of the Creative Commons Attribution (CC BY) license (http://creativecommons.org/licenses/by/4.0/).

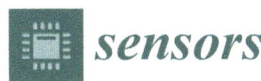

Article

Tracking and Characterization of Spinal Cord-Injured Patients by Means of RGB-D Sensors

Filippo Colombo Zefinetti [1], Andrea Vitali [1,*], Daniele Regazzoni [1], Caterina Rizzi [1] and Guido Molinero [2]

[1] Department of Management, Information and Production Engineering, University of Bergamo, 24044 Dalmine (BG), Italy; filippo.colombozefinetti@unibg.it (F.C.Z.); daniele.regazzoni@unibg.it (D.R.); caterina.rizzi@unibg.it (C.R.)

[2] Azienda Socio Sanitaria Territoriale (ASST) Papa Giovanni XXIII, 24127 Bergamo, Italy; gmolinero@asst-pg23.it

* Correspondence: andrea.vitali1@unibg.it

Received: 23 September 2020; Accepted: 1 November 2020; Published: 4 November 2020

Abstract: In physical rehabilitation, motion capture solutions are well-known but not as widespread as they could be. The main limit to their diffusion is not related to cost or usability but to the fact that the data generated when tracking a person must be elaborated according to the specific context and aim. This paper proposes a solution including customized motion capture and data elaboration with the aim of supporting medical personnel in the assessment of spinal cord-injured (SCI) patients using a wheelchair. The configuration of the full-body motion capturing system is based on an asymmetric 3 Microsoft Kinect v2 sensor layout that provides a path of up to 6 m, which is required to properly track the wheelchair. Data elaboration is focused on the automatic recognition of the pushing cycles and on plotting any kinematic parameter that may be interesting in the assessment. Five movements have been considered to evaluate the wheelchair propulsion: the humeral elevation, the horizontal abduction of the humerus, the humeral rotation, the elbow flexion and the trunk extension along the sagittal plane. More than 60 volunteers with a spinal cord injury were enrolled for testing the solution. To evaluate the reliability of the data computed with SCI APPlication (APP) for the pushing cycle analysis, the patients were subdivided in four groups according to the level of the spinal cord injury (i.e., high paraplegia, low paraplegia, C7 tetraplegia and C6 tetraplegia). For each group, the average value and the standard deviation were computed and a comparison with similar acquisitions performed with a high-end solution is shown. The measurements computed by the SCI-APP show a good reliability for analyzing the movements of SCI patients' propulsion wheelchair.

Keywords: markerless motion capture; automatic pushing analysis; SCI patients; RGB-D sensors

1. Introduction

Spinal cord injury is caused by one or more lesions of the spinal cord. Inside the spinal cord, there is a complex network of neural and vascular connections which can be affected by pathologies and traumatic injuries. In particular, 50% of them are due to road accident, 24% to fall, 17% to other causes, 6% to sports and 3% to extreme sports [1]. The most important classification of spinal cord injury is the International Standard for the Neurological Classification of SCI (ISNCSCI) created by the American Spinal Injury Association (ASIA) [2]. This classification permits us to evaluate the type of injury and the rehabilitation program in order to improve patients' quality of life. Lesions are grouped into levels according to their position along the spinal cord, and each level is correlated to a specific loss of functionality. If the subject loses motor and/or sensitive functions because of a lesion of the spinal cord in the cervical segment, the patient's disability is called tetraplegia. The disability is called paraplegia if the spinal cord-affected areas are the thoracic, lumbar, or sacral segments. When a person is subjected to a spinal cord injury, the wheelchair is the basic support to start the rehabilitation process and recover personal autonomy. The first step of the process with a wheelchair requires a setup made according to the patient's stature and conditions (e.g., muscular force, comorbidities or other impairments). The setup can be also changed according to the level of ability of the user who is learning how to sit and act on the handrims. For the posture analysis and propulsion evaluation, the assessment is still based on direct and qualitative observation, with no standard instruments to measure the improvements in wheelchair use. The observational approach has some limits; in fact, it is subjective and depends on physicians' and physiotherapists' experience. Moreover, data are not stored and only evaluation related to functional scales is recorded. Thus, even if the medical personnel are qualified, a patient's medical history results may be incomplete and accurate monitoring over time is almost impossible.

To overcome these drawbacks, digital technologies for tracking patient's movements can be adopted. Motion capture (Mocap) systems have the potential to track and record real human motion. They allow recognizing, reproducing and analyzing the motion of specific districts or of the entire body. The kinematic data of any action performed during a rehabilitation process can be the basis of an improved way to assess a patient's condition and monitor his/her evolution in the long term. However, Mocap systems require specific technological skills that are challenging for medical personnel, who prefer to continue with the standard and traditional approach based on visual assessment instead of investing resources to introduce new technologies.

The aim of this paper is the creation of a novel procedure to analyze the motion of spinal cord-injured patients using a wheelchair by means of a motion capture system based on inexpensive sensors that is easily usable by physicians and physiotherapists. The design of the procedure has been defined in collaboration with the medical staff of the hospital ASST Papa Giovanni XXIII in Bergamo, which is one of the most important public hospital in Italy. A software application has been developed to automatically execute the pushing cycle analysis and find the key measurements of specific movements which are useful in assessing the patient's performance in a simple way and supporting the medical personnel with objective data during the decision process. The application allows physicians to collect medical information during the patient's rehabilitation process.

For evaluating the reliability of the proposed solution, the research work compares the acquired motion data with those obtained with a professional high-level Mocap solution found in the literature.

In the first part, this paper introduces the state of the art relative to the use of innovative technologies as a new frontier for medical rehabilitation; then, the methodology for developing the whole procedure based on the use of a low-cost Mocap system is described. Finally, the outcomes are discussed and a quantitative analysis is presented comparing the results reached so far with the data available in the literature.

2. State of the Art

The analysis of the propulsion of a wheelchair allows us to assess the correctness of the upper limb movements and loads in spinal cord-injured patients. Actually, the measurement of the upper limb, shoulder and back performance may prevent the risk of patient injury caused by a wrong use of a wheelchair. The correct approach for safe and energy-saving pushing is based on the kinematic data of patient's movements and the forces generated during the propulsion.

Nowadays, rehabilitation centers adopt observational methods to assess the propulsion of a wheelchair. In the scientific literature, several standard protocols have been defined to obtain assessment methods that are as objective as possible for both intra-operator and inter-operator. For example, Gowran et al. [3] propose a list of existing visual standard protocols for the evaluation of wheelchair propulsion. The claimed aim is to find key factors supporting the physiotherapists in defining the best setting of the wheelchair, preventing injury and postural diseases. However, this approach is mainly static and does not consider the movements of patients during the use of the wheelchair. Smith et al. [4] define a specific method, the Wheelchair Propulsion Test (WPT), which relies on the observation of a patient using the wheelchair along a straight path that is 10 m long. The data acquired are the time required, the number of pushes, the identification of the pushing style and a pushing cycle analysis. Even if WPT guarantees an objective approach, still no data about the patient's movements are considered. Other research works have developed the assessment protocol, Wheelchair Skills Test (WST). This defines a set of tasks that the patient has to perform with the wheelchair while one or more physiotherapists visually assess the way the patient performs pushing cycles according to capacity, confidence, performance and training goal. In some research works, such as Lindquist et al. [5] and Askari et. al. [6], physiotherapists use video recordings of the patients' performances for consulting previous assessments. Additionally, WST allows an objective inter-operator and intra-operator approach, but no patient movements are directly measured.

Other research works combine the use of video recording with biomedical signals of muscles using electromyography. The aim is to study what happens to the upper arms during wheelchair propulsion. In particular, Chow et al. [7] use electromyography with recorded video during wheelchair propulsion on a sloped ramp. The result is the correlation of muscular activity of the upper limb with each phase of the pushing cycle. Additionally, in this case no kinematic data are available.

With the aim of detecting and recording the movements and forces generated by the patients during wheelchair usage, innovative technologies have been introduced as tools for assessing the wheelchair propulsion by considering patients' performance.

Some researchers have exploited sensorized wheelchairs. For example, the commercial solution Smartwheel [8] allows measuring the forces and torsions on a wheelchair directly from the wheels. While forces are acquired on the wheels, patients' kinematic data are monitored adding a motion capture (Mocap) system [9,10].

A Mocap system tracks and recognizes the human body shape to reconstruct a virtual skeleton that follows the recorded movements. The virtual skeleton allows directly evaluating the kinematic data of the movement and correlating them to the medical assessment. Three main types of Mocap system can be used: inertial systems and optical marker-based or markerless solutions.

Inertial Mocap systems are based on inertial measurement units (IMUs) applied along the human body to record movements during wheelchair propulsion. Leving et al. [11] show how it is possible to track and record upper limb movements by applying IMUs on patient's shoulders, elbows and wrists. This technology is able to register the position, velocity and acceleration of each IMU sensor; however, no data are directly available that describe the kinematic behaviors of the whole patient's body on the wheelchair. Similarly, Slikke et al. [12,13] show the high accuracy of an IMU motion acquisition system for assessing the wheelchair propulsion of SCI patients in sports. Additionally, in this case data only correlate to a single point along the upper arms. Moreover, IMU sensors can be considered slightly invasive from the patients' point of view, and the eventual slipping of the sensors along the arms during acquisition may affect the final results.

Marker-based Mocap systems are usually expensive but they guarantee a high accuracy and precision. For example, Boninger et al. [14] used the Optitrack system [15] to analyze the kinematics of the upper limb and Smartwheel to measure the forces generated during wheelchair propulsion; this is performed on a propulsion platform in order to execute a large number of pushing cycles in a room. The achieved results show that the main causes of injuries are due to the asymmetry between the right and left upper arm during the pushing cycles. Vegter et al. [10] used a marker-based Mocap system and a sensorized wheelchair for evaluating the mechanical efficiency and the overload of the shoulder articulation. The evaluation takes place during the first part of the rehabilitation process, during which patients learn how to use the wheelchair. The results demonstrate how the kinematic data permit one to optimize the symmetry of the propulsion to reduce the overload on the shoulder and prevent inflammation for a long-lasting period after the initial rehabilitation. Due to their high accuracy and precision, marker-based Mocap systems are usually considered as a reference by which to evaluate other Mocap solutions. Newsam et al. [16] exploited a Vicon system to analyze how SCI patients perform the propulsion step. In particular, the aim was to evaluate a set of specific parameters of arm movements during the pushing cycles to investigate the main differences in performance among patient groups with different levels of spinal cord injury. Eight movements were measured: humeral elevation, horizontal abduction of the humeral, humeral rotation, elbow flexion, forearm pronation, trunk extension, wrist flexion and wrist ulnar deviation. They have been measured in degrees at five specific steps of the pushing cycle: the initial contact of the hand on the pushrim, the hand on the top center of the wheel, the hand off the pushrim, the end of the follow through and the end of the arm return. The results reached can be used as a reference to validate similar research works.

The use of this technology is costly, time-consuming and requires a dedicate room; thus, it is not so widespread in rehabilitation centers.

Markerless Mocap systems instead exploit a set of low-cost portable sensors. The most diffused solutions in the literature adopt RGB-D sensors that combine a standard RGB video with the depth data of the scene. Rammer et al. [17] propose a propulsion platform on which children on a wheelchair perform many pushing cycles. The patient's movements on the wheelchair are acquired by a system composed of three Microsoft Kinect v2 sensors positioned around the wheelchair. The system can detect kinematic metrics relevant in manual wheelchair propulsion. The obtained data are relevant but hardly usable by a medical staff because they are not directly usable for pushing cycle analysis. Furthermore, even if using a platform reduces the volume of acquisition, which is positive, it also obliges the wheels to move on straight binaries, and the pushing movements may be distorted.

Literature contributions are generally focused on the technical feasibility while neglecting the final users' requirements and background. Actually, physicians and physiotherapists must be able at least to set up the hardware devices to track the patients and obtain results in a readable format with a few simple steps. In the last five years, the authors have designed a solution that is patient- and physician-driven to perform pushing cycle analysis by means of a low-cost Mocap system based on three Microsoft Kinect v2 devices. The layout of the Mocap system was optimized to be easily usable, fast to mount and easily replicable in a rehabilitation center [18,19]. Furthermore, a specific application was developed to automatically extrapolate from the acquired data the motion parameters needed to assess the pushing cycle [20].

Concerning the performance of markerless Mocap systems, several research works have compared them with professional marker-based systems. Galna et al. [21] compared the use of a single Microsoft Kinect v1 with the Vicon system [22] to track movements of the upper limbs of patients with Parkinson's disease. The results demonstrate that the Kinect device is an adequate system for acquiring wide movements of the arms with a good accuracy (e.g., abduction, adduction and rotation). Instead, it is not suitable to acquire fine movements of the hands, such as hand clasping. Concerning the use of a wheelchair, Milgrom et al. [23] compared a markerless Mocap system composed of the Microsoft Kinect device with a software development kit (SDK) [24] to acquire the wheelchair propulsion executed by patients on a platform. The results highlight the good accuracy obtained with a Kinect-based Mocap system which is suitable for measuring the key features of pushing cycles.

3. Method

In order to define a technological solution applicable in the medical field, a methodology has been developed by the authors and refined through many years of experience [19]. First, a preliminary study allowed the design of a Mocap layout with 3 Microsoft Kinect v2 sensors to assess the wheelchair propulsion of an SCI patient along a straight path approximatively 6 m long [18]. Then, by involving healthy people, the kinematic data were analyzed in collaboration with medical personnel in order to find a correlation between the movements and the patients' assessment. Starting from medical information described in [19], the goal of the SCI patient analysis was to simplify and organize the acquired biomechanical data in order to make available to medical staff only the information needed for the patient's rehabilitation.

A pushing cycle is subdivided in two main movements of the arms (Figure 1):

- Push: this occurs when the hands grab the wheelchair handrims and move the wheels forward.

- Recovery: this starts when the hands let the handrims go and finishes when the position of pushing is reached.

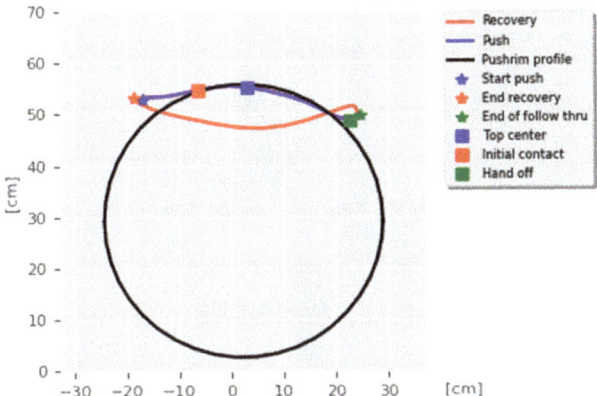

Figure 1. Example of a pushing cycle highlighting the recovery (red line) and push (blue line) movements as well as the considered key points.

The beginning and the end of the push and recovery are very important because they correspond to the extreme reachable positions of the hands and determine the quality and effectiveness of the movements. According to the virtual skeleton describing the human, the hand joint corresponds to the real human wrist. It is connected to the forearm joint that is connected, in turn, to the shoulder joint. This kinematic chain, composed of only two links, is essential for the description of the hand propulsion trajectory. According to the physicians' needs, an optimal pushing cycle analysis can be assessed if the patients can be tracked on a straight path at least 6 m long. Along the propulsion cycle, there are five key points (see Figure 1) that are used to compare the proposed solution with the data available in the literature:

- Top center (TC): the hand reaches the top center position of the pushrim during the push.
- Initial contact (IC): the hand touches the pushrim to start the push.
- Hand off (HO): the hand leaves the pushrim and then the push finishes.
- End of follow through (End FT): the hand finishes going forward before starting the recovery movement.
- End of arm return (End AR): the recovery movement finishes before starting a new pushing cycle.

Table 1 reports the measurements relative to the specific positions of arms, shoulders, and trunk useful for the assessment and also used for comparison with the results found in the literature. Each posture is described by the specific angles that are also shown graphically to permit an easy description and define the orientation.

Figure 2 shows the main phases of the implemented solution. The first is relative to the design of the Mocap procedure to acquire the patient on the wheelchair along the straight path. The second phase is relative to the use of iPiSoft to elaborate the motion-captured data according to the movements useful for the pushing cycles analysis and the final assessment. The third phase is focused on the application named the Spinal Cord Injury APPlication (SCI-APP) that automatically analyzes the acquired data and generates information to support the medical personnel's decisions.

Table 1. Main movements characterizing a patient's posture during wheelchair propulsion. The description is based on four pieces of information: the plane on which the movement is performed, the human articulation performing the movement, an image to visually understand how the movement is assessed and a description of the biomechanics of the movement considered.

Plane Considered	Human Articulation Requested	Position/Movement	Biomechanics Joint Analyzed
Median Plane	Trunk Flection		It contributes to determining the patient stability during wheelchair propulsion. As the angle decreases, the stability increases, but over a threshold angle the wheelchair can overturn during the pushing phase.
Median Plane	Humeral Elevation		The humeral elevation describes the rotation of the shoulder along the median plane during the propulsion of the wheelchair.
Median Plane	Humeral Rotation		The humeral rotation is the rotation around the axes of the humerus.
Transverse Plane	Humeral Horizontal Abduction		The horizontal abduction of the humerus describes the rotation of the shoulder around the transverse plane during the propulsion of the wheelchair.
Median Plane	Elbow Flexion/Extension		The maximum and minimum values of this angle have to stay in an optimum range in order to prevent a problem with the elbow articulation. This angle depends on the seat translation compared to the wheel rotation axle. Right and left angles are compared to assess the symmetric propulsion.

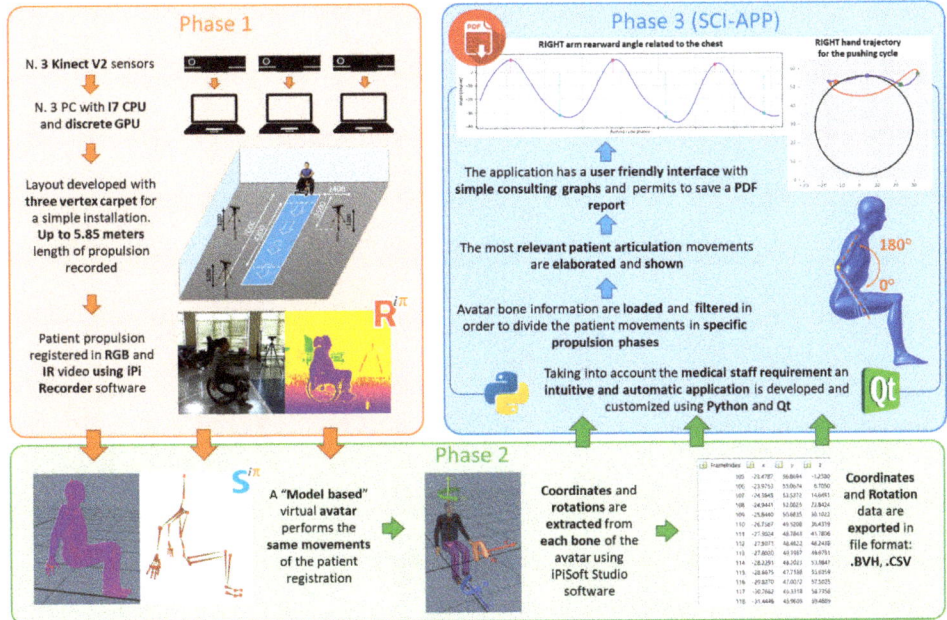

Figure 2. Main technological phases of the developed solution.

3.1. Phase 1: Mocap Acquisition

According to the results reached in previous research works [18,20], the default settings have been modified to improve the maximum performance and give better frame rate parameters. A commercial software solution developed by iPi Soft [25] is used to record the human motion and to extract avatar joint information. The tracked movements and relative skeleton animation have been stored in BVH format.

According to the requirements of the medical staff and the technological limits of the adopted solution, the standard multiple depth sensor configuration of the Mocap software needs to be modified to allow a 5.85 m-long acquisition track and to record three complete propulsion cycles for almost any patient.

The Mocap acquisition was designed in order to establish a checklist to reduce accidental oversights and human errors. In this way, all the patient's actions are taken with the same environmental conditions, hardware setup and software performance. This protocol was developed thanks to the experience gathered with a number of tests at the university laboratory and acquisition sessions. Table 2 describes the sequence of actions grouped according to the three main steps. The first foresees the layout assembly and all the PC connections, the second includes all the actions needed to calibrate the Mocap system and the last concerns how to use iPiSoft recorder.

Table 2. The action checklist for a correct Mocap acquisition of the SCI patients.

	To Do List for SCI Patients' Acquisitions		
LAYOUT	To repeat once a day	1.1	Lay out the three-vertex carpet
		1.2	Check Kinect 1.20 m in height
		1.3	Check Kinect horizontal inclination of −13°
		1.4	Check vertical orientation of Kinect RGB camera field of view
		1.5	Check ambient light source to darken (windows, lamps)
		1.6	Check Kinect - PC USB cable link
		1.7	Check ethernet cable link
		1.8	Setup iPi Soft Recorder Master and Slaves computers
		1.9	Setup new folder of the acquisition day "YYYY-MM-DD"
CALIBRATION 120 [sec]	To repeat for each calibration approx. every 30 min	2.1	Background iPi Soft Recorder 10 sec (with carpet on the floor), the Kinect field of view must be without anyone
		2.2	Setup Kinect with glass filter
		2.3	Spiral movements with light marker + Recording using iPi Soft Recorder
		2.4	Delete PC slave videos -> Button "Merge video" in iPi Soft Recorder
		2.5	Calibration using iPi Soft Studio
		2.6	Take off glass filter from Kinect
		2.7	Take off carpet from the floor
		2.8	Background iPi Soft Recorder 10 [sec] (without carpet on the floor), the Kinect field of view must be without anyone
VIDEO RECORDING	To repeat for each patient	3.1	Setup new patient's folder "No. - Patient Surname"
		3.2	Change folder directory in iPi Soft Recorder
	To repeat for each acquisition	3.3	Registration using iPi Soft Recorder
		3.4	Delete PC slave videos -> Button "Merge video" in iPi Soft Recorder

Further documentation, not reported in this paper, was created to help users in managing files (e.g., about calibration or wheelchair specifications), to check that the lights and patient's clothes are suitable and to properly inform patients about the procedure.

3.2. Phase 2: Data Extraction

This phase has the goal to extract from the acquired data the set of information required by physicians to evaluate the patient and his/her rehabilitation process. A set of correlations was defined between the raw data and the medical evaluation parameters. The adopted human avatar is composed of 29 joints with their associated positions, velocities and accelerations. The evaluated movements are associated with the kinematic data of the virtual joints. Table 3 depicts how medical parameters are quantified according to the tracked data. For the sake of the evaluation, it is also relevant to determine the entire trajectory of the hands during the pushing cycle. The beginning and end of any cycle are automatically identified by the ad hoc developed application. Furthermore, the movements are automatically measured according to the key points of each detected pushing cycle in order to obtain a complete analysis.

3.3. Phase 3: SCI-APP

By starting from the BVH file exported by iPisoft, SCI-APP automatically performs the analysis of the pushing cycles executed by the patients and makes available both linear and angular measurements of the upper limbs. All the information can be automatically exported in PDF and Microsoft Excel file format.

Table 3. Correlations between human articulations and virtual joints. The left column reports the measured human articulations by considering a specific set of virtual joints highlighted in green in the images depicted in the right column. The central column describes how to measure the movements using the virtual joints.

Human Articulation	Data and Information		Virtual Joints and Segments
Elbow Flection	Joints Angle [°] Description	Lower spine, neck. X-axis rotations. The bending of the trunk is measured as the angle between the vertical line and the segment passing between the lower spine and neck.	
Humeral Elevation	Joints Angle [°] Description	R/L shoulder, R/L forearm. X-axis rotations. The humeral elevation is measured as the rotation of the shoulder joint around the X-axis.	
Humeral Rotation	Joints Angle [°] Description	R/L shoulder. X-axis rotations. The humeral rotation is measured as the rotation of the shoulder joint around the axis defined as the vector between the shoulder position and the forearm position.	
Humeral Horizontal Abduction	Joints Angle [°] Description	R/L shoulder, R/L forearm. Y-axis rotations. The humeral horizontal abduction is measured as the rotation of the shoulder joint around the X-axis.	
Elbow Flexion/Extension	Joints Angle [°] Description	L/R forearm. X-axis rotations. During the propulsion phase, the angles considered have periodic movements. Max and min extensions are significant data by which to assess the upper limbs' performance.	

The whole application was developed in Python and is composed of four main modules:

- **Computation of pushing analysis.** This requires as input the kinematic data of the virtual skeleton to automatically detect all the instants relative to the beginning of both phases of the pushing cycle. It automatically checks if there are asymmetries between the left and the right pushing cycles.

- **Data extrapolation of each pushing cycles.** This makes available all the data of a specific pushing cycle. It is used to generate the graphs needed to compare the position of the hand with the position of the handrim and visually evaluates each type of pushing cycle.
- **Measurements of specific patient movements.** This computes the measurements of the human body articulations according to the medical reference system. The computed data are the linear and angular measurements described in Table 3.
- **Generation of the medical reports.** This permits us to automatically generate a report and save the computed data and measurements in a PDF or Excel file.

The medical personnel can access all these data through a user-friendly interface developed by means of Qt [26]. Figure 3 shows the SCI-APP user interface. The upper part is dedicated to the patients' data that have to be filled in by the medical personnel. The bottom part includes three main tabs related to the main system functionalities, each with its graphical area, to show the computed outcomes.

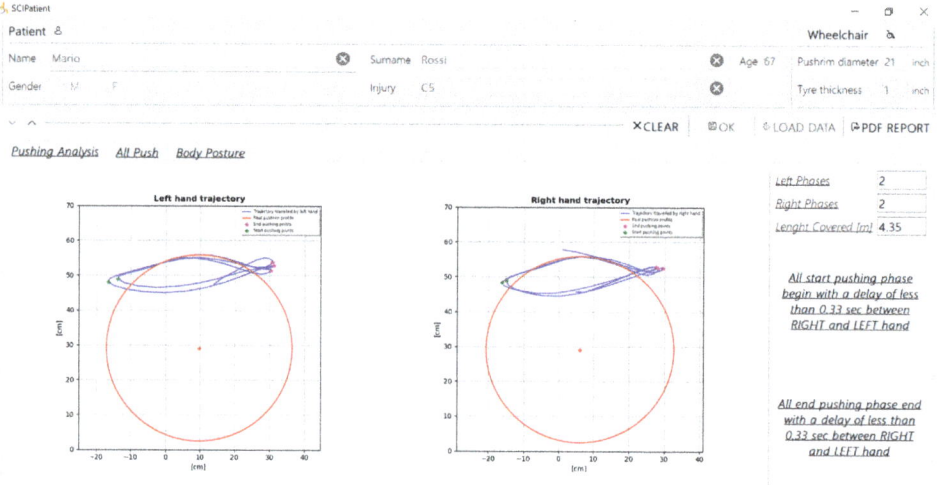

Figure 3. User interface of SCI-APP with an example of pushing analysis with the left and right hand trajectories with an asymmetry warning on the right side.

The first tab, named "Pushing Analysis", contains the data computed using the first module related to the propulsion analysis and its relative key points. In particular, the following information is shown:

- Number of right and left pushing phases made by the patient during wheelchair propulsion.
- Length covered by the patient during the wheelchair propulsion.
- A warning when the application detects symmetry loss during one or more propulsion phases.

Furthermore, it portrays two graphs about the right and left hand trajectory according to the position of the handrim profile (Figure 3). The beginning and the end of the detected pushing phases are highlighted for both the right and left sides. In this way, it is possible to show the extreme positions of upper limbs relative to the handrim during propulsion.

The second tab, entitled "View All Pushes", exploits the second module and shows the graphs of each right and left pushing cycle. Supported by these data, the operator can easily classify each pushing cycle according to the performed trajectory and easily find the difference between the right and left hand gesture during each propulsion movement (Figure 4).

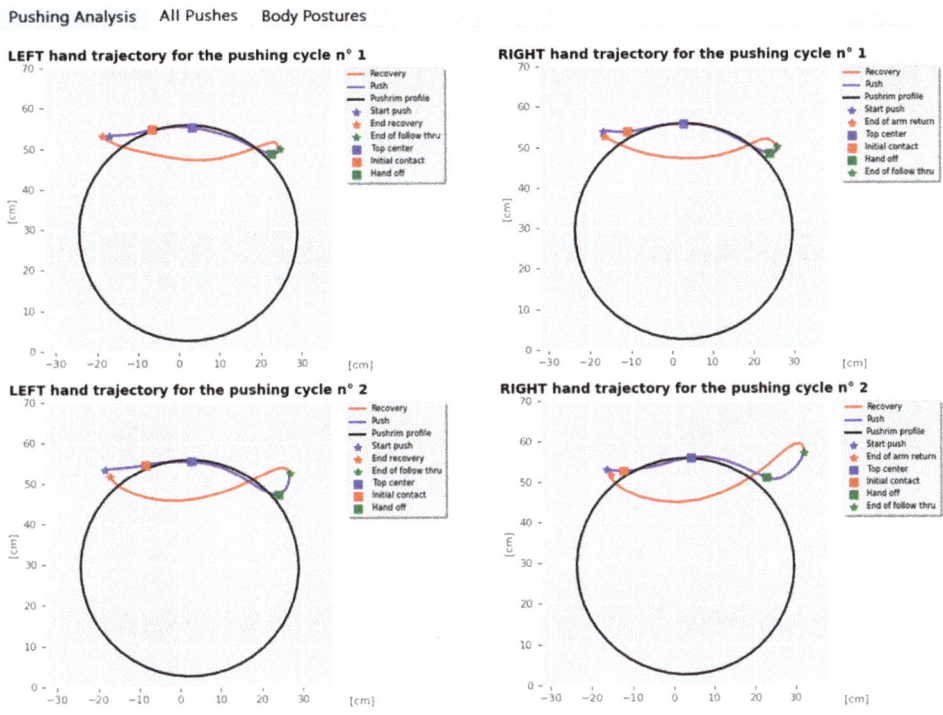

Figure 4. Examples of a trajectory analysis of two pushing cycles for both the left and right hands automatically calculated by SCI-APP.

The third tab, named "Body Posture", makes available graphs plotting the key parameters that describe the patient's motion (Table 2) for the entire acquisition. Furthermore, each graph shows the minimum, maximum and average values of relative parameters; the start and end pushing frames are highlighted in different colors to correlate the pushing cycle phases with the behavior of the evaluated movement (Figure 5). Finally, the operator can generate a pdf report with all the information needed for the medical assessment, as shown in Figure 6.

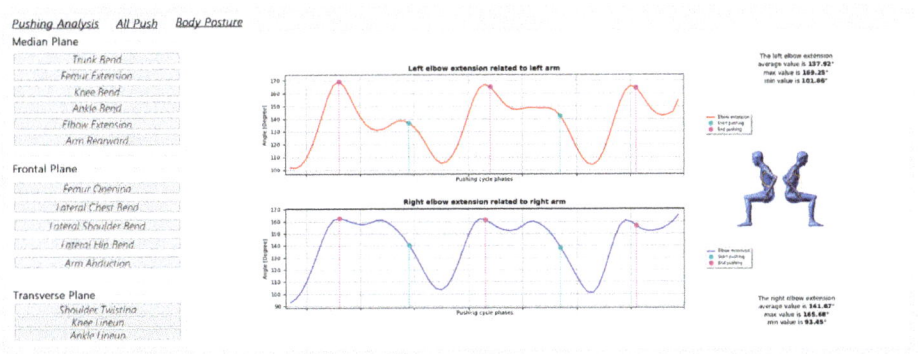

Figure 5. Example of an "Elbow flection" analysis with two graphs related to the specific movements measured according to the median, frontal and transverse planes and a graphical representation.

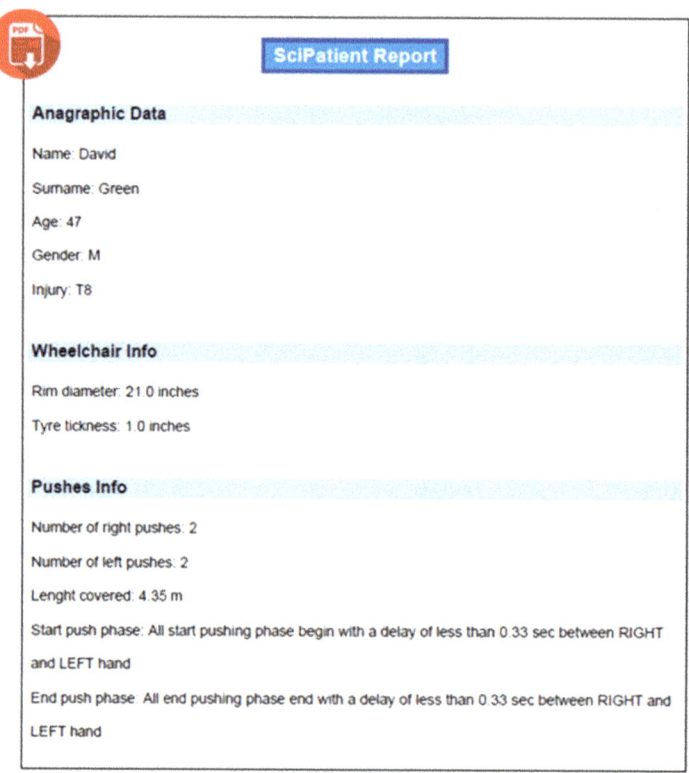
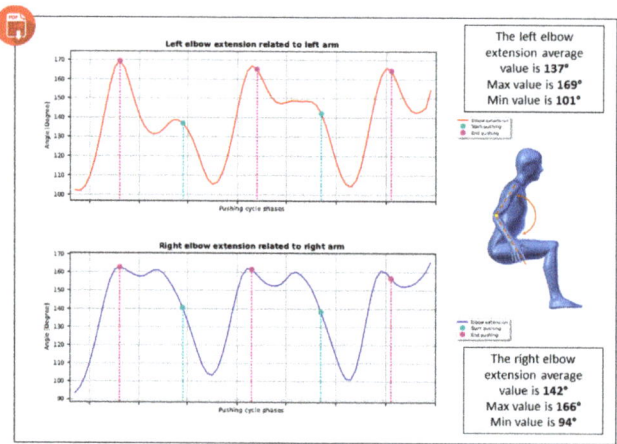

Figure 6. An example of a PDF report generated by SCI-APP including the main patient's data, information about the acquired pushing cycles (upper part) and the results of the analysis with graphical representations (lower part).

In order to evaluate the reliability of the data and the measurements computed with SCI-APP, a comparison must be carried out with similar acquisitions performed with a high-end solution. In this research study, the results of Newsam et al. [16] were chosen as reference data for the comparison.

SCI-APP exports the useful data in Excel file format for each acquisition. In particular, for each pushing cycle the 5 key points shown in Figure 1 are computed and for each of them are shown the measurements of the 5 movements to evaluate the wheelchair propulsion: the humeral elevation, the horizontal abduction of the humerus, the humeral rotation, the elbow flexion and the trunk extension along the sagittal plane. These movements are measured in degrees using the kinematic data of the virtual joints, as depicted in Table 3.

The goal is to investigate if low-cost sensors can track the wheelchair propulsion with an accuracy that can be considered from good to excellent. According to [21–27], a markerless Mocap system can be considered good for the evaluation of medical parameters relative to the movements if the measured movement has either an overestimation or underestimation reasonably smaller than 10°, and excellent when either the overestimation or underestimation is reasonably smaller than 5°.

4. Campaign of Acquisition

The acquisition of the SCI patients was performed at the rehabilitation center of the Hospital ASST Papa Giovanni XXIII, the main public hospital in Bergamo, Italy. Sixty volunteers with spinal cord injury were recorded. They were divided in four groups according to the level of the injury lesion: high paraplegia (n = 15 patients), low paraplegia (n = 15 patients), C6 tetraplegia (n = 13 patients) and C7 tetraplegia (n = 15 patients). Concerning gender, 80% of the patients were male and 20% female.

Figure 7 shows the distribution of the patients by age and height, and Figure 8 shows the distribution of the patients by how many years since the injury occurred and the height of the spinal lesion.

The exclusion criteria are centered on the functional evaluation of patients; age, sex, height or kind of lesion do not limit the patients from being enrolled, but only their ability to use a wheelchair.

Figure 9 shows the rehabilitation gym of the hospital where the experiment was carried out. To avoid variation in the light during long test sessions, artificial lights were preferred to natural light. The three Kinect V2 sensors were placed according to the defined layout using the positioning carpet. Each vertex of the carpet corresponds to the position of a sensor.

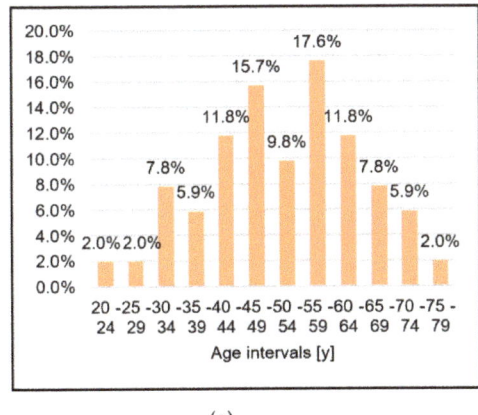
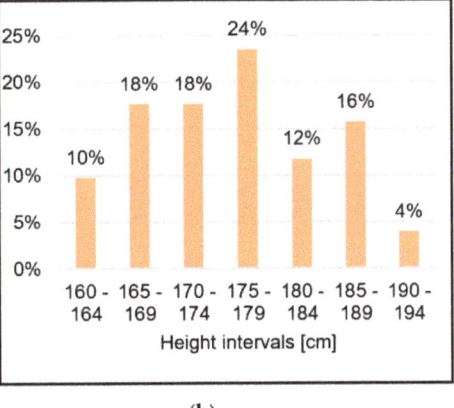

(a)   (b)

Figure 7. Distribution of patients by age (**a**) and height (**b**).

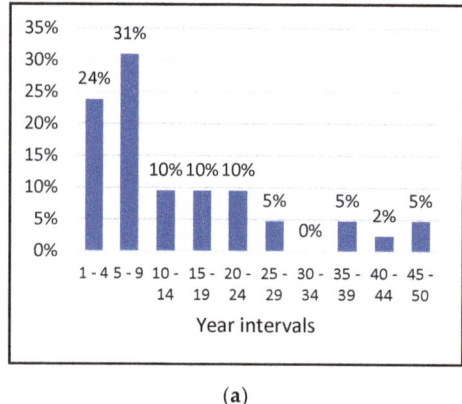
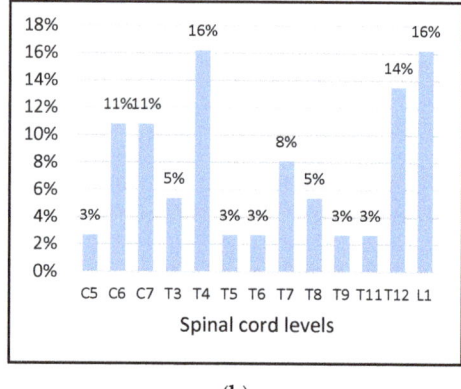

(a)   (b)

Figure 8. Distribution of patients by how many years since the injury occurred (**a**) and height of the spine lesion (**b**).

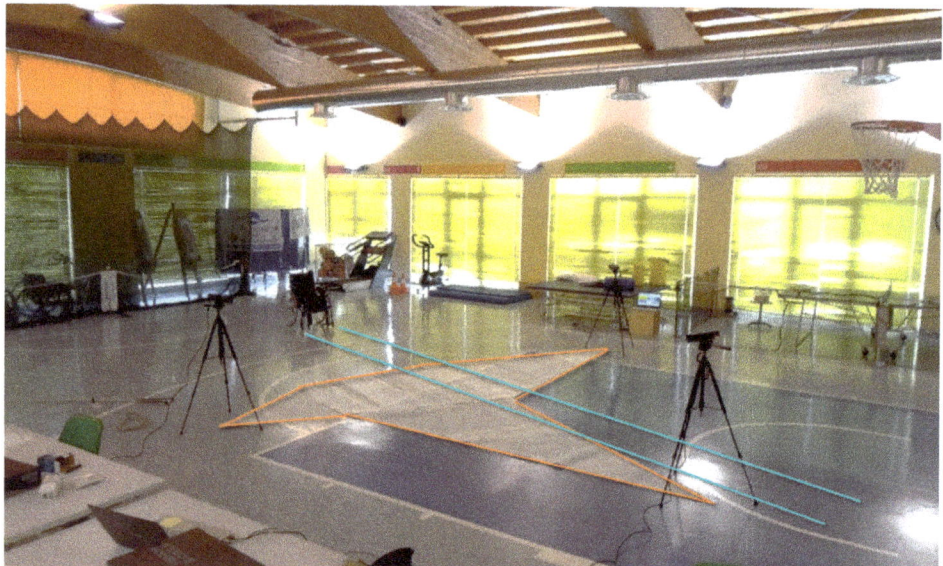

Figure 9. Rehabilitation gym and sensors layout with three-vertex carpet and wheelchair path. This tool allows a faster preparation of the layout of the Mocap system and a reference surface to correctly calibrate the multiple Microsoft Kinect sensors.

Patients are asked to practice on the path before being tracked. Each patient was acquired twice. The generated virtual avatar was exported by iPiSoft in a BVH file (Figure 10), which was used to automatically perform the pushing analysis with the SCI-APP and export the patient's body motions (Table 3) at each key position (i.e., IC, TC, HO, end FT and end AR).

In total, 138 acquisitions have been accomplished. Even if patients have been trained and informed to wear tight clothes, it happened that some acquisitions failed when the data were processed. Unfortunately, it is not possible to check all the parameters in real time and, thus, some acquisitions may fail. Anyway, this could be easily solved if the procedure becomes a routine activity in a rehabilitation center. A total of 116 acquisitions out of 138 (85%) are correct and have been automatically processed by the SCI-APP application.

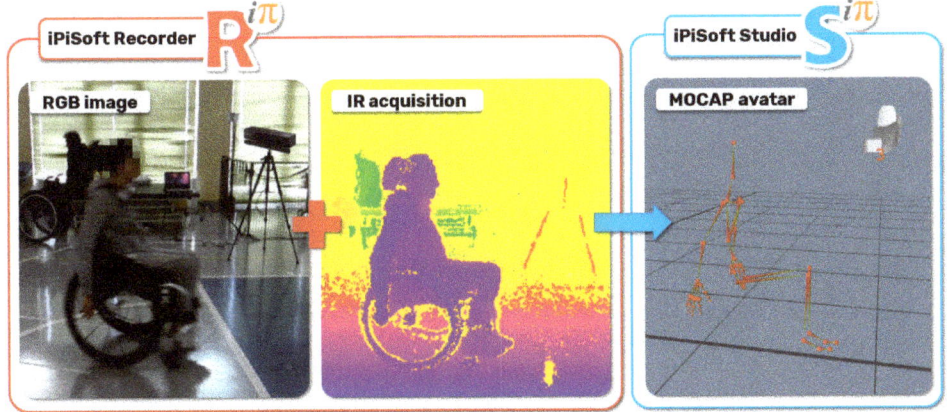

Figure 10. Respectively, RGB image, IR acquisitions and the virtual avatar of the acquired patient.

The average duration of the video acquisition was 105 frames, corresponding to 3.5 s at 30 fps; eventual differences due to slow movements or other conditions can be easily handled. For each acquisition, the SCI-APP application is able to identify, from an average of 4.30 m net acquisition path length, two complete cycles (51%) or three complete cycles (24%). The number of single pushes (i.e., without recovery) goes from two to five in 96% of the cases analyzed. In 9% of the acquisitions analyzed, the SCI-APP detected asymmetric movements between the right and left upper limbs, which involves a different number of pushing phases between the right and the left hands.

There are some drawbacks regarding the use of an optical system to track part of the body—e.g., the pelvis and hips—because they are occluded by the presence of the wheelchair even if these parts are not crucial for patients' assessment.

5. Results and Discussion

In the next subsections, the results reached so far are presented and discussed as follows. For each patient group, the average value and the standard deviation have been computed for each of the five considered movements in each key point and compared with data reported in Newsam et al. [16].

A table is presented for each movement. The table has three rows for each patient group; the first reports the reference data (i.e., the data reported in Newsam et al. [16]), the data computed by the SCI APP and the difference between them. The columns are relative to the five key points of the pushing cycle.

5.1. Humeral Elevation

Table 4 shows the parameters relative to the humeral elevation. The Δ rows show average values very good compared to the reference values for all the key instants in all the groups of patients. In detail, IC, TC and end AR present an optimal measurement using Kinect sensors. This result confirms that the Kinect sensors can track wide movements of the human body as the humeral elevation with a high quality [28,29].

Table 4. Values of the humeral elevation in degrees for each group of patients.

Humeral Elevation	IC		TC		HO		End FT		End AR	
	Avg.	St.D.	Avg.	St.D.	Avg.	St.D.	Avg.	St.D.	Avg.	St.D.
Low paraplegic (Ref. Val.)	55.1	4.4	48.8	4.3	24.2	4.6	22.1	3.9	56.9	4.7
Low paraplegic (Sci App)	52.0	7.3	46.7	8.2	16.7	15.1	11.8	6.5	54.3	9.1
Δ	−3.1		−2.1		−7.5		−10.3		−2.6	
High paraplegic (Ref. Val.)	53.8	7.8	47.1	7.9	23.7	4.3	22.1	4.0	55.7	7.2
High paraplegic (Sci App)	51.3	8.7	45.7	10.4	17.2	14.7	10.0	8.7	50.5	10.2
Δ	−2.5		−1.4		−6.5		−12.1		−5.2	
C7-tetraplegic (Ref. Val.)	49.0	8.9	42.6	9.7	22.1	4.4	21.5	4.2	52.5	7.9
C7-tetraplegic (Sci App)	44.8	6.9	37.7	6.8	7.8	6.6	10.9	8.5	43.4	8.9
Δ	−4.2		−4.9		−14.3		−10.6		−9.1	
C6-tetraplegic (Ref. Val.)	45.4	8.3	41.1	9.2	23.8	6.9	21.6	5.5	49.5	8.0
C6-tetraplegic (Sci App)	41.3	6.8	38.6	5.3	15.0	9.4	13.8	5.7	40.8	5.5
Δ	−4.1		−2.5		−8.8		−7.8		−8.7	

The key points HO and the end FT have the highest Δ. The difference could be due to the fact that Newsam et al. performed the acquisition with a shorter path of 4 m. This may affect the way the patient pushes the wheelchair propulsions [28,29].

5.2. Horizontal Abduction of Humerus

Table 5 shows the parameters relative to the horizontal abduction of the humerus. The Δ rows show the average values optimal for the key points IC, TC, end FT and end AR for all the groups of patients. Additionally, in this case the high similarity confirms the potentialities of Kinect sensors to track wide movements.

Table 5. Values of the abduction of humerus in degrees for each group of patients.

Horizontal Abduction	IC		TC		HO		End FT		End AR	
	Avg.	St.D.	Avg.	St.D.	Avg.	St.D.	Avg.	St.D.	Avg.	St.D.
Low paraplegic (Ref. Val.)	−53.6	8.1	−41.8	8.5	6.8	12.5	21.8	14.8	−55.3	8.3
Low paraplegic (Sci Lab)	−51.7	10.1	−46.7	10.8	−13.9	21.1	22.8	18.8	−51.2	10.2
Δ	1.9		−4.9		−20.7		1.0		4.1	
High paraplegic (Ref. Val.)	−55.5	8.9	−44.8	6.8	0.8	20.7	15.6	24.0	−56.5	8.8
High paraplegic (Sci Lab)	−54.2	9.1	−46.4	9.2	−18.2	18.1	15.1	18.4	−52.1	8.8
Δ	1.3		−1.6		−19.0		−0.5		4.4	
C7-tetraplegic (Ref. Val.)	−58.3	7.7	−48.8	6.8	8.6	17.9	19.6	21.1	−59.3	6.7
C7-tetraplegic (Sci Lab)	−59.2	8.3	−52.8	10.2	−5.4	20.3	23.4	18.7	−57.0	6.1
Δ	−0.9		−4.0		−14.0		3.8		2.3	
C6-tetraplegic (Ref. Val.)	−54.6	8.4	−43.5	13.3	8.2	14.2	9.9	15.4	−55.1	8.4
C6-tetraplegic (Sci Lab)	−56.2	8.3	−51.1	7.8	−9.9	29.3	17.9	11.0	−52.1	7.1
Δ	−1.6		−7.6		−18.1		8.0		3.0	

The key points HO has a very high Δ value. Additionally in this case, the difference could reasonably depend on the length of the acquired path.

5.3. Humeral Rotation

Table 6 shows the parameters relative to the humeral rotation. The Δ rows show average values that are very good for the key points IC, TC and end AR for all groups of patients. Very high Δ values have been computed for HO and end FT. In this case, it is very difficult to understand if the high difference can be correlated with a lower propulsion or if there is a loss of the correct humeral rotation by the Mocap system during tracking in the second part of the propulsion. The loss of tracking may be caused by a type of movement (i.e., the rotation of the humerus around own axis) that can be very hard to detect using optical sensors.

Table 6. Values of the humeral rotation in degrees for each group of patients.

Humeral Rotation	IC		TC		HO		End FT		End AR	
	Avg.	St.D.	Avg.	St.D.	Avg.	St.D.	Avg.	St.D.	Avg.	St.D.
Low paraplegic (Ref. Val.)	78.0	14.8	69.9	14.6	37.0	18.7	24.4	22.2	77.7	14.5
Low paraplegic (Sci Lab)	74.0	3.6	70.6	4.1	53.1	10.4	36.6	10.3	75.0	5.0
Δ	−4.0		0.7		16.1		12.2		−2.7	
High paraplegic (Ref. Val.)	75.6	14.5	67.8	14.4	35.5	26.4	22.4	31.6	76.0	14.2
High paraplegic (Sci Lab)	75.7	4.6	71.8	4.3	57.1	8.5	43.2	7.0	75.5	5.0
Δ	0.1		4.0		21.6		20.8		−0.5	
C7-tetraplegic (Ref. Val.)	73.6	12.9	70.7	12.6	27.2	22.4	17.3	27.5	72.0	12.9
C7-tetraplegic (Sci Lab)	68.7	6.0	63.5	5.2	43.0	9.3	34.6	7.1	67.6	5.8
Δ	−4.9		−7.2		15.8		17.3		−4.4	
C6-tetraplegic (Ref. Val.)	74.6	10.4	69.3	15.2	27.6	18.9	19.1	23.1	72.6	10.2
C6-tetraplegic (Sci Lab)	70.6	5.0	68.1	5.2	52.1	10.6	37.5	8.4	70.3	3.4
Δ	−4.0		−1.2		24.5		18.4		−2.3	

5.4. Elbow Flexion

The evaluation of the elbow flexion/extension is shown in Table 7. The Δ rows show average values good for the key points IC, TC, end FT and end AR for all the groups of patients. There are higher Δ values only for the group with low paraplegia, but the values of their standard deviation permit us to consider the differences negligible. The possibility of shorter propulsions is further confirmed by the Δ values of HO of the elbow flexion/extension. Additionally in this case, the HO values are higher than the reference data and the reason for this could be the same as for the previous cases.

Table 7. Values of the elbow flexion/extension in degrees for each group of patients.

Elbow Flexion	IC		TC		HO		End FT		End AR	
	Avg.	St.D.	Avg.	St.D.	Avg.	St.D.	Avg.	St.D.	Avg.	St.D
Low paraplegic (Ref. Val.)	59.4	10.9	76.4	8.9	43.1	9.8	34.8	9.0	54.3	9.8
Low paraplegic (Sci Lab)	68.2	12.0	72.7	10.1	58.1	19.0	33.6	13.2	64.4	15.1
Δ	8.8		−3.7		15.0		−1.2		10.1	
High paraplegic (Ref. Val.)	59.8	11.6	77.1	11.1	46.1	11.7	37.4	12.7	55.0	11.1
High paraplegic (Sci Lab)	64.2	12.7	74.0	9.5	63.8	14.8	41.8	12.3	57.5	15.1
Δ	4.4		−3.1		17.7		4.4		2.5	
C7-tetraplegic (Ref. Val.)	65.5	8.1	77.1	8.1	42.4	10.1	35.4	10.1	62.9	9.2
C7-tetraplegic (Sci Lab)	62.9	12.4	72.7	6.3	51.7	14.7	35.6	11.8	55.9	17.5
Δ	−2.6		−4.4		9.3		0.2		−7.0	
C6-tetraplegic (Ref. Val.)	62.8	10.0	69.8	10.7	42.8	9.3	41.8	9.3	61.3	10.6
C6-tetraplegic (Sci Lab)	60.9	15.0	71.3	10.0	54.0	15.5	33.4	10.8	58.2	14.4
Δ	−1.9		1.5		11.2		−8.4		−3.1	

5.5. Trunk Flexion/Extension

The trunk flexion/extension along the sagittal plane is very similar for each group of patients. In this case, the data from the literature [16] make available a general average value for all the key instants that have a value between 1 and 7 degrees. According to this range, the values measured with the SCI-APP are very good (Table 8). Furthermore, Newsam et al. highlighted that the subjects with C6 tetraplegia have a total excursion of trunk motion significantly greater than all the other groups (i.e., an average value of 11°), which is confirmed by the data we acquired.

Table 8. Values of the trunk flexion/extension rotation in degrees for each group of patients.

Trunk Extension	IC		TC		HO		End FT		End AR	
	Avg.	St.D.	Avg.	St.D.	Avg.	St.D.	Avg.	St.D.	Avg.	St.D
Low paraplegic	−3.4	4.9	−3.8	5.0	−3.9	5.3	−2.6	5.2	−2.6	5.1
High paraplegic	0.0	7.7	0.0	7.8	0.1	6.8	0.9	6.3	0.3	7.1
C7-tetraplegic	0.7	9.4	0.0	9.1	−0.9	8.7	−0.9	8.8	0.9	8.9
C6-tetraplegic	12.4	5.1	11.0	5.0	9.1	5.1	9.6	5.5	12.4	5.4

5.6. Final Considerations

Concerning the information available in the scientific literature [16,21,27–29], the outcomes reached with the SCI-APP are consistent. Moreover, the long path we are using allows tracking more pushing cycles for each acquisition, making the average values more robust. Actually, tracking patients on a short path, even with top-quality sensors, can influence the way patients behave. This condition may be one of the reasons why the values of movements at key points HO and end FT are not similar to those available in the literature.

The comparison performed so far has been shown to the involved medical personnel and their feedback is positive. Thus, we are confident that the presented markerless Mocap system can be easily adopted as a tool for the medical assessment of pushing cycles.

Further investigations have been planned to analyze in detail the movement of the humerus, since it is the most relevant contribution to the entire pushing. The main weakness of the presented solution seems to be the measurements of the rotations along the axes of virtual bones, as described in § 5.3.

Future developments will be dedicated to tracking the movements of wrists, hands and fingers, which have been neglected in this research work.

6. Conclusions

Paraplegia is mainly due to injuries to the spinal cord and may cause paralysis of the lower limbs; the wheelchair is the best moving solution for most people with this disability. The assessment of posture and the way the wheelchair is used is essential during the rehabilitation process to avoid further ailments or excessive energy expenditure. A structured method has been provided to support the complex issue of evaluating the way a person moves on a wheelchair. The method has been used with 60 patients, whose data have been elaborated by an ad hoc developed application to obtain the required medical parameters. As a result, a simple but flexible user interface allows plotting any translation or rotation of the involved articulations that may be relevant for the assessment. Physiotherapists are provided with automatic alerts to highlight critical conditions, such as asymmetry of the movements, and reports are generated automatically to keep track of the outcomes. The medical knowledge collected and formalized allowed developing a solution that not only provides medical personnel with the exact information they need, but that is also suitable for easy use.

The data generated have been compared with the few references available in the literature, which use costly Mocap systems for tracking. The comparison was conducted on the key movements of the trunk and arms in five specific instants of the pushing cycle. These data were evaluated by subdividing the patients into four groups according to the level of spinal cord injury. The comparison has highlighted mean values very similar to those in the scientific literature. A systematic error for the parameters HO and end-FT was highlighted and the most probable cause is correlated with the procedure of acquisition, which required patients to execute a possible pushing cycle along a straight path. This approach generated a pushing cycle shorter than the natural performance. In general, the results reached confirm that SCI-APP and the proposed markerless solution are useful for an adequate evaluation of propulsion.

Further works will be dedicated to performing a usability test involving personnel who did not participate to the development of the solution in order to highlight the eventual limits. Moreover, a validation campaign will be carried out considering the possibility of using more precise and accurate sensors. After this, the proposed solution will be ready for broad use in rehabilitation centers.

Author Contributions: A.V. and F.C.Z. contributed to the development of the Mocap solution, implementation of SCI-APP, patients' acquisition and data elaboration. D.R. and C.R. contributed to the Mocap system configuration, Knowledge extraction and formalization, and data analysis. G.M. provided the needed medical knowledge, enrolment of patients and data analysis. All authors have read and agreed to the published version of the manuscript.

Funding: This research received no external funding.

Conflicts of Interest: The authors declare no conflict of interest.

References

1. Bickenbach, J.; Officer, A.; Shakespeare, T.; von Groote, P. *International Perspectives on Spinal Cord Injury*; World Health Organization: Geneva, Switzerland, 2013; ISBN 9789241564663.
2. Kirshblum, S.C.; Burns, S.P.; Biering-Sorensen, F.; Donovan, W.; Graves, D.E.; Jha, A.; Johansen, M.; Jones, L.; Krassioukov, A.; Mulcahey, M.J.; et al. International standards for neurological classification of spinal cord injury (Revised 2011). *J. Spinal Cord Med.* **2011**, *34*, 535–546. [CrossRef] [PubMed]
3. Kenny, S.; Gowran, R.J. Outcome measures for wheelchair and seating provision: A critical appraisal. *Br. J. Occup. Ther.* **2014**, *77*, 67–77. [CrossRef]
4. Smith, E.M.; Low, K.; Miller, W.C. Interrater and intrarater reliability of the wheelchair skills test version 4.2 for power wheelchair users. *Disabil. Rehabil.* **2018**, *40*, 678–683. [CrossRef] [PubMed]
5. Lindquist, N.J.; Loudon, P.E.; Magis, T.F.; Rispin, J.E.; Kirby, R.L.; Manns, P.J. Reliability of the performance and safety scores of the wheelchair skills test version 4.1 for manual wheelchair users. *Arch. Phys. Med. Rehabil.* **2010**, *91*, 1752–1757. [CrossRef] [PubMed]
6. Askari, S.; Kirby, R.L.; Parker, K.; Thompson, K.; O'Neill, J. Wheelchair propulsion test: Development and measurement properties of a new test for manual wheelchair users. *Arch. Phys. Med. Rehabil.* **2013**, *94*, 1690–1698. [CrossRef] [PubMed]
7. Chow, J.W.; Millikan, T.A.; Carlton, L.G.; Chae, W.-S.; Lim, Y.-T.; Morse, M.I. Kinematic and Electromyographic Analysis of Wheelchair Propulsion on Ramps of Different Slopes for Young Men With Paraplegia. *Arch. Phys. Med. Rehabil.* **2009**, *90*, 271–278. [CrossRef] [PubMed]
8. Out-Front: The SmartWheel Clinical Tool. Available online: http://www.out-front.com/smartwheel_overview.php (accessed on 24 June 2020).
9. Dellabiancia, F.; Porcellini, G.; Merolla, G. Instruments and techniques for the analysis of wheelchair propulsion and upper extremity involvement in patients with spinal cord injuries: Current concept review. *Muscles Ligaments Tendons J.* **2013**, *3*, 150–156. [CrossRef] [PubMed]
10. Vegter, R.J.K.; Hartog, J.; De Groot, S.; Lamoth, C.J.; Bekker, M.J.; Van Der Scheer, J.W.; Van Der Woude, L.H.V.; Veeger, D.H.E.J. Early motor learning changes in upper-limb dynamics and shoulder complex loading during handrim wheelchair propulsion. *J. Neuroeng. Rehabil.* **2015**, *12*. [CrossRef] [PubMed]
11. Leving, M.T.; Horemans, H.L.D.; Vegter, R.J.K.; De Groot, S.; Bussmann, J.B.J.; van der Woude, L.H.V. Validity of consumer-grade activity monitor to identify manual wheelchair propulsion in standardized activities of daily living. *PLoS ONE* **2018**, *13*. [CrossRef] [PubMed]
12. van der Slikke, R.M.A.; Berger, M.A.M.; Bregman, D.J.J.; Lagerberg, A.H.; Veeger, H.E.J. Opportunities for measuring wheelchair kinematics in match settings; reliability of a three inertial sensor configuration. *J. Biomech.* **2015**, *48*, 3398–3405. [CrossRef] [PubMed]
13. van der Slikke, R.M.A.; Berger, M.A.M.; Bregman, D.J.J.; Veeger, H.E.J. From big data to rich data: The key features of athlete wheelchair mobility performance. *J. Biomech.* **2016**, *49*, 3340–3346. [CrossRef] [PubMed]
14. Boninger, M.L.; Souza, A.L.; Cooper, R.A.; Fitzgerald, S.G.; Koontz, A.M.; Fay, B.T. Propulsion patterns and pushrim biomechanics in manual wheelchair propulsion. *Arch. Phys. Med. Rehabil.* **2002**, *83*, 718–723. [CrossRef] [PubMed]
15. OptiTrack—Motion Capture Systems. Available online: https://optitrack.com/ (accessed on 24 June 2020).

16. Newsam, C.J.; Rao, S.S.; Mulroy, S.J.; Gronley, J.K.; Bontrager, E.L.; Perry, J. Three dimensional upper extremity motion during manual wheelchair propulsion in men with different levels of spinal cord injury. *Gait Posture* **1999**, *10*, 223–232. [CrossRef]
17. Rammer, J.; Slavens, B.; Krzak, J.; Winters, J.; Riedel, S.; Harris, G. Assessment of a markerless motion analysis system for manual wheelchair application. *J. Neuroeng. Rehabil.* **2018**, *15*. [CrossRef] [PubMed]
18. Vitali, A.; Regazzoni, D.; Rizzi, C. Digital motion acquisition to assess spinal cord injured (SCI) patients. *Comput. Aided. Des. Appl.* **2019**, *16*, 962–971. [CrossRef]
19. Regazzoni, D.; Vitali, A.; Rizzi, C.; Colombo, G. A Method to Analyse Generic Human Motion With Low-Cost Mocap Technologies. In Proceedings of the International Design Engineering Technical Conferences and Computers and Information in Engineering Conference, Quebec City, QC, Canada, 26–29 August 2018.
20. Regazzoni, D.; Vitali, A.; Rizzi, C.; Colombo Zefinetti, F. Motion Capture and Data Elaboration to Analyse Wheelchair Set-Up and Users' Performance. In Proceedings of the International Mechanical Engineering Congress and Exposition, Pittsburgh, PA, USA, 9–15 November 2018.
21. Galna, B.; Barry, G.; Jackson, D.; Mhiripiri, D.; Olivier, P.; Rochester, L. Accuracy of the Microsoft Kinect sensor for measuring movement in people with Parkinson's disease. *Gait Posture* **2014**, *39*, 1062–1068. [CrossRef] [PubMed]
22. Vicon|Award Winning Motion Capture Systems. Available online: https://www.vicon.com/ (accessed on 24 June 2020).
23. Milgrom, R.; Foreman, M.; Standeven, J.; Engsberg, J.R.; Morgan, K.A. Reliability and validity of the Microsoft Kinect for assessment of manual wheelchair propulsion. *J. Rehabil. Res. Dev.* **2016**, *53*, 901–918. [CrossRef] [PubMed]
24. Motion Capture Camera & Software Leader|Motion Analysis Corporation. Available online: https://www.motionanalysis.com/ (accessed on 24 June 2020).
25. iPi Soft- Markerless Motion Capture. Available online: http://ipisoft.com/ (accessed on 22 September 2020).
26. Qt|Cross-Platform Software Development for Embedded & Desktop. Available online: https://www.qt.io/ (accessed on 22 September 2020).
27. Otte, K.; Kayser, B.; Mansow-Model, S.; Verrel, J.; Paul, F.; Brandt, A.U.; Schmitz-Hübsch, T. Accuracy and reliability of the kinect version 2 for clinical measurement of motor function. *PLoS ONE* **2016**, *11*. [CrossRef] [PubMed]
28. Stephens, C.L.; Engsberg, J.R. Comparison of overground and treadmill propulsion patterns of manual wheelchair users with tetraplegia. *Disabil. Rehabil. Assist. Technol.* **2010**, *5*, 420–427. [CrossRef] [PubMed]
29. Kwarciak, A.M.; Turner, J.T.; Guo, L.; Richter, W.M. Comparing handrim biomechanics for treadmill and overground wheelchair propulsion. *Spinal Cord* **2010**, *49*, 457–462. [CrossRef] [PubMed]

Publisher's Note: MDPI stays neutral with regard to jurisdictional claims in published maps and institutional affiliations.

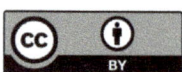

© 2020 by the authors. Licensee MDPI, Basel, Switzerland. This article is an open access article distributed under the terms and conditions of the Creative Commons Attribution (CC BY) license (http://creativecommons.org/licenses/by/4.0/).

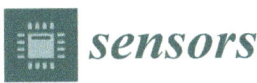

Article

A Game-Based Rehabilitation System for Upper-Limb Cerebral Palsy: A Feasibility Study

Mohammad I. Daoud [1,*], Abdullah Alhusseini [1], Mostafa Z. Ali [2] and Rami Alazrai [1]

1. Department of Computer Engineering, German Jordanian University, Amman 11180, Jordan; abdullah.h.alhusseini@gmail.com (A.A.); rami.azrai@gju.edu.jo (R.A.)
2. Department of Computer Information Systems, Jordan University of Science and Technology, Irbid 22110, Jordan; mzali@just.edu.jo
* Correspondence: mohammad.aldaoud@gju.edu.jo; Tel.: +962-6-429-4444 (ext. 4124)

Received: 17 February 2020; Accepted: 18 April 2020; Published: 24 April 2020

Abstract: Game-based rehabilitation systems provide an effective tool to engage cerebral palsy patients in physical exercises within an exciting and entertaining environment. A crucial factor to ensure the effectiveness of game-based rehabilitation systems is to assess the correctness of the movements performed by the patient during the game-playing sessions. In this study, we propose a game-based rehabilitation system for upper-limb cerebral palsy that includes three game-based exercises and a computerized assessment method. The game-based exercises aim to engage the participant in shoulder flexion, shoulder horizontal abduction/adduction, and shoulder adduction physical exercises that target the right arm. Human interaction with the game-based rehabilitation system is achieved using a Kinect sensor that tracks the skeleton joints of the participant. The computerized assessment method aims to assess the correctness of the right arm movements during each game-playing session by analyzing the tracking data acquired by the Kinect sensor. To evaluate the performance of the computerized assessment method, two groups of participants volunteered to participate in the game-based exercises. The first group included six cerebral palsy children and the second group included twenty typically developing subjects. For every participant, the computerized assessment method was employed to assess the correctness of the right arm movements in each game-playing session and these computer-based assessments were compared with matching gold standard evaluations provided by an experienced physiotherapist. The results reported in this study suggest the feasibility of employing the computerized assessment method to evaluate the correctness of the right arm movements during the game-playing sessions.

Keywords: cerebral palsy; game-based rehabilitation exercises; computerized assessment methods; motion tracking sensors; Kinect sensor

1. Introduction

Cerebral palsy refers to a group of non-progressive neurological disorders that begin at early childhood and can lead, among other limitations, to various degrees of motor impairments, physical disability, postural control, and coordination deficits [1,2]. The worldwide rate of cerebral palsy is around 1 per 500 live births, which makes cerebral palsy the most frequent cause of motor disability in childhood [3]. In fact, many children with cerebral palsy suffer from motor impairments in their upper limbs, which lead to significant impact on their independence in activities of daily living, quality of life, social interaction, and functional abilities [4].

Presently, no cure has been discovered for cerebral palsy [5]. Therefore, the treatment of cerebral palsy is often focused on avoiding complications, enhancing functional independence, managing symptoms, improving motor capabilities, and strengthening weak muscles [6]. One of the most effective and common rehabilitation treatment approaches for patients with cerebral palsy is to participate in task-specific, intensive, and repetitive physical exercises to improve the motor capabilities and reduce the potential of further complications [7,8]. Nevertheless, boredom, lack of motivation, the limited available resources, and high costs are among the key barriers that prevent patients with cerebral palsy from participating in rehabilitation physical exercises as recommended [9,10]. To address the aforementioned limitations, many research groups proposed the use of computer games as a complementary tool for conventional cerebral palsy rehabilitation therapy, with particular focus on children patients [11–16]. The use of computer games in the rehabilitation process has the potential to motivate the patients and increase the frequency and duration of the exercises [9,17,18].

Studies that investigated the use of computer games for cerebral palsy rehabilitation can be broadly classified into two main groups [13,19]. The first group is focused on using off-the-shelf computer games in cerebral palsy rehabilitation, while the second group proposed the use of bespoke computer games that are specifically designed for cerebral palsy rehabilitation [13,19]. Several studies from the first group employed off-the-shelf games that run on the Nintendo Wii game playing system (Nintendo Co., Kyoto, Japan), such as [11,20,21], the Microsoft Kinect system (Microsoft Corporation, Redmond, WA, USA), such as [10,16,22,23], and the Sony PlayStation system (Sony Interactive Entertainment, San Mateo, CA, USA), such as [24]. The use of off-the-shelf games has the advantage of offering high-quality gaming experience for cerebral palsy children at low cost. Nevertheless, such games are designed for typically developing subjects rather than persons with limited motor abilities [11,21]. Hence, the use of off-the-shelf games for cerebral palsy rehabilitation might be limited due to their high complexity and difficulty, the restricted customization options that prevent their adaptation for the rehabilitation process, and the lack of specialized assessment tools to evaluate the performance of the cerebral palsy children during the game-playing sessions [13,19].

Bespoke computer games that are specifically developed for cerebral palsy rehabilitation provide several advantages, including the ability to target physical rehabilitation exercises and the capability of customizing the games to meet the needs of the patients. In fact, one of the widely used commercial bespoke game-based rehabilitation systems is the Immersive Rehabilitation Exercise system (IREX system, GestureTek Health Inc., Toronto, ON, Canada) [25]. The IREX system employs a camera to capture real-time pictures of the patient and embeds the pictures into virtual reality gaming environment. The patient interacts with the virtual reality environment using motion tracking sensors. The study by Bryanton et al. [17] evaluated the use of the IREX system for cerebral palsy rehabilitation, and the results indicated the potential of employing the system to engage children with cerebral palsy in physical exercises within an exciting environment. Despite the improved capability of the IREX system, the high costs associated with the system might restrict its deployment at home as well as therapy centers that have limited budget [26].

Several previous studies investigated the development of non-commercial, low-cost, and effective bespoke computer games to support the rehabilitation of cerebral palsy children. Detailed review about these previous studies is presented in [25]. In fact, a large group of these non-commercial bespoke rehabilitation games employed the Microsoft Kinect sensor for tracking the skeleton joints of the participant to enable him/her to interact with the games [25]. For example, the study in [27] presented a set of Kinect-based games that are developed to engage patients with motor disabilities, including cerebral palsy patients, in physical exercises. Furthermore, several recent studies, such as [13,19,28], proposed Kinect-based games for training the limbs, particularly the upper limbs, of cerebral palsy children. The results reported in these studies suggested the feasibility of using non-commercial, low-cost, bespoke rehabilitation games as adjunct to conventional rehabilitation programs to actively engage cerebral palsy children in physical exercises. Nevertheless, a crucial requirement to enable the use of bespoke computer games as an effective complementary tool for cerebral palsy rehabilitation is to assess the correctness of the movements performed by the patients during the game-playing sessions [13].

The current study contributes to the ongoing efforts to improve the rehabilitation of cerebral palsy by proposing a non-commercial, low-cost, bespoke rehabilitation system. The proposed system aims to engage patients with upper-limb cerebral palsy in game-based physical exercises that target the right arm and assess the correctness of the right arm movements performed during the playing sessions. In particular, the proposed system includes three game-based rehabilitation exercises that are designed under the supervision of a specialized physiotherapist. Human interaction with the game-based exercises is enabled using the Microsoft Kinect sensor (particularly the Kinect v2 sensor). The correctness of the right arm movements during each game-playing session is evaluated using a custom-made computerized assessment method that analyzes the tracking data acquired by the Kinect sensor. To evaluate the performance of the proposed computerized assessment method, two groups of participants volunteered to participate in the three game-based rehabilitation exercises, where the first group included six cerebral palsy children and the second group included twenty typically developing subjects. For every participant, the computerized assessment method was employed to assess the correctness of the right arm movements in each game-playing session and the obtained computer-based assessment was compared with matching gold standard evaluation that is provided by an experienced physiotherapist. The results reported in the current study demonstrate the capability of the proposed assessment method to achieve effective evaluation of the right arm movements during the game-playing sessions.

The remainder of the paper is organized as follows. Section 2 provides an overview of the proposed rehabilitation system as well as detailed description of the three game-based rehabilitation exercises and the computerized assessment method. Section 3 describes the experimental evaluations and results, including the two groups of participants, the experimental protocol, the performance evaluation metrics, and the results obtained for both the cerebral palsy children and the typically developing subjects. The discussion and conclusion are provided in Section 4.

2. Materials and Methods

2.1. Overview of the Proposed Rehabilitation System

The hardware component of our proposed bespoke game-based rehabilitation system consists of a personal computer connected to a 19" liquid crystal display (LCD) and a Microsoft Kinect sensor. The personal computer is employed to perform the computational tasks, the LCD is used to display the game-based rehabilitation exercises, and Kinect sensor is employed to track the skeleton joints of the participant during each game-playing session. The participant was asked to perform the game-based rehabilitation exercises while seating on a chair or a wheelchair. Moreover, the LCD and the Kinect sensor were placed on a table with adjustable height to enable the participant to perform the game-based rehabilitation exercises in a comfortable manner. Figure 1 shows a cerebral palsy patient playing one of the game-based rehabilitation exercises provided by the proposed system.

The Kinect sensor used in the current study is the Kinect for Windows v2 sensor. In fact, this sensor provides a low-cost and effective alternative for high cost reference motion tracking systems, such as the Qualisys motion capture system (Qualisys Inc., Gothenburg, Sweden) [29]. The Kinect v2 sensor is equipped with an RGB camera that has a resolution of 1920×1080 pixels and an infrared camera that has a resolution of 512×424 pixels. Moreover, the sensor can track the 3D positions of twenty five body skeleton joints with a frame rate up to 30 Hz, where each joint position is expressed in the 3D Cartesian coordinate system.

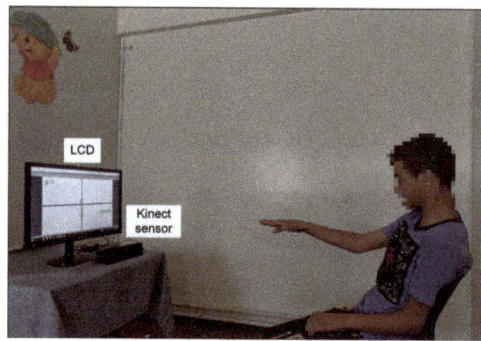

Figure 1. A cerebral palsy patient playing one of the game-based rehabilitation exercises provided by our proposed system.

The software component of our proposed system consists of a set of three game-based rehabilitation exercises that target the right arm and a computerized assessment method that assists the correctness of the right arm movements during the game-playing sessions. In fact, the game-based rehabilitation exercises are developed using the C# programming language and the Unity game development platform (Unity Technologies ApS, San Francisco, CA, USA). The computerized assessment method was implemented using MATALB (MathWorks Inc., Natick, MA, USA) and run offline after completing the playing sessions of the game-based rehabilitation exercises to evaluate the correctness of the right arm movements.

The architecture of the proposed bespoke game-based rehabilitation system is illustrated in Figure 2. As shown in the figure, the system is composed of four phases. The first phase allows the participant, under the supervision of the specialized physiotherapist, to select the game-based rehabilitation exercise. After selecting the game-based exercise, the system proceeds to the second phase. In the second phase, the participant performs the selected game-based exercise under the supervision and vocal guidance of the physiotherapist. In fact, the vocal guidance of the physiotherapist aims to help the participant to perform the game-based exercise in a correct manner. At the beginning of the game-playing session of the selected game-based exercise, the participant starts the exercise with his/her arms relaxed on his/her side and his/her palms facing towards his/her body. Then, the participant moves his/her right arm to perform the movements needed to play the game-based exercise as described in Section 2.2. It is worth noting that the game-playing session refers to the sequence of right arm movements performed by the participant to play the game-based exercise for a single iteration. During the game-playing session, the skeleton joints of the participant are tracked using the Kinect sensor to enable the participant to interact with the game. Moreover, the physiotherapist is asked to monitor the performance of the participant. The second phase ends when the participant completes the game-playing session of the selected game-based exercise. In the third phase, the tracking data of the participant's skeleton joints are recorded. Moreover, the physiotherapist is asked to label the right arm movements during the game-playing session as correct or incorrect based on the evaluation criterion described in Section 3.2. In the fourth phase, the recorded tracking data of the participant's skeleton joints are analyzed using the computerized assessment method, which is described in Section 2.3, to provide a computer-based evaluation of the correctness of the right arm movements during the game-playing session.

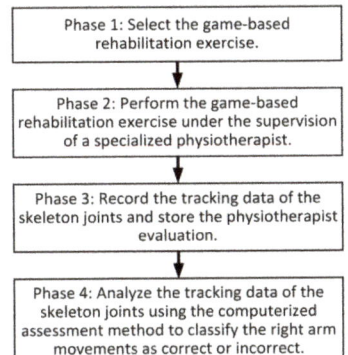

Figure 2. The architecture of the proposed bespoke game-based rehabilitation system.

2.2. The Game-Based Rehabilitation Exercises

The proposed bespoke rehabilitation system includes three game-based exercises that target the right arm. The three game-based exercises are designed under the supervision of a specialized physiotherapist with more than 12 years of experience to increase the range of motion and improve the stability of the right arm. In particular, the three game-based exercises aim to implement the shoulder flexion, shoulder horizontal abduction/adduction, and shoulder adduction physical exercises. Below is a summary of the three game-based exercises.

2.2.1. The Shoulder Flexion Game-Based Exercise

The first game-based exercise aims to engage the participant in the shoulder flexion physical exercise, which is illustrated in Figure 3a. The game-based exercise that is employed to realize the shoulder flexion physical exercise is illustrated in Figure 3b. In this game, a set of nine stars are placed along the central, vertical axis of the screen. The participant is asked to collect the stars using a virtual hand that is controlled using the participant's right hand through the Kinect sensor. In particular, the participant is asked to lift his/her right arm up from the resting position by his/her side (position A in Figure 3a) to his/her front in which the arm is parallel to the floor (position C in Figure 3a). The participant continues the game by lifting his/her arm up from the front position (position C in Figure 3a) to the straight position above the head (position E in Figure 3a). These movements allow the participant to collect the stars located at the screen. The participant maintains his/her arm in the straight position above the head for a predefined time period, which is between 1 and 2 s. At the end of the game, the participant is asked to move his/her arm down from the straight position above the head (position E in Figure 3a) to the resting position by his/her side (position A in Figure 3a), where this movement allows him/her to collect any remaining stars in the screen. The participant is asked to perform all these movements slowly and in a controllable manner in which the arm is kept straight. Moreover, the trunk should be kept straight during the exercise.

To engage the participant in the game in an enjoyable and fun environment, we have added sound effects to the game, such that a cling sound is played each time a star is collected by the participant. In addition, the score of the game is incremented by one point when the participant collects a star. The sound effect and the process of assigning one point for each collected star is applied for the two game-based exercises described below.

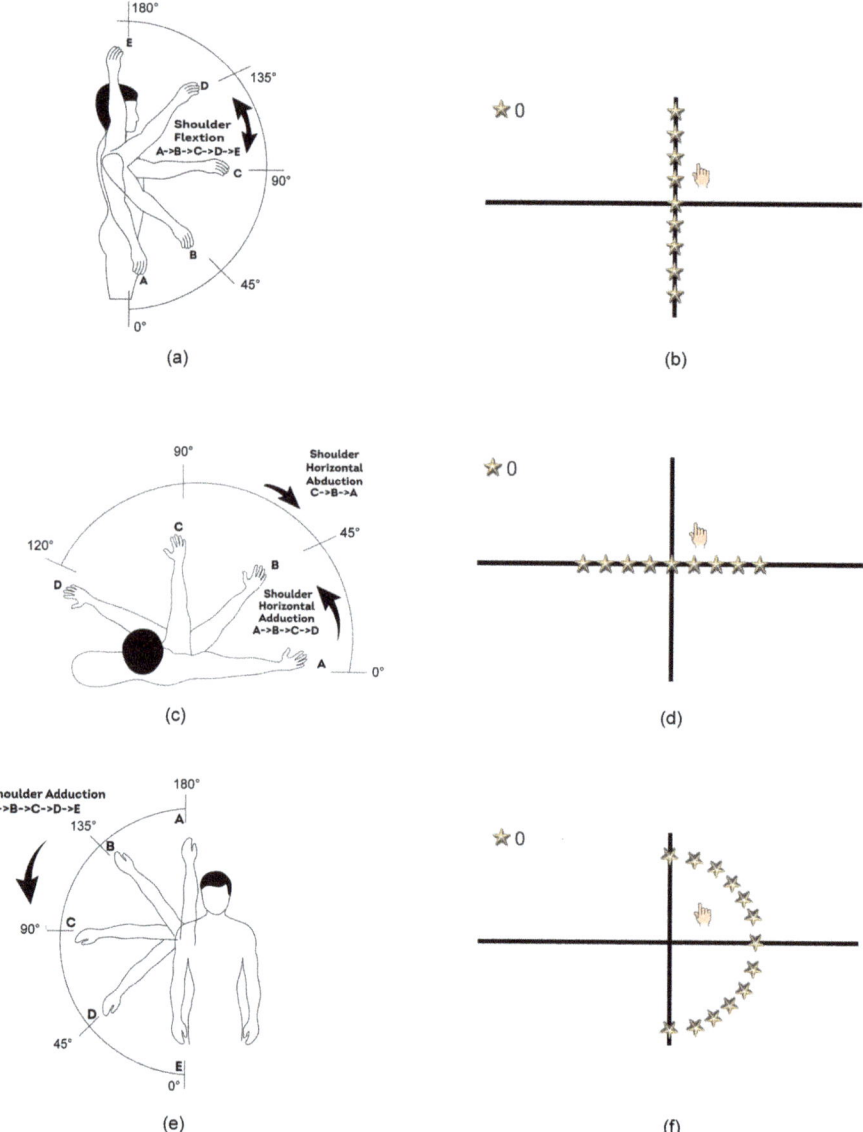

Figure 3. (**a,b**): (**a**) The shoulder flexion physical exercise and (**b**) the corresponding shoulder flexion game-based exercise. (**c,d**): (**c**) The shoulder horizontal abduction physical exercise followed by the shoulder horizontal adduction physical exercise and (**d**) the corresponding shoulder horizontal abduction/adduction game-based exercise. (**e,f**): (**e**) The shoulder adduction physical exercise and (**f**) the corresponding shoulder adduction game-based exercise.

2.2.2. The Shoulder Horizontal Abduction/Adduction Game-Based Exercise

This game-based exercise aims to engage the participant in the shoulder horizontal abduction and shoulder horizontal adduction physical exercises, which are illustrated in Figure 3c. The game-based exercise that is employed to realize these two physical exercises is shown in Figure 3d. In this game, a set of nine stars are placed along the central, horizontal axis of the screen. The participant is asked to collect the stars using a virtual hand that is controlled using the participant's right hand through the Kinect sensor. At the beginning of the game, the participant is asked to lift his/her arm up from the resting position by his/her side to his/her front in which the arm is parallel to the floor (position C in Figure 3c). The participant maintains his/her arm in the front position for a predefined time period, which is between 1 and 2 s. Then, the participant starts playing the game by moving his/her arm to perform the shoulder horizontal abduction movement (positions C to A in Figure 3c), which allows him/her to collect the stars located at the right half of the screen. After that, the participant is asked to move his/her arm to perform the shoulder horizontal adduction movement (position A to D in Figure 3c), which allows him/her to collect any missing star in the right half of the screen and all stars in the left half of the screen. In fact, the participant is asked to perform all these movements slowly and in a controllable manner in which the arm is kept straight and at the height of the shoulder. Moreover, the trunk should be kept straight during the exercise.

2.2.3. The Shoulder Adduction Game-Based Exercise

This game-based exercise aims to engage the participant in the shoulder adduction physical exercise, which is illustrated in Figure 3e. The game-based exercise that is employed to realize the shoulder adduction physical exercise is illustrated in Figure 3f. In this game, a set of thirteen stars are placed along an arc that is located at the right side of the screen and spans 180°. The participant is asked to collect the stars using a virtual hand that is controlled using the participant's right arm through the Kinect sensor. At the beginning of the game, the participant is asked to lift his/her arm up from the resting position by his/her side to a straight position above the head (position A in Figure 3e). The participant maintains his/her arm at this position for a predefined time period, which is between 1 and 2 s. Then, the participant starts playing the game by moving his/her arm to perform the shoulder adduction movement (positions A to E in Figure 3e), which allows him/her to collect the stars located in the arc. In fact, the participant is asked to perform this movement slowly and in a controllable manner in which the arm is kept straight. Moreover, the trunk should be kept straight during the exercise.

2.3. The Computerized Assessment Method

This subsection describes the computerized assessment method that we have developed to achieve automatic evaluation of the right arm movements during the game-based rehabilitation exercises. In fact, this assessment method is based on spatial-temporal analysis of the 3D tracking data of the participant's skeleton joints that is acquired by the Kinect sensor during each game-playing session. To develop the computerized assessment method, the Motion-Pose Geometric Descriptor (MPGD), which was originally introduced by Alazrai et al. to model human movements during human-to-human interactions [30] as well as to detect and predict the fall of elderly people [31,32], is extended in the current study to obtain a view-invariant representation of the pose and motion of the right arm. The extended MPGD, denoted by E-MPGD, aims to extract a set of time-varying features that quantify the pose and motion of the participant's right arm during each game-playing session of the game-based rehabilitation exercises. The extracted features are processed using feature selection and classification analysis to obtain computer-based assessment of the correctness of the right arm movements. In the following subsections, we provide detailed descriptions of the E-MPGD as well as the feature selection and classification analyses employed in the current study.

2.3.1. The Extended Motion-Pose Geometric Descriptor (E-MPGD)

The original formulation of the MPGD [30] used a body-attached 3D coordinate system to compute a set of time-varying features that quantify the pose and motion of the body parts. The body-attached coordinate system is a reference 3D coordinate system that is centered at one of the body joints, denoted by the *origin*, and includes three orthogonal anatomical planes. These anatomical planes are based on the anatomical planes concept described in [33]. A major advantage of the body-attached coordinate system is the capability to obtain view-invariant representation of the 3D positions and movements of the tracked skeleton joints, independently of the location and orientation of the Kinect sensor. Therefore, the locations of the skeleton joints that are tracked by the Kinect sensor are transformed to the body-attached coordinate system to achieve view-invariant analysis of the body movements. The transformed tracking data is then processed to extract a set of time-varying features that describe the pose and motion of the human body.

In the current study, all subjects who participated in the game-based rehabilitation exercises were asked to use their right hands to perform the exercises. Hence, the extended MPGD, denoted by E-MPGD, that we have developed in the current study aims to extend the body-attached coordinate system and the time-varying features of the MPGD to achieve effective representation of the pose and movement of the right arm during the game-based rehabilitation exercises. In the following, we provide detailed description of the body-attached coordinate system and the time-varying features.

E-MPGD: The Body-Attached Coordinate System

The Kinect for Windows v2 sensor employed in the current study has the ability to track the 3D positions of twenty five skeleton joints, which are shown in Figure 4a as red and blue points. In fact, the eight skeleton joints shown as red points, which include the left shoulder (lS) joint, the right shoulder (rS) joint, the spine shoulder (SS) joint, the right hip (rHI) joint, the spine base (SB) joint, the right elbow (rE) joint, the right wrist (rW) joint, and the right hand (rH) joint, are used by the E-MPGD to model the pose and motion of the right arm. The remaining seventeen skeleton joints, which are shown in Figure 4a as blue points, are not considered in the current study as they are not required to model the pose and motion of the right arm.

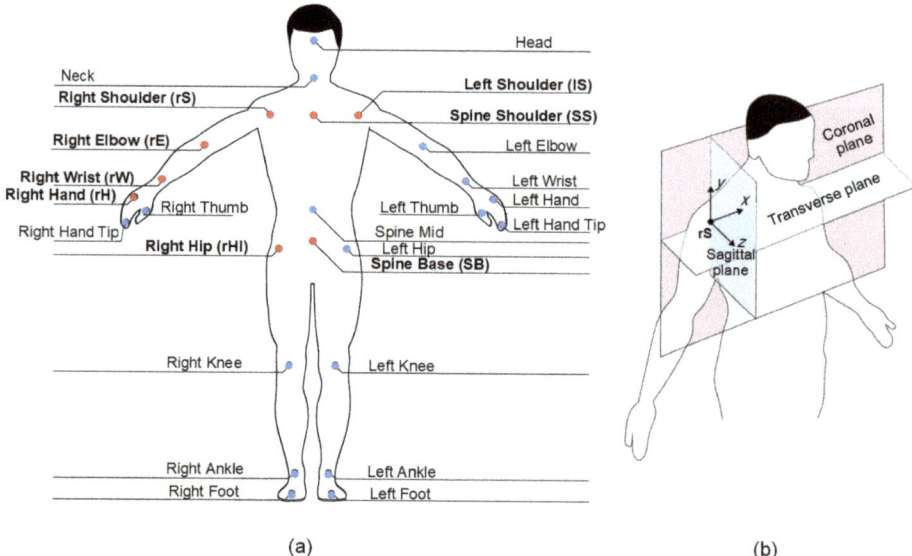

Figure 4. (a) The twenty five skeleton joints that are tracked by the Kinect for Windows v2 sensor. (b) The body-attached coordinate system of the Extended Motion-Pose Geometric Descriptor (E-MPGD).

The body-attached coordinate system of the E-MPGD is configured such that its origin is located at the rS skeleton joint, as shown in Figure 4b. Hence, the 3D locations of the eight skeleton joints considered in the current study, which are shown in Figure 4a as red points, are expressed with respect to the rS joint. In addition, three orthogonal anatomical planes, namely the coronal plane, transverse plane, and sagittal plane, are defined such that these three planes intercept at the origin, as shown in Figure 4b. Each one of these three planes is defined using three non-collinear joints, i.e., joints that are not located along the same line, as described below:

- **The coronal plane (CP):** This plane is defined using the rS, lS, and SB skeleton joints.
- **The transverse plane (TP):** This plane is defined using the rS and lS skeleton joints as well as the $\hat{SS}$ virtual joint. The $\hat{SS}$ virtual joint is obtained by shifting the SS skeleton joint along the direction orthogonal to the coronal plane, denoted by the positive z direction, by a distance of 0.2 m to ensure that the z coordinate of the $\hat{SS}$ joint is different than the rS and lS joints.
- **The sagittal plane (SP):** This plane is defined using the rS skeleton joint as well as the $\hat{rS}$ and $\hat{\hat{rS}}$ virtual joints. The $\hat{rS}$ virtual joint is obtained by shifting the rS skeleton joint along the positive z direction by a distance of 0.2 m. The $\hat{\hat{rS}}$ virtual joints is obtained by shifting the rS skeleton joint along the direction orthogonal to the transverse plane, denoted by the negative y direction, to match the y coordinate of the rHI joint.

E-MPGD: The Time-Varying Features

For all game-based rehabilitation exercises, the tracking data acquired by the Kinect v2 sensor during a particular game-playing session is composed of a series of acquisition frames, where each frame includes the x, y, and z coordinates of the twenty five tracked skeleton joints. For every acquisition frame, which is assumed to have a temporal index k, the coordinates of the skeleton joints are analyzed to synthesize the body-attached coordinate system, as described before. Moreover, the 3D coordinates of the skeleton joints are transformed to the body-attached coordinate system. After that, the coordinates of the rS (i.e., origin), rE, rW, and rH skeleton joins at frame k are analyzed to extract eleven angle-based features and twenty seven joint-based features to quantify the pose and motion of the right arm at that frame. The extraction of the angle-based features is performed by computing three vectors that correspond to the main parts of the right arm. These vectors are the vector that extends from the rS to the rE skeleton joints ($\overrightarrow{SE}$), the vector that extends from the rE to the rW skeleton joints ($\overrightarrow{EW}$), and the vector that extends from the rW to the rH skeleton joints ($\overrightarrow{WH}$). The first nine angle-based features are extracted by computing the angles between each one of these three vectors and the three anatomical planes, i.e., the CP, TP, and SP, at frame k. These nine features are denoted by $\theta_{CP}^{\overrightarrow{SE}}(k)$, $\theta_{TP}^{\overrightarrow{SE}}(k)$, $\theta_{SP}^{\overrightarrow{SE}}(k)$, $\theta_{CP}^{\overrightarrow{EW}}(k)$, $\theta_{TP}^{\overrightarrow{EW}}(k)$, $\theta_{SP}^{\overrightarrow{EW}}(k)$, $\theta_{CP}^{\overrightarrow{WH}}(k)$, $\theta_{TP}^{\overrightarrow{WH}}(k)$, and $\theta_{SP}^{\overrightarrow{WH}}(k)$. The descriptions and mathematical formulations of these nine features are provided in Table 1. The remaining two angle-based features are the angle between the vectors $\overrightarrow{SE}$ and $\overrightarrow{EW}$, denoted by $\theta_{\overrightarrow{SE}}^{\overrightarrow{EW}}(k)$, and the angle between the vectors $\overrightarrow{EW}$ and $\overrightarrow{WH}$, denoted by $\theta_{\overrightarrow{EW}}^{\overrightarrow{WH}}(k)$, at frame k. Table 1 provides the descriptions and mathematical formulations of these two features.

Table 1. The angle- and joint-based features of the E-MPGD.

Type	Features	Description	Mathematical Formulation
Angle-based features	$\theta_{CP}^{\overrightarrow{SE}}(k)$, $\theta_{TP}^{\overrightarrow{SE}}(k)$, $\theta_{SP}^{\overrightarrow{SE}}(k)$	The angles between the vector $\overrightarrow{SE}$ and the CP, TP, and SP at frame k.	$\theta_P^{\vec{V}}(k) = sin^{-1}\left(\frac{|\vec{V} \cdot \vec{n}_P|}{\|\vec{V}\|}\right)$, where $\theta_P^{\vec{V}}$ is the angle between the vector $\vec{V}$ and the plane P at frame k, and $\vec{n}_P$ is the normal vector to the plane P.
	$\theta_{CP}^{\overrightarrow{EW}}(k)$, $\theta_{TP}^{\overrightarrow{EW}}(k)$, $\theta_{SP}^{\overrightarrow{EW}}(k)$	The angles between the vector $\overrightarrow{EW}$ and the CP, TP, and SP at frame k.	
	$\theta_{CP}^{\overrightarrow{WH}}(k)$, $\theta_{TP}^{\overrightarrow{WH}}(k)$, $\theta_{SP}^{\overrightarrow{WH}}(k)$	The angles between the vector $\overrightarrow{WH}$ and the CP, TP, and SP at frame k.	
	$\theta_{\overrightarrow{SE}}^{\overrightarrow{EW}}(k)$	The angle between the vectors $\overrightarrow{SE}$ and $\overrightarrow{EW}$ at frame k.	$\theta_{\vec{U}}^{\vec{V}}(k) = cos^{-1}\left(\frac{|\vec{U} \cdot \vec{V}|}{\|\vec{U}\|\|\vec{V}\|}\right)$, where $\theta_{\vec{U}}^{\vec{V}}(k)$ is the angle between the vectors $\vec{U}$ and $\vec{V}$ at frame k.
	$\theta_{\overrightarrow{EW}}^{\overrightarrow{WH}}(k)$	The angle between the vectors $\overrightarrow{EW}$ and $\overrightarrow{WH}$ at frame k.	
Joint-based features	$p_x^{rE}(k), p_y^{rE}(k), p_z^{rE}(k)$	The x, y, and z components of the rE joint velocity at frame k.	The locations of the rE, rW, and rH skeleton joints at frame k are provided by the Kinect sensor and transformed to the body-attached coordinate system.
	$p_x^{rW}(k), p_y^{rW}(k), p_z^{rW}(k)$	The x, y, and z components of the rW joint location at frame k.	
	$p_x^{rH}(k), p_y^{rH}(k), p_z^{rH}(k)$	The x, y, and z components of the rH joint location at frame k.	
	$v_x^{rE}(k), v_y^{rE}(k), v_z^{rE}(k)$	The x, y, and z components of the rE joint velocity at frame k.	$v_d^p(k) = \frac{p_d^p(k) - p_d^p(k-1)}{\Delta t}$, where $v_d^p(k)$ is the velocity of skeleton joint p along direction d at frame k, $p_d^p(k)$ and $p_d^p(k-1)$ are the locations of p along direction d at frames k and $k-1$, respectively, and Δt is the time step between frames k and $k-1$.
	$v_x^{rW}(k), v_y^{rW}(k), v_z^{rW}(k)$	The x, y, and z components of the rW joint velocity at frame k.	
	$v_x^{rH}(k), v_y^{rH}(k), v_z^{rH}(k)$	The x, y, and z components of the rH joint velocity at frame k.	
	$a_x^{rE}(k), a_y^{rE}(k), a_z^{rE}(k)$	The x, y, and z components of the rE joint acceleration at frame k.	$a_d^p(k) = \frac{v_d^p(k) - v_d^p(k-1)}{\Delta t}$, where $a_d^p(k)$ is the acceleration of skeleton joint p along direction d at frame k, $v_d^p(k)$ and $v_d^p(k-1)$ are the velocities of p along direction d at frames k and $k-1$, respectively, and Δt is the time step between frames k and $k-1$.
	$a_x^{rW}(k), a_y^{rW}(k), a_z^{rW}(k)$	The x, y, and z components of the rW joint acceleration at frame k.	
	$a_x^{rH}(k), a_y^{rH}(k), a_z^{rH}(k)$	The x, y, and z components of the rH joint acceleration at frame k.	

The twenty seven joint-based features aim to quantify the motion of the rE, rW, and rH skeleton joints at frame k. In particular, nine of these features, which are denoted by $p_x^{rE}(k)$, $p_y^{rE}(k)$, $p_z^{rE}(k)$, $p_x^{rW}(k)$, $p_y^{rW}(k)$, $p_z^{rW}(k)$, $p_x^{rH}(k)$, $p_y^{rH}(k)$, $p_z^{rH}(k)$, evaluate the x, y, and z components of the positions of the rE, rW, and rH skeleton joints at frame k. Moreover, nine joint-based features, which are denoted by $v_x^{rE}(k)$, $v_y^{rE}(k)$, $v_z^{rE}(k)$, $v_x^{rW}(k)$, $v_y^{rW}(k)$, $v_z^{rW}(k)$, $v_x^{rH}(k)$, $v_y^{rH}(k)$, and $v_z^{rH}(k)$, quantify the x, y, and z components of the velocities of the rE, rW, and rH skeleton joints at frame k. The last nine joint-based features, which are denoted by $a_x^{rE}(k)$, $a_y^{rE}(k)$, $a_z^{rE}(k)$, $a_x^{rW}(k)$, $a_y^{rW}(k)$, $a_z^{rW}(k)$, $a_x^{rH}(k)$, $a_y^{rH}(k)$, and $a_z^{rH}(k)$, evaluate the x, y, and z components of the accelerations of the rE, rW, and rH skeleton joints at frame k. The descriptions and mathematical formulations of the joint-based features are provided in Table 1.

2.3.2. Features Extraction, Selection, and Classification

Assuming that the tracking data acquired by the Kinect v2 sensor during the game-playing session of a particular participant and a particular game-based exercise is composed of L frames and the goal is to classify the right arm movements during this game-playing session as correct or incorrect. Then, for each frame, we extract a feature vector composed of the eleven angle-based features and the twenty seven joint-based features that are summarized in Table 1. This extraction process generates a series of L feature vectors, where each vector is composed of the angle- and joint-based features. The series of L feature vectors of the game-playing session under consideration is classified to identify if the right arm movements during the game-playing session are performed correctly or incorrectly. The classification process is performed by comparing the series of L feature vectors of the game-playing session under consideration with a set of correct and incorrect gold standard game-playing sessions that are performed by the same participant for the same game-based rehabilitation exercise. Based on this comparison, the game-playing session under consideration can be considered similar to the correct gold standard game-playing sessions, and hence the right arm movements during the game-playing session are classified as correct. Otherwise, the game-playing session under consideration is considered similar to the incorrect gold standard game-playing sessions, and hence the right arm movements during the game-playing session are classified as incorrect.

The comparison process is performed as follows. For the participant and the game-based rehabilitation exercise under consideration, we assume that there is a set of gold standard game-playing sessions, where this set includes N_1 game-playing sessions that are labeled as *correct* and N_2 game-playing sessions that are labeled as *incorrect*. The subset of feature vectors series computed for the correct gold standard game-playing sessions is denoted by $GS_C = \{C\_SFV_1, C\_SFV_2, ..., C\_SFV_{N_1}\}$, where C_SFV_i represents the feature vector of the ith correct gold standard game-playing session. Moreover, the subset of feature vectors series computed for the incorrect gold standard game-playing sessions is denoted by $GS_{IC} = \{IC\_SFV_1, IC\_SFV_2, ..., IC\_SFV_{N_2}\}$, where IC_SFV_i represents the feature vector of the ith incorrect gold standard game-playing session. Assume that the series of feature vectors of the game-playing session under consideration is denoted as SFV. Then, the average distance, $\overline{dist}(SFV, GS_C)$, between SFV and GS_C can be calculated as follows:

$$\overline{dist}(SFV, GS_C) = \frac{\sum_{i=1}^{N_1} dist(SFV, C\_SFV_i)}{N_1}, \quad (1)$$

where $dist(SFV, C\_SFV_i)$ is the distance between SFV and C_SFV_i. The computation of $dist(SFV, C\_SFV_i)$ should consider that fact that the temporal lengths of the game-playing sessions performed by the same participant for a particular game-based rehabilitation exercise varies from time to time due to the intra-personal variations. Hence, the lengths of SFV and C_SFV_i might be different. Moreover, the frames of SFV and C_SFV_i are most likely asynchronous. To address these limitations, the distance between the feature vectors series SFV and the feature vectors series C_SFV_i is computed using the Multidimensional Dynamic Time Warping (MD-DTW) algorithm [34]. In the same manner, the average distance, $\overline{dist}(SFV, GS_{IC})$, between SFV and GS_{IC} is computed as follows:

$$\overline{dist}(SFV, GS_{IC}) = \frac{\sum_{i=1}^{N_2} dist(SFV, IC\_SFV_i)}{N_2}. \quad (2)$$

where $dist(SFV, IC\_SFV_i)$ is the distance between SFV and IC_SFV_i and it is calculated using the MD-DTW algorithm. If the value of $\overline{dist}(SFV, GS_C)$ is greater than or equal to $\overline{dist}(SFV, GS_{IC})$, then the right arm movements of the game-playing session under consideration are labeled as correct. Otherwise, the right arm movements of the game-playing session under consideration are labeled as incorrect.

The performance of the classification algorithm described above depends on the capability of the eleven angle-based features and the twenty seven joint-based features, i.e., thirty eight features in total, to differentiate between the correct and incorrect right arm movements. However, not all angle- and joint-based features described in Table 1 can be considered effective to classify the right arm movements. Moreover, the importance of these features varies depending the participant and the game-based exercises under consideration. To improve the performance of the classification algorithm, the recursive backward elimination procedure [35] is employed to select the features combination that optimizes the capability of classifying the right arm movements. In the first iteration of the recursive backward elimination procedure, one of the features is eliminated, and the remaining features are used to classify the right arm movements. Then, the feature that is eliminated in the previous step is returned and another feature is eliminated before running the classification. This elimination process is repeated until each individual feature of the thirty eight features is eliminated before running the classification. The feature that its elimination leads to the highest improvement in the classification performance is permanently removed to achieve thirty seven features with improved classification performance. In the second iteration of the recursive backward elimination procedure, each individual feature of the thirty seven features is eliminated and the classification is run using the remaining features. This process is repeated until identifying the feature that its removal leads to the highest improvement in the classification performance. The recursive iterations of the backward elimination procedure continue until reaching an optimized features combination in which the removal of any feature leads to a reduction in the classification performance. In the current study, the recursive backward elimination procedure is applied in a participant-specific, game-specific manner, in which the process of selecting the features has been performed for each participant and each game-based exercise. Hence, the right arm movements associated with a particular participant and a particular game-based exercise could be classified using the combination of optimized features that is computed specifically for the participant and game-based exercise under consideration.

3. Experimental Evaluation and Results

3.1. Participants

Two groups of participants volunteered to participate in the experiments to evaluate the performance of the proposed computerized assessment method. The first group included children that are diagnosed with cerebral palsy. These children were recruited from the Model School for Cerebral Palsy, Amman, Jordan to participate in the study during the period between October 2018 and January 2019. The following inclusion criteria have been employed: the participant should be diagnosed with cerebral palsy and his/her age should be 10 years or more. Also, the following exclusion criteria have been applied: the participant cannot perform and interact with the three game-based exercises, he/she do not have the potential to achieve the range of motion targeted by the three game-based exercises as illustrated in Figure 3, and his/her cerebral palsy severity level is classified as severe. Based on these inclusion and exclusion criteria, six cerebral palsy children were selected to participate in the study. The mean ± standard deviation age of the children was 12.7 ± 1.2 years. The gender, the cerebral palsy category, and the cerebral palsy severity of these children are summarized in Table 2. The second group of participants included 20 typically developing subjects (10 females and 10 males) who are undergraduate students at the German Jordanian University, Amman, Jordan. The aim of the second group is to generate additional correct and incorrect game-playing sessions for each one of the three game-based rehabilitation exercises. The typically developing subjects volunteered to participate in the study during the period between August 2018 and September 2018. The mean ± standard deviation age of the typically developing subjects is 20.2 ± 1.2 years. The game-based rehabilitation exercises, which are presented in Section 2.2, and the experimental protocol, which is described below, were explained to the participants in both groups. For the cerebral palsy children, which are younger that 18 years, a signed consent form was collected from the parents of the participants. For the typically developing subjects, which are elder than 18 years, a signed consent form was collected from each subject before participating in the experiments. The experimental protocol employed in the current study was approved by the Ethics Committee at the German Jordanian University, Amman, Jordan and the Ethics Committee at the Model School for Cerebral Palsy, Amman, Jordan.

Table 2. The gender, cerebral palsy category, and cerebral palsy severity of the children included in the first group of participants.

Participant	Gender	Cerebral Palsy Category	Cerebral Palsy Severity
Child 1	Male	Spastic diplegic	Mild
Child 2	Male	Spastic diplegic	Mild
Child 3	Female	Spastic diplegic	Moderate
Child 4	Male	Spastic himiplegic	Moderate
Child 5	Female	Ataxia	Moderate
Child 6	Male	Ataxia	Moderate

3.2. Experimental Protocol

The participants from both groups were asked to perform the three game-based rehabilitation exercises under the supervision of a specialized physiotherapist. For the cerebral palsy children, every participant was asked to play each one of the three game-based rehabilitation exercises and the physiotherapist guided him/her vocally during the game-playing session to do the right arm movements in a correct manner. For both the correct and incorrect game-playing sessions, the participants maintained the trunk straight throughout the game-playing sessions. In each game-playing session, the physiotherapist evaluated the participant's performance and labeled each session as correct or incorrect based on the following subject-specific evaluation criteria:

- The participant should perform the movements associated with the game-based exercise, as described in Section 2.2 and illustrated in Figure 3, in a correct manner. In particular, compensatory movements should be avoided as much as possible.
- The participant should cover the range of motion targeted by the game-based exercise, which is illustrated in Figure 3, as much as possible.
- The participant should perform the movements associated with the game-based exercise slowly and in a controllable and stable manner in which the right arm is kept straight as much as possible.

For the group of typically developing subjects, every participant was asked to perform the game-based rehabilitation exercises both correctly and incorrectly and at various speeds. In particular, the incorrect movements performed by the typically developing subjects were focused on replicating the motion limitations of the cerebral palsy children, which mainly include the limited range of motion, the unstable movement of the right arm, and performing the right arm movements associated with the game-based rehabilitation exercise in wrong manners. At the end of each game-playing session, the physiotherapist evaluated the performance of the typically developing subjects using the same evaluation criterion employed for the cerebral palsy children to label the game-playing session as correct or incorrect.

For every participant, including the cerebral palsy children and the typically developing subjects, we have collected 30 correct game-playing sessions and 30 incorrect game-playing sessions for each one of the three game-based rehabilitation exercises. Hence, the total number of game-playing sessions that have been collected for each participant is equal to 180. The mean ± standard deviation temporal lengths of the game-playing sessions performed by the six cerebral palsy children during their participation in the shoulder flexion, shoulder horizontal abduction/adduction, and shoulder adduction game-based exercises are equal to 6.8 ± 5.1 s, 7.6 ± 4.4 s, and 11.4 ± 5.0 s, respectively. Moreover, the mean ± standard deviation temporal lengths of the game-playing sessions performed by the twenty typically developing subjects during their participation in the shoulder flexion, shoulder horizontal abduction/adduction, and shoulder adduction game-based exercises are equal to 4.4 ± 1.2 s, 4.9 ± 1.6 s, and 6.2 ± 1.5 s, respectively. For each cerebral palsy child, the process of acquiring the 180 game-playing sessions was carried out over 12 to 16 recording periods, where in each period the participant performed 10 to 15 game-playing sessions. For the typically developing subjects, the process of acquiring the 180 game-playing sessions was carried out over 3 recording periods, where in each recording period the participant performed 60 game-playing sessions. For all participants, the game-playing sessions were separated by relaxation periods with a minimum length of 2 min. Moreover, the recording periods of each participant were performed on different days. The acquisition rate of the Kinect v2 sensor was set to 15 frames per second for all game-playing sessions.

3.3. Performance Evaluation

In the current study, we have employed a participant-specific, game-specific approach to evaluate the performance of the proposed computerized assessment method. In this approach, a tenfold cross validation procedure is used to evaluate the capability of the computerized assessment method to classify the right arm movements of every participant during the sixty game-playing sessions that are recorded for each game-based rehabilitation exercise. To carry out the tenfold cross validation procedure, the sixty game-playing sessions are sorted randomly and divided into 10 uniform subsets, such that each subset includes 3 correct and 3 incorrect game-playing sessions. One of these subsets is selected as a testing subset. Moreover, the remaining 9 subsets are combined and employed for constructing the correct and incorrect gold standard game-playing sessions, which are denoted in Section 2.3.2 as GS_C and GS_{IC}, respectively. The proposed computerized assessment method was used to classify the 3 correct and 3 incorrect game-playing sessions included in the testing subset based on GS_C and GS_{IC}, as illustrated in Section 2.3.2. Moreover, the process of selecting one of the subsets as a testing subset and the remaining nine subsets as GS_C and GS_{IC} subsets has been repeated for nine folds to enable the computerized assessment method to classify each one of the sixty game-playing sessions. After applying the tenfold cross validation procedure, the classifications obtained by the proposed computerized assessment method for the sixty game-playing sessions were compared with the matching gold standard labels using four performance metrics. The first three metrics are the classification accuracy, specificity, and sensitivity [36]. The last metric is Cohen's kappa coefficient [37,38]. The kappa coefficient evaluates the agreement between the classifications obtained by the proposed computerized assessment method and the gold standard labels provided by the experienced physiotherapist after considering the agreement occurring by chance. The value of kappa coefficient can be interpreted as follows to quantify the agreement level [39]: $(0.8-1]$ = almost perfect agreement, $(0.6-0.8]$ = substantial agreement, $(0.4-0.6]$ = moderate agreement, $(0.2-0.4]$ = fair agreement, $(0-0.2]$ = slight agreement, and <0 = poor agreement.

For every participant and each game-based rehabilitation exercise, the evaluation process described above, which includes randomly sorting the sixty game-playing sessions performed by the participant, applying the tenfold cross validation procedure, and evaluating the capability of the proposed computerized assessment method to classify the sixty game-playing sessions, was repeated for ten evaluation repetitions. The mean $\pm$ standard deviation values of the accuracy, specificity, sensitivity, and kappa coefficient are computed for the proposed computerized assessment method across the ten evaluation repetitions that are carried out for every participant and each game-based rehabilitation exercise. Furthermore, for every game-based exercise, the mean $\pm$ standard deviation values of the four metrics are computed for all subjects in each one of the two groups of participants.

In addition to evaluating the classification performance of the proposed computerized assessment method, we have analyzed the combinations of angle- and joint-based features that are selected using the features selection approach described in Section 2.3.2 to optimize the classification performance. Particularly, for the first group of participants, which includes six cerebral palsy children, we have computed two metrics: the combination-based occurrence frequency of the features (CBOFF) and the participant-based occurrence frequency of the important features (PBOFIF). For a particular game-based exercise, the two metrics are computed by considering the sixty features combinations that are obtained by combining the optimized features combinations of the ten performance evaluation repetitions performed for each one of the six cerebral palsy children. For each feature, the CBOFF is defined as the number of times the feature appears in the sixty optimized features combinations.

The PBOFIF aims to evaluate the importance of the features with respect to the six cerebral palsy children. To compute the PBOFIF, we have developed a custom-made criterion to determine if a given feature is important to classify the ten performance evaluation repetitions performed for a particular participant and a particular game-based rehabilitation exercise. In this criterion, if the feature appears more than two times in the optimized features combinations that are obtained for the ten performance evaluation repetitions, then the feature is considered important to classify the game-playing sessions associated with the participant and game-based rehabilitation exercise under consideration. For a particular game-based exercise, the PBOFIF is computed by individually considering each one of the angle- and joint-based features listed in Table 1 and counting the number of participants in which the feature is considered important. The metrics CBOFF and PBOFIF have also been computed for the second group of participants, which includes twenty typically developing subjects. However, the computation was based on the ten performance evaluation repetitions that are carried out for each one of the twenty typically developing subjects. Hence, the total number of optimized features combinations that are obtained for all typically developing subjects is equal to 200.

3.4. Results of the Cerebral Palsy Children

The mean ± standard deviation values of the classification accuracy, specificity, and sensitivity as well as kappa coefficient that are obtained using the optimized combinations of angle- and joint-based features for each one of the six cerebral palsy children during their participation in the three game-based exercises are presented in Table 3. As shown in the table, the mean classification accuracy, specificity, and sensitivity values are between 88% and 95% for child 1 and child 2, between 84% and 88% for child 3 and child 4, and between 71% and 80% for child 5 and child 6. The mean kappa coefficient values are between 0.80 and 0.86 for child 1 and child 2, between 0.70 and 0.74 for child 3 and child 4, and between 0.45 and 0.57 for child 5 and child 6. In addition, Table 3 shows that the mean ± standard deviation values of the accuracy, specificity, sensitivity, and kappa coefficient that are obtained for the three game-based exercises by considering all six cerebral palsy children are within the ranges of 83% to 85%, 83% to 86%, 83% to 84%, and 0.66 to 0.70, respectively.

Table 3. The mean ± standard deviation accuracy, specificity, sensitivity, and kappa coefficient values obtained by the computerized assessment method for the six cerebral palsy children.

Participant	Shoulder Flexion				Shoulder Horizontal Abduction/Adduction				Shoulder Adduction			
	Accuracy (%)	Specificity (%)	Sensitivity (%)	Kappa	Accuracy (%)	Specificity (%)	Sensitivity (%)	Kappa	Accuracy (%)	Specificity (%)	Sensitivity (%)	Kappa
Child 1	93 ± 3	91 ± 4	95 ± 3	0.86 ± 0.06	92 ± 4	91 ± 4	92 ± 5	0.83 ± 0.07	90 ± 4	89 ± 6	90 ± 4	0.80 ± 0.09
Child 2	91 ± 3	90 ± 4	91 ± 5	0.81 ± 0.05	92 ± 3	93 ± 3	91 ± 4	0.84 ± 0.05	90 ± 3	88 ± 4	92 ± 6	0.81 ± 0.07
Child 3	87 ± 4	87 ± 6	88 ± 3	0.74 ± 0.07	86 ± 3	85 ± 5	87 ± 5	0.72 ± 0.06	86 ± 2	87 ± 3	84 ± 4	0.72 ± 0.05
Child 4	85 ± 3	86 ± 5	84 ± 4	0.70 ± 0.06	87 ± 4	88 ± 5	85 ± 4	0.73 ± 0.07	85 ± 4	85 ± 5	86 ± 6	0.71 ± 0.09
Child 5	78 ± 4	80 ± 6	76 ± 5	0.57 ± 0.08	77 ± 4	79 ± 5	75 ± 5	0.54 ± 0.08	72 ± 4	73 ± 5	71 ± 6	0.45 ± 0.07
Child 6	75 ± 3	78 ± 4	73 ± 4	0.51 ± 0.06	76 ± 3	80 ± 4	73 ± 4	0.53 ± 0.06	73 ± 2	73 ± 4	72 ± 3	0.46 ± 0.05
All children	85 ± 7	85 ± 7	84 ± 9	0.70 ± 0.14	85 ± 7	86 ± 7	84 ± 9	0.70 ± 0.14	83 ± 8	83 ± 8	83 ± 10	0.66 ± 0.16

The results reported in Table 3 indicate that the performance of the computerized assessment method can be related to the cerebral palsy category and severity of the six cerebral palsy children, which are provided in Table 2. In particular, the first four children (child 1, child 2, child 3, and child 4) have spastic cerebral palsy that is associated with contracted and stiff muscles [40]. The right arms of these four children do not suffer from shaky or uncoordinated movements. However, child 1, child 2, and child 3 have spastic diplegic cerebral palsy that mainly affects the muscles of the legs, with lower effect on the arms [40]. The disorder severity of child 1 and child 2 is lower than child 3. Moreover, child 4 is diagnosed with moderate spastic hemiplegia cerebral palsy that mainly affects one side of the body [40]. For child 4, the disorder involves both the right arm and right leg, but the right arm is more affected. The last two children, i.e., child 5 and child 6, have ataxia cerebral palsy with moderate severity. The ataxia cerebral palsy disorder is characterized by shaky and uncoordinated movements as well as poor balance that affects all body parts [40]. The shaky and uncoordinated movements of the right arm and the poor balance increase the difficulty of differentiating the correct game-playing sessions from the incorrect ones. Therefore, the classification results reported for child 1 and child 2 are higher than the results obtained for child 3. Moreover, the results obtained for child 3 and child 4 have comparable values. Furthermore, the lowest classification results are reported for child 5 and child 6.

Figure 5a–c present the CBOFF values computed for the shoulder flexion game-based exercise, the shoulder horizontal abduction/adduction game-based exercise, and the shoulder adduction game-based exercise, respectively. As described in Section 3.3, for a particular game-based exercise, the CBOFF represents the number of times the feature appears in the sixty optimized features combinations that are obtained by combining the optimized features combinations of the ten evaluation repetitions performed for each one of the six cerebral palsy children. Hence, the highest possible CBOFF value is equal to 60. For the three game-based rehabilitation exercises, the CBOFF results indicate that the commonly selected features in the sixty optimized features combinations include mainly the angle-based features that are related to the $\overrightarrow{EW}$ and $\overrightarrow{SE}$ vectors (i.e., $\theta_{\overrightarrow{SE}}^{\overrightarrow{EW}}(k)$, $\theta_{CP}^{\overrightarrow{EW}}(k)$, $\theta_{TP}^{\overrightarrow{EW}}(k)$, $\theta_{SP}^{\overrightarrow{EW}}(k)$, $\theta_{CP}^{\overrightarrow{SE}}(k)$, $\theta_{TP}^{\overrightarrow{SE}}(k)$, and $\theta_{SP}^{\overrightarrow{SE}}(k)$). In addition, the commonly selected features include some position-based features that quantify the acceleration of the skeleton joints. In particular, the acceleration features $a_y^{rW}(k)$ and $a_z^{rW}(k)$ are among the commonly selected features for the shoulder flexion game-based exercise, the acceleration feature $a_z^{rW}(k)$ is among the features that are commonly selected for the shoulder horizontal abduction/adduction game-based exercise, and the acceleration features $a_z^{rE}(k)$, $a_x^{rW}(k)$, and $a_z^{rW}(k)$ are commonly selected for the shoulder adduction game-based exercise. All optimized features combinations obtained for the three game-based rehabilitation exercises do not include any position-based features related to the position or velocity of the skeleton joints.

The PBOFIF values obtained for the shoulder flexion game-based exercise, the shoulder horizontal abduction/adduction game-based exercise, and the shoulder adduction game-based exercise are presented in Figure 5d–f, respectively. In fact, the PBOFIF quantifies the number of cerebral palsy children in which the feature is considered important. Hence, the highest possible PBOFIF value is equal to 6. As described in Section 3.3, for each game-based exercise, the importance of a given feature for a particular cerebral palsy child is determined by analyzing the optimized features combinations of the ten evaluation repetitions performed for the child under considerations. For the three game-based rehabilitation exercises, the important features obtained by considering the PBOFIF metric, which are shown in Figure 5d–f, are close to the commonly selected features obtained by considering the CBOFF metric, which are presented in Figure 5a–c.

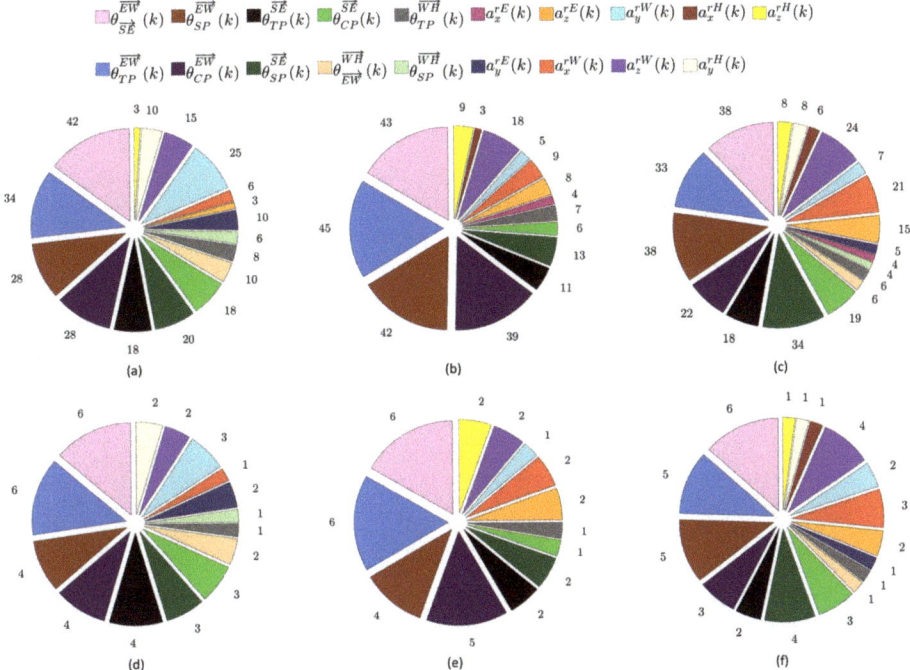

Figure 5. (**a**–**c**) The combination-based occurrence frequency of the features (CBOFF) values computed for the six cerebral palsy children during their participation in (**a**) the shoulder flexion, (**b**) the shoulder horizontal abduction/adduction, and (**c**) the shoulder adduction game-based exercises. (**d**–**f**) The participant-based occurrence frequency of the important features (PBOFIF) values computed for the six cerebral palsy children during their participation in (**d**) the shoulder flexion, (**e**) the shoulder horizontal abduction/adduction, and (**f**) the shoulder adduction game-based exercises.

3.5. Results of the Typically Developing Subjects

For the second group of participants that includes twenty typically developing subjects, the values of the performance metrics computed for the computerized assessment method using the optimized combinations of angle- and joint-based features are presented in Table 4. As shown in the table, the mean classification accuracy, specificity, and sensitivity values that are obtained for the individual typically developing subjects are within the range of 96% to 99%. Moreover, the mean kappa coefficient values achieved for the individual typically developing subjects are between 0.93 and 0.99. When all twenty typically developing subjects are considered, the mean classification accuracy, specificity, and sensitivity values, which are obtained for the three games-based exercises, are within the range of 97% and 98%. Moreover, the mean kappa coefficient values, which are achieved for the three games-based exercises, are between 0.95 and 0.96. These results indicate that the classification performance obtained by the computerized assessment method for the typically developing subjects is higher than the classification performance reported for the cerebral palsy children. This can be attributed to the fact that the typically developing subjects have high control of their right arm movements compared with the cerebral palsy children.

Table 4. The mean ± standard deviation accuracy, specificity, sensitivity, and kappa coefficient values obtained by the computerized assessment method for the twenty typically developing subjects.

Participant	Shoulder Flexion				Shoulder Horizontal Abduction/Adduction				Shoulder Adduction			
	Accuracy (%)	Specificity (%)	Sensitivity (%)	Kappa	Accuracy (%)	Specificity (%)	Sensitivity (%)	Kappa	Accuracy (%)	Specificity (%)	Sensitivity (%)	Kappa
Subject 1	98 ± 2	98 ± 2	98 ± 2	0.96 ± 0.03	98 ± 2	99 ± 2	98 ± 2	0.97 ± 0.03	97 ± 2	98 ± 2	97 ± 3	0.95 ± 0.04
Subject 2	98 ± 2	98 ± 2	97 ± 3	0.96 ± 0.04	99 ± 1	99 ± 1	99 ± 1	0.99 ± 0.03	98 ± 2	97 ± 2	99 ± 2	0.96 ± 0.03
Subject 3	99 ± 1	99 ± 1	99 ± 2	0.98 ± 0.03	99 ± 1	99 ± 1	99 ± 2	0.98 ± 0.03	99 ± 1	99 ± 1	99 ± 1	0.99 ± 0.02
Subject 4	98 ± 2	98 ± 2	98 ± 2	0.97 ± 0.04	99 ± 1	99 ± 2	99 ± 1	0.98 ± 0.03	98 ± 2	97 ± 3	98 ± 3	0.95 ± 0.04
Subject 5	98 ± 2	97 ± 3	99 ± 2	0.96 ± 0.04	98 ± 1	98 ± 2	98 ± 3	0.95 ± 0.03	97 ± 2	97 ± 2	97 ± 2	0.94 ± 0.03
Subject 6	98 ± 2	99 ± 2	98 ± 3	0.96 ± 0.05	98 ± 2	98 ± 2	98 ± 2	0.96 ± 0.04	97 ± 1	97 ± 2	98 ± 2	0.95 ± 0.03
Subject 7	99 ± 2	98 ± 3	99 ± 2	0.97 ± 0.04	99 ± 2	99 ± 2	99 ± 2	0.98 ± 0.03	98 ± 2	98 ± 2	97 ± 3	0.95 ± 0.05
Subject 8	99 ± 1	99 ± 1	99 ± 1	0.99 ± 0.03	99 ± 2	99 ± 2	98 ± 2	0.97 ± 0.04	97 ± 3	97 ± 3	98 ± 3	0.95 ± 0.06
Subject 9	98 ± 3	97 ± 3	98 ± 2	0.95 ± 0.05	97 ± 2	97 ± 3	97 ± 2	0.94 ± 0.04	97 ± 3	96 ± 3	97 ± 3	0.94 ± 0.06
Subject 10	97 ± 3	98 ± 2	97 ± 3	0.95 ± 0.05	97 ± 3	97 ± 2	97 ± 3	0.94 ± 0.05	97 ± 1	96 ± 2	97 ± 2	0.93 ± 0.02
Subject 11	98 ± 2	99 ± 2	97 ± 3	0.96 ± 0.04	98 ± 1	97 ± 2	98 ± 2	0.95 ± 0.03	97 ± 2	97 ± 2	97 ± 3	0.94 ± 0.04
Subject 12	99 ± 2	99 ± 1	98 ± 2	0.98 ± 0.04	99 ± 2	98 ± 3	99 ± 1	0.97 ± 0.04	98 ± 2	97 ± 3	98 ± 2	0.95 ± 0.04
Subject 13	98 ± 3	97 ± 3	98 ± 3	0.95 ± 0.05	98 ± 2	98 ± 2	97 ± 2	0.95 ± 0.04	97 ± 2	97 ± 3	97 ± 3	0.94 ± 0.05
Subject 14	98 ± 1	98 ± 2	99 ± 2	0.96 ± 0.02	98 ± 2	99 ± 2	98 ± 2	0.97 ± 0.03	98 ± 2	98 ± 2	98 ± 3	0.96 ± 0.04
Subject 15	97 ± 2	97 ± 3	97 ± 2	0.95 ± 0.04	98 ± 2	98 ± 2	98 ± 3	0.96 ± 0.05	98 ± 2	97 ± 3	98 ± 2	0.95 ± 0.05
Subject 16	99 ± 1	99 ± 2	98 ± 2	0.97 ± 0.03	98 ± 1	99 ± 2	98 ± 2	0.96 ± 0.02	98 ± 1	98 ± 2	98 ± 2	0.96 ± 0.03
Subject 17	98 ± 2	99 ± 2	98 ± 3	0.97 ± 0.04	99 ± 1	99 ± 2	99 ± 1	0.98 ± 0.02	98 ± 2	97 ± 2	98 ± 3	0.95 ± 0.04
Subject 18	96 ± 2	97 ± 3	96 ± 3	0.93 ± 0.05	98 ± 2	97 ± 3	98 ± 2	0.95 ± 0.05	96 ± 2	97 ± 3	96 ± 3	0.93 ± 0.05
Subject 19	97 ± 3	97 ± 3	96 ± 3	0.94 ± 0.06	97 ± 2	97 ± 3	97 ± 3	0.94 ± 0.05	96 ± 2	97 ± 2	96 ± 3	0.93 ± 0.03
Subject 20	98 ± 1	98 ± 2	97 ± 2	0.95 ± 0.03	98 ± 3	98 ± 3	97 ± 4	0.95 ± 0.06	97 ± 2	97 ± 2	97 ± 3	0.93 ± 0.04
All subjects	98 ± 2	98 ± 2	98 ± 3	0.96 ± 0.04	98 ± 2	98 ± 2	98 ± 2	0.96 ± 0.04	97 ± 2	97 ± 2	97 ± 3	0.95 ± 0.04

Figure 6a–c show the CBOFF values computed for the twenty typically developing subjects during their participation in the shoulder flexion game-based exercise, the shoulder horizontal abduction/adduction game-based exercise, and the shoulder adduction game-based exercise, respectively. As described in Section 3.3, for a particular game-based exercise, the CBOFF represents the number of times the feature appears in the 200 optimized features combinations that are obtained by combining the optimized features combinations of the ten evaluation repetitions performed for each one of the twenty typically developing subjects. Hence, the highest possible CBOFF value is equal to 200. Moreover, the PBOFIF values obtained for the shoulder flexion game-based exercise, the shoulder horizontal abduction/adduction game-based exercise, and the shoulder adduction game-based exercise are presented in Figure 6d–f, respectively. Both the commonly selected features obtained by considering the CBOFF metric and the important features obtained by considering the PBOFIF metric indicate that the right arm movements of the typically developing subjects can be classified using the angle-based features only. This finding is different from the results reported in Figure 5, which indicate that both the angle- and joint-based features are needed to classify the right arm movements of the cerebral palsy children. The difference between the combinations of optimized features of the typically developing subjects and the combinations of optimized features of the cerebral palsy children can be attributed to the fact that the typically developing subjects do not suffer from shaky and uncontrolled right arm movements. Despite this difference, the results in Figure 6 show that the commonly selected features and the important features obtained by considering the CBOFF metric and the PBOFIF metric, respectively, for the twenty typically developing subjects are dominated by angle-based features related to the $\overrightarrow{EW}$ and $\overrightarrow{SE}$ vectors. As described in Section 3.4, the angle-based features that are related to the $\overrightarrow{EW}$ and $\overrightarrow{SE}$ vectors have played also an important role to classify the right arm movements of the six cerebral palsy children.

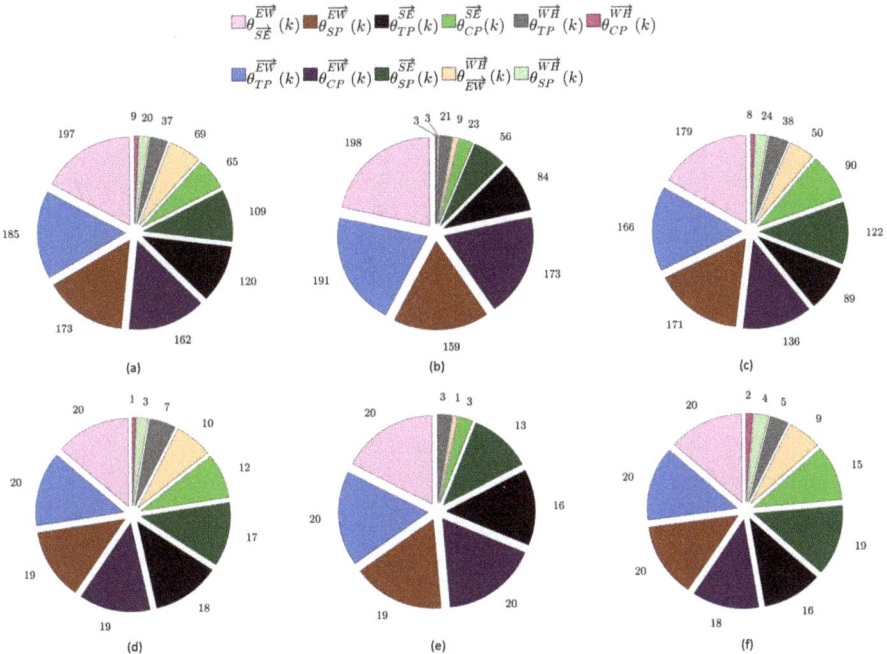

Figure 6. (a–c) The CBOFF values computed for the twenty typically developing subjects during their participation in (a) the shoulder flexion, (b) the shoulder horizontal abduction/adduction, and (c) the shoulder adduction game-based exercises. (d–f) The PBOFIF values computed for the twenty typically developing subjects during their participation in (d) the shoulder flexion, (e) the shoulder horizontal abduction/adduction, and (f) the shoulder adduction game-based exercises.

4. Discussion and Conclusions

The contributions of the current study are three folds. First, a participant-specific, game-specific computerized assessment method is developed to assess the correctness of the right arm movements that are performed during game-based rehabilitation exercises. Second, three game-based rehabilitation exercises, which are designed to target the right arm, have been implemented to evaluate the performance of the proposed computerized assessment method. Third, two groups of participants, which include cerebral palsy children and typically developing subjects, are recruited to perform the game-based rehabilitation exercises and the computerized assessment method is used to assess the correctness of the participants' right arm movements during the game-playing sessions. For the first group of participants that includes six cerebral palsy children, the classification accuracy, specificity, and sensitivity values achieved by the computerized assessment method are within the range of 71% to 95% and the kappa coefficient values are between 0.45 and 0.86, as shown in Table 3. The classification performance of the computerized assessment method varies based on the cerebral palsy category and severity of the cerebral palsy children. For the second group of participants that includes twenty typically developing subjects, the classification accuracy, specificity, and sensitivity values are within the range of 96% to 99% and the kappa coefficient values are between 0.93 and 0.99, as shown in Table 4. The high classification performance results that are obtained for the typically developing subjects can be attributed to the fact that these subjects have high control of their right arm movements. The results reported in the current study suggest the potential of employing the computerized assessment method to assess the correctness of the movements performed by cerebral palsy patients during their engagement in game-based rehabilitation exercises.

Literature reveals that many previous studies that used game-based rehabilitation for cerebral palsy patients evaluated the effectiveness of the game-based exercises using outcome measures that compare the body structure and function, such as range of motion and weakness of muscles, and the level of activity, such as the ability to perform activities of daily living, before and after the game-based rehabilitation [12]. For instance, the study by Hung et al. [19], which employed a set of Kinect-based games to train the upper limbs of cerebral palsy children, evaluated the improvement in the body structure and function and the activity level using the Quality of Upper Extremities Skills Test (QUEST) [41], the Box and Block Test (BBT) [42], the Melbourne Assessment 2 (MA2) [43], and the ABILHAND-kids score [44] outcome measures. In another study, Zoccolillo et al. [10] employed a group of Kinect-based games for the rehabilitation of cerebral palsy patients and used the QUEST and ABILHAND-kids score measures to compare the body structure and function and the activity level before and after the game-based rehabilitation. Acar et al. [45] have also used the QUEST and ABILHAND-Kids score measures as well as the Jebsen Taylor Hand Function Test [46] and the Functional Independence Measure (WeeFIM) [47] to evaluate the enhancement in the body structure and function and the activity level achieved by using a set of Nintendo Wii games as rehabilitation tools for cerebral palsy patients. Compared with these previous studies, the current study is characterized by the use of a computerized assessment method to achieve automatic evaluation of the movements performed by cerebral palsy patients during their engagement in game-based rehabilitation exercises. Such an automatic, computerized assessment approach can be integrated with the outcome measures that evaluate the improvement in the body structure and function and the activity level to analyze the effectiveness of the game-based rehabilitation exercises and improve their utilization as a complementary tool for conventional cerebral palsy rehabilitation therapy.

Despite the promising classification results that are reported in the current study, further studies are required to improve the capabilities of the proposed computerized assessment method. For example, the performance of the computerized assessment method can be improved by employing machine learning technology to classify the movements performed by cerebral palsy patients. For instance, a support vector machine classifier can be used to classify the angle- and joint-based features extracted using the E-MPGD in a manner similar to the procedure proposed by Alazrai et al. [31] to predict the fall of elderly people. The computerized assessment method can also be extended to support the evaluation of the movements performed by the left arm and the legs. In addition, the computerized assessment method can be expanded to provide kinematic-based evaluation metrics to quantify the movements performed by cerebral palsy patients, such as quantifying the smoothness and range of motion of the movements. In fact, such kinematic-based evaluation metrics have been employed by Ding et al. [48] to quantify the smoothness of the movements carried out by stroke patients and Gaillard et al. [49] to quantify the movements performed by unilateral cerebral palsy children based on the "Be an Airplane Pilot" motion analysis protocol.

Although all six cerebral palsy children included in the current feasibility study had the potential to achieve the range of motion targeted by the three game-based exercises as shown in Figure 3, our proposed game-based rehabilitation system can be adapted to support participants that have higher limitations in the range of motion. In particular, the range of motion targeted by the three game-based exercises can be configured to meet the capability of the participant. Moreover, the subject-specific evaluation criteria employed by the physiotherapist to label the game-playing sessions can be adapted to classify the game-playing sessions as correct or incorrect based on the range of motion and physical skills of the participant. This in turn will enable the computerized assessment method, which is trained based on the physiotherapist's labeling of the game-playing sessions, to adapt to the range of motion that can be achieved by the participant. Furthermore, for participants that cannot perform the three game-based exercises included in the current study, the proposed game-based rehabilitation system can be expanded to include additional game-based exercises that meet the capabilities of these participants and the computerized assessment method can be extended to support the additional exercises. However, despite the potential of expanding the proposed game-based rehabilitation system to support a wider range of cerebral palsy cases, the system might not be applied for cerebral palsy cases that have high limitations in their physical skills, such as the severe cases in which the participants cannot move their limbs independently.

The analysis reported in the current feasibility study did not investigate the relationship between the age of the participants and the performance of the computerized assessment method. Such analysis, which requires a large number of participants with different age groups, is planned in the future. Moreover, the current study did not investigate the effect of the clinical or motor function outcome changes of the participant, which might occur due to conventional rehabilitation therapy as well as game-based rehabilitation exercises, on the classification performance of the computerized assessment method. Such analysis requires the recruitment of a large number of cerebral palsy children that participate in the study for an extended period. In fact, we are planning to perform such analysis in the future. Another future direction is to extend the experimental evaluations of the proposed computerized assessment method to include a wider range of cerebral palsy types and severity levels. Furthermore, the computerized assessment method proposed in this study has been implemented using MATLAB, which affects the capability to achieve real-time assessment of the participant's movements during the game-playing sessions. Hence, we are planning to implement the computerized assessment method using the C# programming language or the C++ programming language to achieve real-time, computer-based assessment of the participant's performance.

Despite the fact that our proposed game-based rehabilitation system is configured to use the Kinect for Windows v2 sensor, the system can be easily reconfigured to employ other motion tracking sensors that track the skeleton joints. For example, our game-based system can be easily reconfigured to use the Azure Kinect sensor (Microsoft Corporation, Redmond, WA, USA) that is launched recently as a new generation of the Kinect sensing technology but with improved tracking capabilities. Our system can also be configured to use motion tracking sensors produced by other manufacturers, such as the Orbbec Astra sensor (Orbbec 3D Technology International Inc., Troy, MI, USA).

Author Contributions: Funding acquisition, M.I.D. and R.A.; Investigation, M.I.D. and A.A.; Methodology, M.I.D., A.A., and R.A.; Project administration, M.I.D.; Software, M.I.D. and A.A.; Validation, A.A. and M.I.D.; Visualization, M.I.D., A.A., and M.Z.A.; Writing—original draft preparation, M.I.D.; Writing—review and editing, M.I.D. and R.A. All authors have read and agreed to the published version of the manuscript.

Funding: This research was partially supported by the Scientific Research and Innovation Support Fund—grant number ENG/1/9/2015.

Acknowledgments: The authors would like to acknowledge the physiotherapist, Arwa Al-Otaibi, form the Model School for Cerebral Palsy, Amman, Jordan for her great efforts to acquire the Kinect data of the participants as well as evaluate and guide the participants during their participation in the game-based rehabilitation exercises. Moreover, the authors would like to thank the director of the Model School for Cerebral Palsy, Eiman Bader, for her efforts to recruit the cerebral palsy children to volunteer in this study. This research was partially supported by the Scientific Research and Innovation Support Fund—grant number ENG/1/9/2015.

Conflicts of Interest: The authors declare no conflict of interest.

References

1. Rosenbaum, P.; Paneth, N.; Leviton, A.; Goldstein, M.; Bax, M.; Damiano, D.; Dan, B.; Jacobsson, B. A report: The Definition and classification of cerebral palsy April 2006. *Dev. Med. Child Neurol.* **2007**, *49*, 8–14.
2. Aisen, M.L.; Kerkovich, D.; Mast, J.; Mulroy, S.; Wren, T.A.; Kay, R.M.; Rethlefsen, S.A. Cerebral palsy: Clinical care and neurological rehabilitation. *Lancet Neurol.* **2011**, *10*, 844–852. [CrossRef]
3. Cerebral Palsy Foundation. Key Facts. Available online: http://www.yourcpf.org/statistics/ (accessed on 23 January 2020)
4. Eunson, P. Aetiology and epidemiology of cerebral palsy. *Paediatr. Child Health* **2016**, *26*, 367–372. [CrossRef]
5. Cadwgan, J.; Goodwin, J.; Fairhurst, C. Fifteen-minute consultation: Modern-day art and science of managing cerebral palsy. *Arch. Dis. Childhood Educ. Pract.* **2019**, *104*, 66–73. [CrossRef] [PubMed]
6. Papavasiliou, A.S. Management of motor problems in cerebral palsy: A critical update for the clinician. *Eur. J. Paediatr. Neurol.* **2009**, *13*, 387–396. [CrossRef] [PubMed]

7. Lewis, G.N.; Rosie, J.A. Virtual reality games for movement rehabilitation in neurological conditions: How do we meet the needs and expectations of the users? *Disabil. Rehabil.* **2012**, *34*, 1880–1886. [CrossRef]
8. Novak, I. Evidence-Based Diagnosis, Health Care, and Rehabilitation for Children With Cerebral Palsy. *J. Child Neurol.* **2014**, *29*, 1141–1156. [CrossRef]
9. Green, D.; Wilson, P.H. Use of virtual reality in rehabilitation of movement in children with hemiplegia—A multiple case study evaluation. *Disabil. Rehabil.* **2012**, *34*, 593–604. [CrossRef]
10. Zoccolillo, L.; Morelli, D.; Cincotti, F.; Muzzioli, L.; Gobbetti, T.; Paolucci, S.; Iosa, M. Video-game based therapy performed by children with cerebral palsy: A cross-over randomized controlled trial and a cross-sectional quantitative measure of physical activity. *Eur. J. Phys. Rehabil. Med.* **2015**, *51*, 669–676.
11. Gordon, C.; Roopchand-Martin, S.; Gregg, A. Potential of the Nintendo Wii™ as a rehabilitation tool for children with cerebral palsy in a developing country: A pilot study. *Physiotherapy* **2012**, *98*, 238–242. [CrossRef]
12. Chen, Y.; Fanchiang, H.D.; Howard, A. Effectiveness of virtual reality in children with cerebral palsy: A systematic review and meta-analysis of randomized controlled trials. *Phys. Ther.* **2018**, *98*, 63–77. [CrossRef] [PubMed]
13. Daoud, M.I.; Alazrai, R.; Alhusseini, A.; Shihan, D.; Alhwayan, E.; Abou-Tair, D.I.; Qadoummi, T. ICTs for Improving Patients Rehabilitation Research Techniques. In *Communications in Computer and Information Science*; Chapter Interactive Kinect-Based Rehabilitation Framework for Assisting Children with Upper Limb Cerebral Palsy; Springer: Cham, Switzerland, 2017.
14. Daoud, M.I.; Qadoummi, T.; Abou-Tair, D.I. An interactive rehabilitation framework for assisting people with cerebral palsy. In Proceedings of the 3rd Workshop on ICTs for Improving Patients Rehabilitation Research Techniques (REHAB 15), Lisbon, Portugal, 1–2 October 2015; pp. 46–49.
15. Chang, Y.J.; Han, W.Y.; Tsai, Y.C. A Kinect-based upper limb rehabilitation system to assist people with cerebral palsy. *Res. Dev. Disabil.* **2013**, *34*, 3654–3659. [CrossRef]
16. Luna-Oliva, L.; Ortiz-Gutierrez, R.M.; Cano-de la Cuerda, R.; Piedrola, R.M.; Alguacil-Diego, I.M.; Sanchez-Camarero, C.; Martinez Culebras, M. Kinect Xbox 360 as a therapeutic modality for children with cerebral palsy in a school environment: A preliminary study. *NeuroRehabilitation* **2013**, *33*, 513–521. [CrossRef]
17. Bryanton, C.; Bosse, J.; Brien, M.; Mclean, J.; McCormick, A.; Sveistrup, H. Feasibility, motivation, and selective motor control: Virtual reality compared to conventional home exercise in children with cerebral palsy. *Cyberpsychol. Behav.* **2006**, *9*, 123–128. [CrossRef]
18. Bonnechere, B.; Jansen, B.; Omelina, L.; Da Silva, L.; Mougeat, J.; Heymans, V.; Vandeuren, A.; Rooze, M.; Van Sint Jan, S. Use of serious gaming to increase motivation of cerebral palsy children during rehabilitation. *Eur. J. Paediatr. Neurol.* **2013**, *17*, S12. [CrossRef]
19. Hung, J.; Chang, Y.; Chou, C.; Wu, W.; Howell, S.; Lu, W. Developing a suite of motion-controlled games for upper extremity training in children with cerebral palsy: A proof-of-concept study. *Games Health J.* **2018**, *7*, 327–334. [CrossRef] [PubMed]
20. Jelsma, J.; Pronk, M.; Ferguson, G.; Jelsma-Smit, D. The effect of the Nintendo Wii Fit on balance control and gross motor function of children with spastic hemiplegic cerebral palsy. *Dev. Neurorehabil.* **2013**, *16*, 27–37. [CrossRef]
21. Winkels, D.G.M.; Kottink, A.I.R.; Temmink, R.A.J.; Nijlant, J.M.M.; Buurke, J.H. Wii™-habilitation of upper extremity function in children with cerebral palsy. An explorative study. *Dev. Neurorehabil.* **2013**, *16*, 44–51. [CrossRef] [PubMed]
22. Sevick, M.; Eklund, E.; Mensch, A.; Foreman, M.; Standeven, J.; Engsberg, J. Using free internet videogames in upper extremity motor training for children with cerebral palsy. *Behav. Sci.* **2016**, *6*, 10. [CrossRef]
23. Machado, F.R.C.; Antunes, P.P.; Souza, J.; Dos Santos, A.C.; Levandowski, D.C.; De Oliveira, A.A. Motor improvement using motion sensing game devices for cerebral palsy rehabilitation. *J. Motor Behav.* **2017**, *49*, 273–280. [CrossRef]
24. Sandlund, M.; Domellof, E.; Grip, H.; Ronnqvist, L.; Hager, C.K. Training of goal directed arm movements with motion interactive video games in children with cerebral palsy—A kinematic evaluation. *Dev. Neurorehabil.* **2014**, *17*, 318–326. [CrossRef] [PubMed]

25. Ayed, I.; Ghazel, A.; Jaume-I-Capo, A.; Moyà-Alcover, G.; Varona, J.; Martínez-Bueso, O. Vision-based serious games and virtual reality systems for motor rehabilitation: A review geared toward a research methodology. *Int. J. Med. Inform.* **2019**, *131*, 103909. [CrossRef] [PubMed]
26. Huber, M.; Rabin, B.; Docan, C.; Burdea, G.; Nwosu, M.E.; Abdelbaky, M.; Golomb, M.R. PlayStation 3-based tele-rehabilitation for children with hemiplegia. In Proceedings of the 2008 Virtual Rehabilitation Conference, Vancouver, BC, Canada, 25–27 August 2008; pp. 105–112.
27. Roy, A.K.; Soni, Y.; Dubey, S. Enhancing effectiveness of motor rehabilitation using kinect motion sensing technology. In Proceedings of the IEEE Global Humanitarian Technology Conference: South Asia Satellite (GHTC-SAS), Trivandrum, India, 23–24 August 2013; pp. 298–304.
28. Sinpithakkul, C.; Kusakunniran, W.; Bovonsunthonchai, S.; Wattananon, P. Game-based enhancement for rehabilitation based on action recognition using kinect. In Proceedings of the IEEE Region 10 Conference (TENCON 2018), Jeju, Korea, 28–31 Octorber 2018; pp. 303–308.
29. Vilas-Boas, M.D.C.; Choupina, H.M.P.; Rocha, A.P.; Fernandes, J.M.; Cunha, J.P.S. Full-body motion assessment: Concurrent validation of two body tracking depth sensors versus a gold standard system during gait. *J. Biomech.* **2019**, *87*, 189–196. [CrossRef] [PubMed]
30. Alazrai, R.; Mowafi, Y.; Lee, G. Anatomical-plane-based representation for human-human interactions analysis. *Pattern Recognit.* **2015**, *48*, 2346–2363. [CrossRef]
31. Alazrai, R.; Momani, M.; Daoud, M.I. Fall detection for elderly from partially observed depth-map video sequences based on view-invariant human activity representation. *Appl. Sci.* **2017**, *7*, 316. [CrossRef]
32. Alazrai, R.; Mowafi, Y.; Hamad, E. A fall prediction methodology for elderly based on a depth camera. In Proceedings of the 37th Annual International Conference of the IEEE Engineering in Medicine and Biology Society (EMBC), Milan, Italy, 25–29 August 2015; pp. 4990–4993.
33. Snell, R.S. *Clinical Anatomy by Regions*, 9th ed.; Lippincott Williams & Wilkins: Baltimore, MD, USA, 2011.
34. Wöllmer, M.; Al-Hames, M.; Eyben, F.; Schuller, B.; Rigoll, G. A multidimensional dynamic time warping algorithm for efficient multimodal fusion of asynchronous data streams. *Neurocomputing* **2009**, *73*, 366–380. [CrossRef]
35. Guyon, I.; Weston, J.; Barnhill, S.; Vapnik, V. Gene selection for cancer classification using support vector machines. *Mach. Learn.* **2002**, *46*, 389–422. [CrossRef]
36. Han, J.; Kamber, M.; Pei, J. *Data Mining: Concepts and Techniques*, 3rd ed.; Elsevier: Amsterdam, The Netherlands, 2012.
37. Sim, J.; Wright, C.C. The kappa statistic in reliability studies: Use, interpretation, and sample size requirements. *Phys. Ther.* **2005**, *85*, 257–268. [CrossRef]
38. Cohen, J. A coefficient of agreement for nominal scales. *Educ. Psychol. Meas.* **1960**, *20*, 37–46. [CrossRef]
39. Landis, J.R.; Koch, G.G. The measurement of observer agreement for categorical data. *Biometrics* **1977**, *33*, 159–174. [CrossRef]
40. Cameron, M.H.; Monroe, L. *Physical Rehabilitation for the Physical Therapist Assistant*; Elsevier: Amsterdam, The Netherlands, 2011.
41. DeMatteo, C.; Law, M.; Russell, D.; Pollock, N.; Rosenbaum, P.; Walter, S. The reliability and validity of the quality of upper extremity skills test. *Phys. Occup. Ther. Pediatr.* **1993**, *13*, 1–18. [CrossRef]
42. Mathiowetz, V.; Federman, S.; Wiemer, D. Box and block test of manual dexterity: Norms for 6–19 year olds. *Can. J. Occup. Ther.* **1985**, *52*, 241–245. [CrossRef]
43. Randall, M.; Johnson, L.; Reddihough, D. *The Melbourne Assessment of Unilateral Upper Limb Function: Test Administration Manual*; Royal Children's Hospital: Melbourne, Australia, 1999.
44. Arnould, C.; Penta, M.; Renders, A.; Thonnard, J. ABILHAND-Kids: A measure of manual ability in children with cerebral palsy. *Neurology* **2004**, *63*, 1045–1052. [CrossRef] [PubMed]
45. Acar, G.; Altun, G.P.; Yurdalan, S.; Polat, M.G. Efficacy of neurodevelopmental treatment combined with the Nintendo© Wii in patients with cerebral palsy. *J. Phys. Ther. Sci.* **2016**, *28*, 774–780. [CrossRef]
46. Jebsen, R.H.; Taylor, N.; Trieschmann, R.B.; Trotter, M.J.; Howard, L.A. An objective and standardized test of hand function. *Arch. Phys. Med. Rehabil.* **1969**, *50*, 311–319.
47. Msall, M.E.; DiGaudio, K.; Duffy, L.C.; LaForest, S.; Braun, S.; Granger, C.V. WeeFIM: Normative sample of an instrument for tracking functional independence in children. *Clin. Pediatr.* **1994**, *33*, 431–438. [CrossRef]

48. Ding, W.L.; Zheng, Y.Z.; Su, Y.P.; Li, X.L. Kinect-based virtual rehabilitation and evaluation system for upper limb disorders: A case study. *J. Back Musculoskel. Rehabil.* **2018**, *31*, 611–621. [CrossRef]
49. Gaillard, F.; Cacioppo, M.; Bouvier, B.; Bouzille, G.; Newman, C.J.; Pasquet, T.; Cretual, A.; Rauscent, H.; Bonan, I. Assessment of bimanual performance in 3-D movement analysis: Validation of a new clinical protocol in children with unilateral cerebral palsy. *Ann. Phys. Rehabil. Med.* in Press. [CrossRef]

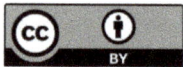

© 2020 by the authors. Licensee MDPI, Basel, Switzerland. This article is an open access article distributed under the terms and conditions of the Creative Commons Attribution (CC BY) license (http://creativecommons.org/licenses/by/4.0/).

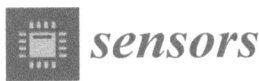

Article

Automatic and Real-Time Computation of the 30-Seconds Chair-Stand Test without Professional Supervision for Community-Dwelling Older Adults

Antonio Cobo [1,2], Elena Villalba-Mora [1,2,*], Rodrigo Pérez-Rodríguez [3], Xavier Ferre [1], Walter Escalante [1], Cristian Moral [1] and Leocadio Rodriguez-Mañas [4,5]

1. Centre for Biomedical Technology (CTB), Universidad Politécnica de Madrid (UPM), Pozuelo de Alarcón, 28223 Madrid, Spain; antonio.cobo@ctb.upm.es (A.C.); xavier.ferre@ctb.upm.es (X.F.); walter.escalante@ctb.upm.es (W.E.); cristian.moral@ctb.upm.es (C.M.)
2. Centro de Investigación Biomédica en Red en Bioingeniería, Biomateriales y Nanomedicina (CIBER-BBN), 28029 Madrid, Spain
3. Fundación para la Investigación Biomédica, Hospital de Getafe, Getafe, 28905 Madrid, Spain; rprodrigo@salud.madrid.org
4. Servicio de Geriatría, Hospital de Getafe, Getafe, 28905 Madrid, Spain; leocadio.rodriguez@salud.madrid.org
5. Centro de Investigación Biomédica en Red en Fragilidad y Envejecimiento Saludable (CIBER-FES), 28029 Madrid, Spain
* Correspondence: elena.villalba@ctb.upm.es; Tel.: +34-910-679-275

Received: 15 September 2020; Accepted: 13 October 2020; Published: 14 October 2020

Abstract: The present paper describes a system for older people to self-administer the 30-s chair stand test (CST) at home without supervision. The system comprises a low-cost sensor to count sit-to-stand (SiSt) transitions, and an Android application to guide older people through the procedure. Two observational studies were conducted to test (i) the sensor in a supervised environment ($n = 7$; m = 83.29 years old, sd = 4.19; 5 female), and (ii) the complete system in an unsupervised one ($n = 7$; age 64–74 years old; 3 female). The participants in the supervised test were asked to perform a 30-s CST with the sensor, while a member of the research team manually counted valid transitions. Automatic and manual counts were perfectly correlated (Pearson's $r = 1$, $p = 0.00$). Even though the sample was small, none of the signals around the critical score were affected by harmful noise; p (harmless noise) = 1, 95% CI = (0.98, 1). The participants in the unsupervised test used the system in their homes for a month. None of them dropped out, and they reported it to be easy to use, comfortable, and easy to understand. Thus, the system is suitable to be used by older adults in their homes without professional supervision.

Keywords: frailty syndrome; sit-to-stand; 30-s chair stand test; wearable sensors; signal processing

1. Introduction

The present paper describes a system for older people to self-administer the 30-s chair stand test (CST) at home without supervision. The system comprises a low-cost sensor that automatically detects and counts sit-to-stand (SiSt) transitions in real-time, and a home care application that guides older people through the whole procedure. Since using novel technologies is not a trivial issue for older adults, we studied whether such a system would be able to match older people's abilities and expectations, so they can use it without supervision. The 30-s CST is a medical exam used to assess older adults' lower-limb strength [1]. It requires a subject to spend thirty seconds repeatedly standing up from, and sitting down on, a chair, with his arms folded on his chest, as fast as possible [1]. The number of times the said subject reached an upright position is then taken as a proxy to lower-limb strength [1]. It is used in combination with other medical exams to assess the functional status of older people.

Depending on the results of such a functional assessment, older people may be diagnosed as robust, pre-frail, or frail [2]. Frailty is a state of increased vulnerability to low power stressors, leading to difficulties in maintaining homeostasis that increases the risk of disability and other adverse outcomes, such as falls, hospitalization, permanent institutionalization, and death [3–6]. In fact, frailty is a major predictor of disability, with frail elders showing twice the risk of disability than non-frail older adults [7].

Disability is one of the major challenges for elderly care, because improvements in life expectancy are not coming together with similar improvements in impairment-free life expectancy (IFLE); on the contrary, a decline in the latter has even been observed in some countries [8]. Disability imposes a heavy psychological and economic burden on older people and their relatives over a long time; fortunately, frailty, which may precede the development of disability by several years [2], can be reversed [9–11]. Hence the paramount role of frailty detection in the prevention of disability. Several models have been proposed to explain frailty, with two of them prevailing as major approaches, namely, Rockwood's deficit accumulation model [12–14] and Fried's phenotypic model [2]. The latter is the most widespread, and identifies the following markers of frailty: (i) weight loss, (ii) exhaustion, (iii) weakness, (iv) slowness, and (v) low physical activity [2]. An older adult is classified as pre-frail if he tests positive to one or two of the frailty components in the phenotypic model, and as frail if he tests positive to three or more of them; otherwise he is classified as robust [2] (see Table 1).

Table 1. The phenotypic model for frailty involves the assessment of five different components (weight loss, exhaustion, weakness, slowness, and low physical activity); and then diagnosing the subject as robust, pre-frail, or frail, according to the number of components that resulted positive in the tests: robust (green rows) for zero components, pre-frail (yellow rows) for 1 or 2 components, or frail (red rows) for 3, 4, or 5 components.

If a Subject Tests Positive to:	He is Diagnosed as:
0 components	Robust.
1 component	Pre-frail.
2 components	
3 components	Frail.
4 components	
5 components	

Frail older adults can reduce their levels of frailty, and even be restored back to robustness, with exercise-based interventions, especially if combined with early diagnosis and continuity of care [9,11,15]. Many different instruments are currently involved in the diagnosis and assessment of frailty. For instance, hand grip strength is used to assess weakness, in fact, the data in the original study of Fried et al. came from hand grip strength measurements [2], but it has also been explored as a measurement of overall frailty on its own; just as the stand up and go (TUG) test, which is a standard test for gait speed [6]. On the other hand, other sources of weakness measurements, such as those based on lower-limb strength, have been observed to be associated with either hand grip strength, gait speed, and even overall frailty [16]. In fact, instruments to assess lower-limb strength, such as the 30-s CST [1], and the STS5 (measuring how long it takes for an older person to repeatedly stand up from a chair five times) [17], are usually included as part of a comprehensive geriatric assessment (CGA). Both early diagnosis and continuity of care require frailty to be frequently assessed in search of early signs of functional decline. For instance, if two consecutive measurements of lower-limb strength taken two weeks apart with the 30-s CST show a decrease bigger that a given threshold, an alarm should be raised. However, it is not feasible to assess every older adult at risk of developing frailty every two weeks with the currently available means to conduct the functional assessment exams. Most of them require the involvement of a specifically trained professional in a geriatrics department to supervise their execution, and compute their corresponding scores. Obviously, a geriatrics department in specialized care cannot afford to undertake such a screening task. In fact, they should be focusing on taking care of the most severe cases. As a result, older people do not have their functional capacity assessed for early signs of frailty very often.

Automatic sensors that do not require the involvement of any specifically trained personnel could help to alleviate this problem. On the one hand, a single staff member in a geriatrics department could supervise several tests on multiple patients simultaneously. On the other hand, and probably involving a bigger potential impact, general practitioners or nurses in primary care could add functional assessment to routine follow-ups of their older adult patients. The potential benefits of such automatic sensors become even more remarkable within the current context of the COVID-19 pandemic. Olde people are at greater risk of developing severe complications and dying from COVID-19 [18]. Therefore, they have been advised to carefully comply with distancing measures to lower the risk of transmission. However, distancing measures favor social isolation and sedentary behaviors. Such sedentary behaviors increase the risk of developing frailty [19], and have been hypothesized to persist and become habits, based on observations from previous natural disasters, in particular, from the three years following the 2011 earthquake and tsunami in East Japan [20]. In such a scenario (i.e., fewer visits to the doctor and increased risk of frailty due to sedentary behavior) older adults would benefit from having automatic sensors to conduct functional assessment exams at home, on their own or helped by their care givers. In the particular case of the 30-s CST, the setup is rather simple; it just requires a regular rigid chair to repeatedly stand-up and sit-down, and a timer to control the duration of the test [1]. Nevertheless, a trained professional is required to judge which SiSt transitions are valid and must be added to the final score. Valid SiSt transitions occur when the subject reaches an upright position [1]. However, some older adults suffer from mobility constraints, and upright positions might differ from one subject to another.

A 30-s CST is not a transparent procedure embedded into people's daily lives. It requires older adults to interrupt their daily activities and go through a specific sequence of actions. Our approach involves a system that comprises an automatic sensor and a home care application to guide older adults through the procedure. One of the determinant factors of such a system is the specifics of the sensing device. According to Millor et al., the study of SiSt and stand-to-sit (StSi) transitions with inertial sensors can be traced back to the mid-1990s [21]; in particular to Kerr et al., in 1994 [22]. Over half of the works that Millor et al. reviewed were based on the assessment of daily life activities [21]. Only a few of them involved the assessment of repeated SiSt/StSi cycles in traditional tests for frailty assessment [21]. While some works relied on the use of multiple devices on different parts of the body, a low number of devices is recommendable to simplify the setup, lower the cost, and eventually improve acceptance and adoption. A very popular approach is to place a single inertial measurement unit (IMU) on the subject's lower back (L3–L5 region), close to the body center of mass, and take advantage of the quasi-periodic nature of the body movement [23,24]. This approach is exemplified in the works of van Lummel et al. (where the authors apply it to the STS5) [23] and Millor et al. (where the authors apply it to the 30-s CST) [24].

In particular, van Lummel et al. developed a fully automated method of processing repeated sit-to-stand-to-sit (STS) cycles [23]. They used triaxial acceleration and triaxial angular velocity signals from a single IMU device (dynaport) on the lower back to compute trunk pitch-angle and vertical velocity signals. They used the morphological properties of the trunk pitch-angle signal to identify and delimit the sub-phases and transitions in repeated STS cycles. They used the vertical velocity signal to spot and discard failed attempts. However, they do not explain which features of the vertical velocity and which criteria were used to classify an attempt as a failure.

On the other hand, Millor et al. developed a fully automated method to process repeated STS cycles in a 30-s CST [24]. They computed vertical velocity and vertical position from the vertical acceleration signal, from a single IMU device (MTx Orientation Tracker—Xsens Technologies B.V. Enschede, Netherlands) on the lower back. They applied double integration, combined with fourth-level polynomial curve adjustment and cubic splines interpolation. They used the morphological properties of the vertical position signal to identify and delimit complete STS cycles. A complete STS cycle can be found between two minima in the vertical position signal. They also used the MTx's onboard Kalman filter estimation for the X-orientation, and combined it with the vertical acceleration, the vertical velocity, and the vertical position signals to identify the sub-phases (i.e., impulse, stand up, and sit down) within each STS cycle. In a subsequent paper Millor, Lecumberri, Gómez, Martínez-Ramírez, and Izquierdo argued that they automatically detected failed attempts "... based on a threshold applied to both the time elapsed between a maximum and a minimum of the Z-position and to their difference." [25], (p. 4). However, they did not clarify what the values for these thresholds were nor how they were computed.

In both cases, the authors complemented their studies by computing multiple kinematic parameters, such as transition duration (TD), maximum and minimum values of the vertical acceleration (max., min., V-acc.), Area Under the Curve (AUC) of V-acc., and roll range, and processed them to obtain additional information beyond the test score [25]. van Lummel et al. were able to identify seat-off and seat-on instants [26], establish a relationship between the subjects' stand up strategies and their overall muscle strength [27], and compare the sensitivity of stair ascending (SA) and Leg-Extension Power (LEP) to detect age-related changes [28]. When they analyzed the associations between clinical outcomes (both health and functional outcomes) and the functional tests results, they observed stronger associations for their instrumented STS5 test than for manual records [29]. On the other hand, Millor et al. were able to detect differences in frailty status (robust, pre-frail, frail) across different subjects directly from their kinematic parameters [25]. They even identified the set of most informative parameters (i.e., anterior-posterior (AP) orientation range during the Imp phase, maximum vertical acceleration and vertical power peaks during SiSt phase, and total impulse during the StSi phase) [30]. In fact, they claimed that these parameters outperformed the number of completed cycles in the 30-s CST, as a criterion for frailty classification [30].

Other locations for the sensing devices, such as the chest, have also been explored [31]. Recently, in that line, Jovanov, Wrigth, and Ganegoda presented some preliminary results from their automated 30-s CST [32]. Instead of attaching a sensor directly to the subject's chest, they took advantage of the fact that the 30-s CST requires the subject to fold his arms over his chest, and used the inertial sensors onboard a smartwatch. They used 3D acceleration signals from two different models (Fossil Gen 4 and Polar M600). They obtained excellent reliability between automated and manual counts, with little processing load. However, their experimental subjects were not older adults (12 subjects, mean age: 39.1 y.o.). They did not provide any explanation of the STS cycle identification and delimitation criteria and algorithms, and they did not mention any mechanism to spot and dismiss failed attempts.

Lately, we have explored a different approach ourselves by using an ambient sensor instead of a body-worn sensor [33]. In our study we explored " ... the feasibility of using the quasi-periodic nature of the distance between a subject's back and the chair backrest during a 30-s CST to carry out unsupervised measurements based on readings from a low-cost ultrasound sensor" [33], (p. 3). Our sensor comprised an ultrasound sensing module, an Arduino controller board, and a wireless communications module. All three of them were integrated into our own design for a portable device that the end-users could attach to the backrest of any regular rigid chair. We observed older people to generate very noisy signals. We applied a moving minimum filter to cancel the effects of said noise and an adaptable threshold to tell the difference between sitting and standing regions in the signal. Even though intra-class correlation coefficients showed good levels of reliability between the sensor outcomes and the trained professional's manual counts, the differences between these outcomes resulted in the performance of some subjects not being correctly classified as average, better than average, or worse than average.

In the present paper we come back to the body-worn sensor approach. We propose to measure the thigh angle with respect to a horizontal plane perpendicular to the direction of gravity (i.e., tilt) with a single device on the subject's thigh itself, and to use the variation of the angle as the subject stands up and down over time to identify SiSt and StSi transitions. Measurements of the thigh angle from a single device have already been used in previous literature to study SiSt and StSi transitions, mostly to identify different postures and activities (sitting, standing, walking, ramp or stair ascending, etc.) while performing activities of daily living (either in controlled lab settings or in free-living conditions) [34–37]. However, we have not found any descriptions of an instrumented version of the 30-s CST based on this approach. The accurate estimation of tilt based on IMU readings relies on the fusion of accelerometer and gyroscope data [38]. Smartphones come equipped with IMUs and relatively high computing power. However, smartphone adoption among the geriatric population (i.e., people over 70 years old) is low, especially among low-income and low-education elders, because they use much simpler and cheaper mobile phones. Smartphones would be too expensive, and oversize, for the single purpose of being used as a sensor; since a home kit for frailty monitoring usually comprises multiple sensors, devices of a much lower cost are required. Kalman and complementary filters are the most widespread data fusion methods for IMU-based applications [38]. Kalman filters are computationally expensive and, as stated by Abhayasinghe, Murray, and Sharif Bidabadi, 32-bit microcontrollers with a digital signal processor (DSP) are necessary to run them in real time [39]. Conversely, the algorithm for the complementary filter is much simpler and, even though it involves the computation of an arc tangent, can be run on much cheaper 8-bit microcontrollers in real time [39]. According to Tognetti et al., making use of a simple accelerometer instead of a complete IMU may contribute to further decreasing the complexity and cost of the sensing device [40]; however, the complementary filter still relies on fusing accelerometer and gyroscope data. Fortunately, tilt can be estimated solely from accelerometry if the main contributor to the accelerometer readings is gravity. During a 30-s CST, however, an accelerometer will be exposed to sudden acceleration and deceleration forces when reaching the upright and sitting positions. Thus, the question remains whether the resulting noise will harm the correct identification of valid transitions.

On the other hand, using novel technologies is not a trivial issue for older adults. Moreover, the sensors described above have been tested in controlled settings, under the supervision of their corresponding research teams. We have found no works reporting older adult's performance when using this kind of automatic sensors on their own. Our approach involves a system that comprises an automatic sensor and a home care application to guide older adults through the procedure. Thus, the question remains whether such a system will match older people's abilities and expectations so they can use it without supervision. We implemented our own design for a low-cost sensor for counting SiSt transitions, which estimates the thigh angle solely form the readings of a single accelerometer. In addition, we implemented a home care app for Android that guides the older adults throughout the whole procedure. We first tested the sensor in a supervised environment, and then we tested the complete system in an unsupervised one. To test the sensor, we studied the impact of noise by analyzing the statistical significance of the estimated probability of finding harmless noise in a valid SiSt transition. We observed the noise in all the valid transitions in the critical scenario (i.e., test scores around the value used to spot patients not fit enough to remain independent) to be harmless. We then delivered the complete system to seven older adults' homes for a month, and conducted an acceptability study. The participants reported finding it easy to use, feeling comfortable using it, understanding the features and functionalities of the app, and feeling able to use it on their own.

2. Materials and Methods

The sensor was tested in an observational study, described in Section 2.1, where the participants used it while taking a 30-s CST, under the supervision of a trained member of the research team. The home care system was tested in another observational study, described in Section 2.2, where the participants used it to take several 30-s CSTs over the course of a month, at their own homes and without any kind of supervision.

2.1. Supervised Validation of the Sensor

2.1.1. Participants

Seven older subjects (age: m = 83.29 years old, sd = 4.19; gender: 5 female and 2 male) were recruited from a pool of participants that expressed a general interest in participating in research studies from the University Hospital of Getafe.

All subjects gave their informed consent for inclusion before they participated in the study. The study was conducted in accordance with the Declaration of Helsinki, and the protocol was approved by the Ethics Committee of the Universidad Politécnica de Madrid on 9 May 2019 (POSITIVE: Maintaining and improving the intrinsic capacity involving primary care and caregivers).

The following inclusion and exclusion criteria were applied:

- A subject COULD ENTER the study if ALL the following INCLUSION CRITERIA applied:

    ○ The subject is willing and able to give written informed consent for participation in the study.
    ○ The subject is 70 years old or older.
    ○ The subject is able to perform the 30-s CST in a safe way.
    ○ The subject has not been diagnosed with cognitive impairment.

- A subject COULD NOT ENTER the study if ANY of the following EXCLUSION CRITERIA applied:

    ○ Subjects suffering from any major disability.
    ○ Subjects suffering from cognitive impairment.

2.1.2. Apparatus

The overall setup is depicted in Figure 1, and consisted of a regular rigid chair with a backrest, an instance of the wearable device under study, and a tablet device. The chair played the same role as usual in any regular 30-s CST. The subjects wore the sensing device on one of their thighs. The sensor is longitudinally aligned with the subject's femur and tightly attached to her thigh with a Velcro strap as shown in Figure 2. Since the sensor is sensitive to orientation, a green sticker was attached to one of its ends to signal which one has to remain closer to the knee. However, it is not visible in Figure 2, because once the sensor is put in place and secured, the Velcro strap covers it. The tablet hosts an app to control the sensor, and it is paired to the latter via Bluetooth. A member of the research team used the app to switch the sensor into either calibration or measurement mode, and to visualize the sensor automatic count at the end of each 30-s CST. In calibration mode, the readings from the accelerometer in the device are used to compute the thigh angle in both a sitting and an upright static posture, as a measurement of the subject's mobility constraints; then, the parameters in the automatic count algorithm are set accordingly to a personalized value. In measurement mode, the subject takes the 30-s CST itself, and the accelerometer readings are processed by the automatic count algorithm (aka STS analysis algorithm). Finally, the sensor sends the automatic count to the tablet via Bluetooth once the test is over. Further details about the sensor hardware, the automatic count algorithm, and the tablet app can be found in Sections 2.1.2.1 to 2.1.2.3, respectively.

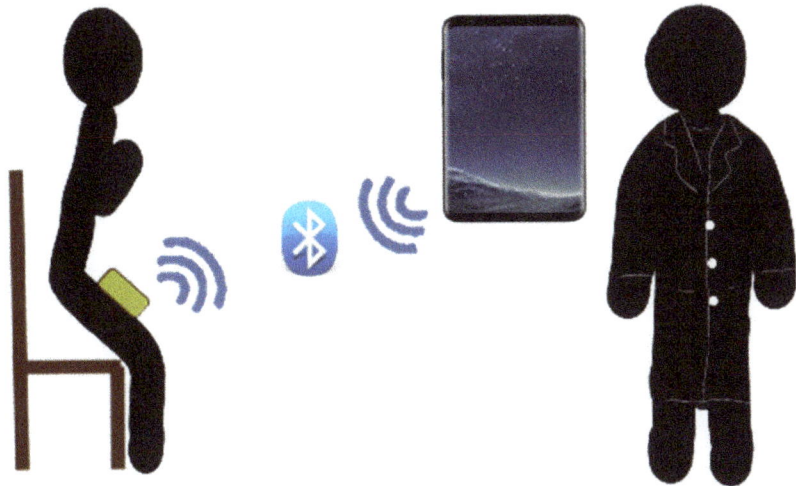

Figure 1. Depiction of the overall experimental setup: The subject stands up from and sits down on a regular rigid chair with the sensing device on one of his thighs; the sensing device is paired with a tablet via Bluetooth; a member of the research team uses the app on board the tablet device to switch the sensor into either calibration or measurement modes, and to visualize the sensor automatic count once the 30-s chair stand test (CST) is over.

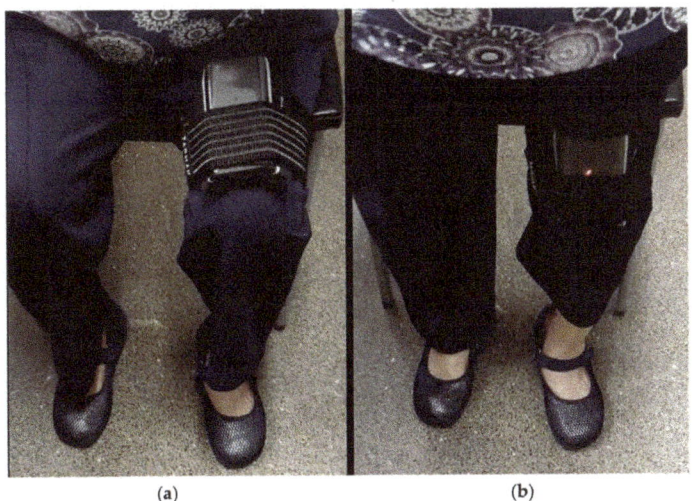

Figure 2. Position and alignment of the sensing device on a subject's thigh. (**a**) The wearable sensor is placed on the subject's thigh longitudinally aligned with her femur. The sensor is tightly attached to the subject's thigh with a Velcro strap to prevent it from sliding. The LED in the sensor is turned off when the subject is sitting; (**b**) and it is turned on every time a valid SiSt transition is detected.

2.1.2.1. The Wearable Sensor Device

The device consists of three main building blocks, as shown in Scheme 1. These blocks are, from left to right:

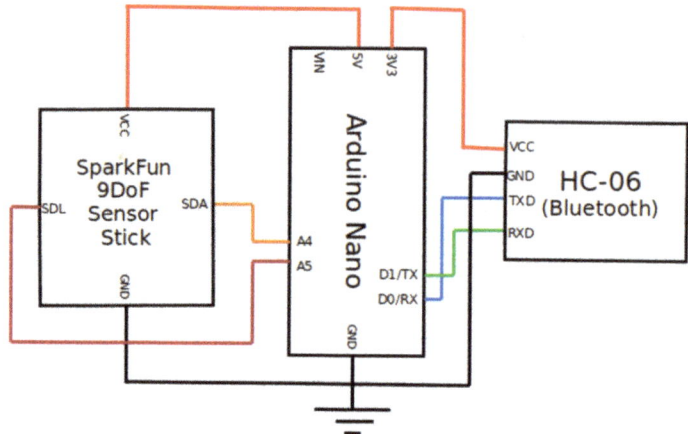

Scheme 1. Schematic block diagram of the interconnection between the device components. The Arduino Nano board (center) acts as the control and processing unit, collecting readings from the accelerometer (SparkFun block on the left), computing the estimations of the thigh angle over time, and analyzing the resulting signal. The Arduino Nano board also makes use of the Bluetooth module (HC-06 block on the right) to exchange messages with the external mobile device over a wireless communication channel. The whole device was powered by a 9V 6LP3146 battery. While the Arduino Nano board was directly powered by the battery, the accelerometer and the Bluetooth boards were indirectly powered by connecting them to the Arduino's 5V and 3.3V DC outputs, respectively. The battery was omitted in this scheme for the sake of clarity.

- An accelerometer (a SparkFun 9DoF Sensor Stick board with an LSM9DS1 IMU chip). This SparkFun board comes with a nine degrees of freedom IMU (i.e., it comprises a triaxial accelerometer, a triaxial gyroscope, and a triaxial magnetometer). However, we did not use the gyroscope and the magnetometer because, as explained in Section 2.1.2.2, acceleration readings are enough to compute an estimation of the thigh angle.
- A control and processing unit (an Arduino Nano board with an ATmega328P microcontroller). The Arduino board acts as the processing unit in the device thanks to its onboard micro-controller. Our processing algorithm runs on board the Arduino, and is responsible for collecting the accelerometer readings, computing the estimations of the thigh angle over time, and analyzing the resulting signal to automatically detect and count SiSt and StSi transitions in real time, without storing or transmitting the individual samples.
- A communications unit: (HC-06 Bluetooth 2.0 + EDR module). End users (in this case, the researcher conducting the experiment) control the behavior of the sensing device by interacting with a mobile app in an external tablet device. This communication unit enables wireless communication between the two devices via Bluetooth. The researcher can issue calibration and measurements commands to the sensing device, and the latter automatically sends the results to the tablet once a 30s-CST is over.

The device is powered by a 9 V battery (6LP3146). However, only the Arduino Nano board was directly powered by this battery. The accelerometer board was powered by connecting it to the Arduino's 5 V DC output, and the Bluetooth board was indirectly powered via the Arduino as well, by connecting the Bluetooth board to the Arduino's 3.3V DC output. The device also has an on/off switch, a LED, and a vibrator. The color of the LED helps to tell the difference between calibration mode and measurement mode. Once the device enters into measurement mode, the vibrator tells the subject when to start and stop the test. All these additional elements (the battery and its corresponding case, the on/off switch, the LED, and the vibrator) were omitted in Scheme 1 for the sake of clarity.

2.1.2.2. The STS Analysis Algorithm

The STS analysis algorithm itself involves two steps. First, the thigh angle is estimated in real-time as the acceleration samples arrive. The thigh angle in the 30-s CST was defined as the angle between the subject's thigh and a horizontal plane perpendicular to gravity (e.g., the seat of the chair), as shown in Figure 3b. During a 30-s CST, this angle is expected to vary over time between 0° in the sitting position (Figure 3a) and 90° in the upright position (Figure 3c).

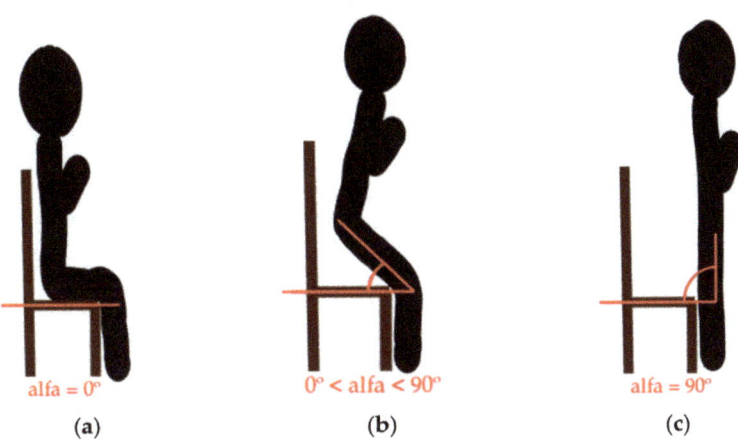

Figure 3. Definition of the thigh angle for the 30-s CST. It is defined as the angle between the subject's thigh and a horizontal plane perpendicular to gravity (e.g., the seat of the chair). It is depicted as the angle (alfa) between the red line along the longitudinal direction of the subject's thigh and the red line on the seat of the chair; therefore, (**a**) the expected value of the thigh angle in the sitting position is 0; (**b**) the value of the thigh angle at any time during SiSt and StSi transitions is bigger than 0 and lower than 90°; and (**c**) the expected value of the thigh angle in the upright position is 90°.

The thigh angle can then be computed from the gravity readings of the accelerometer on the subject's thigh, as demonstrated in Figure 4. The thigh angle (red angle, dubbed as alfa) is equal to the angle between gravity itself and the Z-gravity component of the accelerometer readings (green angle, dubbed as beta) because the gravity is always perpendicular to the horizontal plane (the seat of the chair), and the Z-gravity component is always perpendicular to the thigh.

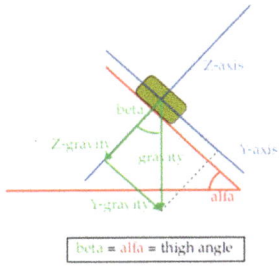

Figure 4. Computation of the thigh angle from the decomposition of gravity into orthogonal components along the axis of the reference system (blue lines) of an accelerometer on the subject's thigh. According to the convention applied in the preceding figure the thigh angle is represented by the red angle (alfa). Gravity and its components are depicted in green. The green angle (beta) between gravity itself and its Z-component is equal to the thigh angle (alfa), because gravity is always perpendicular to the horizontal plane, and the Z-gravity component is always perpendicular to the thigh.

Thus, if the Y-axis of the accelerometer is aligned with the thigh itself, as it is in the case of our experimental setting, the angle value at any given moment can be computed from the accelerometer Z-gravity and Y-gravity readings according to the following expression:

$$\alpha = \arctan(-g_y/g_z) \qquad (1)$$

Obtaining the gravity components from the accelerometer readings would require filtering the raw acceleration signals. However, in order to lower the computational complexity of our algorithm we estimated the thigh angle directly from raw acceleration samples as:

$$\hat{\alpha} = \arctan(-a_y/a_z) \qquad (2)$$

where a_y (i.e., the Y-acceleration component) and a_z (i.e., the Z-acceleration component) include the contribution of both gravity and the forces exerted by the subject to execute the SiSt and StSi transitions. The outcome of the expression above is limited by the fact that the tangent function is a periodic function, and the arc tangent function only returns values for the first period of the angle values, i.e., values between $-p/2$ and $p/2$. Theoretically, this should not be a problem because, as stated before, the value of the thigh angle is expected to oscillate within that range (between 0 and $p/2$ radians, i.e., between 0° and 90°). However, when the subject is close to the upright position, there are some non-ideal behaviors that should result in an angle estimation bigger than 90°, but will not if we applied Equation (2). For instance, the value of the Z-acceleration component is expected to always have a negative sign, except at the upright position where it is expected to be zero. Nevertheless, nearby the upright position, the noise from the acceleration and deceleration forces exerted by the older adult could alter the Z-acceleration sign, and turn it into a positive value. In that case, Equation (2) does not return a value bigger than $p/2$ but a negative value between $-p/2$ and zero. In order to make a correct estimation of the angle, the sign of the accelerometer readings must be taken into account according to the following expression:

$$\hat{\alpha} = \begin{cases} -\arctan(a_y/a_z), & \text{if } a_z \leq 0 \\ \pi - \arctan(a_y/a_z), & \text{if } a_z > 0 \end{cases} \qquad (3)$$

Please note that the sign of the Y-acceleration component cannot be negative while the sign of the Z-acceleration component is positive, unless the device is upside down, because gravity always points downwards.

While the variation of the actual thigh angle over time, and even an estimation based on gravity components, are smooth quasi-periodic signals like the blue line in Figure 5, the values of the thigh angle estimated from raw acceleration readings, and their variation over time, result in a noisy signal like the green line in Figure 5. The said noise is particularly strong close to the maxima and minima of the actual angle, due to the abrupt deceleration forces applied to the sensor upon reaching the upright and sitting positions. Consequently, while the blue signal shows smoothly and clearly defined maxima that can be used to identify the end of a SiSt transition into the upright position, the local maxima and minima in the noisy green signal do not serve that purpose anymore. Which brings us to the second step in the STS analysis algorithm. In the second step, hysteresis thresholding was applied to the signal to remove the effect of the noise in the green signal. The output of such a filter was a binary signal (standing vs. sitting) like the red line in Figure 5. The threshold values and the computational algorithm described below were defined to filter the signal and spot valid SiSt transitions in real time.

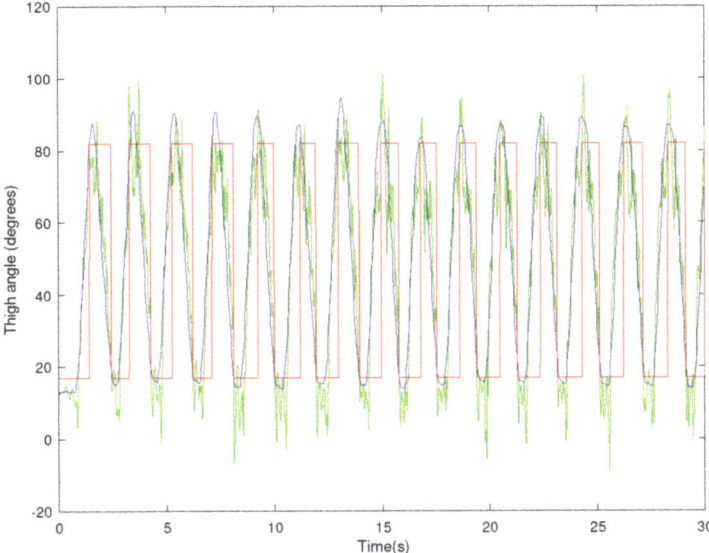

Figure 5. Graphical representation of the outcomes of a 30-s CST. The blue line represents the evolution of the thigh angle over time, computed from the estimation of the gravity components (it is not computed by the device). The green line represents the estimation of the thigh angle used in the device; it is directly computed from raw readings from the accelerometer. The red line represents the output of applying hysteresis thresholding to the green signal.

The output of the hysteresis thresholding algorithm switches between two different states (i.e., sitting and standing) as follows: The estimated value of the thigh angle is compared to two values configured in a previous stage (see the next paragraph). These two values are known as the sitting-threshold and the standing-threshold. If the previous sample was in a standing state and the current estimated thigh angle reaches a value greater than 0°, and lower than the sitting-threshold, the subject is considered to have completed a StSi transition, the state changes to sitting, and the subsequent SiSt transition is an eligible candidate to count as a valid attempt; otherwise the subsequent SiSt transition will not count as a valid attempt no matter what. On the other hand, if the previous sample was in a sitting state and the extension angle reaches a value greater than the standing-threshold, and lower than 90° during an eligible SiSt transition, the state changes to standing, and the transition counts as a valid attempt; otherwise it is dismissed as a failure.

The rationale behind using the sitting-threshold and the standing-threshold comes from the fact that even though the expected angle values theoretically range from 0° (sitting) to 90° (standing), there are two sources of non-ideal behavior that require the definition of more flexible threshold values. First, mobility constraints may narrow this range for some older subjects. A subject's readings whose default standing position does not exceed 80°, will never reach the theoretical 90° standing-angle. Thus, valid standing attempts would be dismissed and the automatic count of valid SiSt transitions would result in a wrong score. Analogously, a subject's readings whose default sitting position does not fall down below 10°, will never reach the theoretical 0° sitting-angle. Thus, subsequent valid standing attempts would be dismissed and the automatic count of valid SiSt transitions would result in a wrong score as well.

The other source of non-ideal behavior is the non-ideal nature of the sensor readings themselves. Even if a subject reaches his default standing position, the sensor might provide a reading slightly lower than the subject's default standing angle. In such a case a valid attempt would be dismissed as a failure, and the automatic count of SiSt transitions would result in a wrong score. The analogous situation applies to the sitting position and the subject's default sitting angle.

To avoid the negative impact of these situations on the sensor performance, the sensor is calibrated before initiating a 30-s CST. The subject's thigh angle in a static sitting position is measured and recorded. In particular, the sitting angle is computed as the mean value of the angle readings collected while the subject is sitting in a static position for four seconds. Then, a correction is applied to allow for some error tolerance. The sitting-threshold is set to its final value by adding 10° to the subject's default sitting angle. Analogously, the subject's thigh angle in a static upright position is measured and recorded, and then the standing-threshold is set to its final value by subtracting 10° from the subject's default standing angle.

2.1.2.3. The Tablet App

The application was developed in Java for Android. The tablet device was a Huawei M2-A01L with Android 5.1.1. The application is used to configure the personalized parameters in the sensor algorithm (i.e., the sitting-threshold and the standing-threshold), to issue a command to the sensor for it to begin the measurement process, and to visualize the test results after completion. The application home screen shows a list of all the sensor devices paired with the tablet so the end-user gets to pick which one to configure. In the case of the data collection stage in the present study, only one device was paired with the tablet. The application has two operation modes, namely, calibration mode and measurement mode. In calibration mode, the values for the sitting-threshold and the standing-threshold are computed and set according to the following process:

1. The researcher puts the sensor into calibration mode by issuing the corresponding command with the app.
2. The researcher asks the sensor to compute sitting angle readings for four seconds and send them back to the app by issuing the corresponding command with the app.
3. The app computes the mean value of these sitting-angle readings and stores them as the subject's default sitting-angle.
4. The researcher asks the sensor to compute standing-angle readings for four seconds and send them back to the app by issuing the corresponding command with the app.
5. The app computes the mean value of these standing-angle readings and stores them as the subject's default standing-angle.
6. The researcher enters an error tolerance value for each default angle.
7. The researcher asks the sensor to set the value of the sitting-threshold and the standing-threshold by issuing the corresponding command with the app. The sitting-threshold is computed as the sum of the subject's default sitting-angle and the error tolerance value for the sitting position. On the other hand, the standing-threshold is computed as the subtraction of the error tolerance value for the standing position from the subject's default standing-angle.

In measurement mode the application waits for the sensor to send the results of the 30-s CST according to the following process:

1. The researcher puts the sensor into measurement mode by issuing the corresponding command with the app.
2. The researcher asks the sensor to start the 30-s CST measurement sequence by issuing the corresponding command with the app.
3. The application waits idle for the results of the 30-s CST.
4. The application shows the results of the 30-s CST on screen.

2.1.3. Procedure

Seven older subjects were administered a 30-s CST each, in accordance with the following procedure. A member of the research team gave instructions to the subjects to guide them through the process. First, a member of the research team paired the wearable sensor with the tablet device via Bluetooth, and asked the subject to put on the wearable device. The subject was then asked to sit down on the chair to calibrate the sensor sitting-threshold. Next, the subject was asked to stand up to calibrate the sensor standing-threshold. After the calibration stage, the subject was asked to repeatedly stand up from, and sit down on, the chair as fast as possible for 30 s. The subject was asked to do so with his arms folded over his chest, and starting from a sitting position. The sensor emitted a short vibration to indicate to the subject when to start. A trained member of the research team manually counted SiSt transitions. Once the 30 s were over, the sensor emitted another short vibration to signal the subject to stop. Then, the sensor sent the outcomes of the automatic count algorithm to the mobile app, which showed them on screen. A member of the research team took note of the values for the manual and automatic counts.

2.1.4. Analysis

The correlation between the manual and the automatic counts were studied. These two variables are of the interval type, therefore we decided to compute their correlation with Pearson's moment-product correlation coefficient. Before applying Pearson's r to the data, the normality of the two data sets (manual vs. automatic counts) was tested. Due to the size of the sample, normality was studied with a Shapiro–Wilk test that resulted not statistically significant in both cases. Therefore, both data sets could be considered to be normally distributed, and we proceeded with Pearson's r. The Shapiro–Wilk test was calculated using the shapiro.test function, and Pearson's r was calculated using the cor.test function; in both cases R statistical software, version 3.6.3, was used. The 95% CI for the Pearson's r estimate was computed by applying Fisher's transformation.

To further characterize the impact of noise on the sensor performance we studied the statistical significance of our estimation for the probability of finding harmless noise levels in a valid SiSt transition. This situation was modeled as a binomial experiment, where each SiSt transition in the data set corresponds to a binomial event, a correct SiSt identification means harmless noise and, therefore, success, and an incorrect SiSt identification means harmful noise and, therefore, failure. The probability of harmless noise was estimated as the number of correct identifications in the data set divided by the total number of SiSt transitions in the data set. The 95% CI for the probability of success was calculated by applying a binomial test with the binom.test function in the R statistical software, version 3.6.3.

2.2. Unsupervised Validation of the Home Care System

2.2.1. Participants

Seven older subjects (3 female and 4 male), between 64 and 74 years old, participated in the unsupervised validation of the home care system. All subjects gave their informed consent for inclusion before they participated in the study. The study was conducted in accordance with the Declaration of Helsinki, and the protocol was approved by the Ethics Committee of the Universidad Politécnica de Madrid on 9 May 2019 (POSITIVE: Maintaining and improving the intrinsic capacity involving primary care and caregivers).

The following inclusion and exclusion criteria were applied:

- A subject COULD ENTER the study if ALL the following INCLUSION CRITERIA applied:

    o The subject is willing and able to give written informed consent for participation in the study.
    o The subject is 64 years old or older.
    o The subject is able to perform the 30-s CST in a safe way.

- The subject has not been diagnosed with cognitive impairment.
- A subject COULD NOT ENTER the study if ANY of the following EXCLUSION CRITERIA applied:
  - Subjects suffering from any major disability.
  - Subjects suffering from cognitive impairment.

2.2.2. Apparatus

2.2.2.1. The Sensor

The sensor hardware was ported to a more ergonomic case which included a sticker with clear instructions about the proper orientation of the ends of the device, with the help of two tags, namely, "Rodilla", which is the Spanish word for knee, and "Cabeza", which is the Spanish word for head (see Figure 6).

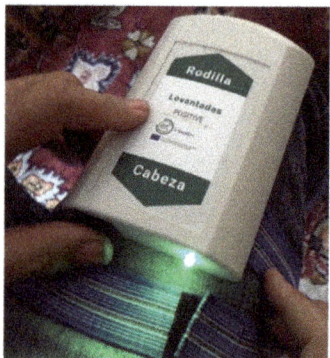

Figure 6. Second version of the sensor casing. The sticker on the sensor reports the correct orientation of the sensor with the help of two tags: "Rodilla", which is the Spanish word for knee, and "Cabeza", which is the Spanish word for head.

2.2.2.2. The Home Care Application

The home care application was developed in Java for Android and was a user friendly evolution of the application in Section 2.1.2.3. The application included a user-friendly interface specifically designed for older adults. Once the default and the threshold values of the participants sitting and standing angles were calibrated for the first time, the application recorded the outcomes so it was not necessary to re-calibrate every time the participant took a test. The app provided explanatory pictures, audio, and video to help the participant in preparing for taking a test, and audio instructions were also available to guide him through the whole procedure.

2.2.2.3. The Acceptability and General Impressions Questionnaires

In order to assess the system acceptability, a semi-structured interview comprising the questions in the second column in Table 2 was conducted. Furthermore, the participants' general impressions were also collected by conducting another semi-structured interview, comprising the questions in the third column in Table 2. The first three questions in each questionnaire are related to the participant's opinions on the sensor. The remaining ones are related to the participant's opinions on the application in the tablet.

Table 2. List of questions in the acceptability and general impressions questionnaires. The first three questions in each questionnaire ask about the participant's experience while using the sensor. Whereas, the remaining ones ask about the participant's experience while using the home care application on the tablet.

Type of Question	Acceptability Questionnaire	General Impressions Questionnaire
Related to the sensor	1. What difficulties did you find while using the sensor? 2. What is your opinion on the sensor? 3. How did you feel while using the sensor?	1. Was the device easy to put on? 2. Do you find the device comfortable? 3. Do you think you would be able to use the device at home on your own?
Related to the application	4. What difficulties did you find while using the tablet? 5. What is your opinion on the tablet? 6. How did you feel while using the tablet?	4. Which activities did you find the most difficult to achieve while using the tablet? 5. Which features did you find the hardest to understand in the tablet? 6. What are your general impressions on the tablet? 7. Do you think you would be able to use the app at home on your own?

2.2.3. Procedure

A trained technician went to the participants' homes to set up the system and explain to them how to use it (only one user per home was configured). The technician delivered a tablet device with the home care application pre-installed. Once in the participant's dwelling, the technician paired the sensor and the tablet via Bluetooth and proceeded to calibrate the participant's default sitting and standing angles as described in Section 2.1.2.3. The application recorded the values so the participant did not have to repeat this step every time he took a 30-s CST. The participants could contact the technician to get help to fix any technical issues that could arise over the course of the study.

The participants used the system for a month. The participant initiates a test by entering into the "My medical tests" in the app. The participants had to follow the instructions of the home care application to complete a 30-s CST, without any supervision or further assistance, and according to the following procedure. The participant put the tablet on a nearby surface. The participant then had to put the device on over his knee, secure it with the strap, and click next on the tablet. Then the participant had to switch on the device and click next on the tablet. After that, the participant had to fold his arms over his chest and wait for the start signal. Then he had to stand up and sit down repeatedly until the stop signal. After that, the participant could switch the device off and take it off. Once the 30-days period of study was over, a member of the research team went to the participants' homes to pick up the equipment and to conduct an interview to evaluate acceptability and general impressions by administering the corresponding questionnaires.

2.2.4. Analysis

The results of the acceptability and general impressions questionnaires were qualitatively assessed.

3. Results

3.1. Supervised Validation of the Sensor

Table 3 summarizes the outcomes from the data collection process. Most of the people in older populations are female, and this pattern was also reflected in the composition of the sample of volunteers recruited for the present study (5 female and 2 male).

Table 3. Data collected during the experimental procedure. Each row in the table holds the data for one of the seven older adults in the experiment (age: m = 83.29 years old, sd = 4.19; gender: 5 female and 2 male). Each participant took a single 30-s CST. The outcomes from the sensor automatic count match the outcomes from the trained professional's manual count for all the seven participants. All the 67 SiSt transitions that took place were correctly identified, and the mean absolute error was equal to zero.

Participant ID	Gender	Age	Default Sitting-Angle	Default Standing-Angle	30 s CST Result (Manual Count)	30 s CST Result (Automatic Count)
1	male	88	25°	55°	5	5
2	female	87	25°	70°	6	6
3	male	81	27°	87°	13	13
4	female	79	25.5°	84°	8	8
5	female	79	18.7°	85°	8	8
6	female	81	44°	81°	9	9
7	female	88	19°	82°	18	18

The mean absolute error for the automatic count of SiSt transitions was computed, as usual, according to the following expression:

$$\text{error} = \frac{1}{7} \cdot \sum_{i=1}^{7} |\text{manualCount}_i - \text{autoCount}_i|. \tag{4}$$

The mean absolute error was equal to zero because the sensor output was error-free in all the seven 30-s CSTs, i.e., all the 67 SiSt transitions were correctly identified. This means the high frequency noise in the estimated angle signal was not larger than the gap between the sitting and the standing thresholds for any of the SiSt transitions in the data set. Therefore, the hysteresis thresholding mechanism had not been affected by said noise and no spurious transitions between states had taken place.

Additionally, the correlation between the manual and the automatic counts was studied to test the statistical significance of the perfect match in our observations. Being two variables of the interval type, we chose Pearson's r to study their correlation. Before computing Pearson's r, the normality of the two variables (manual count vs. automatic count) was studied with a Shapiro–Wilk test, as shown in Table 4.

Table 4. Results of the normality test for the manual count data set (left) and the automatic count data set (right). None of the tests were statistically significant. Thus, we did not find statistical significance to state that any of the data sets were not normally distributed. Therefore, we considered that they complied with the bivariate normality assumption, and proceeded to study their correlation with Pearson's r.

Manual Count	Automatic Count
W = 0.88227, p-value = 0.2367	W = 0.88227, p-value = 0.2367

The data set complies with the bivariate normality assumption because the Shapiro–Wilk test resulted not statistically significant for both variables. Therefore, we proceeded to study their correlation with Pearson's moment–product correlation (r = 1, p = 0.00). This correlation estimate showed full correlation between the sensor automatic count and the manual count. The 95% CI was computed as a means to measure the accuracy of our estimation. The cor.test function in R computes the CI by applying Fisher's transformation, and returned a 95% CI = (1, 1). This result suggests that our observation was indistinguishable from a perfect correlation. However, the Fisher transformation defines the lower and upper limits of the 95% CI as:

$$\tanh\left(\text{artanh}(\rho) \pm 1.96/\sqrt{(n-3)}\right), \tag{5}$$

where r is the Pearson correlation coefficient and n is the sample size, which in this case equals the number of participants recruited for the study. The hyperbolic arc tangent function is defined only within the open interval (−1, 1), but not for the case when r equals one. Since the hyperbolic arc tangent function tends to infinity as r tends to one, the contribution of the sample size to the value of the upper and lower values in Fisher's expression becomes irrelevant. Therefore, we think we are not getting much information about the impact of our sample size on the accuracy of our estimation.

In order to tackle this issue and study the accuracy of our sensor, we studied the probability of finding a SiSt transition with harmless levels of noise; because the higher the number of transitions with harmless levels of noise, the more accurate the sensor outcomes will be. The situation was modeled as a binomial experiment (as described in Section 2.1.4), which resulted in an estimated probability of success $p = 1$ with a 95% CI = (0.96, 1). Therefore, the older adults in our sample are expected to produce SiSt transitions with harmless levels of noise at least 96% of the time. Therefore, our sensor would need to observe 25 SiSt transitions in order to make a mistake due to a high level of noise. Since the mean number of SiSt transitions per 30-s CST in our sample is 9.57, the sensor would make a mistake once every 2.61 tests; thus, in order to observe one wrong score, you need to conduct three tests. In other words, according to our estimated 95% CI, in the worst case scenario, our sensor would provide an error free score for at least 67% of the tests conducted, while the remaining 33% would miss the correct score by one SiSt transition. These results show our sensor to be very accurate, however, it could be argued that a sample of seven older adults is too small to be representative of the many interpersonal differences in the general older population and, therefore, the results might have been poorer if the device had been tested on a wider variety of cases.

A larger sample might have shown cases with higher levels of noise; so we analyzed under which conditions angle signals would be noisier, and tested our algorithm behavior in those conditions. The noise in the angle signal is the result of the acceleration and deceleration forces applied to the sensor, especially upon reaching the upright and sitting positions. The faster, and the more sudden, the stand up and sit down moves are, the stronger these forces will be. On the one hand, subjects would have moved faster if they have completed a higher number of SiSt transitions within the 30 s in the test. On the other hand, given a fixed number of transitions, subjects need a larger momentum for those transitions with a wider range. Therefore, the angle signal is expected to be noisier for 30-s CSTs with a higher number of SiSt transitions and a wider range for the thigh angle. Rikli and Jones identified the normative standard values to use the 30-s CST outcomes to compare an older adult's performance with the average population [41]. According to these standards, a subject's performance might be considered to be (i) within, (ii) below, or (iii) over the reference range of the average population [41]. However, the reference ranges have different values depending on gender and age [41]. Thus, two people of the same gender with the same test score but belonging to different age groups need not be considered to have the same level of physical decline; and the same applies to two people of different gender but belonging to the same age group. According to these standards 90% of the men in the younger age group (between 60 and 64 years old) score below 22 [41]. The analogous scores for the remaining age groups in the case of men are lower than 22; as they are in the case of women of all age groups. On the other hand, Rikli and Jones also identified the critical values that predict physical independence until late in life [42]. An older adult scoring above the critical value is considered to be fit enough to remain independent until late in life; conversely an older adult scoring below the critical value is considered to be at risk of becoming dependent and requires taking action. These critical values depend on gender and age as well [42]. The critical value for men in the younger group (between 60 and 64 years old) is 17 [42]. The critical values for the remaining age groups in the case of men are lower than 17; as they are in the case of women for all age groups. Thus, we took 22 SiSt transitions as a reference value for an extreme and highly demanding scenario, and 17 SiSt transitions for a critical and likely scenario. Then, we conducted an exploratory study to inquire about the performance of our approach under those two scenarios.

A member of the research team took ten 30-s CSTs scoring 22 or above (highly demanding scenario) and another ten 30-s CSTs scoring around 17 (critical scenario). The data for this exploratory study were collected with a smartphone (Nokia 6 TA-1021 with Android 9) on the subject's thigh and were processed with GNU Octave 5.2.0; this was because the researchers were locked down at their homes, due to the COVID-19 pandemic, and did not have access to the prototypes of the sensor devices. The experiment in the highly demanding scenario resulted in a total of 230 SiSt transitions. Of which, 15 showed harmful noise. All 15 behaved like the transitions depicted around Time = 20 and Time = 25 s in Figure 7. Both transitions show a strong and narrow inverse peak of noise (green line in Figure 7) that tricks the algorithm into detecting a spurious StSi transition, and another spurious SiSt transition (red line in Figure 7). Thus, an extra SiSt transition was detected for each valid transition affected by this kind of noise; in the case of Figure 7, the final score was overestimated by two points, i.e., 25 SiSt transitions were reported instead of 23. All the signals collected, and the code to process and visualize them, are available as Supplementary Materials.

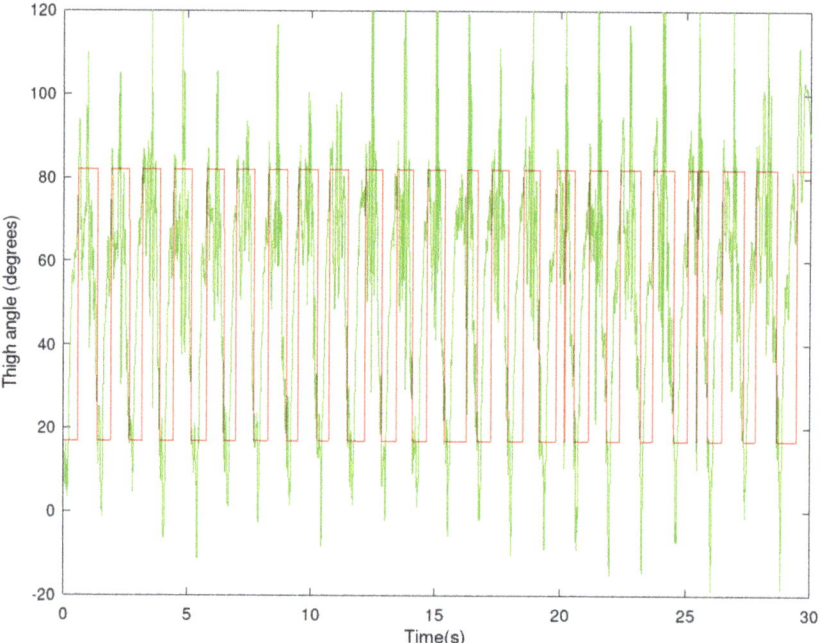

Figure 7. Graphical representation of the outcomes of a 30-s CST in the presence of some transitions with harmful levels of noise. The green line represents the estimation of the thigh angle over time, while the red line represents the transitions detected by the hysteresis algorithm. The transitions around Time = 20 and Time = 25 show a strong and narrow inverse peak of noise that tricks the algorithm into detecting a spurious StSi transition, and then another spurious SiSt transition. Thus, an extra SiSt transition was detected for each of them, and the final score was overestimated by two points; 25 SiSt transitions were reported instead of 23.

Like in the case of the older adults' data set, we studied the probability of finding a SiSt transition with harmless levels of noise. Again, it was modeled as a binomial experiment (as described in Section 2.1.4) and the experiment resulted in an estimated probability of success p = 0.93, with a 95% CI = (0.89, 0.96). According to the lower limit of this CI, it would be necessary to observe 10 SiSt transitions in order to observe one of them with a high level of noise. The mean number of SiSt transitions per 30-s CST in our sample is 23; thus, between two and three high level noise transitions would be observed per test. On the other hand, according to the upper limit of the 95% CI, i.e., p (harmless noise) = 0.96, only one in two tests would miss the correct score, and would do so by a single point.

Finally, the experiment in the critical scenario resulted in a total of 173 SiSt transitions. The algorithm successfully identified all of them. In this case, the estimated probability of success is $p = 1$ with a 95% CI = (0.98, 1). Therefore in the worst case (lower limit of the CI), it is necessary to observe 50 SiSt transitions in order to observe one error. Since the mean number of SiSt transitions in our sample is 17.3, an error would be observed every 2.89 tests. Thus, in order to observe one wrong score, you need to conduct three tests. Therefore, according to the 95% CI, the noise pattern around the critical value would result in a single wrong transition in only one in three tests. Under such a noise pattern our sensor would remain very accurate around the target critical value.

3.2. Unsupervised Validation of the Home Care System

3.2.1. The Acceptability Questionnaire

3.2.1.1. Question #1: What Difficulties Did You Find While Using the Sensor?

All but one of the participants declared they did not find any major problems while using the device. One participant declared having experienced some pain in his knee due to osteoarthritis. The same participant also declared being worried about the possibility of the device falling out during the course of the 30-s CST.

3.2.1.2. Question #2: What is Your Opinion on the Sensor?

All the participants provided favorable answers to this question. They highlighted that the sensor is comfortable and easy to use. They also remarked that the labels on the sensor sticker were easy to follow and helped them to know how to correctly put the device on the leg.

3.2.1.3. Question #3: How Did You Feel While Using the Sensor?

The participants declared that they felt comfortable using the device, and that they felt motivated to improve their performance over time. In line with the answers to Question #1, one participant declared to be worried about the possibility of the device falling out during the course of the tests.

3.2.1.4. Question #4: What Difficulties Did You Find While Using the Tablet?

Some participants struggled to understand the video instructions, and some participants faced a few technical issues, however, they declared not to have experienced any major problems once those issues were fixed.

3.2.1.5. Question #5: What is Your Opinion on the Tablet?

Most users reported satisfactory experiences and good opinions on the tablet.

3.2.1.6. Question #6: How Did You Feel While Using the Tablet?

Some participants experienced some technical issues that made them feel uncomfortable. However, their experience and feelings became more satisfactory once these issues were solved.

3.2.2. The General Impressions Questionnaire

3.2.2.1. Question #1: Was the Device Easy to Put on?

Six participants reported they found the device easy to put on. None of the participants reported that they did not find it easy, however, one of them reported the strap did not fit very well around his leg.

3.2.2.2. Question #2: Do You Find the Device Comfortable?

Six participants reported they found the device comfortable. In line with the answers to Question #1, one of them reported some issues regarding the length of the strap.

3.2.2.3. Question #3: Do You Think You Would Be Able to Use the Device at Home on Your Own?

All the participants felt able to use the device at home on their own.

3.2.2.4. Question #4: What Activities Did You Find the Most Difficult to Achieve While Using the Tablet?

Some participants detected some discrepancies between the explanatory videos and the textual description of the exercise, which made them have some doubts. The rest of the application features were reported to be easy to understand.

3.2.2.5. Question #5: Which Features Did You Find the Hardest to Understand in the Tablet?

In line with the answers to Question #4, all of the application functionality was reported to be easy to understand.

3.2.2.6. Question #6: What are Your General Impressions on the Tablet?

All the participants reported favorable opinions about the tablet. They highlighted the motivating potential of such an app and the subsequent health benefits.

3.2.2.7. Question #7: Do You Think You Would Be Able to Use the App at Home on Your Own?

All the participants felt able to use the app at home on their own. However, one of them highlighted that he would be able to do so as long as the application did not become more complex, and another one highlighted that technical support would be required.

4. Discussion

Our sensor took advantage of the quasiperiodic variation of the thigh angle over time (i.e., the angle between the longitudinal axis of the subject's thigh and a horizontal plane perpendicular to gravity, e.g., the seat of the chair). The thigh angle was computed from acceleration readings from an accelerometer on the subject's thigh. Previous works found in the literature have taken advantage of the quasiperiodic variation of some other variables such as the trunk pitch-angle [23], vertical velocity [23,24], and vertical position [24] to study repetitive STS cycles in STS5 and 30-s CST tests. They estimated the values of these variables from the readings of an IMU on the L3 region of the subject's lumbar spine. We think the thigh angle is a more convenient approach for two reasons. On the one hand, we think that older people might find it easier to correctly place the sensor on their thighs than on their lower backs, especially if they do not have any help to put them on. However, none of the papers studied their algorithm's sensitivity to misplacing of the sensor. The procedure for the estimation of the thigh angle described in the present paper (i.e., estimating the angle from the Y-acceleration and Z-acceleration components) requires the sensor X-axis to be aligned with the knee rotation axis. However, this constraint is easy to overcome by extending the angle estimation expression to its three-dimensional form. On the other hand, computing trunk pitch-angle, vertical velocity, and vertical position require integration and even double integration of the IMU readings. Due to the noisy nature of the latter, the result is distorted by drift and requires a lot of effort to estimate the original signal with computationally complex algorithms. Millor et al., for instance, applied double integration, combined with fourth-level polynomial curve adjustment and cubic splines interpolation [24]. Conversely, it is not necessary to integrate the acceleration readings to make an estimation of the thigh angle. Such an estimation can be computed from the values of the different components of gravity in the accelerometer reference system; and these values can be estimated by filtering raw acceleration readings.

We did not include any Kalman or complementary filters in our design to avoid the extra hardware and computational load. Instead, we estimated the thigh angle directly from raw acceleration readings; which resulted in noisy but drift-free angle estimations. In spite of the noisy nature of the angle estimations, the device showed an excellent performance. All the SiSt transitions were correctly identified in real time, and the device provided error-free outcomes for all the seven 30-s CST conducted with older adults. The narrow CI returned by the cor.test function in R suggests this observation is indeed statistically indistinguishable from a perfect correlation. However, the limitations described for the Fisher transformation in Section 3, to accommodate such an extreme value for Pearson's r, make us think we are not getting much information about the impact of our sample size on the accuracy of our estimated correlation.

Looking at the results of our study from a different perspective, we studied the accuracy of our device based on the probability of observing noise levels high enough to exceed the gap between their personalized upper and lower thresholds in the hysteresis stage. Since all the transitions were correctly identified in real time, we concluded that the participants in the study did not generate any transitions with such high levels of noise. According to the narrow 95% CI in our estimation, low levels of noise are expected to happen at least 96% of the time. Which would result in very accurate sensor outcomes. This result can be generalized to the SiSt transitions generated by any population represented by our sample. However, our sample is limited because it could be argued that seven older adults are too few to be representative of the many interpersonal differences in the general older population and, therefore, signals with a higher level of noise might have been observed if the device had been tested on a wider variety of cases. Nevertheless, we did not find any SiSt transitions with harmful levels of noise in our exploratory study for the critical scenario (around 17 transitions with high momentum). According to the narrow 95% CI obtained for that critical scenario (0.98, 1), even if any high noise transitions were to be observed, a single wrong transition would be observed in only one in three tests. Since the 30-s CST is expected to be scheduled to be taken once or twice a week in a home care scenario, we did not observe any risks of missing anyone not fit enough due to sustained overestimated scores over time. We observed that a frequent overestimation of the scores is likely to happen in the highly demanding scenario (over 22 transitions with high speed and high momentum). However, we think that this result does not have a strong impact on the utility of our approach for two reasons. First, less than 10% of the older population are able to reach such high scores, and second, even in case of overestimation, people scoring over 22 are far away from the critical threshold, and therefore are undoubtedly fit enough not to require any immediate intervention. Anyway, further experiments may be useful to characterize the noise profile between the scores of 17 and 22.

We integrated the sensor into a home care app that guides the user throughout the process of taking a 30-s CST, and conducted an acceptability study with older adults in free-living conditions (i.e., using a home care app at home for several weeks to interact with the device without any assistance). All the participants kept using the system throughout the course of the study and none of them dropped out. This observation is in line with their favorable opinions about both the sensor and the application; and, in particular, corroborates the participants' positive answers to whether they feel able to use the system at home on their own. Despite the excellent results of this acceptability study, further studies will be necessary to test, on the one hand, the long-term acceptability and adoption by older adults and their caregivers, and, on the other hand, to test the feasibility of this novel home care model for frailty in accommodating end-users' needs and expectations, not just on the older adults' side, but also on the health care professionals' side.

5. Conclusions

We developed a system for older people to self-administer the 30-s chair stand test (CST) at home without supervision. The system comprises a low-cost sensor that automatically detects and counts sit-to-stand (SiSt) transitions in real time, and a home care application that guides older people through the whole procedure. We studied whether such a system was able to match older people's abilities and expectations so they can use it at home on their own without any supervision. The sensor automatic counts were perfectly correlated to the researcher's manual count, so we concluded that the signals generated by the participants did not push the device to its operational limits. This observation is supported by a very narrow 95% CI for the probability of finding a SiSt transition with a low level of noise. The small size of our sample limits our ability to generalize this result to the general older population because more demanding signals might have been observed if the device had been tested on a larger sample. However, we did not find harmful levels of noise in any of the signals in our exploratory study around the critical score. Thus, we did not observe any risks of missing anyone not fit enough due to sustained overestimated scores over time. None of the participants in the unsupervised study of the complete system dropped out, and at the end of the study none of them reported any major problems in understanding the system and interacting with it. They declared they felt comfortable using it, and felt able to use it on their own. Thus, the system is suitable to be used by older adults in their homes without professional supervision.

Supplementary Materials: The data collected for the exploratory study on the demanding and the critical scenarios, together with the code used to process and plot the corresponding signals, are available online at http://www.mdpi.com/xxx/s1.

Author Contributions: Conceptualization, E.V.-M., R.P.-R., X.F., and L.R.-M.; methodology, E.V.-M., R.P.-R., X.F., and L.R.-M.; software, W.E. and A.C.; validation, C.M.; formal analysis, A.C. and W.E.; investigation, W.E., A.C., and C.M.; resources, E.V.-M., X.F., R.P.-R., L.R.-M., W.E., and A.C.; data curation, W.E., and A.C.; writing—Original draft preparation, A.C.; writing—Review and editing, E.V., A.C., X.F., R.P.-R., and L.R.-M.; visualization, A.C.; supervision, E.V.-M., X.F., R.P.-R., and L.R.-M.; project administration, E.V., X.F., R.P.-R., and L.R.-M.; funding acquisition, L.R.-M., E.V., R.P.-R., and X.F. All authors have read and agreed to the published version of the manuscript.

Funding: This research was funded by EIT-Health, grant number 19091 (POSITIVE project).

Acknowledgments: We would like to thank FEDER funds for co-financing our home institutions. The authors would like to specially thank the volunteers in the study for their unselfish collaboration, enthusiasm, and dedication.

Conflicts of Interest: The authors declare no conflict of interest. The funders had no role in the design of the study; in the collection, analyses, or interpretation of data; in the writing of the manuscript, or in the decision to publish the results.

References

1. Jones, C.J.; Rikli, R.E.; Beam, W.C. A 30-s Chair-Stand Test as a Measure of Lower Body Strength in Community-Residing Older Adults. *Res. Q. Exerc. Sport* **1999**, *70*, 113–119. [CrossRef]
2. Fried, L.P.; Tangen, C.M.; Walston, J.; Newman, A.B.; Hirsch, C.; Gottdiener, J.; Seeman, T.; Tracy, R.; Kop, W.J.; Burke, G.; et al. Frailty in Older Adults: Evidence for a Phenotype. *J. Gerontol. Ser. A Biol. Sci. Med. Sci.* **2001**, *56*, M146–M157. [CrossRef]
3. Campbell, A.J.; Buchner, D.M. Unstable disability and the fluctuations of frailty. *Age Ageing* **1997**, *26*, 315–318. [CrossRef]
4. Rockwood, K.; Ehogan, D.B.; Macknight, C.; Rockwood, P.K. Conceptualisation and Measurement of Frailty in Elderly People. *Drugs Aging* **2000**, *17*, 295–302. [CrossRef]
5. Walston, J.; Fried, L.P. Frailty and the Older MAN. *Med. Clin. N. Am.* **1999**, *83*, 1173–1194. [CrossRef]
6. Clegg, A.P.; Young, J.; Iliffe, S.; Rikkert, M.O.; Rockwood, K. Frailty in elderly people. *Lancet* **2013**, *381*, 752–762. [CrossRef]
7. Kojima, G. Frailty as a predictor of disabilities among community-dwelling older people: A systematic review and meta-analysis. *Disabil. Rehabil.* **2016**, *39*, 1897–1908. [CrossRef]
8. Zheng, Y.; Cheung, K.S.L.; Yip, P.S. Are We Living Longer and Healthier? *J. Aging Health* **2020**, 0898264320950067. [CrossRef]

9. Cesari, M.; Vellas, B.; Hsu, F.-C.; Newman, A.B.; Doss, H.; King, A.C.; Manini, T.M.; Church, T.; Gill, T.M.; Miller, M.E.; et al. A Physical Activity Intervention to Treat the Frailty Syndrome in Older Persons–Results From the LIFE-P Study. *J. Gerontol. Ser. A Biol. Sci. Med. Sci.* **2014**, *70*, 216–222. [CrossRef]
10. Rodríguez-Mañas, L.; Fried, L.P. Frailty in the clinical scenario. *Lancet* **2015**, *385*, e7–e9. [CrossRef]
11. Fairhall, N.; Langron, C.; Sherrington, C.; Lord, S.R.; Kurrle, S.E.; Lockwood, K.A.; Monaghan, N.; Aggar, C.; Gill, L.; Cameron, I.D. Treating frailty-a practical guide. *BMC Med.* **2011**, *9*, 83. [CrossRef]
12. Mitnitski, A.B.; Mogilner, A.J.; Rockwood, K. Accumulation of Deficits as a Proxy Measure of Aging. *Sci. World J.* **2001**, *1*, 323–336. [CrossRef]
13. Rockwood, K.; Mitnitski, A. Frailty in Relation to the Accumulation of Deficits. *J. Gerontol. Ser. A Biol. Sci. Med. Sci.* **2007**, *62*, 722–727. [CrossRef]
14. Rockwood, K.; Mitnitski, A. Frailty Defined by Deficit Accumulation and Geriatric Medicine Defined by Frailty. *Clin. Geriatr. Med.* **2011**, *27*, 17–26. [CrossRef]
15. Ko, F. The Clinical Care of Frail, Older Adults. *Clin. Geriatr. Med.* **2011**, *27*, 89–100. [CrossRef]
16. Batista, F.S.; Gomes, G.A.D.O.; Neri, A.L.; Guariento, M.E.; Cintra, F.A.; Sousa, M.D.L.R.D.; D'Elboux, M.J. Relationship between lower-limb muscle strength and frailty among elderly people. *Sao Paulo Med. J.* **2012**, *130*, 102–108. [CrossRef]
17. Guralnik, J.M.; Simonsick, E.M.; Ferrucci, L.; Glynn, R.J.; Berkman, L.F.; Blazer, D.G.; Scherr, P.A.; Wallace, R.B. A Short Physical Performance Battery Assessing Lower Extremity Function: Association with Self-Reported Disability and Prediction of Mortality and Nursing Home Admission. *J. Gerontol.* **1994**, *49*, M85–M94. [CrossRef]
18. Zhou, F.; Yu, T.; Du, R.; Fan, G.; Liu, Y.; Liu, Z.; Xiang, J.; Wang, Y.; Song, B.; Gu, X.; et al. Clinical course and risk factors for mortality of adult inpatients with COVID-19 in Wuhan, China: A retrospective cohort study. *Lancet* **2020**, *395*, 1054–1062. [CrossRef]
19. Song, J.; Lindquist, L.A.; Chang, R.W.; Semanik, P.A.; Ehrlich-Jones, L.S.; Lee, J.; Sohn, M.-W.; Dunlop, D.D. Sedentary Behavior as a Risk Factor for Physical Frailty Independent of Moderate Activity: Results from the Osteoarthritis Initiative. *Am. J. Public Heal.* **2015**, *105*, 1439–1445. [CrossRef]
20. Hall, G.; Laddu, D.R.; Phillips, S.A.; Lavie, C.J.; Arena, R. A tale of two pandemics: How will COVID-19 and global trends in physical inactivity and sedentary behavior affect one another? *Prog. Cardiovasc. Dis.* **2020**. [CrossRef]
21. Millor, N.; Lecumberri, P.; Gomez, M.; Martinez-Ramirez, A.; Izquierdo, M. Kinematic Parameters to Evaluate Functional Performance of Sit-to-Stand and Stand-to-Sit Transitions Using Motion Sensor Devices: A Systematic Review. *IEEE Trans. Neural Syst. Rehabil. Eng.* **2014**, *22*, 926–936. [CrossRef]
22. Kerr, K.; White, J.; Barr, D.; Mollan, R. Standardization and definitions of the sit-stand-sit movement cycle. *Gait Posture* **1994**, *2*, 182–190. [CrossRef]
23. Van Lummel, R.C.; Ainsworth, E.; Lindemann, U.; Zijlstra, W.; Chiari, L.; Van Campen, P.; Hausdorff, J.M. Automated approach for quantifying the repeated sit-to-stand using one body fixed sensor in young and older adults. *Gait Posture* **2013**, *38*, 153–156. [CrossRef]
24. Millor, N.; Lecumberri, P.; Gómez, M.; Martínez-Ramírez, A.; Rodríguez-Mañas, L.; García-García, F.J.; Izquierdo, M. Automatic Evaluation of the 30-s Chair Stand Test Using Inertial/Magnetic-Based Technology in an Older Prefrail Population. *IEEE J. Biomed. Heal. Inform.* **2013**, *17*, 820–827. [CrossRef]
25. Millor, N.; Lecumberri, P.; Gómez, M.; Martínez-Ramírez, A.; Izquierdo, M. An evaluation of the 30-s chair stand test in older adults: Frailty detection based on kinematic parameters from a single inertial unit. *J. Neuroeng. Rehabil.* **2013**, *10*, 86. [CrossRef]
26. Van Lummel, R.C.; Ainsworth, E.; Hausdorff, J.M.; Lindemann, U.; Beek, P.J.; Van Dieën, J.H. Validation of seat-off and seat-on in repeated sit-to-stand movements using a single-body-fixed sensor. *Physiol. Meas.* **2012**, *33*, 1855–1867. [CrossRef]
27. Van Lummel, R.C.; Evers, J.; Niessen, M.; Beek, P.J.; Van Dieën, J.H. Older Adults with Weaker Muscle Strength Stand up from a Sitting Position with More Dynamic Trunk Use. *Sensors* **2018**, *18*, 1235. [CrossRef]
28. Van Roie, E.; Van Driessche, S.; Huijben, B.; Baggen, R.; Van Lummel, R.C.; Delecluse, C. A body-fixed-sensor-based analysis of stair ascent and sit-to-stand to detect age-related differences in leg-extensor power. *PLoS ONE* **2019**, *14*, e0210653. [CrossRef]

29. Van Lummel, R.C.; Walgaard, S.; Maier, A.B.; Ainsworth, E.; Beek, P.J.; Van Dieën, J.H. The Instrumented Sit-to-Stand Test (iSTS) Has Greater Clinical Relevance than the Manually Recorded Sit-to-Stand Test in Older Adults. *PLoS ONE* **2016**, *11*, e0157968. [CrossRef]
30. Millor, N.; Lecumberri, P.; Gomez, M.; Martinez, A.; Martinikorena, J.; Rodríguez-Mañas, L.; García-García, F.J.; Izquierdo, M. Gait Velocity and Chair Sit-Stand-Sit Performance Improves Current Frailty-Status Identification. *IEEE Trans. Neural Syst. Rehabil. Eng.* **2017**, *25*, 2018–2025. [CrossRef]
31. Regterschot, G.R.H.; Zhang, W.; Baldus, H.; Stevens, M.; Zijlstra, W. Sensor-based monitoring of sit-to-stand performance is indicative of objective and self-reported aspects of functional status in older adults. *Gait Posture* **2015**, *41*, 935–940. [CrossRef]
32. Jovanov, E.; Wright, S.; Ganegoda, H. Development of an Automated 30 Second Chair Stand Test Using Smartwatch Application. In Proceedings of the 2019 41st Annual International Conference of the IEEE Engineering in Medicine and Biology Society (EMBC), Berlin, Germany, 23–27 July 2019; Volume 2019, pp. 2474–2477.
33. Cobo, A.; Villalba-Mora, E.; Hayn, D.; Ferre, X.; Pérez-Rodríguez, R.; Sánchez-Sánchez, A.; Bernabé-Espiga, R.; Sánchez-Sánchez, J.-L.; López-Diez-Picazo, A.; Moral, C.; et al. Portable Ultrasound-Based Device for Detecting Older Adults' Sit-to-Stand Transitions in Unsupervised 30-Second Chair–Stand Tests. *Sensors* **2020**, *20*, 1975. [CrossRef]
34. Abhayasinghe, N.; Murray, I. Human activity recognition using thigh angle derived from single thigh mounted IMU data. In Proceedings of the 2014 International Conference on Indoor Positioning and Indoor Navigation (IPIN), Busan, Korea, 27–30 October 2014; pp. 111–115.
35. Steeves, J.A.; Bowles, H.R.; McClain, J.J.; Dodd, K.W.; Brychta, R.J.; Wang, J.; Chen, K.Y. Ability of Thigh-Worn ActiGraph and activPAL Monitors to Classify Posture and Motion. *Med. Sci. Sports Exerc.* **2015**, *47*, 952–959. [CrossRef]
36. Martinez-Hernandez, U.; Dehghani-Sanij, A.A. Probabilistic identification of sit-to-stand and stand-to-sit with a wearable sensor. *Pattern Recognit. Lett.* **2019**, *118*, 32–41. [CrossRef]
37. Pickford, C.G.; Findlow, A.H.; Kerr, A.; Banger, M.; Clarke-Cornwell, A.M.; Hollands, K.L.; Quinn, T.; Granat, M.H. Quantifying sit-to-stand and stand-to-sit transitions in free-living environments using the activPAL thigh-worn activity monitor. *Gait Posture* **2019**, *73*, 140–146. [CrossRef]
38. Gui, P.; Tang, L.; Mukhopadhyay, S. MEMS based IMU for tilting measurement: Comparison of complementary and kalman filter based data fusion. In Proceedings of the 2015 IEEE 10th Conference on Industrial Electronics and Applications (ICIEA), Auckland, New Zealand, 15–17 June 2015; pp. 2004–2009.
39. Abhayasinghe, N.; Murray, I.; Bidabadi, S.S. Validation of Thigh Angle Estimation Using Inertial Measurement Unit Data against Optical Motion Capture Systems. *Sensors* **2019**, *19*, 596. [CrossRef]
40. Tognetti, A.; Lorussi, F.; Carbonaro, N.; De Rossi, D. Wearable Goniometer and Accelerometer Sensory Fusion for Knee Joint Angle Measurement in Daily Life. *Sensors* **2015**, *15*, 28435–28455. [CrossRef]
41. Rikli, R.E.; Jones, C.J. Functional Fitness Normative Scores for Community-Residing Older Adults, Ages 60–94. *J. Aging Phys. Act.* **1999**, *7*, 162–181. [CrossRef]
42. Rikli, R.E.; Jones, C.J. Development and Validation of Criterion-Referenced Clinically Relevant Fitness Standards for Maintaining Physical Independence in Later Years. *Gerontologist* **2012**, *53*, 255–267. [CrossRef]

Publisher's Note: MDPI stays neutral with regard to jurisdictional claims in published maps and institutional affiliations.

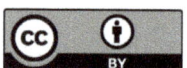

© 2020 by the authors. Licensee MDPI, Basel, Switzerland. This article is an open access article distributed under the terms and conditions of the Creative Commons Attribution (CC BY) license (http://creativecommons.org/licenses/by/4.0/).

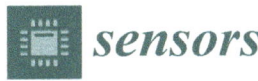

Article

The Danger of Walking with Socks: Evidence from Kinematic Analysis in People with Progressive Multiple Sclerosis

Su-Chun Huang [1], Gloria Dalla Costa [1,2], Marco Pisa [1,2], Lorenzo Gregoris [2], Giulia Leccabue [2], Martina Congiu [1], Giancarlo Comi [1,2] and Letizia Leocani [1,2,*]

1. Neurorehabilitation Department and Experimental Neurophysiology Unit, INSPE-Institute of Experimental Neurology, San Raffaele Hospital, 20132 Milan, Italy; huang.suchun@hsr.it (S.-C.H.); dallacosta.gloria@hsr.it (G.D.C.); pisa.marco@hsr.it (M.P.); congiu.martina@hsr.it (M.C.); comi.giancarlo@hsr.it (G.C.)
2. Vita-Salute San Raffaele University, Via Olgettina, 58, 20132 Milan, Italy; gregorislorenzo96@gmail.com (L.G.); giulialeccabue95@gmail.com (G.L.)
* Correspondence: letizia.leocani@hsr.it

Received: 4 September 2020; Accepted: 12 October 2020; Published: 29 October 2020

Abstract: Multiple sclerosis (MS) is characterized by gait impairments and severely impacts the quality of life. Technological advances in biomechanics offer objective assessments of gait disabilities in clinical settings. Here we employed wearable sensors to measure electromyography (EMG) and body acceleration during walking and to quantify the altered gait pattern between people with progressive MS (PwPMS) and healthy controls (HCs). Forty consecutive patients attending our department as in-patients were examined together with fifteen healthy controls. All subjects performed the timed 10 min walking test (T10MW) using a wearable accelerator and 8 electrodes attached to bilateral thighs and legs so that body acceleration and EMG activity were recorded. The T10MWs were recorded under three conditions: standard (wearing shoes), reduced grip (wearing socks) and increased cognitive load (backward-counting dual-task). PwPMS showed worse kinematics of gait and increased muscle coactivation than controls at both the thigh and leg levels. Both reduced grip and increased cognitive load caused a reduction in the cadence and velocity of the T10MW, which were correlated with one another. A higher coactivation index at the thigh level of the more affected side was positively correlated with the time of the T10MW (r = 0.5, $p < 0.01$), Expanded Disability Status Scale (EDSS) (r = 0.4, $p < 0.05$), and negatively correlated with the cadence (r = −0.6, $p < 0.001$). Our results suggest that excessive coactivation at the thigh level is the major determinant of the gait performance as the disease progresses. Moreover, demanding walking conditions do not influence gait in controls but deteriorate walking performances in PwPMS, thus those conditions should be prevented during hospital examinations as well as in homecare environments.

Keywords: multiple sclerosis; gait analysis; kinematics; surface EMG; accelerator; inertial sensor; T10MW

1. Introduction

Multiple sclerosis (MS) is a complex autoimmune disease characterized by multifocal and recurrent formation of demyelinating plaques possibly involving every area of the central nervous system (CNS) [1]. The disease usually affects multiple domains, but the motor pathway is constantly involved and usually it follows a disto-proximal gradient of severity with lower limbs being more precariously and severely impaired than the upper limbs [2]. Gait is one of the most disabling neurological symptoms in people with MS [3]. In the most advanced phases of the disease, gait dysfunction is typically due to pyramidal deficits, and sensory and cerebellar disturbances also coexist with variable extents [4].

Technological advances in biomechanics offer possibilities to objectively estimate gait disabilities such as joint kinematics, kinetics, and patterns of muscle activations during walking [5]. Non-invasive wireless wearable devices for the recording of surface electromyography and kinematics are commercially available [6]. These devices can be placed on different parts of the body based on clinical needs and they are capable of measuring gait quality in an everyday environment. For example, belt-mounted devices are used routinely in the clinical setting as they provide information on gait parameters such as cadence and velocity. The results of these simple techniques are highly consistent with more sophisticated laboratory equipment used in the research setting [7]. However, for people with MS the ideal conditions under which gait should be tested need to be better explored. Although for one of the most widely used walking tests, the 25 foot walk test, it is recommended to use comfortable shoes, in the clinical setting it can be useful to observe gait patterns without shoes in order to better appreciate subtle abnormalities in ankle or toe movements, and in order to reduce variability at longitudinal assessments due to changes of shoes. Even in research settings, gait parameters are collected during barefoot walking [8]. Sometimes, the barefoot condition is not fully reached and the patient is allowed to wear socks for better comfort. However, walking while wearing socks may be dangerous. Walking in socks without shoes or in slippers without a sole has been associated with falls in women [9]. Being barefoot or wearing socks without shoes may also increase the risk of falls from slipping or trauma from unexpected contact [10]. Older people going barefoot, wearing socks without shoes, or wearing slippers have an increased risk of serious injury at home due to a fall [11]. Falls are a common cause of harm in people with MS; it has been described that 50% of patients report falls in a 3-month period [12]. Walking under more demanding conditions, such as during cognitive loads, greatly influences motor performance [13]. Worsening of gait during a dual-task situation is also associated with an increased risk of falls in people with MS [8]. The aim of the current study was to explore whether walking with socks may be associated with a worsening in gait performance in people with progressive MS (PwPMS), similarly to what was already described for cognitive load.

2. Materials and Methods

2.1. Subjects

We examined gait performance in 40 consecutive patients attending the Department of Neurorehabilitation of San Raffaele Hospital (Milan, Italy), with a confirmed diagnosis of MS based on the 2017 McDonald criteria [14], age 18–65 years old, Expanded Disability Status Scale (EDSS) up to 6.5 (able to walk for at least 10 min safely with or without aids), absence of orthopedic pathologies that might influence walking performances, without depression nor cognitive involvements as per routine neurological and cognitive examinations at entry (token test, symbol digit modalities test, Beck Depression Inventory-II). All patients' data were collected as part of their clinical care according to the Guideline of Good Clinical Practice [15]; all patients provided written informed consent to the use of their data for research. Fifteen healthy subjects were enrolled as the control group with similar age and sex distribution; they first provided written informed consent to participate in the study, that was approved by our Institutional Ethics Committee (approval number: N13/2017) and all data were anonymized prior to analysis.

2.2. Gait Analysis

Gait analysis was assessed using a G-Walk (BTS bioengineering, Italy), an inertial sensor which measures tri-axial accelerations, while performing a timed 10 min walking test (T10MW). The subject was asked to walk straight for 10 min with the sensor attached to the waist with a belt, covering the lower lumbar area (L4–L5). Body accelerations along the anterior-posterior, medio-lateral, and vertical axes during the T10MW were recorded with a sampling frequency of 100 Hz. According to standard

T10MW procedure, patients were asked to complete the test at the maximum speed they could safely walk. A counting dual-task (DT) condition was also tested by adding a mental tracking cognitive task in which the subject was asked to count backward by 3 from 100 while performing the T10MW. As the dual task is routinely performed to test interference on gait by cognitive load, it was performed only in the more frequently used condition, while wearing shoes. Therefore, the T10MW was assessed in three different conditions: (1) walking with shoes on (2) walking with only socks on and (3) walking with shoes on while performing DT.

The acceleration data were analyzed with G-Studio (G-Studio software, BTS bioengineering, Milan, Italy) for the three conditions. Time, cadence, velocity, and step length were calculated for further analyses.

2.3. sEMG Recording

Surface EMG was used to record muscular activity simultaneously with the acceleration measurement. Eight wireless electrodes (FREEEMG-1000, BTS bioengineering, Milan, Italy) were attached directly to the skin overlying the Rectus Femoris (RF), long head of Biceps Femoris (BF), Tibialis Anterior (TA) and Medial Gastrocnemius (GM) bilaterally. EMG data were sampled at a rate of 1000 Hz and signals were remotely transferred to a USB receiver.

The sEMG data were processed with self-developed Matlab scripts (Matlab 2016b, MathWorks, Natickm, MA). The raw sEMG data were first band-pass filtered between 10 to 500 Hz, full-wave rectified, then smoothed with a low pass filter (3.5 Hz cut-off frequency). The averaged amplitude of the resting EMG (before the subject started walking) was subtracted from the smoothed EMG for each muscle. This subtracted data were then normalized to the largest recorded value of each muscle (max. EMG). Coactivation between each agonistic-antagonistic muscle pairs (RF-BF and TA-GM) were quantified as the coactivation index (CoI). The CoI was calculated as the overlap areas of the normalized EMG data divided by the duration of the overlapping, a higher CoI indicates more coactivation between the muscle pairs [16]. However, the length of the EMG data differs between subjects since it depends on the walking speed. In order to obtain a more stable CoI and enable the comparisons between subjects, CoI was calculated from five consecutive steps of the T10MW.

2.4. Clinical Assessment

The EDSS score was evaluated by the treating neurologist at hospital admissions. All patients also underwent a clinical evaluation of spasticity according to the Modified Ashworth Scale (MAS) on bilateral RF, BF, TA and GM. On the same muscular groups, strength was measured with Medical Research Council Scale (MRC) [17,18]. These scores were used to define the less affected (LA) and more affected (MA) side in each patient. Static balance performance was assessed with the Berg Balance Scale (BBS) [19].

Patient reported outcomes were also added to the clinical evaluation. The walking status of PwPMS was measured with a 12-Item MS Walking Scale (MSWS-12) [20]; fatigue was assessed with the Fatigue Severity Scale (FSS) [21]; the MS Spasticity Scale-88 (MSSS-88) and the Numeric Rating Scale of Spasticity (NRS) were used for estimating the impact of spasticity [22] on physical performances [23]. The risk of falls was evaluated with Conley scale [24]. The disability is evaluated using the Functional Independence Measure (FIM) [25] and the Barthel Index [26].

2.5. Statistics

For data demographics, the data are expressed in mean and standard deviations (SD). Independent t-test and chi-square tests were used to compare age, gender, and body mass index (BMI) distributions between PwPMS and healthy controls (HCs) respectively.

The spatiotemporal parameters and CoI from both PwPMS and HCs for all three conditions (shoes, socks, DT) were used for further statistics. Mixed two-way ANOVA (group x conditions) were employed to test significant differences between PwPMS and HCs under the three conditions.

The analyses of CoI were performed in less and more affected side (LA/MA), respectively. If the ANOVA model was significant, turkey post-hoc analysis with Bonferroni correction ($p < 0.01$) was used to search the difference between (1) shoes and socks condition and (2) shoes and the DT condition, while the difference between PwPMS and HCs were tested with the independent t-test.

Correlations were performed among the kinematic parameters, sEMG recording, and clinical assessments. The alpha-level was corrected with Bonferroni correction and set at 0.017 for two tails as the correlations were performed in three major categories. Spearman's correlation was used to explore the relationship between the quantitative data (spatiotemporal parameters and CoI) and the clinical assessment (EDSS, MSWS-12, FSS, MSSS-88, Conley, Barthel, FIM, BBS, and NRS). Pearson's correlation was used to examine the relationship between spatiotemporal parameters and CoI. All the statistical analyses were performed with Prism 5 (GraphPad Software, Inc., San Diego, CA).

3. Results

3.1. Subjects Demographics

Forty people with progressive MS (20 males; mean age: 51.0 ± 9.8 years; mean BMI = 24.0 ± 4.6) with a mean EDSS score of 5.5 ± 1 (ranging from 1.5 to 6.5) were examined and fifteen HCs (4 males; mean age: 52.7 ± 4.4 years; mean BMI = 24.0 ± 2.2) were enrolled. The characteristics and results of clinical assessments of the two groups are shown in Table 1. No significant difference was found in age ($p = 0.4971$), sex ($p = 0.3381$), nor BMI ($p = 0.9448$) distributions between the groups.

Table 1. Data demographics of the subjects and clinical assessments. No significant difference was found in gender ($p = 0.3381$), age ($p = 0.4971$) nor in body mass index (BMI, $p = 0.9448$) between groups. Data are shown in mean ± standard deviation format. PwPMS: patients with progressive multiple sclerosis; HCs: healthy controls. MAS: Modified Ashworth Scale; MRC Scale: Medical Research Council Scale; MSWS-12: 12-Item MS Walking Scale; FSS: Fatigue Severity Scale; MSSS-88: MS Spasticity Scale-88; FIM: Functional Independence Measure; BBS: Berg Balance Scale; NRS: Numeric Rating Scale of Spasticity.

Characteristics	PwPMS (n = 40)	HC (n = 15)
Gender (M/F)	20 / 20	4 / 9
Age (years)	50.9 ± 9.8	52.7 ± 4.4
BMI	24.0 ± 4.6	24.0 ± 2.2
EDSS	5.5 ± 1.1	-
More Affected Side (R/L)	23 / 17	-
MAS (more affected side)	2.4 ± 2.0	-
MRC scale (more affected side)	13.1 ± 3.2	-
MSWS-12	38.6 ± 9.7	-
FSS	39.5 ± 15.0	-
MSSS-88	188.6 ± 52.7	-
Conley scale	2.9 ± 1.8	-
Barthel scale	88.4 ± 10.3	-
FIM	112.5 ± 9.0	-
BBS	40.5 ± 7.7	-
NRS	3.9 ± 2.6	-

3.2. Comparisons of Spatiotemporal Parameters

Significant differences in both groups (PwPMS and HCs) and conditions (shoes, socks, and DT) were found in time (group: $p < 0.0001$; condition: $p = 0.0032$), cadence (group: $p < 0.0001$; condition: $p = 0.0032$), velocity (both $p < 0.0001$) and step length (both $p < 0.0001$). Interactions between group and conditions were only significant in time ($p = 0.0277$) and step length ($p = 0.0105$). Post-hoc analyses revealed that compared with the HCs, the PwPMS showed longer time, lower cadence, slower velocity, and shorter step length while performing T10MW in all three conditions ($p < 0.01$ for all post-hoc comparisons).

For intra-group comparisons, when wearing shoes, PwPMS showed shorter time ($p < 0.0001$), higher cadence ($p = 0.0005$), higher velocity ($p < 0.0001$), and longer step length ($p < 0.0001$) than walking with socks. On the other hand, HCs showed only smaller step size when wearing socks compared to shoes ($p = 0.0142$).

For the comparison between single and dual tasks, longer time ($p < 0.0001$), lower velocity ($p = 0.0002$), and shorter step length ($p = 0.0003$) was found in PwPMS while performing a counting DT, while cadence was not significantly different ($p = 0.09$). Interestingly, significantly reduced cadence during the DT compared to a single task was found in HCs ($p = 0.014$).

The results of spatiotemporal parameters are shown in Figure 1.

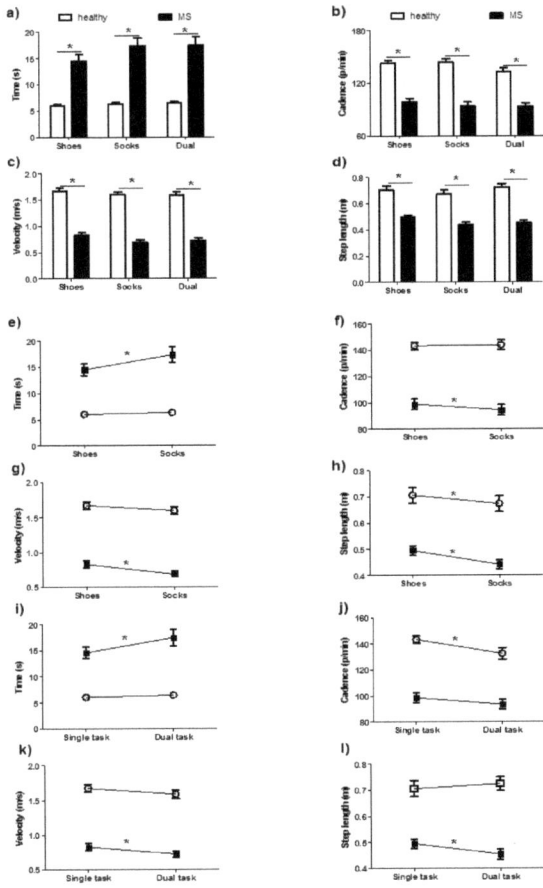

Figure 1. Inter- and intra group comparisons of spatiotemporal parameters. Significant group differences in time (**a**), cadence (**b**), velocity (**c**) and step size (**d**) were found in all three conditions. Intra-group comparison between shoes and socks conditions also showed significant differences in time (**e**), cadence (**f**), velocity (**g**), and step length (**h**) in PwPMS, while only step length in the HCs. For the comparison of single and dual tasks, longer time (**i**), lower velocity (**k**), and shorter step length (**l**) was found when PwPMS were performing a DT compared to performing a single task, while in the HCs only significantly reduced cadence (**j**) was found. *: $p < 0.01$ in post hoc analysis ((**a**–**d**): between-group comparison; (**j**–**l**): within-group comparisons).

3.3. Comparisons of Coactivation Index

Two-way ANOVA showed significant group differences of coactivation in both the MA and LA side in RF-BF ($p = 0.0007$ for both) and GM-TA (MA: $p = 0.0144$; LA: $p = 0.0047$) pairs, while no significant difference were found among conditions. Post-hoc analyses revealed that compared with HCs, PwPMS showed higher coactivation in the MA and LA sides for both antagonistic pairs among all three conditions ($p < 0.01$ for all).

For intra-group comparisons, in both PwPMS and the HC, no difference of the CoI was found when comparing between shoes and socks conditions, nor in shoes and with DT conditions. The results are shown in Figure 2.

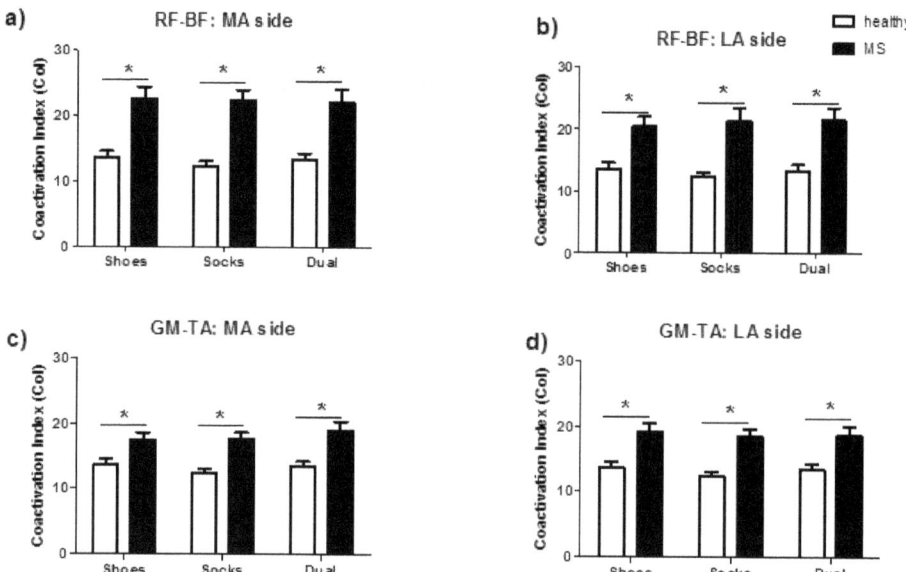

Figure 2. The inter-group difference of the coactivation index. Two-way ANOVA showed significant group difference of coactivation in both the MA and LA side in RF-BF (**a,b**) and GM-TA (**c,d**), while no significant difference was found among conditions. *: $p < 0.01$ in posthoc analyses.

3.4. Correlations among Measurements

For correlation between clinical assessments and spatiotemporal parameters, the EDSS score was correlated with time (shoes: $r = 0.4785$, $p = 0.0018$; socks: $r = 0.4984$, $p = 0.0011$; DT: $r = 0.4006$, $p = 0.0104$), cadence (shoes: $r = -0.4932$, $p = 0.0012$; socks: $r = -0.4995$, $p = 0.0010$; DT: $r = -0.4270$, $p = 0.0060$), and velocity (shoes: $r = -0.4790$, $p = 0.0018$; socks: $r = -0.4967$, $p = 0.0011$; DT: $r = -0.4225$, $p = 0.0066$) in all three conditions. On the other hand, with EMG results, the EDSS correlated with the CoI in the RF-BF pair of the MA side in socks ($r = 0.4237$, $p = 0.0169$) and with DT ($r = 0.4761$, $p = 0.0078$) conditions, also a trend correlation was found in the shoes condition ($r = 0.3828$, $p = 0.0368$). The FSS was correlated with the CoI in the RF-BF pair in both the MA and LA side in the socks condition (MA: $r = -0.4953$, $p = 0.0054$; LA: $r = -0.5457$, $p = 0.0105$). The FIM scores was correlated with time in shoes ($r = -0.4026$, $p = 0.0100$) and with the DT ($r = -0.3875$, $p = 0.0135$), and with velocity in all three conditions (shoes: $r = 0.4080$, $p = 0.0090$; socks: $r = 0.4011$, $p = 0.0103$; DT: $r = 0.4235$, $p = 0.0065$). The BBS correlated with time ($r = -0.3961$, $p = 0.0126$) and velocity ($r = 0.3957$, $p = 0.0127$) in shoes condition. The correlation results are summarized in Tables 2 and 3.

Table 2. Spearman's correlation coefficient between spatiotemporal parameters and clinical assessments in all the conditions. Spearman's correlation was performed to explore the relationship between kinematics and clinical measurements.

Variables	Conditions	EDSS	MSWS-12	FSS	MSSS-88	Conley	Barthel	FIM	BBS	NRS
Time (N = 40)	shoes	0.48 **	0.22	−0.23	−0.01	−0.07	−0.11	−0.40 *	−0.40 *	0.05
	socks	0.50 **	0.22	−0.27	−0.04	−0.08	−0.01	−0.35	−0.32	0.06
	DT	0.40 *	0.15	−0.16	0.03	−0.16	−0.00	−0.39 *	−0.29	−0.03
Cadence (N = 40)	shoes	−0.49 **	−0.20	0.31	0.08	0.11	0.08	0.33	0.36	0.07
	socks	−0.50 **	−0.21	0.32	0.06	0.13	0.02	0.33	0.35	0.07
	DT	−0.43 **	−0.13	0.15	−0.09	0.14	−0.07	0.29	0.27	0.16
Velocity (N = 40)	shoes	−0.48 **	−0.22	0.23	0.02	0.06	0.10	0.41 **	0.40 *	−0.05
	socks	−0.50 **	−0.20	0.27	0.03	0.11	0.03	0.40 *	0.36	−0.07
	DT	−0.42 **	−0.13	0.18	0.01	0.11	0.06	0.42 **	0.34	−0.08
Step Length (N = 40)	shoes	−0.27	−0.03	0.24	0.13	0.08	0.06	0.32	0.24	−0.13
	socks	−0.18	−0.06	0.14	0.03	−0.01	−0.04	0.11	0.04	−0.21
	DT	−0.15	−0.08	0.11	0.02	0.12	0.03	0.30	0.14	−0.13

The significance level was set to $p < 0.017$. *: $p < 0.017$; **: $p < 0.001$.

Table 3. Spearman's correlation coefficient between the coactivation index and clinical assessments in all the conditions. Spearman's correlation was performed to explore the relationship between sEMG recording and clinical exams.

Variables	Conditions	EDSS	MSWS-12	FSS	MSSS-88	Conley	Barthel	FIM	BBS	NRS
RF-BF MA (N = 31)	shoes	0.38	0.06	−0.27	−0.03	−0.10	−0.13	−0.30	−0.15	−0.41
	socks	0.42 *	−0.10	−0.50 **	−0.11	−0.18	−0.02	−0.14	−0.12	−0.30
	DT	0.48 **	−0.04	−0.38	−0.13	−0.05	0.05	−0.08	0.02	−0.35
RF-BF LA (N = 22)	shoes	0.12	−0.28	−0.46	−0.21	−0.09	−0.02	−0.13	0.02	−0.22
	socks	0.21	0.07	−0.55 *	−0.18	0.03	−0.05	−0.12	0.02	−0.02
	DT	0.26	−0.32	−0.41	−0.13	−0.08	−0.01	−0.00	0	−0.05
GM-TA MA (N = 40)	shoes	0.13	−0.04	0.02	0.16	−0.06	0.20	−0.03	0.10	0.17
	socks	0.07	0.02	−0.01	0.07	0.06	0.14	−0.08	0.01	0.13
	DT	0.17	−0.02	0.01	0.02	−0.05	0.22	−0.07	0.01	0.12
GM-TA LA (N = 40)	shoes	0.22	0.07	−0.09	0.07	0.11	0.12	−0.34	−0.39	0.18
	socks	0.16	0.10	0.13	0.18	0.33	0	−0.28	−0.30	0.22
	DT	0.02	−0.10	−0.11	−0.01	0.22	0.03	−0.14	−0.18	0.27

The significance level was set to $p < 0.017$. *: $p < 0.017$; **: $p < 0.001$.

Finally, when we compared the changes from the standard shoe condition to the two challenging conditions (i.e., socks or DT), we found significant positive correlations between the reduction in velocity (r = 0.3662, p = 0.0141) and cadence (r = 0.4158, p = 0.0076) when walking with socks versus shoes and when performing the dual versus simple task for PwPMS. A negative correlation was found between lower score of the BBS and the time increases from shoe condition to the socks condition (r = −0.3901, p = 0.0141) and a trend of negative correlation with the time increases from a single to a DT condition (r = −0.3247, p = 0.0437). The results are shown in Figure 3. No such correlations were found in HCs.

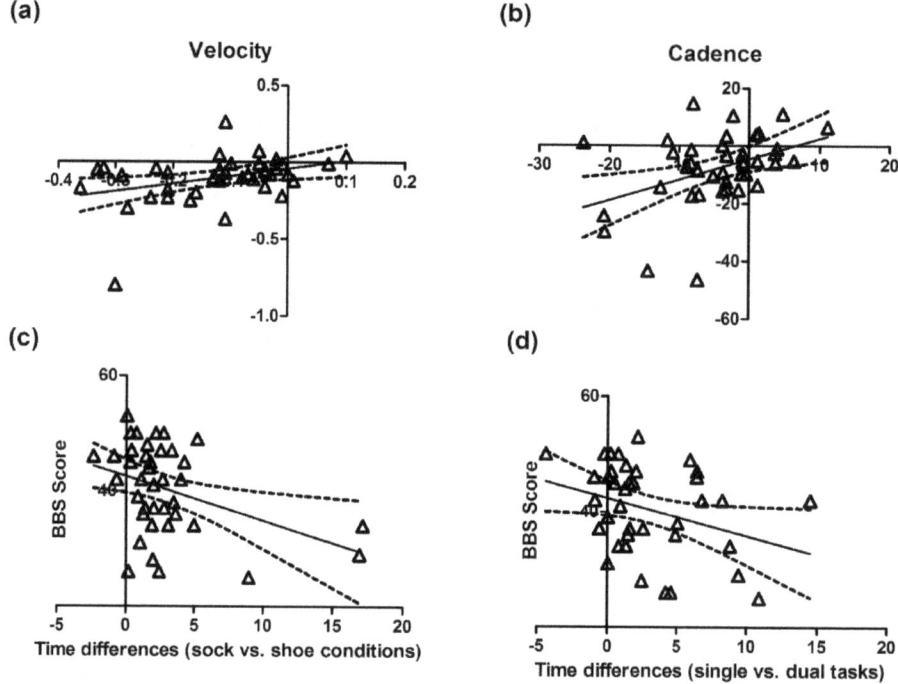

Figure 3. The correlations among kinematics and clinical assessments when the walking conditions changed for PwPMS. (**a**,**b**): x-axis: the difference between the shoes and the socks conditions (socks minus shoes); y-axis: the difference between the single task and DT conditions (single minus DT, both performed with shoes). Positive correlations were found in velocity (r = 0.3662, p = 0.0141) and cadence (r = 0.4158, p = 0.0076) between the differences of the shoes vs. socks condition and the single vs. DT conditions. (**c**,**d**): A significant negative correlation was found between the BBS scores and the time increases from shoe to sock conditions (r = −0.3901, p = 0.0141), and a trend correlation was found with time increases of single versus dual tasks (r = −0.3247, p = 0.0437).

4. Discussion

In the present study we employed wireless wearable devices to examine changes in gait control in demanding conditions. The T10MW was tested under three conditions (shoes, socks, and the counting DT) with the combined use of an accelerator and sEMG monitoring. As expected, PwPMS showed worse gait performance in kinematics and higher coactivation in antagonistic muscle pairs at thigh and leg levels than HCs. We found that only in the PwPMS, the kinematic measures changed when walking was performed under demanding conditions, while the pattern of coactivation remained the same. Further, the kinematic changes between the socks versus shoes conditions were positively correlated with those found between the single versus dual task condition. This result indicates that for PwPMS, the impact on gait performance when walking with socks without shoes, is correlated with that introduced by a cognitive load; similar findings were not present in the HC group. Both walking with socks and with a cognitive load were associated with increased risk of falls in women, elder people, or in people with MS [8–11].

A score of less than 45 in the Berg Balance Scale exposes one to a greater risk of falling [27]. We found that in the PwPMS group, lower scores of the Berg Balance Scale were related to worse gait control when walking in socks or performing a counting DT. No difference nor correlation was found regarding gender, age, nor BMI in different conditions. Therefore, for tests such as the T10MW or the timed 25 foot walk test, performing with socks should be avoided for all PwPMS.

The sEMG results showed increased coactivation in both the MA and LA side of the lower limbs during total stance in PwPMS compared with the HCs. However, due to the limitation of the devices used, the stance cannot be further separated into sub-phases. Boudarham et al. reported higher coactivation during the whole stance at the leg level, while at the thigh level only during the single support phase [28]. Compared with their group, our PwPMS group has a higher disability (mean EDSS: 5.5 vs. 3.8) and worse spasticity (MAS of MA side: 2.2 vs. 1), which could explain why we found excessive coactivation in the whole lower limbs. Also, in Budarham's study, no correlation between the EDSS and the CoI was found, while in our study the CoI of RF-BF at the MA side was correlated with the EDSS in more challenging walking conditions (i.e., with socks or the counting DT). Furthermore, the CoI of RF-BF at both the MA and LA side were correlated with worsening of most kinematic measurements. These results suggest that as the disease progresses, higher coactivation at the thigh level is the major source of the increasing walking impairment.

It is important to combine the information regarding muscle activation and joint kinematics to have a more comprehensive view of gait performance, which is fundamental for the clinicians to design more tailored rehabilitation protocols [29]. Thanks to the advance of technology, both sEMG and kinematics can be measured with wearable devices in the clinical setting. Additionally, wireless communication allows the remote transfer of data to laboratories and clinics for further analysis. This approach paves the way for remote assessment, as it is able to provide real-time information for both the patient and the clinician [6]. The costs for wearable devices used routinely in the clinical setting are usually lower compared with more sophisticated non-wearable equipment reserved to research laboratory environment [6]. These potential advantages make wearable devices a good candidate to be incorporated into home care and remote medicine, besides the hospital settings.

There are some limitations of the current study. First, the inertial sensor is not sensitive enough to reliably distinguish sub-phases of the stance cycle. All the data were reported as the performance of a whole gait cycle. However, for patients with a milder disability, the differences may only appear during the sub-phases. Second, as our cohort of patients was already characterized by moderate EDSS severity already indicating involvement of gait, we could not test whether kinematic parameters in the present study may be more sensitive than a clinical examination. Third, as the dual task has been performed with shoes, it is not possible to explore possible further worsening of gait measures under the combination of the two more difficult conditions (i.e., dual task with socks). Last, as the majority of our cohort included subjects with normal BMI, our results may not fully reflect the whole BMI variability.

5. Conclusions

Walking tests wearing socks should be discouraged to prevent falls for PwPMS. This concern should be embedded into guidelines for future remote medicine when these measurements can be performed during home care instead of hospital settings. The combined use of wearable accelerators and sEMG provide quantitative measurements of muscle activity and kinematics during walking, which can benefit future remote medicine programs, offering the opportunity to monitor disease progression and evaluate the efficiency of rehabilitation for PwPMS remotely.

Author Contributions: L.L.: Conceptualization, study design, method implementation, data collection supervision, analysis and interpretation, manuscript revision; L.G., G.L., M.C.: data collection; S.-C.H.: Data analysis; M.P.: data interpretation and manuscript revision; G.D.C.: statistical analysis and manuscript revision; S.C.H., L.G., G.L.: manuscript preparation; G.C.: manuscript revision for intellectual content. All authors have read and agreed to the published version of the manuscript.

Funding: This research received no external funding, while S.C.H. is supported by a senior research fellowship FISM–Fodazione Italiana Sclerosi Multipla–cod. 2018/B/4, and FISM is financed or co-financed with the "5 per mille" public funding.

Conflicts of Interest: The authors declare no conflict of interest.

References

1. Lassmann, H.; Bruck, W.; Lucchinetti, C.F. The immunopathology of multiple sclerosis: An overview. *Brain Pathol.* **2007**, *17*, 210–218. [CrossRef] [PubMed]
2. Institute of Medicine (US) Committee on Multiple Sclerosis. *Current Status and Strategies for the Future. Multiple Sclerosis: Current Status and Strategies for the Future*; Joy, J.E., Johnston, R.B., Jr., Eds.; National Academies Press: Washington, DC, USA, 2001.
3. Heesen, C.; Böhm, J.; Reich, C.; Kasper, J.; Goebel, M.; Gold, S.M. Patient perception of bodily functions in multiple sclerosis: Gait and visual function are the most valuable. *Mult. Scler. J.* **2008**, *14*, 988–991. [CrossRef] [PubMed]
4. Kalron, A.; Givon, U. Gait characteristics according to pyramidal, sensory and cerebellar EDSS subcategories in people with multiple sclerosis. *J. Neurol.* **2016**, *263*, 1796–1801. [CrossRef] [PubMed]
5. Lizama, L.E.C.; Khan, F.; Lee, P.V.; Galea, M.P. The use of laboratory gait analysis for understanding gait deterioration in people with multiple sclerosis. *Mult. Scler. J.* **2016**, *22*, 1768–1776. [CrossRef]
6. Shanahan, C.J.; Boonstra, F.M.C.; Lizama, L.E.C.; Strik, M.; Moffat, B.A.; Khan, F.; Kilpatrick, T.; Van Der Walt, A.; Galea, M.P.; Kolbe, S.C. Technologies for Advanced Gait and Balance Assessments in People with Multiple Sclerosis. *Front. Neurol.* **2018**, *8*, 708. [CrossRef] [PubMed]
7. Vítečková, S.; Horáková, H.; Poláková, K.; Krupička, R.; Růžička, E.; Brožová, H. Agreement between the GAITRite®System and the Wearable Sensor BTS G-Walk®for measurement of gait parameters in healthy adults and Parkinson's disease patients. *PeerJ* **2020**, *8*, e8835. [CrossRef]
8. Etemadi, Y. Dual task cost of cognition is related to fall risk in patients with multiple sclerosis: A prospective study. *Clin. Rehabil.* **2016**, *31*, 278–284. [CrossRef]
9. Larsen, E.R.; Mosekilde, L.; Foldspang, A. Correlates of falling during 24 h among elderly Danish community residents. *Prev. Med.* **2004**, *39*, 389–398. [CrossRef] [PubMed]
10. Menz, H.B.; Morris, M.E.; Lord, S.R. Footwear Characteristics and Risk of Indoor and Outdoor Falls in Older People. *Gerontology* **2006**, *52*, 174–180. [CrossRef]
11. Kelsey, J.L.; Procter-Gray, E.; Nguyen, U.-S.D.T.; Li, W.; Kiel, D.P.; Hannan, M.T. Footwear and falls in the home among older individuals in the MOBILIZE Boston Study. *Footwear Sci.* **2010**, *2*, 123–129. [CrossRef]
12. Coote, S.; Sosnoff, J.J.; Gunn, H. Fall Incidence as the Primary Outcome in Multiple Sclerosis Falls-Prevention Trials: Recommendation from the International MS Falls Prevention Research Network. *Int. J. MS Care* **2014**, *16*, 178–184. [CrossRef]
13. Leone, C.; Patti, F.; Feys, P. Measuring the cost of cognitive-motor dual tasking during walking in multiple sclerosis. *Mult. Scler. J.* **2014**, *21*, 123–131. [CrossRef] [PubMed]
14. Thompson, A.J.; Banwell, B.L.; Barkhof, F.; Carroll, W.M.; Coetzee, T.; Comi, G.; Correale, J.; Fazekas, F.; Filippi, M.; Freedman, M.S.; et al. Diagnosis of multiple sclerosis: 2017 revisions of the McDonald criteria. *Lancet Neurol.* **2018**, *17*, 162–173. [CrossRef]
15. ICH Harmonised Tripartite Guideline: Guideline for Good Clinical Practice. *J. Postgrad. Med.* **2001**, *47*, 199–203.
16. Unnithan, V.B.; Dowling, J.J.; Frost, G.; Ayub, B.V.; Bar-Or, O. Cocontraction and phasic activity during GAIT in children with cerebral palsy. *Electromyogr. Clin. Neurophysiol.* **1996**, *36*, 487–494. [PubMed]
17. Bohannon, R.W.; Smith, M.B. Interrater Reliability of a Modified Ashworth Scale of Muscle Spasticity. *Phys. Ther.* **1987**, *67*, 206–207. [CrossRef]

18. Hermans, G.; Clerckx, B.; Vanhullebusch, T.; Segers, J.; Vanpee, G.; Robbeets, C.; Casaer, M.P.; Wouters, P.; Gosselink, R.; Berghe, G.V.D. Interobserver agreement of medical research council sum-score and handgrip strength in the intensive care unit. *Muscle Nerve* **2011**, *45*, 18–25. [CrossRef]
19. Toomey, E.; Coote, S. Between-Rater Reliability of the 6-Minute Walk Test, Berg Balance Scale, and Handheld Dynamometry in People with Multiple Sclerosis. *Int. J. MS Care* **2013**, *15*, 1–6. [CrossRef]
20. Hobart, J.C.; Riazi, A.; Lamping, D.L.; Fitzpatrick, R.; Thompson, A.J. Measuring the impact of MS on walking ability: The 12-Item MS Walking Scale (MSWS-12). *Neurology* **2003**, *60*, 31–36. [CrossRef]
21. Krupp, L.B.; LaRocca, N.G.; Muir-Nash, J.; Steinberg, A.D. The fatigue severity scale. Application to patients with multiple sclerosis and systemic lupus erythematosus. *Arch. Neurol.* **1989**, *46*, 1121–1123. [CrossRef]
22. Hobart, J.C.; Riazi, A.; Thompson, A.J.; Styles, I.M.; Ingram, W.; Vickery, P.J.; Warner, M.; Fox, P.J.; Zajicek, J. Getting the measure of spasticity in multiple sclerosis: The Multiple Sclerosis Spasticity Scale (MSSS-88). *Brain* **2005**, *129*, 224–234. [CrossRef]
23. Farrar, J.T.; Troxel, A.B.; Stott, C.; Duncombe, P.; Jensen, M.P. Validity, reliability, and clinical importance of change in a 0–10 numeric rating scale measure of spasticity: A post hoc analysis of a randomized, double-blind, placebo-controlled trial. *Clin. Ther.* **2008**, *30*, 974–985. [CrossRef]
24. Guzzo, A.; Meggiolaro, A.; Mannocci, A.; Tecca, M.; Salomone, I.; La Torre, G. Conley Scale: Assessment of a fall risk prevention tool in a General Hospital. *J. Prev. Med. Hyg.* **2015**, *56*, E77–E87.
25. Ottenbacher, K.J.; Hsu, Y.; Granger, C.V.; Fiedler, R.C. The reliability of the functional independence measure: A quantitative review. *Arch. Phys. Med. Rehabil.* **1996**, *77*, 1226–1232. [CrossRef] [PubMed]
26. Mahoney, F.I.; Barthel, D.W. Functional Evaluation: The Barthel Index. *Md. State Med. J.* **1965**, *14*, 61–65. [PubMed]
27. Berg, K.O.; Wood-Dauphinee, S.L.; Williams, J.I.; Maki, B. Measuring balance in the elderly: Validation of an instrument. *Can. J. Public Health* **1992**, *83*, S7–S11.
28. Boudarham, J.; Hameau, S.; Zory, R.; Hardy, A.; Bensmail, D.; Roche, N. Coactivation of Lower Limb Muscles during Gait in Patients with Multiple Sclerosis. *PLoS ONE* **2016**, *11*, e0158267. [CrossRef]
29. Papagiannis, G.I.; Triantafyllou, A.I.; Roumpelakis, I.M.; Zampeli, F.; Eleni, P.G.; Koulouvaris, P.; Papadopoulos, E.C.; Papagelopoulos, P.J.; Babis, G.C. Methodology of surface electromyography in gait analysis: Review of the literature. *J. Med. Eng. Technol.* **2019**, *43*, 59–65. [CrossRef]

Publisher's Note: MDPI stays neutral with regard to jurisdictional claims in published maps and institutional affiliations.

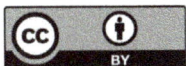

© 2020 by the authors. Licensee MDPI, Basel, Switzerland. This article is an open access article distributed under the terms and conditions of the Creative Commons Attribution (CC BY) license (http://creativecommons.org/licenses/by/4.0/).

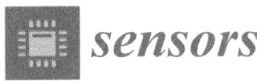

Article

Towards a Simplified Estimation of Muscle Activation Pattern from MRI and EMG Using Electrical Network and Graph Theory

Enrico Piovanelli [1,*], Davide Piovesan [2], Shouhei Shirafuji [3,5], Becky Su [1], Natsue Yoshimura [4,5,6], Yousuke Ogata [4,5] and Jun Ota [3]

1. Department of Precision Engineering, The University of Tokyo, Hongo, Tokyo 113-8656, Japan; su@race.t.u-tokyo.ac.jp
2. Department of Biomedical, Industrial and Systems Engineering, Gannon University, Erie, PA 16541, USA; piovesan001@gannon.edu
3. Research Into Artifacts Center for Engineering (RACE), School of Engineering, The University of Tokyo, Tokyo 113-8656, Japan; shirafuji@race.t.u-tokyo.ac.jp (S.S.); ota@race.t.u-tokyo.ac.jp (J.O.)
4. Institute of Innovative Research, Tokyo Institute of Technology, Midori-ku, Yokohama 226-8503, Japan; yoshimura@pi.titech.ac.jp (N.Y.); ogata@cns.pi.titech.ac.jp (Y.O.)
5. Integrative Brain Imaging Center, National Center of Neurology and Psychiatry (NCNP), Kodaira,Tokyo 187-0031, Japan
6. Precursory Research for Embryonic Science and Technology (PRESTO), Japan Science and Technology Agency (JST), Kawaguchi, Saitama 332-0012, Japan
* Correspondence: piovanelli@race.t.u-tokyo.ac.jp

Received: 27 December 2019; Accepted: 26 January 2020; Published: 28 January 2020

Abstract: Muscle functional MRI (mfMRI) is an imaging technique that assess muscles' activity, exploiting a shift in the T2-relaxation time between resting and active state on muscles. It is accompanied by the use of electromyography (EMG) to have a better understanding of the muscle electrophysiology; however, a technique merging MRI and EMG information has not been defined yet. In this paper, we present an anatomical and quantitative evaluation of a method our group recently introduced to quantify its validity in terms of muscle pattern estimation for four subjects during four isometric tasks. Muscle activation pattern are estimated using a resistive network to model the morphology in the MRI. An inverse problem is solved from sEMG data to assess muscle activation. The results have been validated with a comparison with physiological information and with the fitting on the electrodes space. On average, over 90% of the input sEMG information was able to be explained with the estimated muscle patterns. There is a match with anatomical information, even if a strong subjectivity is observed among subjects. With this paper we want to proof the method's validity showing its potential in diagnostic and rehabilitation fields.

Keywords: MRI; EMG; graph theory; electrical network; muscle activity; forearm

1. Introduction

In the study of neuromuscular degenerative disease and in the development of rehabilitation therapies to treat them, monitoring the activity of muscles is crucial to better understand the nature of the impairment and to have a feedback about the changes occurring after applied treatments. As a consequence of pathological conditions, it is also not so uncommon to observe changes occurring in the physical structure and in the behaviour of muscles of impaired individuals [1–3]. It is, therefore, crucial to have a full vision that simultaneously encloses the underlying morphology and the muscle activation pattern, in order to have a full understanding of the impairment status. This overall vision would allow clinicians to have a wider picture of the pathological status, potentially being able to provide a targeted treatment.

The gold standard method to acquire morphological information is to use Magnetic Resonance Imaging (MRI). MRI is a diagnostic imaging technique that is widely used to depict the anatomy and the dynamics of physiological processes happening in the body. For muscle studies in particular, a prolongation in T2 relaxation time between rest and intensive muscle activity has been reported to be useful for a quantitative evaluation of muscle activity [1]. This technique is referred as muscle functional MRI (mfMRI) and has been used in studies on lower back [3–6], lower limbs [7,8], upper limbs [9,10], shoulder [11], hip abductors [12] and plantar flexion movements [13]. It allowed the estimation of the activity of all muscles in the considered field of view with a single scan, showing particular advantage for the study of deeper muscles that have usually prohibitive access with other methods.

However, since a considerable time span is necessary between two T2-relaxation time measurements, the temporal resolution of mfMRI is low and therefore it is not possible to have reliable information about the activation dynamics of contracting muscles. Additionally, mfMRI has shown limitation in the evaluation of task at low level force [1], because of a lower activity threshold compared to other technique used to study muscle activity such as electromyography (EMG). EMG is a medical signal acquisition technique that read the potential variation caused by contracting muscles and it can be invasive (needle EMG) or non invasive (surface EMG). Usually surface EMG (sEMG) is collected with single or bipolar electrodes placed above the target muscles; however, the recent introduction of High Density sEMG (HD-sEMG) [14] allowed the collection of a significantly higher volume of data with the use of electrodes matrices placed above an area covering multiple muscles. Due to the higher number of electrodes however, the information is highly redundant and noisy and therefore a burdening post processing is usually needed.

Estimation of muscle activation using only sEMG was proposed and several works were presented with the use of HD-sEMG [15–17]. However, an important limitation of these studies relies on the fact that deep muscle activation cannot be estimated. Furthermore, these methods estimate the motor units' activity ignoring morphological information about the person's anatomy.

To cope with the limitations of mfMRI and sEMG, studies tried to merge the two techniques [5,9]. However, the outcomes were not always in agreement, and a direct relationship between increase in T2 value and in muscle activity was not always observable [1]. The reason for this discrepancy is alleged to reside in the nature of the information that is collected by the MRI and the sEMG, respectively. The information reflects the metabolic activity within the muscle for the MRI and records the neural electrical activity for the EMG. Thus, the need for a better merging of the two techniques to obtain significant information has emerged while overcoming the underlying conflict. Alternative hybrid MRI-EMG approaches in the literature are lacking and only a few works could be found [18,19]. However, these solutions required the use of discretized models and of heavy optimization which make them not suitable for clinical application due to the processing and computational time required.

To find a better symbiosis of the information provided by MRI and EMG, our group recently proposed an alternative methodology that provides an estimation of the forearm muscle activity. The method exploits the morphological information contained in the MRI scan to build an electrical lumped model of the conductive volume. Such model is then used to solve an inverse problem starting from the sEMG collected from a dense array of electrodes around the forearm [20,21]. The method, unlike previously proposed methods, provide an estimation of all muscles' activation with a value for each muscle that lump its activity. With this paper, we evaluate the method on a group of participants performing different tasks involving different muscles, in order to observe how the method perform. An electromyographic dataset of four healthy subjects performing wrist and finger isometric tasks, has been studied. Since a direct validation of the estimated activities via needle EMG is impossible due to the difficulties and discomfort that it would entail for the subject, the performance was evaluated using specialized literature and quantifying the fitting of the sEMG with the projection of the estimated currents on the electrodes space. The study was conducted on the average muscles behaviour, therefore any time dynamics has been ignored and the root mean square (RMS) of the sEMG data was considered during each of the contraction tasks.

The results shows that, for four isometric contractions at different force level, our method is able to provide sets of muscles' current that explain over 90% of the average sEMG information. The currents' time profiles have a physiological explanation in most of the studied case and the method highlights subjective difference in the activation pattern for each subject given the same task. Furthermore, different level of force do not change the muscle activation profile in accordance to what is reported in the literature.

The details of the method in all its parts along with the description of the experimental setup is reported in the Material and Methods section. In particular, how the MRI and the EMG are collected and how the model is constructed from this information is described. The results are reported and discussed in the Results and Discussion section, respectively. Final comments and considerations about possible development and future application are then described in the Conclusion section.

2. Experimental Procedure

2.1. Subjects

Four healthy subjects (2 males and 2 females, average age = 27.3 ± 2.3 years old) volunteered for this study. All the subjects gave their consent to take part to the experiment. The experimental protocol was approved by ethics committee of the University of Tokyo. None of the subject had any reported history of neuromuscular impairment at the time of the experiment.

2.2. MRI Acquisition

A T1-weighted MRI of the forearm has been acquired for all the subjects with a 3T Siemens Verio (Siemens, Germany) scanner at the National Center of Neurology and Psychiatry (Tokyo, Japan). The slice resolution was set to 0.2×0.2 mm while the resolution along the longitudinal axis i.e., slice thickness, has been set to 3 mm. Repetition time was 11 ms, Echo time was 4.92 ms and a 448×448 matrix has been considered. The forearm was held in supinated position for consistency with the setup during sEMG data. Vitamin E capsules were attached to bony reference point on the wrist and on the elbow as contrast markers for subsequent registration purposes.

2.3. Experimental Setup and HD-sEMG Acquisition

The experimental setup is depicted in Figure 1. The subject lay supine. A real time visual feedback of the exerted force was given with a monitor mounted over the subject's face. The right forearm of the subject was then positioned on a custom made alloy frame that sustained the forearm and the hand horizontally aligned along the body. The wrist was in supinated position with the hand facing upwards in order to avoid crossing between the ulna and radius bone.

The hand was sustained with a 3D printed cage connected to force sensors in lateral and palmar position to measure the lateral and vertical forces, respectively. During the finger contractions the setup was slightly changed. The target finger was constrained inside an additional 3D printed structure connected to another force sensor to measure the exerted force along the direction normal to the surface of the finger tip (Figure 1a,b). Forces were measured with an Arduino board sampling at 10 Hz.

Each subject had to perform five different isometric tasks at two levels of force, 25% and 50% of maximum voluntary contraction (MVC). The isometric tasks executed were the following:

1. Middle finger metacarpophalangeal joint (MCP) extension
2. Wrist flexion
3. Wrist extension
4. Ulnar deviation
5. Index finger MCP extension

Each of the listed tasks was repeated 15 times. Each repetition consisted of a 2 s force raising, 5 s force holding, 2 s release and 15 s of rest. For the purpose of this analysis, the first two and the last two contractions has not been considered to avoid effect of adaptation and fatigue, therefore all the analysis was conducted on 11 repetitions. An additional contraction at maximum force has been done prior to each type of task, in order to set the MVC force value.

Since the main responsible for index finger MCP extension, extensor indicis muscle, is located in a more distal section of the forearm compared to the muscles involved in the other considered task, in this work, the index finger MCP extension was not considered.

The HD-sEMG has been acquired with four custom designed electrodes' sheets wrapped around the forearm at different lengths around the forearm, so to cover as much of it as possible. The forearm skin was cleaned with alcohol previous to attach the HD-sEMG sheets. Each electrodes' sheet had 16 × 4 electrodes and a total of 256 channels were acquired on the forearm. Two different sized sheets were used depending on the size of the subject's forearm: a shorter sheet of 195 mm × 52 mm size with 10 mm × 19.5 mm inter-electrode spacing, and a longer sheet of 270 mm × 52 mm size with 15 mm × 19.5 mm inter-electrode spacing. For the purpose of this work a single row of electrode properly selected around the forearm was considered.

The signal was acquired with a RHD2000 Evaluation System (Intan Technology, Los Angeles, CA, USA) with a 2500 Hz sampling frequency with no prior analog filtering. Additional adhesive electrodes were placed on the radial styloid and at the metacarpophalangeal joint level of the thumb as, respectively, ground and reference (Figure 1).

The position of the electrodes and of the anatomical references marked in the MRI were recorded with a Polhemus Fastrak 3D digitizer system (Polhemus, Colchester, VT, USA). The forearm was susequently wrapped with an elastic bandage to keep the electrodes sheet adherent to the skin.

The sEMG measurements were collected for all tasks in a single session, a few days after the MRI acquisition.

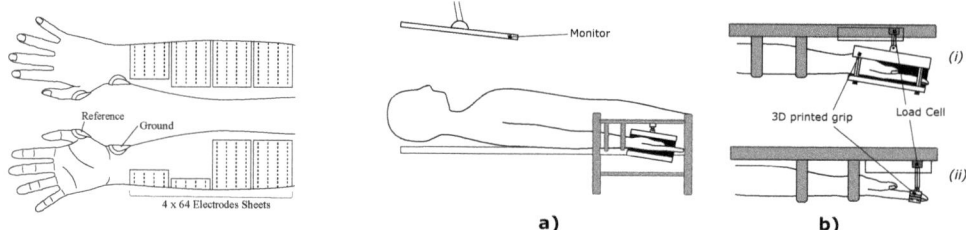

Figure 1. *Left* : Top and bottom view of electrodes positioning on the forearm. Four sheets of 64 electrodes were wrapped around the forearm in order to cover the maximum amount of its surface. A reference electrode was positioned on the metacarpophalangeal joint of the thumb. A ground electrode was sticked to the radial styloid. *Right* : Experimental setup. (**a**) Position of the subject during data acquisition. The subject was lying down facing a monitor through which a visual feedback was given of the applied force. The forearm was held in supine position, with the hand palm facing upward. (**b**) Force measuring structure for wrist movements (i) and for finger tasks (ii). The hand/finger was enclosed in a custom 3D printed structured coupled with a load cell to measure the force amplitude.

3. Proposed Method

We propose a method that allows the estimation of the muscle activation pattern from a selected MRI slice and the EMG signals collected from electrodes around the selected section. The conductive volume and the interaction between the different tissues is described with a lumped parameter model that can be represented with a graph.

The method simplify the solution of the inverse problem for the identification and the quantification of the activity of muscles involved. The conductive properties in a selected section of the arm is described with a resisitive network connecting the different tissue elements and the electrodes. The MRI section is chosen in order to include the muscles responsible for the target movements.

Muscles are identified with a segmentation step and, along with the electrodes, identify the nodes of a graph which edges are defined based on the anatomy observable from the MRI slice. The model is then solved assuming the muscles as current generators placed on muscle nodes to obtain an estimation of muscles activity.

The model construction process can be separated into three main sections (Figure 2) which will be explained in detail within the next subsections:

1. MRI segmentation and electrodes' registration
2. Construction of the electrical Network
3. Muscle currents estimation.

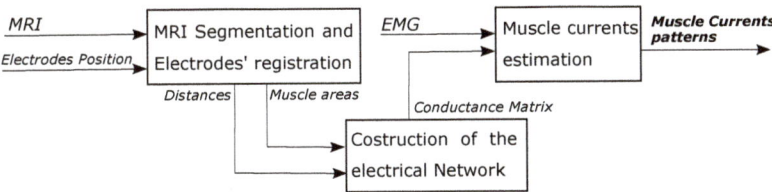

Figure 2. Diagram of the proposed approach. Three main parts can be identified, MRI segmentation and electrodes' registration, Construction of the electrode network and muscle currents estimation. From the left, the MRI segmentation and electrodes' registration block process the information in the MRI and about the electrodes' position to estimate the distance between the elements (muscles and electrodes) in the MRI and the muscles' cross section areas. This information is then used to create and weight the edges of a graph describing the interaction between the nodes representing muscles and electrodes. In the Muscle current estimation block, the EMG is exploited to obtain an estimation of the muscle activation patterns solving an inverse problem using the conductance matrix that describes the graph and the related electrical network.

3.1. MRI Segmentation and Electrodes Registration

To discriminate the different tissues and the different muscles within the selected MRI slice, a segmentation process is necessary. Segmentation is the imaging process through which the different anatomical structures are identified on a diagnostic image. In the forearm it is possible to mainly identify four types of tissues: bone, skin, fat, and muscular tissue.

While the skin, fat and bones can be easily identified due to their different contrast in the T1-weighted MRI image, muscle tissue needs to be subdivided into the different muscles that compose it. The forearm contains about 20 muscles which are responsible for forearm pronation/supination, wrist radial/ulnar deviation and flexion/extension, and for finger flexion/extension. It is possible to roughly divide the forearm's muscles into two groups based on their function: extensors along the posterior side and flexors on the anterior side. Additionally, extensor and flexors can be further divided into superficial and deep muscles depending on their positioning in the cross-section. Muscles delineate complex paths along the forearm. Cross sections at different longitudinal coordinate of the forearm can therefore be identified as different muscle sets. The segmentation process allows for the identification and definition of the muscle's position, cross sectional areas, and boundaries (Figure 3).

For all subjects a single slice was selected. The selected slice contains for every subject the same set of muscles, which were identified using the imaging software ImageJ [22]. The considered set of muscles was the following: Abductor Pollicis Longus (APL), Extensor Pollicis Longus (EPL), Brachioradialis (BR), Extensor Digitorum (ED), Extensor Carpi Radialis Longus (ECRL), Extensor Carpi Radialis Brevis (ECRB), Extensor Carpi Ulnaris (ECU), Extensor Digiti Minimi (EDM), Flexor Digitorum Profundis (FDP), Flexor Digitorum Superficialis (FDS), Flexor Carpi Ulnaris (FCU), Flexor Carpi Radialis (FCR).

The skin layer has been ignored for the purpose of this work and its thickness has been included into fat layer thickness. Fat layer thickness is estimated as the average value of electrode-muscle distance along the arm circumference.

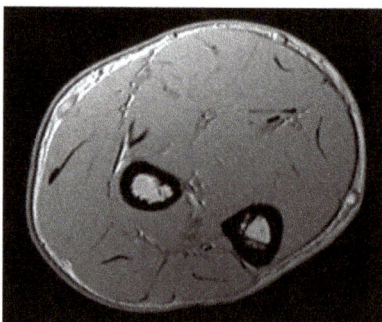 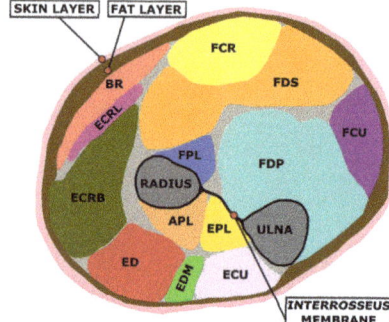

Figure 3. Example of segmentation on an MRI slice. On the left the original MRI is depicted, on the right its segmentation is reported. Muscles are represented with different colors, the radius and ulna bones are reported in gray. It is possible to observe the interosseus membrane connecting ulna and radius and dividing the posterior and the anterior side muscles. Skin and fat layers are colored respectively in pink and brown.

To correctly place the electrodes on the MRI volume a registration step has been done prior to the creation of the model, since electrodes' coordinates and MRI anatomy have been acquired with different reference frames. Registration estimates the optimal transformation to match the coordinate system of the electrodes to the coordinate system of the MRI. The registration has been done using 3D slicer [23,24], minimizing the distance between the anatomical markers on the MRI and the markers acquired with the electrodes coordinates using the digitizer. The electrodes around the arm that were closest to the chosen slice were selected and their 2D projection on the MRI section was calculated (Figure 4a). The position of the electrodes on the slice was set as the closest point on the skin of the projected electrodes (Figure 4b). The mean and the maximum distance error made during electrodes' projections steps are reported in Table 1 for all subjects. On the upper rows the errors for the projection on the selected slice are reported while on lower rows the errors on the projection on the skin surface are reported. On average the error during the projection on the selected slice is between 3 and 4.2 mm, with maximum values ranging from 7.5 to 11 mm. The distance errors on the projection on the skin surface was lower, with an average error smaller than 1 mm for all subjects and maximum values going from 1.5 to 3 mm.

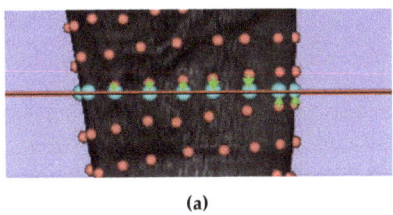 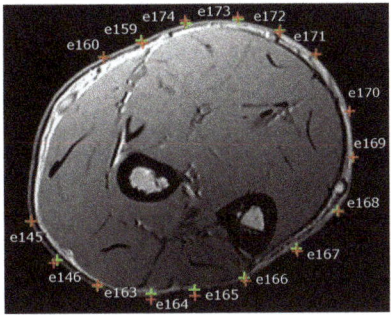

Figure 4. (a) The projection of the electrodes closest to the selected slice plane. The real electrodes position is indicated with a red sphere, the MRI plane is indicated with a red line and the projected position is indicated with a light blue sphere. The projection is depicted with a green arrow. (b) Section of the MRI with the position and the number of the electrodes. The projection of the electrode 3D position on the 2D slice is represented with a red cross. Such points are further projected on the skin (green cross) to find the closest position on the forearm surface.

Table 1. Distance error in the projection of the electrodes' positions. The distance errors in the projection on the selected slice as shown in Figure 4a are reported on first two rows of the table. The distance errors during the projection of the position on the skin surface as shown in Figure 4b are reported on the bottom two rows. For each of the subjects, the mean and the maximum distance errors are reported.

		Subject 1	Subject 2	Subject 3	Subject 4
On the slice	Mean distance [mm]	4.121	3.848	3.167	3.540
	Max distance [mm]	11.829	9.029	8.818	7.521
On the skin	Mean distance [mm]	0.890	0.862	0.789	0.620
	Max distance [mm]	2.217	1.980	3.085	1.570

Once muscles and electrodes are correctly positioned and identified on the MRI slice plane, it is possible to measure the relative distance between muscles and electrodes. In particular, it is possible to identify three type of distance:

- electrode-electrode (e-e) distance
- muscle- electrode (m-e) distance
- muscle-muscle (m-m) distance

Distances have been calculated from the centroid of the segmented cross sectional area for muscles. Electrodes' distances were calculated from the projection of the electrode position on the skin. In an MRI slice it is possible to identify n_m muscles and n_e electrodes on the skin surface.

3.2. Construction of the Electrical Network

The anatomical information extracted with the segmentation can be described with a topology. A topology can define the connections between the different elements identified in the segmentation. One of the most common way to describe a topology is a graph, a mathematical discrete structure constructed with a set of nodes and a set of edges. A node represent an object of the structure that carry a different meaning depending on the application. Edges describe a relationship between a pair of nodes. To describe the anatomical information contained in the MRI slice it is possible to model muscles and electrodes as nodes of a graph, with edges that describe connections that are defined with a set of custom rules based on several assumptions and prior anatomical information. The rules used in this work are listed as follows:

i. Each electrode defines a sector of the forearm section bounded by the lines going from the centroid of the MRI section to the two adjacent electrodes as shown in Figure 5.
ii. All muscles included in a sector with a fraction of their area greater than 5% of their cross sectional area are connected to the electrode that defines that sector.
iii. If between the fraction of the muscle in a sector and the electrode defining that sector there is a bone structure, that edge is not considered.
iv. In general a muscle node is connected to another muscle node only if they are adjacent on the segmented image. Exception are considered to take into account specific anatomical structure that are known to alter the currents flow in the volume. In particular the effect of the interosseus membrane between the ulna and the radius has been considered.
v. The fat layer is assumed to be of constant thickness around the section circumference. Such thickness is set to be the average obtained from the segmentation and it includes the skin thickness.
vi. Since it is an electrical network and additional node has to be added to model the ground.

This set of rules allows the definition of a graph with N nodes and E edges that specifically describes the anatomy of the subject and the electrodes setup for a specific cross section of the forearm. Each edge is weighted based on the nodes pair (n_1, n_2) that defines it. The weight is set to be the electric conductivity $G_{n_1 n_2}$ between the nodes pair obtained as

$$G_{n_1 n_2} = g \cdot r(n_1, n_2) \tag{1}$$

where g is the conductance of the tissue interposed between the 2 nodes and $r(n_1, n_2)$ is the distance between the nodes n_1 and n_2. The conductance for the considered tissues (i.e., muscle, fat and skin) are those reported by Lowery et al. in [25]: $g_{skin} = 4.3 \cdot 10^{-1} S/m$ for the skin, $g_{fat} = 0.04 S/m$ for the fat and $g_{muscle} = 0.09 S/m$ for muscle along the transverse direction.

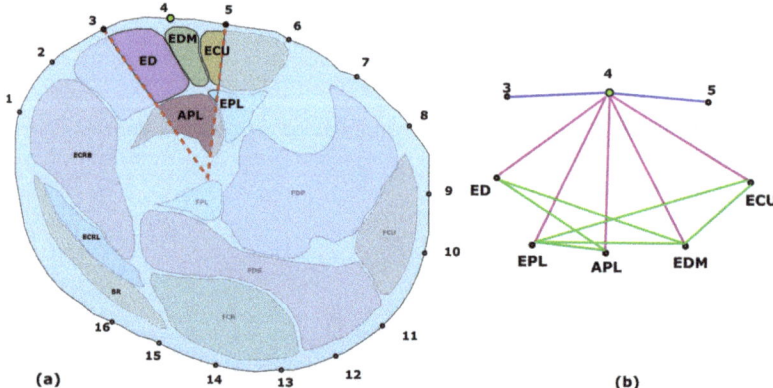

Figure 5. Example of one step of the graph creation. (a) Sector belonging to one of the electrodes, indicated with a green dot. The muscles that are included (ED, EDM, ECU, APL, and EPL) are highlighted with the area that is accounted for. (b) Graph created from the section considered in (a). e-e edges are indicated in blue, e-m edges are indicated in purple and m-m edges are indicated with green lines.

The nature of the node pair in the edges define the type of conductance that is chosen. As described for the measured distance, it is possible to identify electrode-electrode(e-e), muscle-muscle(m-m) and electrode-muscle(e-m) type of edges. For (e-e) and (m-m) edges, they can be directly weighted using Equation (1), assuming that the current between two adjacent electrodes flow through the skin and that the current between two muscles flow through only muscle tissue:

$$G_{ee} = g_{skin} \cdot d_{ee}$$
$$G_{mm} = g_{muscle} \cdot d_{mm}. \qquad (2)$$

In the case of (e–m) edges the conductance to weight the edge has been set to the series of two resistive elements in order to consider that current flow from muscle to electrode passing through muscle and fat tissue:

$$G_{em} = \frac{G_{fat} \cdot g_{muscle}(d_{em} - D_{fat})}{G_{fat} + g_{muscle}(d_{em} - D_{fat})}. \qquad (3)$$

To consider the effect of partial inclusion in the sector, the conductance of the (e-m) edges were weighted with the normalized area:

$$\hat{G}_{em} = G_{em} * \left(\frac{A_{em}}{A_m}\right) \qquad (4)$$

where A_{em} indicates the area of the muscle m included in the sector defined by the electrode e, and A_m is the total area of the muscle m.

Each of the muscle nodes was modelled as a current generator to represent the active muscle behaviour. Finally, all the nodes were connected to the ground node with a shunt resistance. The shunt resistance has been set to $D_{skin} \cdot G_{el-el}$ and $D_{muscle-bone} \cdot G_{muscle}$, respectively for electrode nodes and muscle nodes, where D_{skin} is the average distance between electrodes and $D_{muscle-bone}$ is the average distance between the centroid of muscles and the closest bone (ulna or tibia).

The electrical model so built can be described exploiting the principles of graph theory. Under the assumption of no external power injection and in static condition the current of the generators can be described with the following relationship [26]:

$$I = (\mathcal{L}_R + G)V \qquad (5)$$

where $I \in \mathbb{R}^{N \times 1}$ is the vector of currents, $V \in \mathbb{R}^{N \times 1}$ is the vector of node potentials, $\mathcal{L}_R \in \mathbb{R}^{N \times N}$ is the conductance matrix and $G \in \mathbb{R}^{N \times N}$ is the shunt conductance matrix. If G has at least one non-negative element, Equation (5) can be inverted:

$$V = (\mathcal{L}_R + G)^{-1}I = FI \qquad (6)$$

where $F = (\mathcal{L}_R + G)^{-1}$ is the matrix describing the system. Using Equation (6) it is possible to estimate the potential of the nodes with respect to the reference value, which is usually set to $V_0 = 0V$.

3.2.1. Muscle Currents Estimation

Using the built model, the muscle activities are estimated solving an inverse problem. Equations (5) and (6) describe the linear relationship that relate the currents and the voltages in the network. Equation (5) describes the relationship from the potentials and the currents on the node. Since we are only interested in how the muscles' current are reflected on the electrodes potentials it is possible to further simplify the problem reducing the dimension of the system matrix, i.e., selecting the row corresponding to electrodes nodes and columns corresponding to muscle nodes from the matrix F. The resulting matrix is a matrix $\tilde{F} \in \mathbb{R}^{n_e \times n_m}$ where the ith column is the potential that would be present on the n_e electrodes if the ith muscle is activated with unitary current.

With this notation it is possible to describe the transformation from muscles currents to electrodes' potentials as follows

$$V_e = \tilde{F}I_m \qquad (7)$$

where V_e is the $n_e \times 1$ electrode potential vector and I_m is the $n_m \times 1$ muscle current vector.

Since the number of electrodes is always higher than the number of muscles, the problem is over-determined. A minimum norm approach would therefore lead to unstable solutions. To find a unique solution, a regularization is needed. We assumed that the voltage measured at the sEMG is caused mainly by the activities of big muscles, therefore the regularization is penalizing the activation of muscles with small cross sectional area. The resulting estimated muscles current $\hat{I}_m$ has been therefore calculated as follows:

$$\hat{I}_m = \check{F}^T(\check{F}\check{F}^T + \lambda I)^{-1} V_e \tag{8}$$

where λ is a regularization vector that has been set to the inverse of the cross sectional area of all the muscles.

3.2.2. Validation

A direct evaluation of forearm's muscle activity would entail the use of invasive probe directly inserted on each of the considered muscles. This is obviously practically impossible because of the pain and the discomfort that it would cause to the subject. Therefore, to validate the results indirect methods must be used. In this work we considered two criteria, one qualitatively based on functional prior knowledge and the other quantitatively measuring the fitting on the measured sEMG data on the electrodes' space. To qualitatively evaluate the results from an anatomical point of view, the muscles involved in the examined motor task has been compared to those reported in the literature. In particular the muscles involved in each of the movements are the following:

— Middle finger extension : ED, EDM
— Wrist flexion : FCU, FCR, APL, EDM
— Wrist extension: ECU, ECRL, ECRB, ED
— Ulnar deviation: FCR, FCU, ECR, ECU

The method was evaluated comparing the estimated active muscles with those reported as main responsible by specialized literature [27,28]. A quantitative performance evaluation of the method is conducted comparing the projection of the estimated muscle on the electrode space with the measured sEMG, to express the amount of the sEMG information that is explained by the estimated activity. The Goodness of Fit (GOF) is evaluated using the Normalized Root Mean Square Error (NRMSE) defined as follows:

$$GOF = 1 - NRMSE = \frac{RMSE}{max - min}. \tag{9}$$

With this definition, a value of GOF close to 1 indicates a higher fitting on the experimental sEMG data, with 1 indicating a perfect fit. Lower values indicates lower fitting performance.

4. Results

The results of the segmentation and registration process are represented in Figure 6. Each muscle is represented with a different color and the projection of the electrodes on the skin is represented with a dot and a number indicating the sequential order of the electrodes.

The RMS profile of the sEMG for the studied isometric tasks at 50% of the MVC are depicted with polar plots in Figure 7. Each tasks is shown with different line color. For the sake of clarity the polar plots were created assuming that the arm section is circular and that it is divided into $n_e + 1$ sectors by n_e electrodes arranged with equal space between each other. The value of the RMS voltage is represented with a circle on the line. Each subject has a different number of electrodes depending on the size of the forearm. To better identify the position of the electrodes, the portion of the cross section area with extensor muscles (posterior side) and flexor muscles (anterior side) are depicted with a different background color on the section, respectively with in red and green.

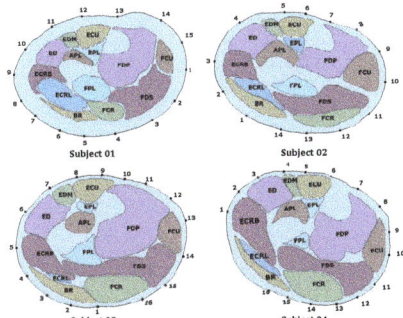

Figure 6. Results of the segmentation on muscles and registration of electrodes position on the 2D image plane of the MRI slice. In each MRI slice the following muscles can be identified: Abductor Pollicis Longus (APL), Extensor Pollicis Longus (EPL), Brachioradialis (BR), Extensor Digitorum (ED), Extensor Carpi Radialis Longus (ECRL), Extensor Carpi Radialis Brevis (ECRB), Extensor Carpi Ulnaris (ECU), Extensor Digiti Minimi (EDM), Flexor Digitorum Profundis (FDP), Flexor Digitorum Superficialis (FDS), Flexor Carpi Ulnaris (FCU), Flexor Carpi Radialis (FCR).

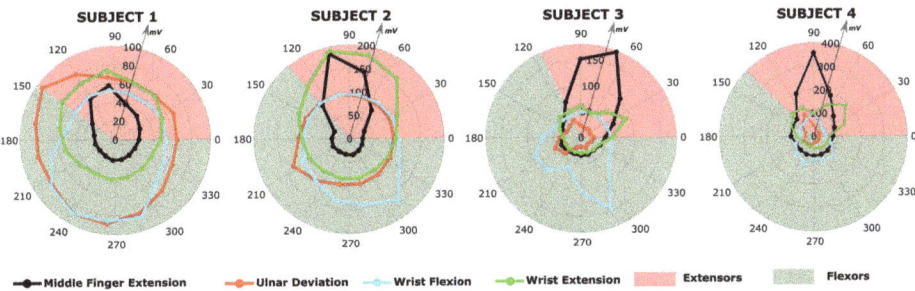

Figure 7. sEMG RMS profile for the four considered tasks at 50% MVC for all the subjects. Each isometric task profile is represented with a different color with a circle indicating the local value measured on the electrode. The electrodes are assumed to be equally distributed around the circumference of the cross section of the forearm. The posterior and anterior side, corresponding to the sectors where extensor and flexors muscles are located, are represented with different background color.

The first two subjects have similar RMS values with similar RMS sEMG profiles along the circumference, while subject 3 and 4 have a higher RMS value for the middle finger extension. For each of the tasks it is possible to observe a subjective sEMG profile around the arm.

The results of the current estimation procedure and the relative voltages reprojected on the electrodes' space are reported in Figure 8 and in Figure 9 for tasks at 25% MVC and 50% MVC, respectively. For each subject and given task, the top graph represents the estimated currents generated by each of the muscle node, while the lower graph represents the reprojected voltage on the electrode space compared to the measured sEMG. The bar on the top graph represents the average current estimated for the generators on each muscle node for all the 11 contractions considered and are coloured based on their function. On the lower plot, the black dotted line represents the projection of the estimated currents on the voltage space whereas the measured sEMG is represented with a dashed red line. The background color is represented with red for electrodes on the anterior side, i.e., electrodes over flexor muscles, and green for electrodes on the posterior side, i.e., electrodes over extensor muscles. The number of electrodes is different for each subject and the number of electrodes of the anterior or posterior side changes depending on the subject.

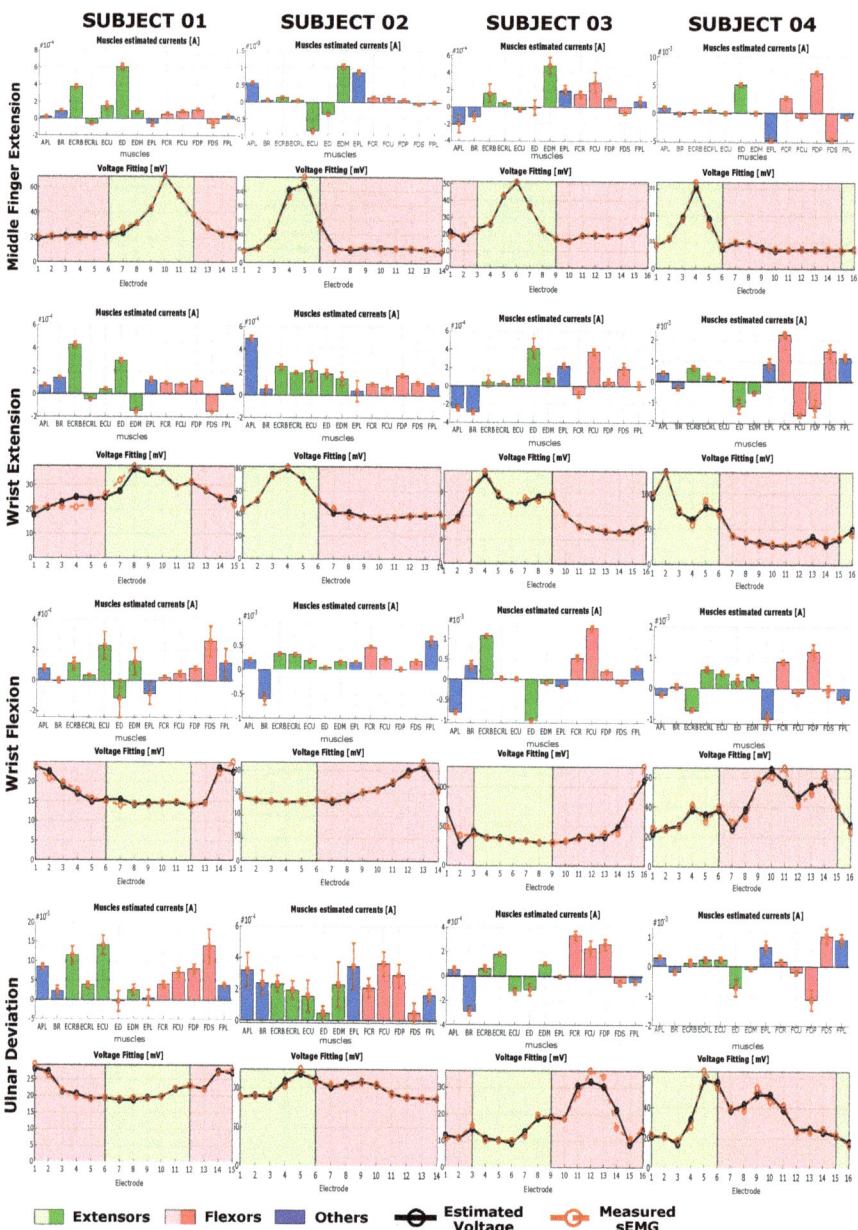

Figure 8. Estimated currents and voltage fitting on the electrodes space for all the tasks considered at 25% of MVC. Each bar represents the average current estimated for a muscle for 11 repetitions. The bar is coloured in green for extensors and in red for flexors. Muscles that are not mainly involved in the considered movements according to anatomy are colored in blue. On the electrodes space, the measured sEMG is represented with a red dotted line, whereas one example of the estimated value is represented with a solid black line. The background color is green for electrodes over the posterior side of the forearm (extensors) and is red for electrodes over the anterior side of the forearm (flexors). For further information on the meaning of the abbreviation of the muscles and their position refer to Figure 6.

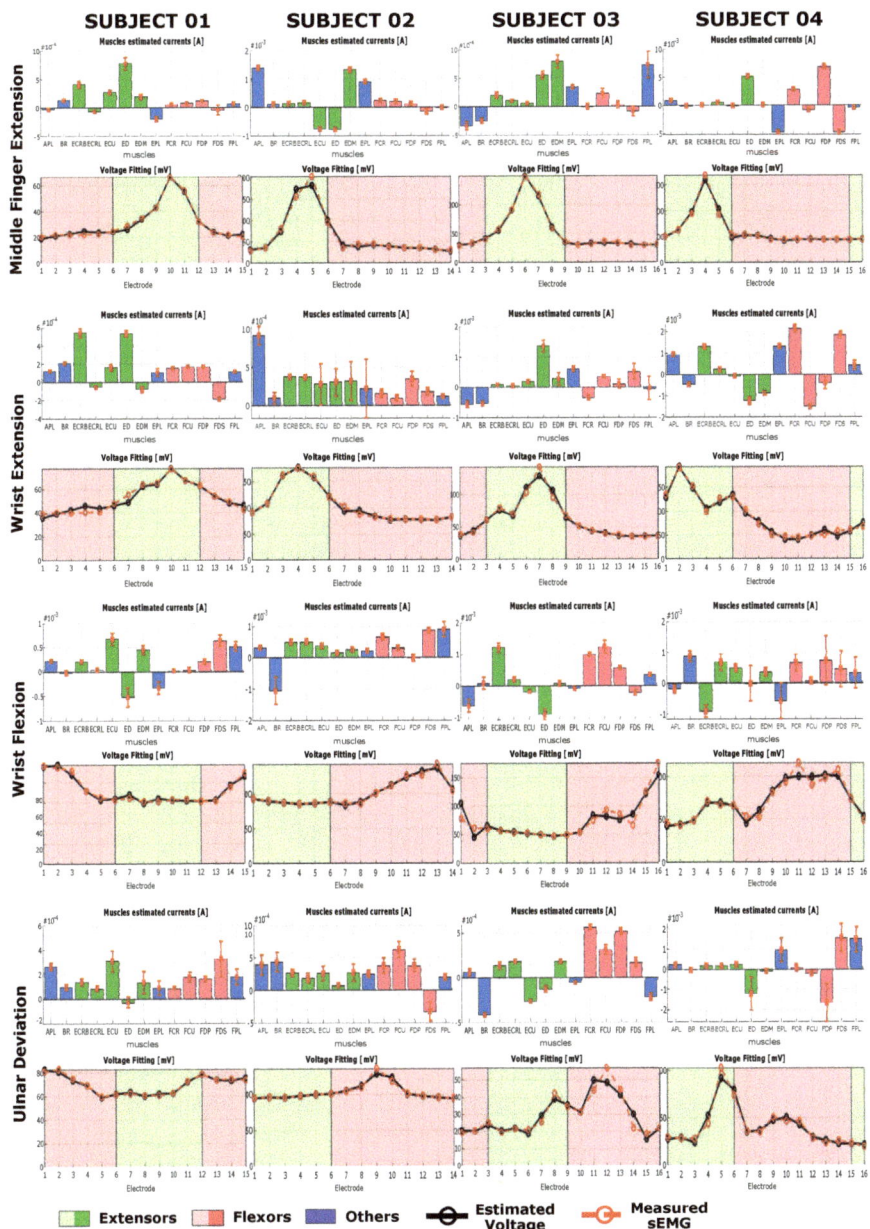

Figure 9. Estimated currents and voltage fitting on the electrodes space for all the tasks considered at 50% of MVC. Each bar represents the average current estimated for a muscle for 11 repetitions. The bar is coloured in green for extensors and in red for flexors. Muscles that are not mainly involved in the considered movements according to anatomy are colored in blue. On the electrodes space, the measured sEMG is represented with a red dotted line, whereas one example of the estimated value is represented with a solid black line. The background color is green for electrodes over the posterior side of the forearm (extensors) and is red for electrodes over the anterior side of the forearm (flexors). For further information on the meaning of the abbreviation of the muscles and their position refer to Figure 6.

A quantitative evaluation of the voltage fitting onto the electrodes space is reported with GOF values in Table 2 with the average value and the standard deviations over the 11 tasks considered.

Table 2. Goodness of Fit (GOF) value of the reconstructed sEMG value on the electrode space in terms of Normalized Root Mean Square Error (NRMSE).

	Subject 01	Subject 02	Subject 03	Subject 04
middle fing. ext (25% MVC)	96.64 ± 0.41%	95.95 ± 0.39%	96.22 ± 1.27%	97.90 ± 0.17%
middle fing. ext (50% MVC)	97.06 ± 0.55%	95.81 ± 0.34%	98.18 ± 0.26%	98.01 ± 0.09%
ulnar deviation (25% MVC)	94.18 ± 0.57%	94.32 ± 1.60%	90.51 ± 0.43%	95.45 ± 0.53%
ulnar deviation (50% MVC)	96.27 ± 1.34%	95.45 ± 0.84%	89.63 ± 0.67%	96.80 ± 0.53%
wrist ext (25% MVC)	88.94 ± 0.73%	96.43 ± 0.74%	94.55 ± 1.42%	96.27 ± 0.23%
wrist ext (50% MVC)	92.48 ± 0.67%	96.37 ± 0.60%	95.11 ± 1.73%	97.00 ± 0.40%
wrist flex (25% MVC)	93.05 ± 1.67%	95.45 ± 0.44%	91.25 ± 0.45%	90.91 ± 0.90%
wrist flex (50% MVC)	92.91 ± 1.08%	94.78 ± 0.50%	89.25 ± 0.96%	91.46 ± 0.72%

5. Discussion

Observing the plots in Figures 8 and 9 for each of the tasks, the inter-subject and inter-task differences can be seen [29–31]. For a given task, however, the group of muscles involved is not significantly changing between subjects, but it is possible to observe subjective characteristics in muscle activation. No significant changes can be observed in the activation pattern between different force level.

Each of the tasks shows specific muscle activation pattern that are in most of the case in agreement with what is reported in the anatomical literature. Each of the subject shows a subjective variation on the task activation pattern, especially for middle finger extension, (MFE), wrist extension (WE) and wrist flexion (WF) (Figures 8 and 9). Ulnar deviation (UD) shows a higher variability among subjects in both the estimated muscle pattern and in the input sEMG. UD could have a marked variability between subject depending upon the prono-supination and wrist flexion extension angle at which the subject have their neutral position. For a slightly flexed wrist, activation of the flexor muscles will be higher during ulnar deviation when compared to slightly extended wrist.

During middle finger extension (MFE), for all subjects and in both force conditions a clear peak activity was registered on one or two extensor muscles, and for all subjects there was at least one muscle active among ED and EDM, indicated in the literature as major responsible for that task. In particular, looking at both Figures 8 and 9, for subject 1 there is a peak on ED with a lower peak on ECRB, on subject 2 there are peaks on EDM and EPL and a negative peak also on ECU, on subject 3 there is a clear peak on EDM, while on subject 4 the peaks are on ED and EPL, with this last one negative. During WE it is possible to observe a general activation of extensor muscles on all subject, with subject 1 showing a peak activation of ECRL and ED, subjects 2 showing a more homogenous activation among all extensors and subject 3 and 4 showing a sparse activation with clear peaks on, respectively ED for subject 3 and on ED and EDM for subject 4. On subject 2 a peak on APL can be observed as well. APL is not actively involved in the extension task but its activation can be due to the fact that the subject tried to spread the hand fingers, including the thumb, during the extension of the wrist. The fact that the activation pattern for subject 2, unlike the other subjects, is homogeneous among all extensors might indicates that the subject extended the fingers while trying to extend the wrist.

During WF, it is possible to observe a peak activation on FDS on subject 1, peaks on FCR, FCU, and FPL on subject 2, peaks on FCR and FCU for subject 3 while for subject 4 there is only a peak on FCR and FPD. These results are in accordance to the anatomical knowledge, and each of the subject uses a different muscle among the possible ones to perform the same task. Subject 2 shows an additional significant activation of BR, indicating that, probably, during the flexion of the wrist the subject also tried to flex the forearm around the elbow joint.

For ulnar deviation (UD) results are according to anatomical knowledge in the case of subject 1, 2, and 3. In fact it is possible to observe peaks on either one or both of ECU and FCU. Subject 4 presents an activation on ED, EPL and FDP, while muscles that are indicated as main responsible for UD i.e., ECU, FCU, FCR, ECRL, ECRB, show a lower activation level. Observing the measured sEMG of UD for subject 4, it shows a different shape compared to the other subjects, indicating that the difference might be due to a subjective muscle activation pattern characteristic of that subject.

Observing both the estimated muscle activation profile (Figures 8 and 9) and the measured sEMG profile (Figure 7) around the forearm, each of the subjects perform each of the task in a characteristic way. Observing the input sEMG profiles it can be noted that for a chosen task there are important differences among subjects. The difference in the morphology of the forearm could explain different muscle patterns estimation. In the case of MFE, observing the sEMG profiles in Figure 7, it can be noticed that a similar profile shape among subjects is shared, where a single peak in the posterior side of the forearm muscles is present. For subject 2 the activation peak is shifted more toward the muscles on the anterior side, which might justify higher peaks on EDM and EPL. This means that all subjects performed the MFE in approximately the same way, activating either the same muscles or group of muscles around the same section of the forearm. On the other hand, a different relative activation is present, based on how the neural system of each subject adapted to perform that specific task. In the case of WE and WF, subject 1 and 2 show a measured voltage with a smoother profile around the arm, whereas subject 3 and subject 4 present a more irregular profile with a biphasic behaviour. An even bigger difference can be observed for UD, where subject 1 and 2 present a rather smooth and flat sEMG with a peak on the flexor side of the arm, while subject 3 and 4 presents clear peaks. In particular subject 4 showed a biphashic sEMG profile with voltage peaks measured around electrodes 5 and 10 (Figures 8 and 9). Since UD, due to the nature of the movement, involves both extensor and flexor muscles, it can be seen that in general the peaks in the sEMG profiles are around the boundary area between extensor and flexors. However, each of the subjects present a characteristic shape, indicating that for this movement the muscle pattern might change significantly between subjects. The reason behind this apparent difference in the sEMG profile might be the position of the forearm with respect to the neutral position of each subject during the experiment. The supination angle of the forearm during the data collection might not have been perfectly horizontal causing a different activation of muscles.

Comparing the muscle signal patterns between 25% and 50% MVC conditions (Figures 8 and 9), they remain almost unchanged. This means that each subject maintain their specific muscle activation strategy among different force conditions. Each of the subjects therefore keeps activating the same muscles with the same strategy at different force levels, increasing the overall muscle activity of the involved muscles, without using other muscles or changing activation pattern. The method is therefore robust to different force conditions for the same task. However, it is important to notice that the force conditions and the choice of ignoring the first and the last repetition were meant to minimize the risk of having adaptation and fatigue effects. In fact, in case of adaptation and fatigue conditions the activated muscle pattern might undergo changes due to a varying muscle recruitment pattern from the CNS [32–35].

The projection of the estimated current on the electrodes potential space fits the measured sEMG with a GOF over 90% for almost all of the task considered in both force conditions (Table 2). Thus, the currents estimated with the proposed model are able to explain on average more than 90% of the information enclosed in the RMS of the measured sEMG. Exceptions are WE for subject 1 at 25% MVC and WF and UD at 50%MVC for subject4, where GOF is slightly under 90%.

In different cases it is possible to observe a simultaneous activation of both agonist and antagonistic muscles, i.e., flexors and extensors, thus co-contraction is happening. Furthermore, it is worth noting that in several cases, such as MFE, WE, UD for subject 4, MFE and WE for subject 1 or WE, WF, and UD for subject 3, currents with opposite signals are estimated for antagonistic muscles. Therefore, we hypothesised that the sign of the current is indicating the direction of the power exerted by the muscles. That would mean that the sign of the current is giving mechanical information of the system, such as the type of contraction of the muscles, which can be concentric or eccentric. The estimated voltages at the muscles nodes were all positive, therefore the sign of the electrical power of the network was defined by the sign of the currents. This is however, does not seem to be valid in general, probably because of the fact that for this work only an average behaviour has been considered. A study on the time series estimation of muscle pattern would help supporting this hypothesis and it will be further considered in the future.

Overall the results show that, for a chosen task, a small signal variance is estimated among tasks repetition. Thus, on average, each of the task has been performed in the same manner by the subject. However, such as for UD at 50% MVC for subject 2 or WF at 50% MVC for subject 4, the estimated patterns show a higher variability, indicating that at each of the repetition significant differences in the contraction were happening.

The number of electrodes was different for all the subjects because of the different circumferences of each of the subject's forearms. The electrode sheets were therefore able to cover a different amount of the forearm circumference as it can be observed in Figure 6. Subject 1 and subject 3 show a uniform coverage of the forearm surface with 15 and 16 electrodes respectively. Subject 2 and subject 4 present regions that are not covered with electrodes. In particular, for subject 2 the density of electrodes is lower over the extensor side of the forearm, while for subject 4 there were fewer than two electrodes directly over BR, ECRL, and ECRB. For subject 2, the lower electrode density over the extensor side of the forearm might be responsible for the higher activation of APL observed during WE. The fact that only one electrode is collecting the information above ED and APL might have mislead the inverse algorithm in the estimation of the activation pattern. On subject 4, the width of the area not covered with electrodes is bigger than that of other subjects. In particular, between the electrodes 1 and 16, no electrodes is directly over ECRL. This does not seem to influence too much the estimation of the results for MFE, WF and UD, since, observing Figures 8 and 9, the sEMG values on electrodes 1 and 16 are low and of similar values. Since anatomically BR, ECRB and ECRL are not involved in these tasks, we can assume that the sEMG values in the electrode missing would be similar to that measured on electrodes 1 and 16. However, in the case of WE, ECRB and ECRL are muscles involved in the task. Observing the sEMG values on electrodes 1 and 16, they show a different amplitude. Therefore, it may be presumed that between electrode 1 and 16 the sEMG value is not low. As a consequence, the lack of electrodes in that forearm portion might have caused a loss of information that influenced the muscle pattern estimation for WE.

Finally, it is important to notice that in this work, the role of the skin conductance was ignored. Skin is known to have a strong low-pass filtering effect on the sEMG signal. Since only the average behaviour was considered, we think that for the purpose of this paper, this did not have a big influence on the results. However, it is important to notice that it might have an influence on the general amplitude of the estimated currents, since the conductivity value of the skin is significantly lower than that of muscles and of fat tissue. For this reason, the value of the single muscle current cannot be considered a precise estimation of the muscle activity. However, the relative activation among muscles remain unvaried in the estimation process. With this work, we rather want to show new simple way to estimate the activation pattern of a set of muscles rather than focusing on the single muscles.

6. Conclusions

We presented a novel method for the estimation of muscle activity. The activity was quantified using the muscle current estimated in an electrical system created from subject specific MRI images. The model is able to provide an estimation of the relative activation for a set of muscles identified within an MRI section of the forearm, through the construction of a purely resistive electrical model of the conductive volume depicted in the slice. The results highlighted some interesting properties of the method in the estimation of subject muscle activation patterns for potential rehabilitation applications. For the same task the estimated pattern were similar among subjects, but subjective activation features can still be observed among subjects, showing that the proposed method is able to capture anatomically valid muscle activation maintaining a subjectivity in the results that allows a comparison between different subjects. The input sEMG profiles changed with subject, reflecting the fact that each of the subject has a personal signature in the activation pattern, even if each of the single muscle maintain its properties and role. The proposed method is able to cope with this variability rearranging the muscle activation pattern to explain the input sEMG with a valid current pattern. Furthermore, the muscle patterns are not changing between different force levels, indicating that changes in the signal amplitude are not perturbing the estimated pattern. The estimated currents are able to explain over 90% of the input sEMG and the results have an anatomical meaning based on specialized literature and physiological consideration. The number of electrodes and their distribution might have had an influence in the estimation results. For two of the subjects the electrode density was lower in particular sections and this might have lead to different interpretation of the sEMG in the solution of the inverse problem.

With this work we wanted to introduce a novel idea for solving the problem of estimating deep muscle activities. We used a simple electrical model, providing results obtained using a dataset acquired from healthy subjects. The proposed model inherently includes information about each of the subject inner morphology described in a simple and intuitive way. Furthermore, the rules defined for the model construction and for the estimation can be easily automatized making the translation of the presented logic into a software routine with a low number of parameters.

The results shows that, for most of the task considered, the estimated muscle patterns are anatomically plausible. For simple static tasks, such as MFE, the estimated pattern, even if with a clear difference among subjects, provides an activation pattern that matches what is reported in the literature. In case of WE and WF, most of the case considered are anatomically consistent. However, some isolated results are uncertain. For UD, subject 1 and 2 shows valid results, while subject 4 shows different results, most likely due to a different sEMG profile around the arm, which indicate a different overall muscle activation, or an insufficient number of electrodes.

Several aspects of the model can still be improved, starting from the modeling to the estimation algorithm. In this work, we rather wanted to focus on the presentation of a different approach to exploits both information from MRI and sEMG to build a model able to solve the problem of muscle activity estimation, with a validation on a pool of healthy subject and with different movements in order to assess the performance that can be achieved with a simple and intuitive modeling. The impossibility to have a ground truth remain a challenging part for the validation of the method and it will be addressed in subsequent works with the aid of tools such as musculoskeletal modeling and simulations, even if the strong subjectivity of the muscle pattern activation is a point that makes the problem of a solid validation very challenging. A possible solution would be the use of ultrasound imaging during the execution of tasks. Using the ultrasounds it would be in fact possible to capture the thickness changes in all muscles, including deep ones. The thickness of muscles is related to its activation [36,37] providing a direct mean to validate the results. The RMS of the sEMG during contraction was considered for this work in order to give an average estimation of the behaviour of the muscles during the selected tasks. The introduction of the study on the time dimension would allow observing the contraction strategies of the muscles during the task execution. Furthermore, the subject pool was limited to four participants in this work. All these issues will be addressed in future developments of the proposed method.

We believe that this method can be a valid way for overcoming the limitations of the mfMRI, allowing the estimation of muscle activation with a temporal resolution that would improve the information quality for clinicians in the diagnostic process. In particular, we believe that the proposed method can make an important contribution in the field of rehabilitation allowing to track muscle activation pattern on impaired subject during rehabilitative cycles considering the underlying morphology of the patient and eventual changes that might happen over time due to a pathological situation. The proposed model relies completely on anatomical and physiological information and is therefore easy to understand for clinical personnel, providing results that are giving a direct quantification of the muscle activation. The dimensions of the model are low and this allow a fast estimation process, potentially allowing a real time tracking of the muscle activity, once the model is created from the subject MRI. For this reason, it is a suitable method to acheive a general overview of the neuromuscular system activation status during rehabilitative exercises and therapies, potentially allowing therapists to assess the reaction and the effectiveness of the rehabilitation strategy on the patients.

Author Contributions: Conceptualization and Methodology, E.P., D.P. and S.S.; Software and Analysis, E.P.; Experiment Design: B.S., MRI dataset: N.Y. and Y.O.; sEMG data collection: B.S. and S.S.; writing—original draft preparation, E.P.; Supervision, J.O. All authors have read and agreed to the published version of the manuscript.

Funding: This work was partially supported by JSPS KAKENHI "Modelling of hyper adaptability in human postural control considering the role of neurotransmitters" Grant Number 19H05730.

Conflicts of Interest: The authors declare no conflict of interest.

References

1. Cagnie, B.; Elliott, J.; O'Leary, S.; D'Hooge, R.; Dickx, N.; Danneels, L. Muscle functional MRI as an imaging tool to evaluate muscle activity. *J. Orthop. Sport. Phys. Ther.* **2011**, *41*, 896–903. [CrossRef]
2. Franettovich Smith, M.; Collins, N.; Vicenzino, B. Intrinsic foot muscle atrophy in individuals with chronic plantar heel pain: a cross-sectional investigation using ultrasound imaging. *J. Sci. Med. Sport* **2019**, *22*, S17. [CrossRef]
3. Goubert, D.; De Pauw, R.; Meeus, M.; Willems, T.; Cagnie, B.; Schouppe, S.; Van Oosterwijck, J.; Dhondt, E.; Danneels, L. Lumbar muscle structure and function in chronic versus recurrent low back pain: A cross-sectional study. *Spine J.* **2017**, *17*, 1285–1296. [CrossRef]
4. Mayer, J.M.; Graves, J.E.; Clark, B.C.; Formikell, M.; Ploutz-Snyder, L.L. The use of magnetic resonance imaging to evaluate lumbar muscle activity during trunk extension exercise at varying intensities. *Spine* **2005**, *30*, 2556–2563. [CrossRef]
5. Dickx, N.; D'Hooge, R.; Cagnie, B.; Deschepper, E.; Verstraete, K.; Danneels, L. Magnetic resonance imaging and electromyography to measure lumbar back muscle activity. *Spine* **2010**, *35*, 836–842. [CrossRef]
6. De Ridder, E.M.; Van Oosterwijck, J.O.; Vleeming, A.; Vanderstraeten, G.G.; Danneels, L.A. Muscle functional MRI analysis of trunk muscle recruitment during extension exercises in asymptomatic individuals. *Scand. J. Med. Sci. Sport.* **2015**, *25*, 196–204. [CrossRef] [PubMed]
7. Fernandez-Gonzalo, R.; Tesch, P.A.; Linnehan, R.M.; Kreider, R.B.; Di Salvo, V.; Suarez-Arrones, L.; Alomar, X.; Mendez-Villanueva, A.; Rodas, G. Individual Muscle use in Hamstring Exercises by Soccer Players Assessed using Functional MRI. *Int. J. Sports Med.* **2016**, *37*, 559–564. [CrossRef] [PubMed]
8. Kinugasa, R.; Akima, H. Neuromuscular activation of triceps surae using muscle functional MRI and EMG. *Med. Sci. Sports Exercise* **2005**, *37*, 593–598. [CrossRef] [PubMed]
9. Adams, G.R.; Duvoisin, M.R.; Dudley, G.A. Magnetic resonance imaging and electromyography as indexes of muscle function. *Eur. J. Appl. Physiol.* **1992**, *73*, 1578–1583. [CrossRef] [PubMed]
10. Drew, M.K.; Trease, L.; Caneiro, J.P.; Hooper, I.; Ooi, C.C.; Counsel, P.; Connell, D.A.; Rice, A.A.; Knight, E.; Hoy, G.; et al. Normative MRI, ultrasound and muscle functional MRI findings in the forearms of asymptomatic elite rowers. *J. Sci. Med. Sport* **2016**, *19*, 103–108. [CrossRef]
11. Castelein, B.; Cools, A.; Parlevliet, T.; Cagnie, B. The influence of induced shoulder muscle pain on rotator cuff and scapulothoracic muscle activity during elevation of the arm. *J. Shoulder Elb. Surg.* **2017**, *26*, 497–505. [CrossRef] [PubMed]
12. Kumagai, M.; Shiba, N.; Higuchi, F.; Nishimura, H.; Inoue, A. Functional evaluation of hip abductor muscles with use of magnetic resonance imaging. *J. Orthop. Res.* **1997**, *15*, 888–893. [CrossRef] [PubMed]
13. Price, T.B.; Kamen, G.; Damon, B.M.; Knight, C.A.; Applegate, B.; Gore, J.C.; Eward, K.; Signorile, J.F. Comparison of MRI with EMG to study muscle activity associated with dynamic plantar flexion. *Magn. Reson. Imaging* **2003**, *21*, 853–861. [CrossRef]
14. Merletti, R.; Botter, A.; Troiano, A.; Merlo, E.; Minetto, M.A. Technology and instrumentation for detection and conditioning of the surface electromyographic signal: State of the art. *Clin. Biomech.* **2009**, *24*, 122–134. [CrossRef] [PubMed]

15. Farina, D.; Holobar, A.; Merletti, R.; Enoka, R.M. Decoding the neural drive to muscles from the surface electromyogram. *Clin. Neurophysiol.* **2010**, *121*, 1616–1623. [CrossRef] [PubMed]
16. Holobar, A.; Minetto, M.A.; Farina, D. Accurate identification of motor unit discharge patterns from high-density surface EMG and validation with a novel signal-based performance metric. *J. Neural Eng.* **2014**, *11*. [CrossRef] [PubMed]
17. Holobar, A.; Farina, D.; Gazzoni, M.; Merletti, R.; Zazula, D. Estimating motor unit discharge patterns from high-density surface electromyogram. *Clin. Neurophysiol.* **2009**, *120*, 551–562. [CrossRef]
18. Nakajima, Y.; Keeratihattayakorn, S.; Yoshinari, S.; Tadano, S. An EMG-CT method using multiple surface electrodes in the forearm. *J. Electromyogra. Kines.* **2014**, *24*, 875–880. [CrossRef]
19. Su, B.; Shirafuji, S.; Oya, T.; Ogata, Y.; Funato, T.; Yoshimura, N.; Pion-Tonachini, L.; Makeig, S.; Seki, K.; Ota, J. Source separation and localization of individual superficial forearm extensor muscles using high-density surface electromyography. In Proceedings of the 2016 International Symposium on Micro-NanoMechatronics and Human Science (MHS), Nagoya, Japan, 28–30 November 2016; pp. 1–7. [CrossRef]
20. Piovanelli, E.; Piovesan, D.; Shirafuji, S.; Ota, J. A Simple Method to Estimate Muscle Currents from HD-sEMG and MRI using Electrical Network and Graph Theory. In Proceedings of the 2019 41st Annual International Conference of the IEEE Engineering in Medicine and Biology Society (EMBC), Berlin, Germany, 23–27 July 2019; pp. 2657–2662. [CrossRef]
21. Piovanelli, E.; Piovesan, D.; Shirafuji, S.; Ota, J. Estimating Deep Muscles Activation from High Density Surface EMG using Graph Theory. In Proceedings of the 2019 IEEE 16th International Conference on Rehabilitation Robotics (ICORR), Toronto, ON, Canada, 24–28 June 2019; pp. 3–8.
22. Schneider, C.A.; Rasband, W.S.; Eliceri, K.W. NIH Image to ImageJ: 25 years of Image Analysis. *Nat. Methods* **2012**, *9*, 671–675. [CrossRef]
23. Kikinis R, Pieper S.; Vosburgh, K.G. 3D Slicer: A platform for subject-specific image analysis, visualization, and clinical support. In *Intraoperative Imaging Image-Guided Therapy*; Jolesz, F.A., Ed.; ; Springer Science & Business Media: Berlin, Germany, 2014; 277–289
24. Horn, B.K.P. Closed-form solution of absolute orientation using unit quaternions. *J. Opt. Soc. Am. A* **1987**, pp. 629–642. [CrossRef]
25. Lowery, M.M.; Stoykov, N.S.; Dewald, J.P.A.; Kuiken, T.A. Volume Conduction in an Anatomically Based Surface EMG Model. *IEEE Trans. Biomed. Eng.* **2004**, *51*, 2138–2147. [CrossRef] [PubMed]
26. Dorfler, F.; Simpson-Porco, J.W.; Bullo, F. Electrical Networks and Algebraic Graph Theory: Models, Properties, and Applications. *Proc. IEEE* **2018**, *106*, 977–1005, . [CrossRef]
27. Kapandji, A.I. *The Physiology of the Joints*, 7th ed.; Handspring Publishing: Scotland, UK, 2019.
28. Platzer, W. *Color Atlas of Human Anatomy, Vol.1 Locomotor System*, 7th ed.; Thieme Medical Publishers: Stuttgart, Germany, 2015.
29. Kristiansen, M.; Madeleine, P.; Hansen, E.A.; Samani, A. Inter-subject variability of muscle synergies during bench press in power lifters and untrained individuals. *Scand. J. Med. Sci. Sport.* **2015**, *25*, 89–97. [CrossRef] [PubMed]
30. Hug, F.; Bendahan, D.; Le Fur, Y.; Cozzone, P.J.; Grélot, L. Heterogeneity of muscle recruitment pattern during pedaling in professional road cyclists: A magnetic resonance imaging and electromyography study. *Eur. J. Appl. Physiol.* **2004**, *92*, 334–342. [CrossRef] [PubMed]
31. Araujo, R.C.; Duarte, M.; Amadio, A.C. On the inter- and intra-subject variability of the electromyographic signal in isometric contractions. *Electromyogr. Clin. Neurophysiol.* **2000**, *40*, 225–230.
32. Edwards, R.G.; Lippold, O.C. The Relation Between Force and Electrical Activity in Fatigued Muscle. *J. Physiol.* **1956**, 677–681. [CrossRef]
33. Naeije, M.; Zorn, H. Relation between EMG power spectrum shifts and muscle fibre action potential conduction velocity changes during local muscular fatigue in man. *Eur. J. Appl. Physiol. Occup. Physiol.* **1982**, *50*, 23–33. [CrossRef]
34. Moritani, T.; Nagata, A.; Muro, M. Electromyographic manifestations of muscular fatigue. *Med. Sci. Sports Exerc.* **1982**, *14*, 198–202 [CrossRef]
35. Gandevia, S.C. Spinal and supraspinal factors in human muscle fatigue. *Physiol. Rev.* **2001**, *81*, 1725–1789. [CrossRef]

36. Colby Mangum, L.; Henderson, K.; Murray, K.P.; Saliba, S.A. Ultrasound assessment of the transverse abdominis during functional movement. *J. Ultrasound Med.* **2018**, *37*, 1225–1231. [CrossRef]
37. Fukunaga, T.; Miyatani, M.; Tachi, M.; Kouzaki, M.; Kawakami, Y.; Kanehisa, H. Muscle volume is a major determinant of joint torque in humans. *Acta Physiol. Scand.* **2001**, *172*, 249–255. [CrossRef] [PubMed]

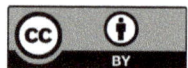

© 2020 by the authors. Licensee MDPI, Basel, Switzerland. This article is an open access article distributed under the terms and conditions of the Creative Commons Attribution (CC BY) license (http://creativecommons.org/licenses/by/4.0/).

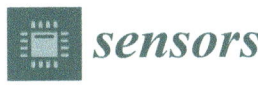

Article

Automated Home Oxygen Delivery for Patients with COPD and Respiratory Failure: A New Approach

Daniel Sanchez-Morillo [1,2,*], Pilar Muñoz-Zara [1,3], Alejandro Lara-Doña [1,2] and Antonio Leon-Jimenez [1,3]

1. Biomedical Research and Innovation Institute of Cadiz (INiBICA), 11009 Cadiz, Spain; pilarmz89@gmail.com (P.M.-Z.); alejandro.lara@uca.es (A.L.-D.); anleji@hotmail.es (A.L.-J.)
2. Biomedical Engineering and Telemedicine Research Group, Department of Automation Engineering, Electronics and Computer Architecture and Networks, University of Cadiz, 11519 Puerto Real, Cadiz, Spain
3. Pulmonology, Allergy and Thoracic Surgery Unit, Puerta del Mar University Hospital, 11009 Cadiz, Spain
* Correspondence: daniel.morillo@uca.es

Received: 3 January 2020; Accepted: 18 February 2020; Published: 20 February 2020

Abstract: Long-term oxygen therapy (LTOT) has become standard care for the treatment of patients with chronic obstructive pulmonary disease (COPD) and other severe hypoxemic lung diseases. The use of new portable O_2 concentrators (POC) in LTOT is being expanded. However, the issue of oxygen titration is not always properly addressed, since POCs rely on proper use by patients. The robustness of algorithms and the limited reliability of current oximetry sensors are hindering the effectiveness of new approaches to closed-loop POCs based on the feedback of blood oxygen saturation. In this study, a novel intelligent portable oxygen concentrator (iPOC) is described. The presented iPOC is capable of adjusting the O_2 flow automatically by real-time classifying the intensity of a patient's physical activity (PA). It was designed with a group of patients with COPD and stable chronic respiratory failure. The technical pilot test showed a weighted accuracy of 91.1% in updating the O_2 flow automatically according to medical prescriptions, and a general improvement in oxygenation compared to conventional POCs. In addition, the usability achieved was high, which indicated a significant degree of user satisfaction. This iPOC may have important benefits, including improved oxygenation, increased compliance with therapy recommendations, and the promotion of PA.

Keywords: COPD; oxygen concentrator; oxygen therapy; automatic oxygen concentrator; physical activity; machine learning; respiratory medicine; portable oxygen concentrator; oxygen delivery

1. Introduction

Oxygen is a substantial element in the sustenance of human life. Of the hundreds of tasks that oxygen performs in the human body, two stand out for their importance: detoxification and energy production. However, some diseases affect the ability of the lungs to perform the gas exchange necessary to incorporate oxygen into the bloodstream and to release carbon dioxide. In many situations, extra oxygen is needed when the respiratory system cannot maintain an adequate pulmonary exchange of physiological gases. This therapeutic use of supplemental oxygen is defined as oxygen therapy and it aims at increasing the inspired oxygen fraction (FiO_2). Therefore, when medically prescribed, oxygen is a drug. Oxygen therapy is an established treatment, and it continues to be one of the most important measures in the management patients with progressing chronic respiratory disease. In this case, the main objective of oxygen therapy is to improve tissue oxygenation and to correct the severe hypoxemia that these patients usually present with in the advanced stages of the disease [1,2]. The goal is to maintain oxygenation levels above the range of respiratory failure, defined by an O_2 blood partial pressure [PaO_2] > 60 mmHg, and an oxygen saturation measured by pulse oximetry [$SpO2$] > 90%.

Currently, clinical applications for the use of oxygen have extended beyond the hospital setting. When patients receive oxygen supplementation at home, the therapy is referred to as home oxygen therapy (HOT). HOT provided as long-term oxygen therapy (LTOT), that is, used on a daily basis and at least by 15 h per day, is recommended by current treatment guidelines since it has been shown to be effective in increasing survival in patients with chronic obstructive pulmonary disease (COPD) and respiratory failure [3–6]. In addition, ambulatory oxygen therapy improves physical performance in patients with COPD [7].

Despite all these benefits of HOT for patients with respiratory failure, evidence that supports the prescription of HOT in other chronic conditions associated with hypoxemia is limited [8]. While supplemental oxygen is valuable in clinical situations such as those aforementioned, the inappropriate use of this therapy can be detrimental. Hypoxemia is defined as the decrease in PaO_2 below the normal limits, variable for the subject's age (normal PaO_2 ranges from 80 to 100 mmHg [9]). There is evidence that both hypoxemia and hyperoxemia, which results from exposure to excessive O_2 flows for a prolonged period of time, can have serious consequences for patients with acute and chronic respiratory failure [10,11]. Although the risks for hypoxemia are well known [12], there is growing evidence that excessive oxygen flow can be potentially harmful. In this regard, hyperoxemia has been associated with increased hospital mortality among patients admitted to intensive care units (ICUs) following cardiac arrest resuscitation [13]. In this regard, hyperoxemia may be especially problematic in patients with COPD in the acute phase of exacerbation, because of its association with hypercapnia [14,15] and its potential to mask the onset of a worsening in lung function [10]. In addition, toxicity caused by hyperoxemia in some patients with COPD receiving LTOT has received attention from researchers [16].

Notwithstanding this, all the scientific evidence supports the idea that the proper use of supplemental oxygen therapy is an important factor that can positively influence clinical outcomes in patients with respiratory failure and severe hypoxemia [17].

The administration of LTOT requires devoted delivery devices. The source of oxygen and the equipment for its administration, which will depend on the patient's profile, his/her movability, the flow required, the time needed for oxygen therapy sessions, and above all, the proper correction of SpO_2 both at rest and during sleep or effort are also important factors [18].

Until recently, the most common way to deliver LTOT to patients has been by using static sources, such as stationary oxygen concentrators or high-pressure cylinders. The shortcoming of such devices is that they prevent the patient from wandering or leaving home while therapy is being received. The heightened mobility and physical activity of these patients have resulted in the need for smaller, lighter, and more autonomous portable oxygen devices [19]. For those reasons, a new generation of portable, lightweight devices has emerged in recent years. These devices, known as portable oxygen concentrators (POCs), have sufficient autonomy to enable the patient to live an active life outside the home. Unlike classical gaseous or liquid oxygen devices, POCs produce their own oxygen by removing nitrogen from atmospheric air. Before it goes into the concentrator through the inlet filter, air is composed of 80% nitrogen and 20% oxygen. Firstly, the POC compresses the oxygen using a compressor. The compressed air moves to a sieve bed of filters that separate the nitrogen from the oxygen. Then, the oxygen, now at around 90%–95% purity, is stored in a product tank within the device and is delivered to the patient via a delivery device (i.e., a nasal cannula).

POCs can deliver oxygen via continuous flow or pulse flow. Continuous flow units put out a specific adjustable dose measured in litres per minute. Pulse units pulse air through a cannula with each breath and their output is determined by the size of the individual pulse (millilitres per pulse) and the patient's respiratory rate.

It is accepted that the oxygen flow, normally delivered in fixed doses to patients in oxygen therapy, is not always optimized [19]. In fact, the oxygen requirements of patients under LTOT vary depending on the type, intensity and duration of the physical activity that is being carried out. Low blood oxygen levels may cause short-term symptoms, such as dyspnoea, and physio-pathological organic changes, such as tachycardia, increased respiratory rate, arterial hypertension and, in the long term, serious problems such as pulmonary hypertension and cor pulmonale, among others. On the other hand, excessive levels of blood oxygen can cause hypercapnic encephalopathy in some patients. In this regard, the patients receiving LTOT are generally instructed to adjust the oxygen flow according to the activities of daily living. Oxygen flow is therefore routinely targeted to maintaining the desired oxygenation range. However, this task places a burden on patients that often affects adherence to therapy, and the existing methods of oxygen delivery may not be sufficient when the patient's activity, and therefore the demand of oxygen, increases [20]. It has been reported that patients with COPD and moderate hypoxemia have frequent and eventually significant desaturations during activities of daily living and at night [21].

Adapting oxygen therapy to dynamic patients' needs appears to be a key challenge. Among the primary goals of the dynamic and adaptive oxygen flow adjustment are: (a) the optimization of therapy and safety by minimizing the number of desaturation episodes, preventing periods of hyperoxia and hyperoxia [12]; (b) the customization of the oxygen flow to the individual needs of patients; and (c) oxygen consumption optimization.

In traditional flow oxygen delivery, the titration of oxygen therapy is generally performed manually by selecting the level of oxygen flow [22]. In LTOT, this manual adjustment of oxygen flow is carried out by patients themselves to meet their changing needs. The current POCs have a manual flow regulator that is adjusted by prescription to a specific level of flow measured in litres or pulses. Existing flow regulators modify the flow mechanically, by manipulating a valve, or electronically, by means of a keypad integrated into the device. However, the manually continuous adjustment of the oxygen flow rate is a time-consuming task that requires experienced and trained patients [23], and this can lead to the improper use of the device and consequently to a poor quality flow adjustment during the changing daily activities, which is usually linked to unintended delays and periods of desaturation [24,25]. Given the advanced average age of patients with COPD under LTOT [26], the probability of inadequate use of the device is significant.

Very recently, the abovementioned limitations led to the search for new physiological closed-loop devices (PCLC) that timely adjust oxygen flow rates to the needs of patient automatically [22]. PCLC medical devices use one or several physiological sensors to manipulate a physiological variable autonomously according to the guidelines given by clinicians [27]. Exponents of PCLC in respiratory medicine are the novel intelligent portable oxygen concentrators. Most of the published articles on technologies for PCLC in oxygen therapy for adults are from post-2010, indicating that these devices are a relatively new field in the respiratory speciality. These devices may potentially optimize oxygen therapy, reduce the workload of health professionals, minimise medical error, shorten health care costs, and decrease mortality and morbidity [28,29].

Intelligent POCs include three main components: a system for monitoring the patient's oxygenation, an algorithm to estimate the O_2 flow settings to achieve the targeted oxygenation level, and an O_2 source [20]. Figure 1 depicts the global architecture of a PCLC oxygen therapy device.

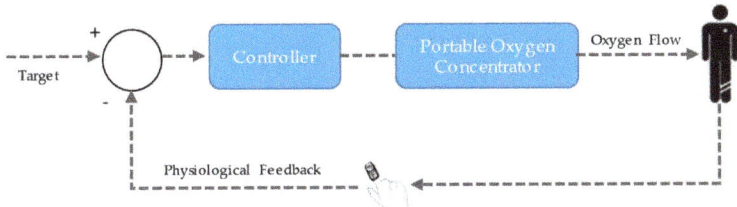

Figure 1. Common architecture of mostly proposed closed-loop portable oxygen concentrators.

In the most common approach, the process variable is selected to be SpO_2, since it is a non-invasive measure that does not require calibration. A recent systematic review reported that SpO_2 (pulse oximeter) was used in 100% of studies on PCLC systems for automatic oxygen delivery in patients with COPD [25]. Concerning the algorithms, the review concluded that continuous control by applying conventional classical proportional-integral-derivative (PID), proportional-integral (PI), and rule-based controllers have been proposed in the context of LTOT systems [30–33]. In these studies, the most significant findings were related to the shortening of hypoxemia and hyperoxemia episodes when PCLCs were used. However, a challenge in these algorithms is related to stability and robustness, associated with the system capacity to discriminate between real abnormal oxygenation events and ghost episodes caused by motion artefacts or a poor-quality oximetry signal. This major challenge has not been overcome, and, at present, there are only a few commercial systems available (i.e., Optisat AccuO2® [34], the O2 Flow Regulator® [33], and the FreeO2® [19]). The existing systems require the patients to be continuously connected to a pulse oximeter, which becomes the primary source of information for the algorithm. Current pulse oximetry technology is marked by the instability of the sensor relating to movements or by the physiological delay in the measurements, which may reduce its clinical effectiveness. Additionally, this technology presents very limited effectiveness in assessing hyperoxia and promptly detecting respiratory depression [22]. Moreover, pulse oximeters are known to be inaccurate in conditions that decrease arterial blood perfusion or cause the presence of elevated concentrations of carboxyhaemoglobin (CoHb) and methaemoglobin (metHb).

As a consequence, the development of innovative physiological sensors and predictors of oxygen desaturations to enable autonomous therapy and support its clinical validity is still an on-going challenge [35].

In addition to technological matters, patient perceptions on usability and adequacy of POCs is an issue. In a recent study, 51% of the patients under LTOT consulted reported oxygen problems related to equipment malfunction, a lack of physically manageable portable systems, and a lack of portable systems with high flow rates [36]. In that study, 44% of respondents referred to the limitations in activities outside the home imposed by inadequate portable oxygen systems.

In summary, despite their potential and the existing end-users (patients) demand, PCLC oxygen therapy devices are scarcely found in real clinical applications. The robustness of control algorithms, the limited reliability of sensors, safety and usability issues, among others, can underlie this lack of clinical implementation [25].

In this work, we propose an alternative approach that enables a POC to be transformed into an intelligent POC (iPOC) to adjust the oxygen flow automatically in patients with COPD and respiratory failure that receive LTOT. The proposed system is based on the automatic classification of the intensity of the patient's physical activity and can adjust the oxygen flow to individual real-time needs autonomously. It is a transdisciplinary work, rooted in the field of respiratory medicine, with contributions from electronics, control theory, computer science and artificial intelligence.

An external portable electronic system was designed and integrated into a commercially available POC. The system comprised two units: 1) a sensor unit attached to the patient, that classifies the physical activity in real-time; and 2) a receiver unit, interfaced to the POC, that adjusts the oxygen flow according to the input from the sensor unit automatically. The algorithm for the automatic recognition of physical activity was trained and validated using machine learning techniques. A circuit was designed to gather data for personalizing models and to evaluate the system performance in a group of patients with COPD and respiratory failure receiving LTOT.

The rest of the paper is organised as follows. Section 2 details the participants, materials, devices and methodology applied to develop the iPOC system and to conduct the experiments. In Section 3, the results achieved are presented and discussed. Finally, Section 4 captures the conclusions and future works.

2. Materials and Methods

2.1. System Architecture and Working Principle

Figure 2 shows the general outline of the proposed iPOC. The closed-loop control was implemented using a SISO (Single Input - Single Output) controller [37]. The control law is defined by a lookup-table controller. The oxygen flow level (output) corresponding to each state of physical activity intensity (y_n) was defined by the pulmonologists and personalised to the needs of each patient according to conventional clinical assessment procedures [38]. The system automatically identifies the intensity of the patient's physical activity by classifying it into one of a 3-class scheme (sedentary, light, and moderate). The intensity of physical activity detected in real-time is communicated to a control unit connected to the POC, which is responsible for adapting the oxygen flow to the level previously calibrated by the physician for each situation. Therefore, when an increase in the intensity of the patient's physical activity is detected, the system manages the automatic increase in oxygen flow. Conversely, when the patient lowers the intensity of the physical activity, the device orders the flow to be decreased to the predetermined level for that new condition. In addition, the automatic dosing device can be deactivated by switching the system to the conventional manual mode. The proposed system comprises a unit for estimating the intensity of the patient's physical activity (sensor unit) and unit for controlling the oxygen supplied flow (control unit). These units where designed iteratively using a patient-centred approach. Each of these elements will be described in more detail in the next subsections.

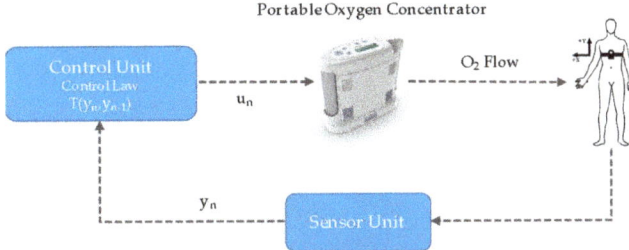

Figure 2. The architecture of the proposed intelligent closed-loop portable oxygen concentrator (*iPOC*).

2.1.1. Sensor Unit

The sensor unit is a portable module placed on the patient's chest. Accelerometer- and gyroscope-based physical monitoring systems have been shown to be able to discriminate between different daily activities [39–42]. Each of these physical activities leads to a different level of energy expenditure, and in patients under LTOT, to different oxygen flow requirements. For the estimation of the intensity of physical activity, an inertial measurement unit (IMU) based on MEMs technology was used. This IMU included a three-axis accelerometer, a triple-axis gyroscope, and a barometer. The signals acquired by the IMU were processed using a microcontroller (MCU) and digital signal processing techniques to extract features useful for discrimination. A classification model, trained and validated using machine learning algorithms, automatically classified the intensity of the activity and transmitted this information wirelessly to the control unit.

The sensor unit incorporated a Mealy finite-state machine (FSM) after the classification stage as a safety mechanism (Figure 3) to prevent abrupt changes in the flow of oxygen (e.g., change of state from a sedentary level to a moderate one or vice versa).

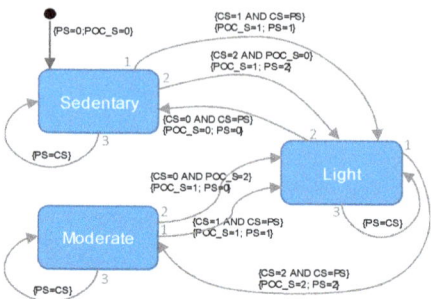

Figure 3. The Mealy finite-state machine included as output layer to provide a supplementary safety mechanism in the automatic delivery of oxygen flow. PS: Previous state; POC_S: Portable Oxygen Concentrator State; CS: Current state.

In order to conduct the research, two prototypes of the sensor unit were developed, each with different purposes and requirements. The first prototype was designed to perform raw-data collection using a μSD card during the training and internal validation of the machine learning models (Figure 4). It was equipped with a SAM-D21 (ARM M0+ 32bits, 256KB Flash, 32KB RAM) microcontroller. An RGB LED was added to show the device state (e.g., error state, standing state, starting data recording state and recording data state).

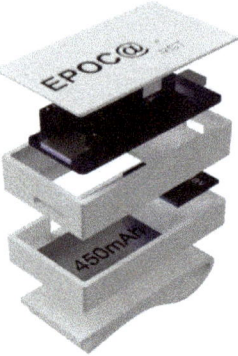

Figure 4. The sensor unit implemented for data logging in the first design stage.

The second prototype was implemented to host the final trained classification model including the FSM. It featured an ARM M0 (32bits, 128KB Flash and 24KB RAM) and wireless Bluetooth Low Energy (BLE) communications. Both prototypes were equipped with the 9-axis MEMS sensor LSM9DS1, which includes 3 digital acceleration channels (±2/±4/±8/±16 g linear acceleration full scale), 3 angular rate channels (±245/±500/±2000 dps angular rate full scale), SPI/I2C serial interfaces, 16-bit data output and programmable interrupt generators. In addition, an LPS25HB MEMS piezo-resistive pressure sensor was used. The PS25HB barometer measurement range is from 260 to 1260 hPa. Pressure sensor information showed poor sensitivity for real-time classification purposes and was not used in the study. Both PCBs incorporated a 600 mAh lithium polymer (LiPo) battery, management connectors and circuits. The housing of the final prototype was designed with a double patient fixation option: nasal cannula tube fixation (Figure 5a) and thoracic elastic band fixation (Figure 5b).

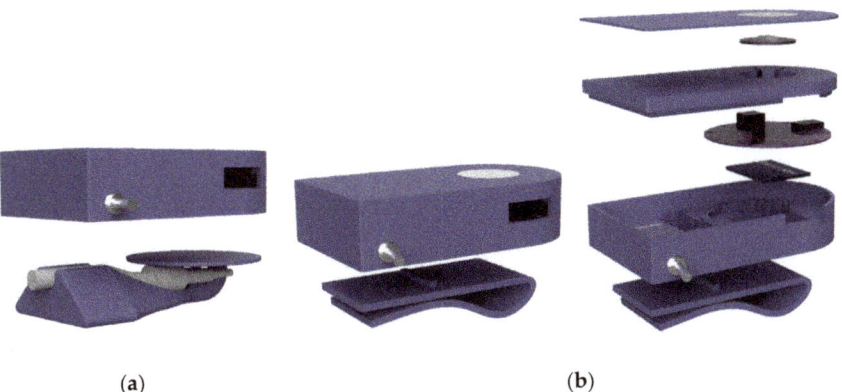

Figure 5. Three-dimensional design of the embodiment of the final prototype of the sensor unit including: (**a**) an adapter to the nasal cannula; (**b**) an adapter for a chest-band.

The sensor unit draws around 10 mA with 60 mA peaks when Bluetooth communications are used. In the worst scenario, considering an average consumption of 30 mA and the 600 mAh battery, the unit performs monitoring for about 14 h using the 600 mAh battery. This operating time is significantly longer than that of the oxygen concentrator, which ranges from 2 to 5 h.

The sensor unit was placed in the chest of the user, just at the end of the sternum. It has been reported that this location generates fewer motion artefacts due to movements compared to systems placed on the wrist, ankle or the belt [43]. The unit was mounted to ensure that the Y-axis of the IMU pointed at the head of the subject, and the Z-axis in the walking course. (Figure 6).

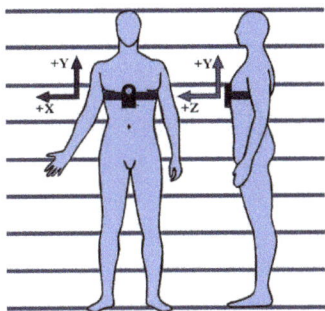

Figure 6. Preferred placement of the sensor unit on the subject's body.

2.1.2. Control Unit

The control unit receives the estimate of the intensity of the patient's physical activity and is responsible for adjusting the oxygen flow supplied to the patient according to the instructions established during the process of tuning of the therapy. The control unit includes an MCU and wireless communication capabilities, and interfaces directly with the POC. It was equipped with an ARM M0 (32bits, 128KB Flash and 24KB RAM), wireless BLE communications, an RGB LED, and a push-button to activate the automatic mode in the POC (Figure 7). The unit was directly powered from the POC.

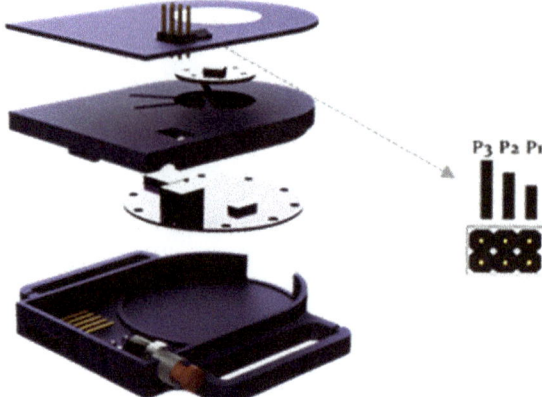

Figure 7. The control unit implemented for communication with the sensor unit and for controlling the portable oxygen concentrator. Header jumpers were used to personalize oxygen therapy settings and push button to switch the portable oxygen concentrator operating mode (manual or automatic).

The control of the concentrator by the control unit was carried out by simulating physical pulses to the increase and decrease buttons in the touch keyboard of the POC. As a consequence, the interface between the control unit and the POC was implemented using a 5-pin connector that enabled the power supply of the unit and the switching of the signals to increase or decrease the flow. In addition, a 6-pin male connector was included to enable the personalisation of different oxygen levels settings using header jumpers (see Table 1 and Section 2.1.2). As an example, the setting number 2 should be selected (jumper P2 on) for a patient who requires, at 15 breaths per minute, a bolus volume of 12 mL at rest, of 36 mL while doing light intensity activity, and of 60 mL when doing moderate intensity activity.

Table 1. Personalisation of oxygen therapy in the control unit. Seven different options were available. Bolus volume (pulse setting 1 to 5) delivered to patient depending on the intensity of physical activity ranges from 180 mL (pulse setting 1) to 900 mL (pulse setting 5).

Setting	Pulse Setting according to Physical Activity			Jumpers Setting		
	Sedentary	Light	Moderate	P3	P2	P1
1	1	2	4			X
2	1	3	5		X	
3	1	4	5		X	X
4	2	4	5	X		
5	3	4	5	X		X
6	0	2	5	X	X	
7	0	1	4	X	X	X

The control unit presents the same power consumption as the sensor unit. It is powered from the POC and causes a battery drain of 214 mAh, what supposes a decrease of about 12 min in the concentrator operating time.

2.1.3. Portable Oxygen Concentrator

Inogen One G2 POC was used in the study (Figure 8). The Inogen One G2 delivers up to 900 mL/min of 90% oxygen and supports pulsed dose delivery [44]. This concentrator has five levels for the adjustment of the oxygen needs. The oxygen dose applied to each patient in each situation depended on the previous titration by the specialist.

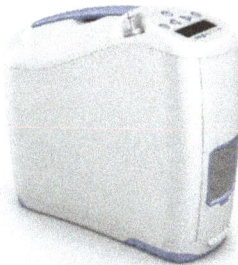

Figure 8. Inogen One G2 Portable Oxygen Concentrator used in the study.

In general, this POC delivers 12 mL per bolus per flow setting at 15 breaths per minute (180 mL/min per-flow setting). Table 2 summarizes the bolus volumes delivered at reference environmental conditions. Slower breathing patients will receive larger boluses, and faster breathing patients will receive smaller boluses.

Table 2. Bolus volumes delivered by Inogen One G2 at 20 °C at sea level at different breathing frequencies.

Pulse Setting	Pulse Volume (ml ± 10%)		
	15 Breaths per Minute	20 Breaths per Minute	25 Breaths per Minute
1	12	9	7.2
2	24	18	14.4
3	36	27	21.6
4	48	36	28.8
5	60	45	36.0

2.1.4. Communication Protocol

The units were programmed using the Arduino Integrated Development Environment (IDE). The bidirectional communication between the sensor unit and the control unit takes place using low-latency Bluetooth 4.0 (BLE) with 128-bit AES CCM (counter with cypher block chaining message authentication code CBC-MAC) encryption/decryption without pairing. The messages are sent encrypted with the serial number of the sending microcontroller and it is the receiver that uses the serial number to decrypt the messages. The wireless control can be authenticated through toasts for the confirmation of the desired operations and also tracked through timestamps. BLE remains in sleep mode at all times, except when participating in a data exchange, which reduces overall energy consumption. In this manner, the sensor unit only sends messages when there is a change in physical activity intensity.

2.2. Study Design and Participants

A total of 18 volunteers (Table 3) were recruited for this study at the Pneumology, Allergy, and Thoracic Surgery Unit of the University Hospital Puerta del Mar de Cadiz (Spain) (14 male, average age 66.9 ± 12.8 years, range 60–93 years, average body mass index (BMI) 27.00 ± 3.6 kg/m^2). The participants selected had a diagnosis of COPD and stable chronic respiratory failure, and were receiving LTOT and using a POC.

Table 3. Demographic and clinical data for patients in the internal validation group.

Characteristics	Data *
N	18
Male/Female	14/4 (77.7%/22.3%)
Age (years)	66.9 ± 12.8 (60–93)
51–60	5.6% (1)
61–70	44.4% (8)
71–80	16.7% (3)
81–90	33.3% (6)
BMI (Kg/cm^2)	27.0 ± 3.6
LTOT history (months)	22.1 ± 18.1
POC history (months)	19.5 ± 13.2
Daily hours using the POC	2.3 ± 1.0
mMRC dyspnoea baseline level	2.6 ± 0.5
FEV1/FVC	0.5 ± 0.2

BMI: Body mass index; LTOT: long term oxygen therapy; POC: portable oxygen concentrator; mMRC: Modified Medical Research Council scale; FEV_1/FVC: forced expiratory volume in 1-s to forced vital capacity ratio. * Results expressed as mean ± SD, except where otherwise indicated.

Exclusion criteria included any organic comorbidity that could cause or contribute to exertional dyspnoea that would hinder the realization of the circuit (cardiovascular diseases, metabolic or other associated respiratory diseases), COPD exacerbation within the six weeks before the enrolment or any disease that could limit the physical activity of the patient (e.g., neuromuscular or skeletal diseases). The general fragility (i.e., difficulty in walking or lack of autonomy) that could substantially prevent the patient's participation in the study was also considered an exclusion criterion, as well as the diagnosed mental incapacity. Prior to enrolment, all participants signed an informed consent form. The local ethics committee approved the study protocol.

In order to train and validate the machine learning models, an accurate reference (gold standard) was required. For this reason, the experiments were carried out in the hospital, where it was possible to observe participants closely, perform accurate references and do it under medical and technical supervision.

During a single visit to the hospital, participants were first interviewed. The Mini-Mental state examination (MMSE) was conducted and dyspnoea was measured before and after the test using the Modified Medical Research Council scale (*mMRC*). Then, subjects were fitted with the designed sensor unit and the Inogen One G2 portable oxygen concentrator. The participants followed the designed study protocol that started with an initial period of three minutes at rest, in a seated position. Next, participants were asked to walk, following the circuit illustrated in Figure 9, for 12 min.

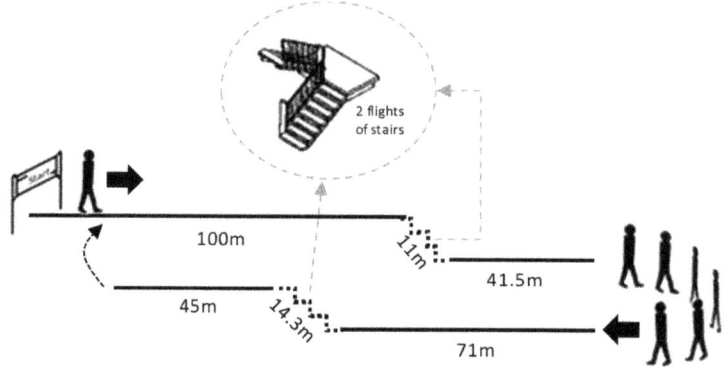

Figure 9. Walk-through circuit designed to acquire data for training and system validation.

The circuit included sections for walking, climbing and descending stairs. Participants were asked to exercise a gait pattern similar to that maintained in their daily activity in order to capture representative conditions of the activities performed in daily free-living conditions. Along the route, chairs were arranged for the subject to make stops when he/she considered necessary. Throughout the experiment, there were no restrictions on the participant's body movements. The final activity consisted of sitting for three minutes.

During each test, the stop and start times of each activity were noted and a label was assigned to each period of time. In addition, the number of user interactions with the POC, the flow level selected by the patient in each section of the circuit, the number of rest episodes (seated) of the participant, the oxygen saturation and the heart rate (measured using a Nonin WristOx$_2$® Model 3150 pulse-oximeter), and the distance walked were recorded.

2.3. Automatic Classification of the Intensity of Physical Activity

2.3.1. Daily Activities in Patients with COPD

The metabolic equivalent of tasks (MET) expresses the energy cost of physical activities and is defined as the ratio of the work metabolic rate to the resting metabolic rate, expressed in kcal/kg/hour. One MET is considered to be equivalent to the energy cost during quiet sitting. In addition, a MET can also be defined as the amount of oxygen consumed while sitting at rest, measured in ml/kg/min. In this case, one MET is equal to the oxygen cost of sitting quietly, equivalent to 3.5 mL/kg/min. A third definition relates MET to the rate of energy produced per unit surface area of an average person seated at rest, expressed in W/m^2 [45].

Different intensity physical activities entail different energy costs and therefore require varying levels of oxygen consumption. Table 4 describes the physical activities considered in this study. High intensity physical activities were not addressed since they are not expected in patients with COPD and respiratory failure. As described above, the amount of oxygen supplement required for each patient according to the intensity of the physical activity is titrated by the specialist at the initiation of therapy. A change in the intensity of the physical activity performed by the patient poses a need for updating the amount of oxygen provided by the POC [46].

Table 4. Activities, grouped by intensity, associated MET, and the number of instances.

Intensity	Activity	METs (W/kg)	Number of Instances
Sedentary	Sitting Standing Lying	1.3	2160
Light	Walking	2	3115
Moderate	Walking upstairs Walking downstairs	3.5–5	550
Total			5825

MET: The metabolic equivalent of task.

2.3.2. Data Processing and Features Extraction

The data from the accelerometer and from the gyroscope (X, Y and Z axes) were collected at a sampling rate of 25 Hz. The acceleration signals were divided into windows of 3 s (75 samples) without overlap, which was considered enough to capture significant properties of the signal. Activities of different intensity were identified from annotated labels.

In order to remove the DC component in the IMU signals, a high-pass filter with a cut-off frequency of 0.15 Hz was applied. The filtering was implemented using a low-pass IIR filter whose output was subtracted from the original signal.

For each of the time windows, 98 time-domain features were extracted from the six filtered acceleration and gyroscope signals. The explored features are detailed in Table 5. Features from the frequency and non-linear domains were excluded to reduce the computational burden in the microprocessor when implementing the real-time classification model.

Table 5. Initial feature set.

Feature Set (Accelerometer + Gyroscope)	Features
RMS, standard deviation, absolute mean	18
Mean of the derivative	6
Pairwise correlations	6
Simplified energy	6
Moments (skewness, kurtosis, median)	18
Min, max, difference between max and min	18
Interquartile range	6
Signal magnitude vector (mean, standard deviation, median, skewness, kurtosis)	10
Signal magnitude vector (interquartile range, max, min, the difference between max and min)	8
Signal magnitude area	2
Total	98

RMS: Root mean squared.

2.3.3. Features Selection

In order to improve the computational efficiency and reduce the generalization error of the model by removing irrelevant features, a wrapper feature selection approach was followed. The space of attribute subsets was searched by greedy hill-climbing augmented with a backtracking facility [47]. The search started with an empty set of attributes and search forward. The number of consecutive non-improving nodes allowed before terminating the search was 5. The feature selection algorithm operated in tandem with different machine learning classifiers and classification accuracy at each step was compared. The entire training-internal validation process is shown in Figure 10.

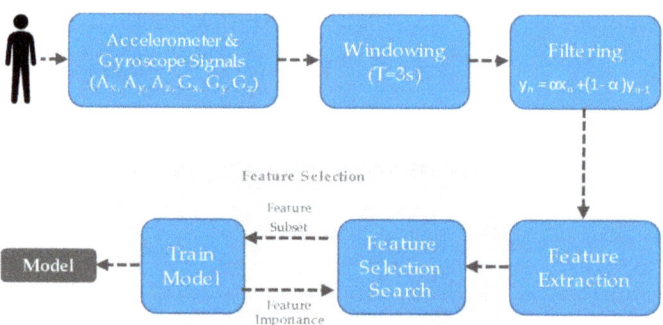

Figure 10. Wrapper approach to feature subset selection. A search algorithm was used through the space of possible features and evaluate each subset by training and cross-validation a model.

2.3.4. Classification and Internal Validation

A binary hierarchical classification structure (BHC) with two classifiers was chosen due to its computational simplicity [48]. Figure 11 shows the proposed architecture of a hierarchical classifier that requires two pairwise classifiers arranged as a binary tree with three leaf nodes, one for each class, and two internal nodes, each with its own feature space. Each of the two internal nodes consisted of a classifier and a set of features specific to it. The coarse separation between classes (sedentary vs active intensity of physical activity) occurred at the upper level in the hierarchy and a finer classification decision (light vs moderate intensity) at a lower level [49]. The architecture had a balanced binary hierarchical structure, in which the two meta-classes at each node had the same number of classes. For this study, decision trees (DT), Linear Discriminant Analysis (LDA), Logistic Regression Classifier (LR), Support Vector Machines (SVM), and Radial Basis Function (RBF) classifiers were evaluated as candidates for each of the internal nodes.

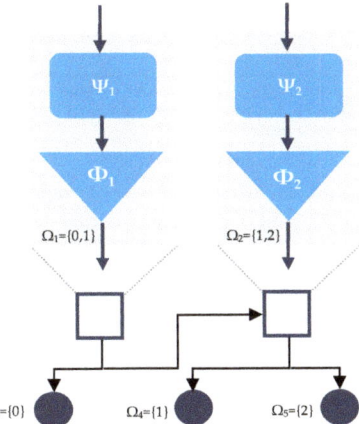

Figure 11. The proposed binary hierarchical classifier (BHC) applied to the classification of the intensity of physical activity. Given that the classifier operates with three classes, its structure has 2 internal nodes and 3 leaf nodes. Each internal node is comprised of a set of features (ψ_i) and a classifier (ϕ_i). Each node n is associated with a set of classes. In this study, classes are defined as: 0 = sedentary physical activity; 1 = light-intensity physical activity; and 3 = moderate-intensity physical activity.

The FSM machine described in Section 2.1.1 was added to the BHC as an output layer to enhance safety. Each classifier was trained with leave-one-subject-out cross-validation (LOSO-CV) scheme, where data from 17 participants were used for training the classifier, and the remaining participant data for evaluating the model performance. This process was repeated 18 times so that each participant was used once for validation.

Several weighted metrics were used to measure model performance: precision, recall, and F1-measure, defined as the weighted average of precision and recall. Additionally, sensitivity (Se), specificity (Sp), and the geometric mean of sensitivity and specificity (G) were estimated. Finally, the receiver operating characteristic (ROC) curve was computed and the area under the curve (AUC) for each class was estimated. Signal processing and model training and validation were performed using MATLAB software (Mathworks Inc., Natick, MA, USA) and DTREG predictive modelling software.

2.4. Technical Pilot Test

In the final stage, five participants went through the circuit designed during the previous phase, using the POC in automatic mode (iPOC). Demographic and clinical data for these patients are shown in Table 6.

Table 6. Demographic and clinical data for patients in the technical pilot test.

Characteristics	Data *
N	5
Male	5 (100 %)
Age (years)	72.2 ± 6.5
BMI (Kg/cm^2)	28.4 ± 6.0
LTOT history (months)	27.6 ± 25.7
POC history (months)	22.8 ± 15.5
Daily hours using the POC	4.2 ± 2.4
mMRC (baseline dyspnoea index)	2.6 ± 0.5
FEV$_1$/FVC	0.5 ± 0.2

BMI: Body mass index; *LTOT*: long term oxygen therapy; *POC*: portable oxygen concentrator; *mMRC*: Modified Medical Research Council scale; *FEV$_1$/FVC*: forced expiratory volume in 1-s to forced vital capacity ratio. * Results expressed as mean ± SD, except where otherwise indicated.

This feasibility pilot was conducted with the purpose of examining technical and usability issues, and the differences in the changes in blood oxygen saturation with respect to the circuit performed in manual mode. Special attention was paid to the number of oxygen desaturation episodes and to the maximum and minimum SpO$_2$ values during the test.

2.5. Usability

After each experiment, a semi-structured interview was conducted with the involved patient, in order to obtain information regarding the usefulness, ease of use and expectations of the participant.

In addition to the 18 patients enrolled, 15 additional patients under LTOT were interviewed by phone, in order to have a more significant sample.

Three main questions were asked in the interview:

1. Do you consider a system such as the one proposed to be necessary?
2. Would the automatic concentrator promote your out-of-home activities?
3. In your daily use of the concentrator, do you forget to adjust the recommended dose of O$_2$ when the intensity of your physical activity varies?

In questions 1 and 2, the subject was asked to describe his/her degree of agreement on a Likert scale from 1 through to 5, with the strongest positive agreement being 5. To assess usability, the System Usability Scale (SUS) was used in the technical pilot test. SUS is a 10-item questionnaire with 5 response options ranging from strong agreement to strong disagreement. The SUS possible values range from 0 to 100 [50].

3. Results and Discussion

3.1. Model Training and Internal Validation

The dataset used in this study phase included 18 patients, and three different classes with 2160 epochs of sedentary, 3115 epochs of light activity and 550 epochs of moderate activity. Figure 12 illustrates the signals acquired in a time window during different activities along with a test.

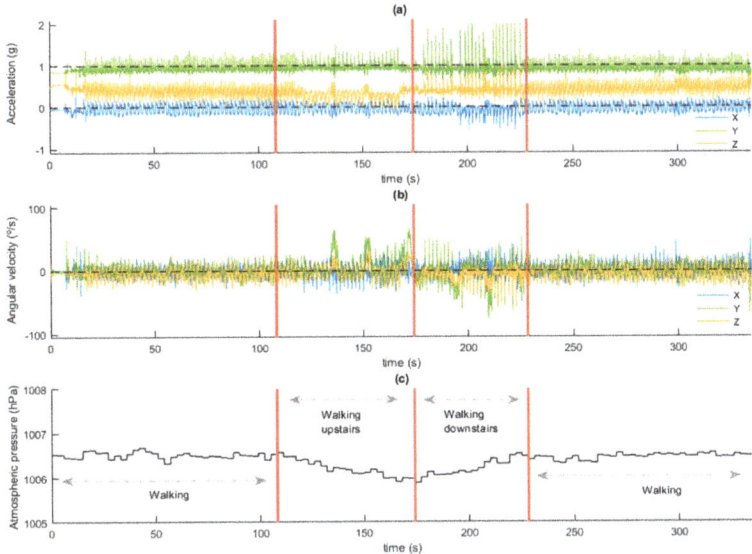

Figure 12. Signals acquired during one of the experiments in the hospital, with the patient walking the circuit designed for the physical test. (**a**) 3-axis accelerometer signals; (**b**) 3-axis gyroscope signals; (**c**) barometer signal. Red vertical lines indicate changes in activity (walking on level, going upstairs, going downstairs).

Table 7 shows the dimensions of the feature set that resulted from the wrapper-based Sequential Feature Selection (SFS) approach for each of the explored models and classifiers.

Table 7. The optimal feature set obtained from Wrapper-based feature selection for the classifiers ϕ_1 and ϕ_2.

Method	Selected Features for ϕ_1	Selected Features for ϕ_2
LR	8	17
J48	4	14
SVM	15	14
LDA	9	20
MLP	11	12

LR: logistic regression; J48: C4.5 decision tree; SVM: support vector machines; LDA: linear discriminant analysis; MLP: multilayer perceptron.

Table 8 shows the model performance achieved by classifiers ϕ_1 and ϕ_2, respectively, using the selected feature set for each trained and validated algorithm. In the case of ϕ_2, and given the large imbalance between classes, instances of light activity were weighted in order to balance target categories. The weights were adjusted so that the sum of the weights for the instances within each target category was the same.

Table 8. Performance metrics of classifiers ϕ_1 and ϕ_2 for each cross-validated machine learning algorithm.

Method	Accuracy		F1-Measure		Se		Sp		G		AUC	
	ϕ_1	ϕ_2	ϕ_1	ϕ_2	ϕ_1	ϕ_2	ϕ_1	ϕ_2	ϕ_1	ϕ_2	ϕ_1	ϕ_2
LR	94.54	91.86	95.60	64.71	95.70	51.16	93.38	98.81	94.53	71.10	0.98	0.85
J48	96.45	74.72	96.98	74.15	96.76	72.55	95.97	76.89	96.36	74.69	0.98	0.74
SVM	97.13	88.49	97.92	61.18	97.44	35.82	96.62	97.78	97.03	59.18	0.99	0.81
LDA	95.30	84.01	95.93	79.25	93.87	75.09	97.36	85.59	95.60	80.17	0.99	0.88
MLP	96.02	77.24	96.62	77.58	96.31	78.73	95.60	75.76	95.95	77.23	0.99	0.85

LR: logistic regression; J48: C4.5 decision tree; SVM: support vector machines; LDA: linear discriminant analysis; MLP: multilayer perceptron; Se: Sensitivity; Sp: specificity; G: geometric mean of sensitivity and specificity; AUC: area under the receiver operating characteristic curve (ROC) curve.

The results show that the ϕ_1 classifier implemented using SVM was able to discriminate between sedentary and active physical activity with a maximum value of F1-measure, G, and AUC of 97.92%, 97.03% and 0.99 respectively. In the case of the ϕ_2 classifier, designed to discriminate between light and moderate-intensity physical activities, maximum F1-measure, G and AUC were 79.25% (LDA), 97.13% (SVM) and 0.99 (SVM, LDA, MLP) respectively. The lower performance shown by classifier ϕ_2 is explained by the difficulty in discriminating between up and downstairs activities, which has already been reported in other studies.

According to the results found, the LDA model, which demonstrated a better compromise between sensitivity and specificity, and the higher AUC, was chosen for implementing the classifier ϕ_2 in the hardware. For classifier ϕ_1, the J48 decision tree was chosen for the hardware deployment. Although the SVM algorithm obtained better results in terms of G, it was discarded given that the differences in performance were minimal and the computational cost of the SVM and its associated feature space was significantly higher.

Figure 13 shows the Receiver Operation Characteristics (ROC) curves for each class and both classifications approaches.

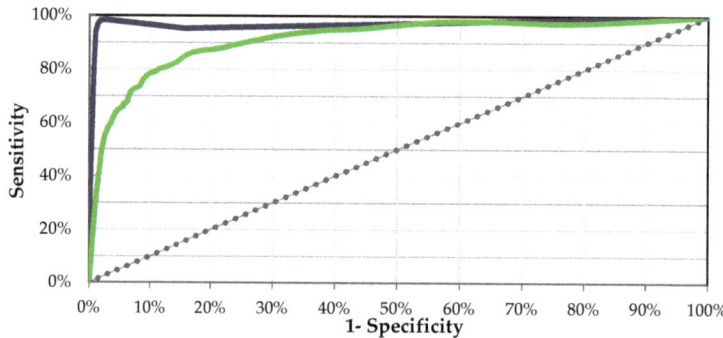

Figure 13. Receiver Operating Characteristics (ROC) Curves for selected models. The blue line represents the ROC curve for the J48 model. The green line shows the ROC curve for the J48 classifier.

Table 9 illustrates the confusion matrix and the performance metrics for the build two stages of classification procedure (BHC). The BHC was able to achieve a weighted-F1 measure of 85.9% with weighted-precision and weighted-recall of 85.9%, and 86.1%, respectively.

During the completion of the circuit, the participants had to manually adjust the oxygen flow several times during the route. The total number of adjustments required for the rounds completed was 96. By contrast, participants only manipulated the oxygen concentrator to suit the needs of O_2 demanded by the physical activity performed on 17 occasions, which showed underuse (only 17.7% of needed adjustments were carried out) of the device that could potentially lead to oxygen desaturation events.

Table 9. Performance metrics for the binary hierarchical classification structure for each of the levels of intensity of physical activity.

		Predicted		Performance			
		S	Other	Precision	Recall	Accuracy	F1-Measure
True	S	2073	77	95.4%	96.4%	97.0%	95.9%
	Other	101	3666				
		L	Other				
	L	1569	335	76.1%	82.4%	85.9%	79.1%
	Other	493	3466				
		M	Other				
	M	1393	470	82.9%	74.8%	86.9%	78.6%
	Other	288	3642				

S: Sedentary; L: light intensity of physical activity; M: moderate intensity of physical activity.

3.2. Technical Pilot Test

The technical pilot test was carried out in a controlled environment in the hospital. The participants walked the same circuit designed for data collection for model training and internal validation.

Figure 14 shows one of the participants during the test carrying the POC and the auxiliary units designed for its automation.

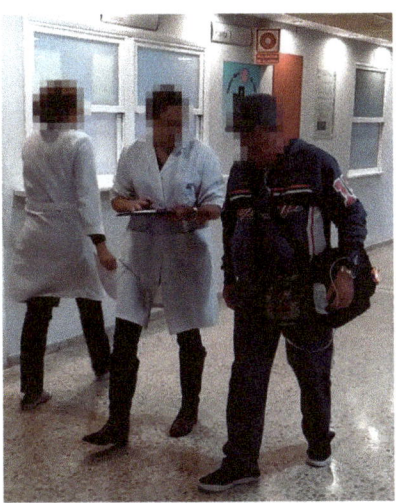

Figure 14. A participant using the automatic portable oxygen concentrator during the technical pilot test.

Table 10 synthesizes the results obtained by the BHC using the same performance metrics applied for internal validation.

Table 10. Weighted performance metrics of the binary hierarchical classification structure in the technical pilot test.

Accuracy	F1-Measure	Precision	Recall
91.1%	76.6%	74.9%	83.6%

Again, the accuracy achieved is high (91.1%) but conditioned by the errors in the classification of the activities up/downstairs. These errors are caused by the inherent difficulty in classifying these tasks, and by the different pattern in each patient's gait, which depends on their physical condition.

As a general rule, patients with COPD and respiratory failure who are receiving LTOT avoid using long flights of stairs, thus errors made in this regard cannot be considered critical in a real-life scenario.

Table 11 shows a comparison of the results for changes in blood oxygen saturation for each of the five participants during manual mode (conventional use of the device) and automatic mode tests (proposed iPOC).

Table 11. Changes in blood oxygen saturation levels during the tests performed using the conventional portable oxygen concentrator (POC) and the proposed intelligent POC (iPOC).

Mode	Automatic POC (iPOC)					Manual POC				
Subject	S1	S2	S3	S4	S5	S1	S2	S3	S4	S5
SpO$_2$ events	2	1	1	2	3	3	3	6	1	2
Mean SpO$_2$	89.5	92.2	89.1	94.7	87.1	88.6	90.4	86.1	91.5	89.5
min (SpO$_2$)	77.0	87.0	85.0	89.0	81.0	80.0	86.0	75.0	81.0	93.0
CT90	50.1	18.8	70.9	8.4	73	62.9	33.1	91.7	20.9	60.6
CT85	34.9	0.0	0.0	0.0	27.6	17.4	0.0	33.9	2.8	6.3

CTxx: time spent with SpO$_2$ < xx%.

An overall reduction in the number of desaturation events can be appreciated in four out of the five subjects. In the same four patients, the average blood oxygen saturation values were increased with respect to the POC test in manual mode. In the same way, the minimum blood saturation values were also improved. The cumulative time spent with SpO$_2$ below 90% (CT90) and 85% (CT85) again showed a generally better response when the iPOC was used.

Subject 5 deserves a special mention. He went around the circuit with reduced mobility due to the use of a crutch as a result of an episode of low back pain. Additionally, he showed signs of exacerbation within few days after the test. Some authors have detected significantly decreased saturation in the period of seven days preceding exacerbation [51], so we think that the result of the test could have been biased by these factors.

Figure 15 illustrates the change in blood oxygen saturation pattern on exertion for one of the participants. The stabilization of SpO$_2$ values, the reduction in the number of desaturation events, and the higher mean value obtained with the use of the proposed system can be clearly observed.

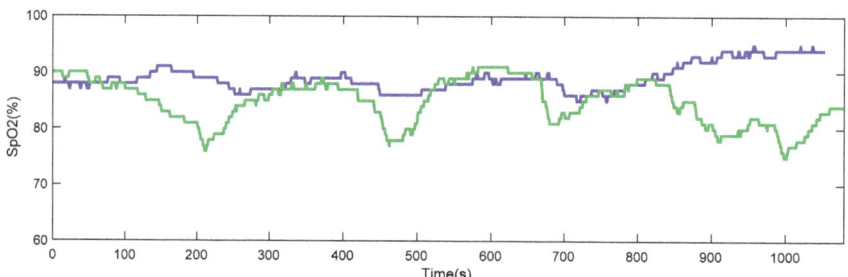

Figure 15. SpO$_2$ patterns of a participant during the technical pilot test. The blue line refers to SpO$_2$ values while using the portable oxygen concentrator with the proposed automatic mode. The green line refers to SpO$_2$ values using the POC in manual (conventional) mode.

Improvement in oxygenation is attributable to the fact that the adjustment of oxygen flow during daily living activities in response to higher oxygen demand is done, in conventional POCs, manually by the patient. Incorrect use in the oxygen flow adjustment or adjustment made with a delay relative to the change in physical activity intensity often leads to desaturation episodes [24].

3.3. Usability

Table 12 presents a synthesis of the results obtained in the semi-structured interview with the participants in the initial phase.

Table 12. Results from the semi-structured interview.

Question	Average Likert Score
1. Do you consider a system such as the one proposed to be necessary?	5 ± 0 (33)
2. Would you the automatic concentrator promote your out-of-home activities?	5 ± 0 (33)
3. In your daily use of the concentrator, did you forget to adjust the recommended dose of O2 when your degree of physical activity varies?	
• Yes	51.5% (17)
• The patient consciously does not adapt the flow	30.3% (10)
• The patient ignores that he has to adjust it	18.2% (6)

All the patients interviewed considered that a system capable of automatically regulating the oxygen flow in the concentrator was necessary. They also felt that such a system would help increase physical activity outside the home. The high percentage of patients who admit to forgetting to adjust the concentrator when faced with changes in physical activity intensity (51.5%) is noteworthy. Similarly, the percentage of patients who consciously skip the adjustment of the oxygen flow is outstanding. Finally, the average SUS score calculated after the technical pilot test was 79 ± 11.4. There was one participant that had an average SUS score of 95, followed by scores of 85 (1/5), 75 (2/5), and 65 (1/5). In the research, the average SUS value is 68, which can be considered a benchmark. The achieved value of 79 indicates significantly better usability than average [52].

4. Conclusions

The long-term benefits of oxygen have been proven since the 1980s in certain respiratory conditions such as COPD. Very recently, future research in oxygen therapy has been pointed at developing and evaluating new models for therapeutic oxygen patient education and improving portable oxygen devices [53]. It has been reported that, when compared to the conventional POCs, the closed-loop POCs can maintain higher saturation levels, spend less time below the target saturation, and save O_2 resources [25]. The correction of exercise hypoxemia in lung diseases like COPD is crucial and challenging [54], and automatic POCs can contribute to the individualized adjustment of oxygen flow.

Currently, the challenge of designing closed-loop portable devices which are able to adjust O_2 flow automatically is being faced by mainly using indirectly measured blood oxygen saturation as a process variable to close the loop. However, the robustness of control algorithms and the limited reliability of current oximetry sensors are hindering the effectiveness of this approach.

In line with all the above-mentioned factors, this study presents the proof of concept of an alternative approach: a system to transform a conventional POC into a closed-loop controlled device capable of automatically self-adjusting, in real time, the oxygen flow supplied to the patient according to the intensity of the physical activity carried out by the user under LTOT.

A sensor unit capable of detecting the physical intensity developed by the patient (in real time) has been developed and evaluated. This sensor unit can wirelessly connect to the POC for the self-adjustment of the oxygen flow. The system has been designed with the flexibility to customize up to seven different oxygen therapy profiles. The developed iPOC was tested with a widely used commercial POC unit. For this purpose, a treadmill circuit was designed that included basic physical activities most common in the daily practice of elderly patients with respiratory disorders. Different models were trained and validated using artificial intelligence techniques, a wrapper approach, 98 time-domain features, and data from 18 patients with COPD and respiratory failure. A final meta-classifier (BHC) was designed and deployed in the sensor unit to operate in real-time. A weighted accuracy of 91.1% was achieved in the technical pilot test with five patients. A reduction in the number of desaturation events was achieved in 80% of patients as well as improved minimum and average blood oxygen saturation values compared to the POC in manual operating mode. In these cases, CT90 and CT85 also showed a promising better response when the iPOC was used. Finally, all interviewed patients (N = 33) considered that the proposed iPOC satisfied them, and could promote their physical activity outside the home.

Among the limitations of this study were those related to hypoxia. In this regard, the combination of the proposed system with the novel oxygen reserve index (ORI) included in the new generation of pulse oximeters that use multi-wavelength pulse co-oximetry might improve oxygen titration and enable the prevention of unintended hyperoxia [55].

A closed-loop control system, like the proposed iPOC, has clear potential benefits, including improved oxygenation regardless of physical activity and enhanced patient follow-up and compliance with therapy recommendations. In addition, closed-loop oxygen supply systems have shown that they can potentially reduce medical error, improve morbidity and mortality, and reduce care costs [22].

Future research steps include the miniaturization of the sensor unit, expanding the study sample, and the home monitoring of the patients while using IPOC during daily tasks in an unsupervised environment, in order to obtain clinical evidence of the impact that this approach may have on the targeted patient population.

5. Patents

DSM and ALJ are the inventors of the utility model ES U201831680 with the title 'Automatic flow-metering device for oxygen therapy equipment'.

Author Contributions: Conceptualization, D.S.-M. and A.L.-J.; methodology, D.S.-M. and A.L.-J.; software, A.L.-D. and D.S.-M.; validation, P.M.-Z., A.L.-J., A.L.-D and D.S.-M.; formal analysis, A.L.-D. and D.S.-M.; investigation, A.L.-J., P.M.-Z., A.L.-D. and D.S.-M.; writing—original draft preparation, D.S.-M.; writing—review and editing, A.L.-J., A.L.-D., and D.S.-M.; visualization, A.L.-D. and D.S.-M.; supervision, D.S.-M.; project administration, D.S.-M.; funding acquisition, D.S.-M. All authors have read and agreed to the published version of the manuscript.

Funding: This research was funded by grants from "Consejería de Salud y Familias de la Junta de Andalucía" and "Iniciativa Territorial Integrada [ITI] 2014-2020 para la provincia de Cádiz" (PI-0006-2017); and by "Consejería de Salud y Familias de la Junta de Andalucía" (PIN-0053-2017).

Acknowledgments: We want to thank the company Nippon Gases for the loan of the portable oxygen therapy concentrator to carry out some of the experiments conducted in this research.

Conflicts of Interest: DSM and A.L.-J. are inventors of the utility model ES U201831680 with the title 'Automatic flow-metering device for oxygen therapy equipment'. A.L.-D. and P.M.-Z. have no conflict of interest.

Ethical Statement: All subjects gave their informed consent for inclusion before they participated in the study. The study was conducted in accordance with the Declaration of Helsinki and the protocol was approved by the Research Ethics Committee of Cadiz.

References

1. Lacasse, Y.; Tan, A.-Y.M.; Maltais, F.; Krishnan, J.A. Home Oxygen in Chronic Obstructive Pulmonary Disease. *Am. J. Respir. Crit. Care Med.* **2018**, *197*, 1254–1264. [CrossRef] [PubMed]
2. O'Driscoll, B.R.; Howard, L.S.; Earis, J.; Mak, V. BTS guideline for oxygen use in adults in healthcare and emergency settings. *Thorax* **2017**, *72*, ii1–ii90. [CrossRef] [PubMed]
3. From the Global Strategy for the Diagnosis, Management and Prevention of COPD, Global Initiative for Chronic Obstructive Lung Disease (GOLD). Available online: http://goldcopd.org/ (accessed on 1 January 2020).
4. Celli, B.R.; MacNee, W. Standards for the diagnosis and treatment of patients with COPD: A summary of the ATS/ERS position paper. *Eur. Respir. J.* **2004**, *23*, 932–946. [CrossRef] [PubMed]
5. Nocturnal Oxygen Therapy Trial Group. Continuous or Nocturnal Oxygen Therapy in Hypoxemic Chronic Obstructive Lung Disease. *Ann. Intern. Med.* **1980**, *93*, 391. [CrossRef]
6. Medical Research Council Working Party. Long term domiciliary oxygen therapy in chronic hypoxic cor pulmonale complicating chronic bronchitis and emphysema. Report of the Medical Research Council Working Party. *Lancet* **1981**, *317*, 681–686. [CrossRef]

7. Bradley, J.M.; Lasserson, T.; Elborn, S.; MacMahon, J.; O'Neill, B. A Systematic Review of Randomized Controlled Trials Examining the Short-term Benefit of Ambulatory Oxygen in COPD. *Chest* **2007**, *131*, 278–285. [CrossRef]
8. Casaburi, R. Long-Term Oxygen Therapy: The Three Big Questions. *Ann. Am. Thorac. Soc.* **2018**, *15*, 14–15. [CrossRef]
9. Samuel, J.; Franklin, C. Hypoxemia and Hypoxia. In *Common Surgical Diseases*; Springer: Berlin/Heidelberg, Germany, 2008.
10. Branson, R.D.; Robinson, B.R.H. Oxygen: When is more the enemy of good? *Intensive Care Med.* **2011**, *37*, 1–3. [CrossRef]
11. Mach, W.J.; Thimmesch, A.R.; Pierce, J.T.; Pierce, J.D. Consequences of Hyperoxia and the Toxicity of Oxygen in the Lung. *Nurs. Res. Pract.* **2011**, *2011*, 1–7. [CrossRef]
12. Cameron, L.; Pilcher, J.; Weatherall, M.; Beasley, R.; Perrin, K. The risk of serious adverse outcomes associated with hypoxaemia and hyperoxaemia in acute exacerbations of COPD. *Postgr. Med. J.* **2012**, *88*, 684–689. [CrossRef]
13. Kilgannon, J.H. Association Between Arterial Hyperoxia Following Resuscitation From Cardiac Arrest and In-Hospital Mortality. *JAMA* **2010**, *303*, 2165. [CrossRef] [PubMed]
14. Austin, M.A.; Wills, K.E.; Blizzard, L.; Walters, E.H.; Wood-Baker, R. Effect of high flow oxygen on mortality in chronic obstructive pulmonary disease patients in prehospital setting: Randomised controlled trial. *BMJ* **2010**, *341*, c5462. [CrossRef] [PubMed]
15. Sassoon, C.S.; Hassell, K.T.; Mahutte, C.K. Hyperoxic-induced hypercapnia in stable chronic obstructive pulmonary disease. *Am. Rev. Respir Dis* **1987**, *135*, 907–911. [CrossRef] [PubMed]
16. Croxton, T.L.; Bailey, W.C. Long-term oxygen treatment in chronic obstructive pulmonary disease: Recommendations for future research: An NHLBI workshop report. *Am. J. Respir. Crit. Care Med.* **2006**, *174*, 373–378. [CrossRef]
17. Brill, S.E.; Wedzicha, J. A Oxygen therapy in acute exacerbations of chronic obstructive pulmonary disease. *Int. J. Chron. Obstruct. Pulmon. Dis.* **2014**, *9*, 1241–1252.
18. McCoy, R.W. Options for home oxygen therapy equipment: Storage and metering of oxygen in the home. *Respir. Care* **2013**, *58*, 65–81. [CrossRef]
19. Lellouche, F.; L'Her, E. Automated Oxygen Flow Titration to Maintain Constant Oxygenation. *Respir. Care* **2012**, *57*, 1254–1262. [CrossRef]
20. Claure, N.; Bancalari, E. Automated closed loop control of inspired oxygen concentration. *Respir. Care* **2013**, *58*, 151–161. [CrossRef]
21. Casanova, C.; Hernández, M.C.; Sánchez, A.; García-Talavera, I.; De Torres, J.P.; Abreu, J.; Valencia, J.M.; Aguirre-Jaime, A.; Celli, B.R. Twenty-four-hour ambulatory oximetry monitoring in COPD patients with moderate hypoxemia. *Respir. Care* **2006**, *51*, 1416–1423.
22. Mayoralas-Alises, S.; Carratalá, J.M.; Díaz-Lobato, S. New Perspectives in Oxygen Therapy Titration: Is Automatic Titration the Future? *Arch. Bronconeumol.* **2019**, *55*, 319–327. [CrossRef]
23. Dunne, P.J. Long-term oxygen therapy (LTOT) revisited: In defense of non-delivery LTOT technology. *Rev. Port. Pneumol.* **2012**, *18*, 155–157. [CrossRef] [PubMed]
24. Dunne, P.J.; MacIntyre, N.R.; Schmidt, U.H.; Haas, C.F.; Jones-Boggs Rye, K.; Kauffman, G.W.; Hess, D.R. Respiratory Care Year in Review 2011: Long-Term Oxygen Therapy, Pulmonary Rehabilitation, Airway Management, Acute Lung Injury, Education, and Management. *Respir. Care* **2012**, *57*, 590–606. [CrossRef] [PubMed]
25. Sanchez-Morillo, D.; Olaby, O.; Fernandez-Granero, M.A.; Leon-Jimenez, A. Physiological closed-loop control in intelligent oxygen therapy: A review. *Comput. Methods Programs Biomed.* **2017**, *146*, 101–108. [CrossRef] [PubMed]
26. British Lung Foundation: Chronic Obstructive Pulmonary Disease (COPD) Statistics. Available online: https://statistics.blf.org.uk/copd (accessed on 1 January 2020).
27. International Electrotechnical Commission. *IEC 60601-1-10 Medical Electrical Equipment–Part 1-10: General Requirements for Basic Safety and Essential Performance–Collateral Standard: Requirements for the Development of Physiologic Closed-Loop Controllers*; International Electrotechnical Commission: Geneva, Switzerland, 2007.
28. Dumont, G.A. Feedback control for clinicians. *J. Clin. Monit. Comput.* **2014**, *28*, 5–11. [CrossRef]

29. Lellouche, F.; Lipes, J.; L'Her, E. Optimal oxygen titration in patients with chronic obstructive pulmonary disease: A role for automated oxygen delivery? *Can. Respir. J.* **2013**, *20*, 259–261. [CrossRef]
30. Iobbi, M.G.; Simonds, A.K.; Dickinson, R.J. Oximetry feedback flow control simulation for oxygen therapy. *J. Clin. Monit. Comput.* **2007**, *21*, 115–123. [CrossRef]
31. El Adawi, M.I.; El-garhy, A.M.; Sawafta, F.O. Design of Fuzzy Controller for Supplying Oxygen in Sub-acute Respiratory Illnesses. *Int. J. Comput. Sci. Issues* **2012**, *9*, 192–206.
32. Lellouche, F.; Bouchard, P.; Roberge, M.; Simard, S.; L'Her, E.; Maltais, F.; Lacass, Y. Automated oxygen titration and weaning with FreeO2 in patients with acute exacerbation of COPD: A pilot randomized trial. *Int. J. COPD* **2016**, *11*, 1983–1990. [CrossRef]
33. Cirio, S.; Nava, S. Pilot study of a new device to titrate oxygen flow in hypoxic patients on long-term oxygen therapy. *Respir. Care* **2011**, *56*, 429–434. [CrossRef]
34. Rice, K.L.; Schmidt, M.F.; Buan, J.S.; Lebahn, F.; Schwarzock, T.K. AccuO2 Oximetry-Driven Oxygen-Conserving Device Versus Fixed-Dose Oxygen Devices in Stable COPD Patients. *Respir. Care* **2011**, *56*, 1901–1905. [CrossRef]
35. Chan, E.D.; Chan, M.M.; Chan, M.M. Pulse oximetry: Understanding its basic principles facilitates appreciation of its limitations. *Respir. Med.* **2013**, *107*, 789–799. [CrossRef] [PubMed]
36. Jacobs, S.S.; Lindell, K.O.; Collins, E.G.; Garvey, C.M.; Hernandez, C.; McLaughlin, S.; Schneidman, A.M.; Meek, P.M. Patient perceptions of the adequacy of supplemental oxygen therapy: Results of the American thoracic society nursing assembly oxygen working group survey. *Ann. Am. Thorac. Soc.* **2018**, *15*, 24–32. [CrossRef] [PubMed]
37. Lara-Doña, A.; Sanchez-Morillo, D.; Pérez-Morales, M.; Fernandez-Granero, M.Á.; Leon-Jimenez, A. A Prototype of Intelligent Portable Oxygen Concentrator for Patients with COPD Under Oxygen Therapy. In *XV Mediterranean Conference on Medical and Biological Engineering and Computing–MEDICON 2019*; Henriques, J., Neves, N., de Carvalho, P., Eds.; Springer: Berlin/Heidelberg, Germany, 2020.
38. Branson, R.D. Oxygen therapy in copd. *Respir. Care* **2018**, *63*, 734–748. [CrossRef] [PubMed]
39. Dutta, A.; Ma, O.; Toledo, M.; Pregonero, A.; Ainsworth, B.; Buman, M.; Bliss, D. Identifying Free-Living Physical Activities Using Lab-Based Models with Wearable Accelerometers. *Sensors* **2018**, *18*, 3893. [CrossRef]
40. Tedesco, S.; Barton, J.; O'Flynn, B. A Review of Activity Trackers for Senior Citizens: Research Perspectives, Commercial Landscape and the Role of the Insurance Industry. *Sensors* **2017**, *17*, 1277. [CrossRef]
41. Rosenberg, D.; Godbole, S.; Ellis, K.; Di, C.; Lacroix, A.; Natarajan, L.; Kerr, J. Classifiers for Accelerometer-Measured Behaviors in Older Women. *Med. Sci. Sports Exerc.* **2017**, *49*, 610–616. [CrossRef]
42. Farooq, M.; Sazonov, E. A Novel Wearable Device for Food Intake and Physical Activity Recognition. *Sensors* **2016**, *16*, 1067. [CrossRef]
43. Yang, C.-C.; Hsu, Y.-L. A review of accelerometry-based wearable motion detectors for physical activity monitoring. *Sensors* **2010**, *10*, 7772. [CrossRef]
44. Inogen One G2 Oxygen Concentrator Technical Manual. Available online: https://www.inogen.com/pdf/Inogen_One_G2_Technical_Manual.pdf (accessed on 11 October 2019).
45. Mortazavi, B.; Alsharufa, N.; Lee, S.I.; Lan, M.; Sarrafzadeh, M.; Chronley, M.; Roberts, C.K. MET calculations from on-body accelerometers for exergaming movements. In Proceedings of the 2013 IEEE International Conference on Body Sensor Networks, Cambridge, MA, USA, 6–9 May 2013.
46. Ainsworth, B.E.; Haskell, W.I.L.; Whitt, M.C.; Irwin, M.L.; Swartz, A.M.; Strath, S.J.; O'Brien, W.I.L.; Bassett, D.R., Jr.; Schmitz, K.H.; Emplaincourt, P.O.; et al. Compendium of physical activities: An update of activity codes and MET intensities. *Med. Sci. Sports Exerc.* **2000**, *32*, S498–S504. [CrossRef]
47. Kohavi, R.; John, G.H. Wrappers for feature subset selection. *Artif. Intell.* **1997**, *97*, 273–324. [CrossRef]
48. Casasent, D.; Wang, Y.C. A hierarchical classifier using new support vector machine for automatic target recognition. *Neural Netw.* **2005**, *18*, 541–548. [CrossRef] [PubMed]
49. Wang, Y.-C.F.; Casasent, D. A support vector hierarchical method for multi-class classification and rejection. In Proceedings of the 2009 International Joint Conference on Neural Networks, Atlanta, GA, USA, 14–19 June 2009.
50. Brooke, J. SUS-A quick and dirty usability scale. *Usabil. Eval. Ind.* **1996**, *189*, 4–7.
51. Miłkowska-Dymanowska, J.; Białas, A.J.; Obrębski, W.; Górski, P.; Piotrowski, W.J. A pilot study of daily telemonitoring to predict acute exacerbation in chronic obstructive pulmonary disease. *Int. J. Med. Inform.* **2018**, *116*, 46–51. [CrossRef] [PubMed]

52. Brooke, J. SUS: A Retrospective. *J. Usabil. Stud.* **2013**, *8*, 29–40.
53. Jacobs, S.S.; Lederer, D.J.; Garvey, C.M.; Hernandez, C.; Lindell, K.O.; McLaughlin, S.; Schneidman, A.M.; Casaburi, R.; Chang, V.; Cosgrove, G.P.; et al. Optimizing Home Oxygen Therapy. An Official American Thoracic Society Workshop Report. *Ann. Am. Thorac. Soc.* **2018**, *15*, 1369–1381. [CrossRef]
54. Marti, S.; Pajares, V.; Morante, F.; Ramon, M.-A.; Lara, J.; Ferrer, J.; Guell, M.-R. Are Oxygen-Conserving Devices Effective for Correcting Exercise Hypoxemia? *Respir. Care* **2013**, *58*, 1606–1613. [CrossRef]
55. Scheeren, T.W.L.; Belda, F.J.; Perel, A. The oxygen reserve index (ORI): A new tool to monitor oxygen therapy. *J. Clin. Monit. Comput.* **2018**, *32*, 379–389. [CrossRef]

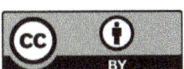

© 2020 by the authors. Licensee MDPI, Basel, Switzerland. This article is an open access article distributed under the terms and conditions of the Creative Commons Attribution (CC BY) license (http://creativecommons.org/licenses/by/4.0/).

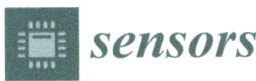

Letter

A Dual-Padded, Protrusion-Incorporated, Ring-Type Sensor for the Measurement of Food Mass and Intake

Wonki Hong, Jungmin Lee and Won Gu Lee *

Department of Mechanical Engineering, Kyung Hee University, Yongin 17104, Korea; wk.hong@khu.ac.kr (W.H.); mudoosan@khu.ac.kr (J.L.)
* Correspondence: termylee@khu.ac.kr

Received: 3 August 2020; Accepted: 28 September 2020; Published: 1 October 2020

Abstract: Dietary monitoring is vital in healthcare because knowing food mass and intake (FMI) plays an essential role in revitalizing a person's health and physical condition. In this study, we report the development of a highly sensitive ring-type biosensor for the detection of FMI for dietary monitoring. To identify lightweight food on a spoon, we enhance the sensing system's sensitivity with three components: (1) a first-class lever mechanism, (2) a dual pad sensor, and (3) a force focusing structure using a ring surface having protrusions. As a result, we confirmed that, as the food arm's length increases, the force detected at the sensor is amplified by the first-class lever mechanism. Moreover, we obtained 1.88 and 1.71 times amplification using the dual pad sensor and the force focusing structure, respectively. Furthermore, the ring-type biosensor showed significant potential as a diagnostic indicator because the ring sensor signal was linearly proportional to the food mass delivered in a spoon, with $R^2 = 0.988$, and an average F_1 score of 0.973. Therefore, we believe that this approach is potentially beneficial for developing a dietary monitoring platform to support the prevention of obesity, which causes several adult diseases, and to keep the FMI data collection process automated in a quantitative, network-controlled manner.

Keywords: dietary monitoring; healthcare; ring-type biosensor; personalized digital medicine

1. Introduction

The intake amount of food is a critical factor in determining the state of the body's health because overeating can cause obesity, diabetes, and high blood pressure [1–3]. Patients who die from diseases such as cardiovascular disease, diabetes, and cancer account for more than 70% of deaths worldwide. The WHO reports that obesity due to an unhealthy diet and lack of physical activity is one of the leading causes of death [4]. In particular, obesity in children leads to obesity in adults and causes hyperinsulinemia, hyperlipidemia, glucose intolerance, and decreased growth hormone [5]. Moreover, the increase in social costs due to obesity is an economic burden for every country. Therefore, dietary monitoring is necessary for societal, economic and public health reasons. The need for food mass and intake (FMI) information has been increasing because of the knowledge that FMI plays an essential role in revitalizing a person's health and physical condition.

A wearable type of sensing system is required to detect and analyze intake in real-time throughout the day. In previous research, devices such as a mouthpiece, a skin patch, a wristband, a neckband, a microphone, a camera, and smart glasses were used. Among the previous studies, there was a study to detect food intake patterns using an accelerometer mounted on a mouthpiece [6]. There was also a dietary monitoring method using a skin attachment sensor [7]. Moreover, monitoring FMI has been analyzed using an attachment on a tooth. Although the attachment had an ultra-thin design, it still gave the user a negative perception due to the electrical current flowing in the mouth [8]. Additionally, rejection of the attachment by the body is also a problem to be solved. Separately, there is an indirect dietary monitoring method that measures the freshness of food by the detection of bacteria in tuna broth [9]. Dietary monitoring has also been attempted by sound discrimination using a microphone in a headset. In this case, the reduction of accuracy caused by ambient noise can be an issue [10,11]. In a different example, a sensing method was developed that monitored the swallowing motion using a piezoelectric element or an EGG (electroglottography) sensor in the neckband. This sensor approach focused on only intake pattern, limiting the use of the actual dietary monitoring [12,13].

Dietary monitoring may also be performed by using a smartphone camera to detect the food volume and pattern of intake. However, there is the inconvenience of carrying a camera and the requirement of taking an accurate picture according to instructions in a manual [14–20]. The eating pattern can also be detected through a wrist-type inertial sensor, such as a watch [21]. There is also a method for detecting the movement of facial muscles, including the oral cavity, with a piezoelectric sensor attached to the side of eyeglasses. However, that system has a problem in that it is difficult to identify the correct pattern because the force recognized by the sensor is insensitive. There is also an issue that the volume of the glasses at the temple increase [22,23]. In summary, the existing dietary monitoring studies had limitations in accurately measuring FMI, which is the core of dietary monitoring. In addition, there was an issue of users not wanting to wear the sensors due to the non-compact form factor.

In this study, we present a new dietary monitoring method using a compact, ring-type sensor on the hands, the final body part involved in eating prior to intake. We develop a highly sensitive finger sensing system using a ring-type flexible force sensor, with data connectivity via Bluetooth. We introduce three factors to enhance the sensitivity of the sensing system for detecting lightweight food. We validate our sensing system via experiments focused on the usability and accuracy of the device. Our results indicate that a wireless, ring-type finger sensing system can measure FMI with high sensitivity and accuracy for dietary monitoring.

2. Materials and Methods

2.1. Design and Fabrication of the Ring Sensing System

The composition layers of the ring sensing system and the flexible sensor are shown in Figure 1A. The layers of the sensing system start from the bottom, consisting of the ring, and include a flexible sensor, a printed circuit board, a battery in a holder, and the housing. The flexible sensor is composed of a cover lens, a polyethylene terephthalate (PET) substrate, a conductive polymer, an electrode, a substrate, and a pressure-sensitive adhesive (PSA). The layer on the top of the electrodes is a high-resistance material in which conductive particles are dispersed in a polymer such as polycarbonate (PC) or poly (methyl methacrylate)(PMMA), and pressure is detected by the contact area's change with the electrode according to the applied force. The cover lens protects the sensor. The electrodes and conductive polymers are deposited and patterned with a screen printing process.

As shown in Figure 1B, the ring sensor is placed on the bottom of the thumb, the typical contact point when holding a spoon. Here, the ring sensor uses a flexible force-sensing resistor, which detects the resistance change caused by the contact area's change when pressure is applied. We used a ring apparatus with a unique pattern that can focus the pressure from the spoon contact. The structure is made from polylactic acid and is fabricated using a 3D-printed, fused deposition method. The flexible force sensor is then placed on the structure. The driving voltage, 3 V, is applied to the sensor through two coin LR44 batteries in the battery holder layer, and the system communicates wirelessly with a smartphone via a field-programmable gate array (FPGA) board with a Bluetooth module. We used the compact module, Steval stlcs01v1 by STMicronics(Geneva, Switzerland), for Bluetooth low energy connectivity and pressure sensing. For the smartphone operating system, we used Android version 9(Mountain View, CA, USA). Finally, we confirmed the signal of no spoon mass by taking a new baseline using filtering, and then monitored the signal generated by food mass on the spoon using the wireless system, as shown in Figure 1C,D.

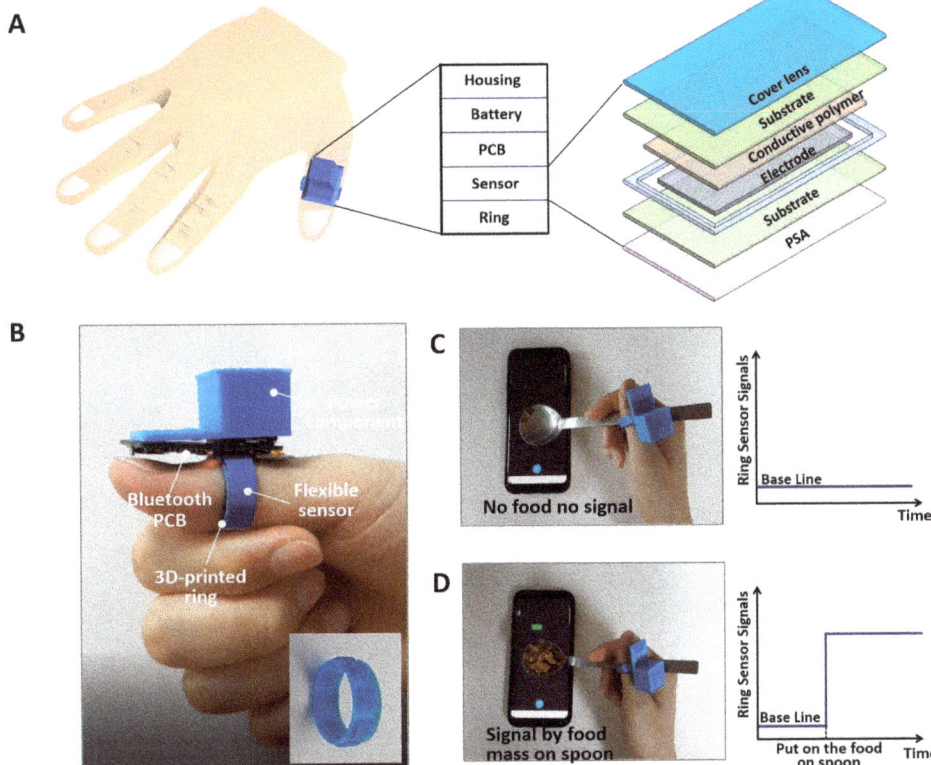

Figure 1. Schematic illustration and photograph of the ring-type biosensor for dietary monitoring via a smartphone. (**A**) Composition layer of ring sensing system: ring, sensor, printed circuit board, battery and housing, and flexible sensor: cover lens, substrate, conductive polymer, electrode, substrate, and pressure-sensitive adhesive. (**B**) Ring-type biosensing system mounted on the thumb and component unit: flexible tactile sensor, 3D-printed ring, power component and circuit board for wireless communication and battery. (**C**) Establishment of a baseline signal for a spoon with no food mass, taken using filtering. (**D**) Signal generated by food mass on the spoon.

2.2. Principle and Theory

The actual weight of the food placed on the spoon is minuscule, so highly sensitive detecting sensors and systems are absolutely required. The sensing mechanism of the ring sensor is shown in Figure 2a. When the sensor is pressed, contact between the pressure-sensitive material and the electrode occurs. As the pressure increases, the contact area increases, and the total resistance decreases. This resistance change is detected through the voltage distribution principle. The overall mechanism for sensor operation is described as shown in the flowchart in Figure 2b.

We enhance the sensitivity of the sensing system with three mechanical factors: (1) a first-class lever modified mechanism; (2) a force focusing structure consisting of protrusions of the ring surface; and (3) a dual pad sensor. First, the lever effect can improve the sensitivity of the system [24–26]. There are three classes of levers, and among them, we use the first-class lever mechanism to enhance the sensitivity. The first-class lever is used to create a large force at the load point by applying a small force to the effort point on the other side of the fulcrum. The advantage of the general lever law is that a small force can be used at the effort point. In the case of the ring sensor, when lightweight food is placed at the effort point, a large force is applied to the ring sensor, which corresponds to the load force position of the first-class lever. Thus, we can amplify the force applied to the ring sensor via the first-class lever mechanism.

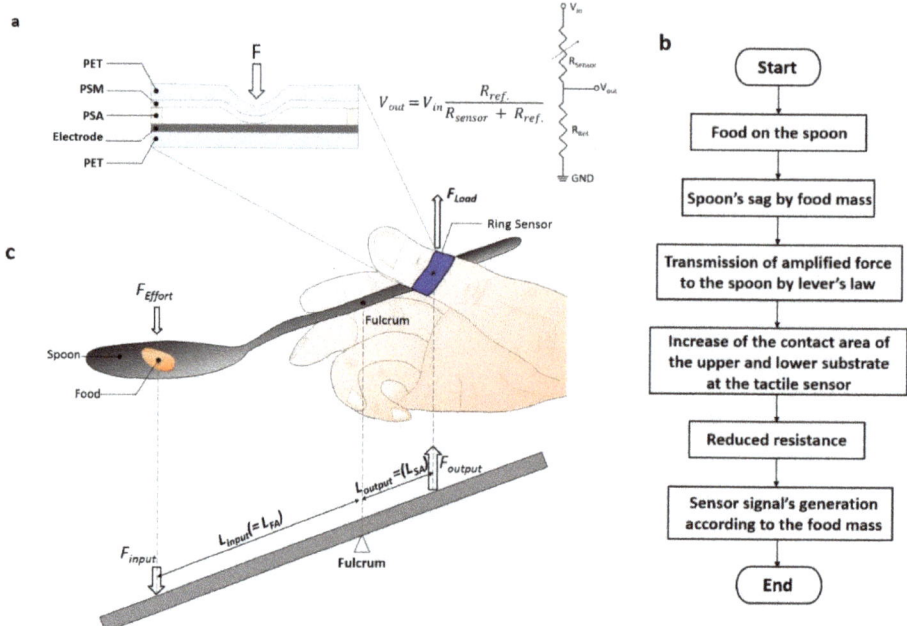

Figure 2. Schematic illustration of the ring-type sensing system's principle. (**a**) Schematic illustration of the force-sensitive layers of the ring sensor with voltage in-and-out relation. (**b**) Flow chart of the operation mechanism. (**c**) Schematic diagram of the ring-type biosensor using the first-class lever mechanism: L_{input} means the length of food arm (L_{FA}) and L_{output} means the length of the sensor arm (L_{SA}).

The specific details of the force amplification are shown in Figure 2c. The food mass is the input force and the force detected by the ring sensor is the output force. Here, L_{input} is the length of the food arm (L_{FA}), and L_{output} is the length of the sensor arm (L_{SA}). Also, the position where the spoon is pressed and fixed by the thumb serves as a support point. The magnitude of the force amplification is calculated by the lever equation, $F_{output} = F_{input} (L_{input}/L_{output})$. This lever effect depends on where the spoon is held. We also use a dual pad sensor, and it is expected that the dual effect will be obtained by applying the dual pad sensor in the same limited area. We use a unique structure that focuses the force on the sensor node by using protrusions on the ring. On a flat surface, force is dispersed globally, so there is a loss of force at the sensor node, whereas protrusions concentrate the force on the sensor node. We anticipate that the pressing region is limited to an active area, so it generates high pressure even if the force is the same.

3. Results

3.1. Characteristic Analysis of Sensor Signals to Spoon Arm Ratios for Different Sensor Grip Positions

We experimentally validated the influence of the three components that provided sensitivity enhancement. First, we verified the effects of the first-class lever mechanism. For proof-of-concept, the sensor was wound and tested as a sticker directly on the finger without the ring apparatus. Before loading food, the baseline was reset to take into account the spoon's own weight. The distance of the food arm, which is the distance between the middle finger of fulcrum and food that acts as the input force, was set to 4.5, 6, 7.5, and 9 cm. The sensor arm's length, which is the distance between the fulcrum and the sensor of the output force point, was fixed at 1.5 cm. The mass of food was set at 5 g. As shown in the graph of Figure 3, we confirmed that, as the food arm increased, the signal of the sensor was amplified by the first-class lever mechanism. It was confirmed that the minuscule mass of the food could be sensed through the amplified signal provided by the first-class lever mechanism using a sensing system located on the thumb. The reason the amplification was larger in the real environment than the ratio from the lever formula is that the inclination of the spoon naturally increases as the fulcrum point moves toward the ring sensor. Therefore, even with the same food mass on the spoon, the ring sensor is stimulated with a greater force when the spoon is tilted.

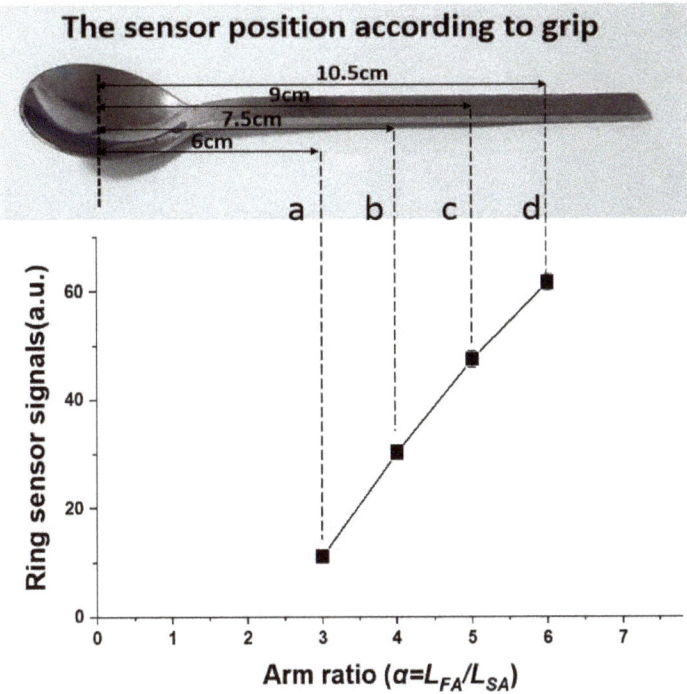

Figure 3. Experimental verification result of the first-class lever mechanism through ring sensor signals according to the gripped position of the spoon ($n = 15$). The sensor signal increases in proportion to the arm ratio, where the sensor position is the position of the thumb when holding the spoon and L_{SA} is fixed at 1.5 cm.

3.2. Effect of the Number of Ring Sensor Pads on Ring Sensor Signals: Single Versus Dual

Here we aimed to show the effect of the number of ring sensor pads. The sensor was overlapped and wound directly on the finger to show only pure pad number effects in the limited area. The food mass and arm ratio were set at 5 g and 6.0, respectively. The dual pad's signal intensity was significantly different from that of the single pad (p-value = 2.0×10^{-10}). We confirmed the ring sensor signal on the dual pad was 1.88 times that of the single pad, as shown in Figure 4.

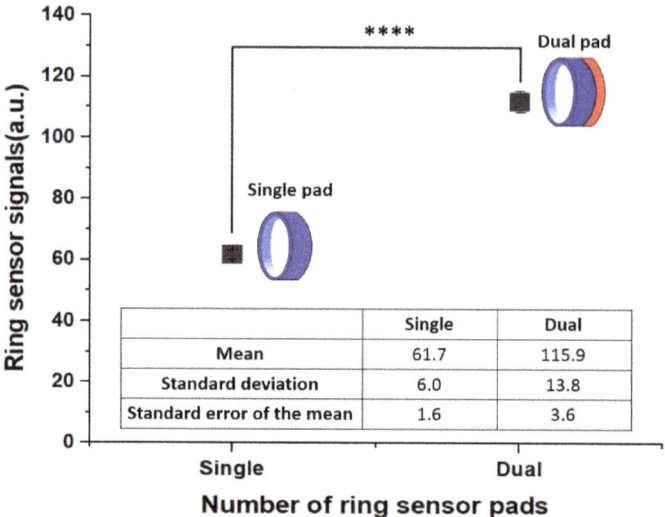

Figure 4. Experimental results for the ring sensor signals according to the number of sensor pads ($n = 15$). The sensor's signal strength of the dual pad was almost twice that of the single pad. Asterisks are denoting the statistical significance, ranging from significant (*) to extremely significant (****).

3.3. Effect of the Ring Surface Structure on Ring Sensor Signals: Plain Versus Protrusions

We also confirmed the effect of protrusions relative to a flat structure. First, as shown in Figure 5A we simulated the protrusion effect with finite element analysis using the Ansys mechanical tool (Canonsburg, PA, USA). The simulations suggested a 1.88 times performance increase of the protrusion structure compared to the flat structure. To verify this, we experimentally compared the protrusion structure and planar structure on the ring apparatus. The protrusion structure on the ring surface consisted of seven protrusion arrays that were 5×4 mm^2 in size with an array pitch of 7.45 mm, which is the pitch of the sensor node. The protrusion size was set based on force propagation and the sensor node size (5×6 mm^2).

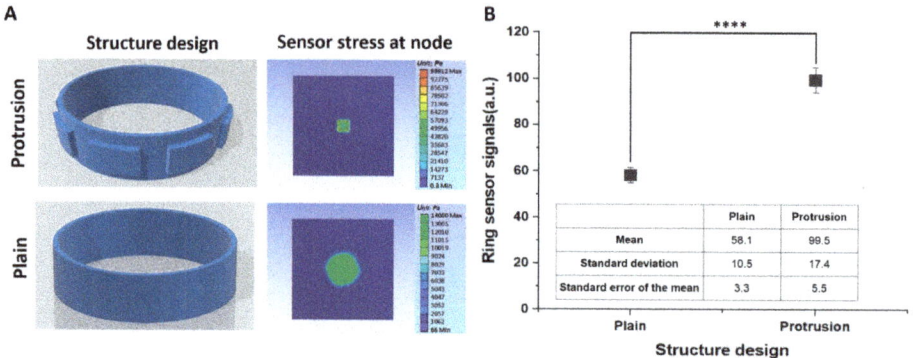

Figure 5. Numerical simulations and experimental results for the effect of the protrusion structure on ring sensor signals ($n = 10$). (**A**) Analysis of the finite element simulation of the protrusion and plain structures, where the white dashed line denotes the size of the protrusion. (**B**) The effect of the protrusion structure in comparison to the planar surface, with a p-value of 1.5×10^{-5}.

The food mass and arm ratio were set at 10 g and 6.0, respectively. As shown in Figure 5B, the sensor's signal strength of the protrusion and plain structure was significantly different, with a p-value of 1.5×10^{-5}. The sensitivity of the protrusion structure was 1.71 times that of the flat structure. The increased sensitivity was caused by protrusions locally concentrating the force on the sensor node.

3.4. Ring Sensor's Performance Analysis for Food Detection Using the F_1 Score

We checked the classification results on the eating behavior using a confusion matrix to grasp the ring sensor system's performance. For the test, we used a mass of 5 g. Accuracy was computed as the following Equation (1), and the F_1 score was calculated using a harmonic mean of Precision and Recall from Equations (2)–(4).

$$Accuracy = (TP + TN)/(TP + FN + TN + FP) \tag{1}$$

$$Precision = TP/(TP + FP) \tag{2}$$

$$Recall = TP/(TP + FN) \tag{3}$$

$$F_1 = (2\ Precision \cdot Recall)/(Precision + Recall) \tag{4}$$

where TP (true positive) means that when there was a 5 g mass on the spoon, a signal above the threshold was generated, and the FP (false positive) was defined as when a signal above the threshold was generated when there was no mass on the spoon. The experiment was conducted by dividing it into a vertical movement and a circular movement on a plane, a typical case where the spoon moves without food. As shown in Table 1, an accuracy of 0.963 and an F_1 score of 0.962 were calculated for vertical movement. Accuracy of 0.983 and an F_1 score of 0.983 were obtained for circular motion on a plane. In the case of food with vertical movement, the rate of misrecognition, that is, the frequency in which actual food was present but not detected was relatively high. It was determined that in case of vertical motion without mass on the spoon, the spoon's weight stimulates the sensor of the finger when the vertical motion stops, due to effect of acceleration. For this reason, an error occurred even when there was no mass on the spoon.

Table 1. Confusion matrix for accuracy and F_1 score analysis of food detection.

Movement Categories		Actual Activities	
		Food on Spoon	No Food on Spoon
Category I (Vertical movement)	Food on spoon	141	2
	No food on spoon	9	148
	Accuracy	0.963	
	F_1 score	0.962	
Category II (Circular movement on the plane)	Food on spoon	148	3
	No food on spoon	2	147
	Accuracy	0.983	
	F_1 score	0.983	

3.5. Correlation Analysis between Food Mass and Signal of the Ring Sensor

We confirmed the device's accuracy with the dual-padded sensor and the protrusion structures using a correlation of the ring sensor signal and the food mass. When masses of 3, 6, 9, 12, 15, 18, or 21 g were placed on a spoon, the corresponding analog signal of the sensor was measured. The experiment was performed for three users, with the results shown in the graph in Figure 6. We believe that the difference between the graphs occurred due to the sensors' deviation and the users' proficiency. However, the R^2 values were very high, with an average value of 0.988. Finally, we verified the detection of a signal proportional to the mass of food on a spoon and showed the feasibility of a personalized digital medicine solution capable of quantitative intake sensing.

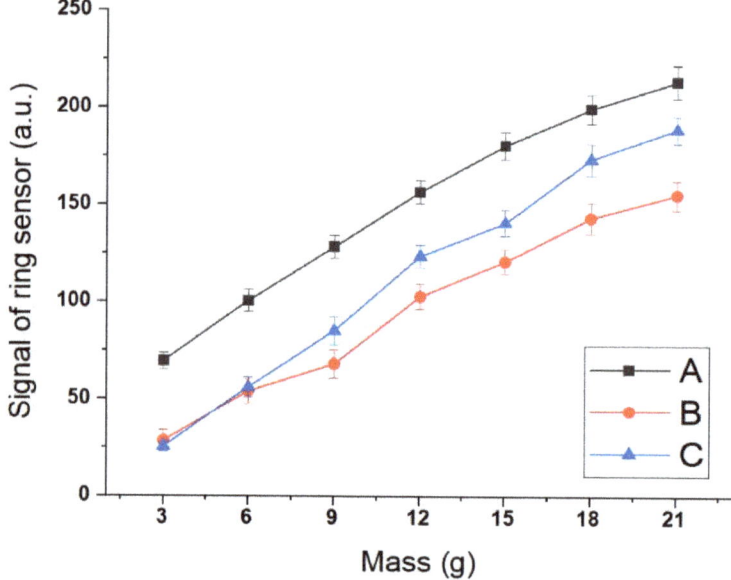

Figure 6. Correlation between the sensor signal and food mass on spoon using a ring sensor system ($n = 15$). The experiment was conducted by three users, and ring sensor signals increase proportionally according to the mass placed on the spoon. For A, B, and C the R^2 values were 0.986, 0.989, and 0.990, respectively. The spoon arm ratio was set to 6.0. The error bar indicates the standard error of the mean.

4. Discussion

4.1. Supplementary Needs of the Ring Sensor System as a Food Mass and Intake Detector

A few complementary additions could add to the quality of the ring sensor as a useful healthcare application for real-life dietary monitoring. In the protrusion structure experiment, complete contact between the spoon and the ring sensor was not possible due to the ring's thickness and the ring's and spoon's rigidity. Therefore, if the modulus of the ring material was tuned, it is expected that improved results could be obtained. Also, in the current system, it is necessary to locate the finger grip position manually. Therefore, it is also necessary to insert the touch sensor so that the position of the spoon grip can be automatically known. Through the finger's gripping position, the signal intensity as it is changed by the lever law could be calculated to determine the actual FMI. Furthermore, in the future it will be necessary to determine the amount of food when using different tools, such as forks and chopsticks.

4.2. Synergy Effect of Combining the Ring Sensor with Different Fields

The ring sensor system has the attractive ability to measure accurately the mass of food consumed with a spoon. To achieve the ultimate goal of dietary monitoring, a hybrid approach is required that will combine different fields beyond the mixture of sensors to identify the types and mass of foods ingested. For example, in the case of liquid and solid foods, a sensing error can occur due to the difference in the center of mass when placed on a spoon even when the weight is the same. This difference can be compensated by merging the spoon sensor with smart glasses to analyze intake patterns such as chewing and drinking [24–26]. The combination with smart glasses would make it possible to reduce the error through mass calibration based on the spoon shape and the center of gravity by determining whether the form of the ingested food is solid or liquid. Smart glasses will also be useful for continuous monitoring. Using smart glasses makes it possible to clearly distinguish whether or not the actual food is ingested. Through this, it is possible to continuously monitor the intake amount through an automatic baseline adjustment and calculation process when food intake is completed.

5. Conclusions

The essence of this study is that it provided a direct and objective measurement method for FMI. Moreover, we developed a highly sensitive dual-padded ring-type sensor with a protrusion structure to detect and monitor FMI. The improved sensitivity of the system was based in part on its use of a lever mechanism. The sensitivity could be increased by 1.88 and 1.71 times by using a double layer and protrusion structures, respectively. The sensor accuracy shows a high correlation of ring sensor signal to food mass, with $R^2 = 0.988$ and an average F_1 score of 0.973.

The previous method only determined the intake pattern and the amount of chewing, so there was a limit to the practical dietary information that could be obtained. However, we demonstrated the feasibility of FMI analysis using a ring-type bio-sensing system for actual dietary monitoring. Therefore, we believe that this approach is potentially beneficial for developing a wearable platform to support the prevention of obesity, which causes a number of adult diseases. Furthermore, metabolic syndrome can be prevented, and physical activity can be revitalized through dietary monitoring. Therefore, a dietary monitoring system using a ring sensor is expected to be useful as a diagnostic indicator that identifies physiological signals based on the individual's dietary behavior.

Author Contributions: Conceptualization, W.H.; Data curation, W.H.; Formal analysis, W.G.L.; Funding acquisition, W.H. and W.G.L.; Investigation, W.G.L.; Methodology, W.H. and J.L.; Project administration, W.G.L.; Supervision, W.G.L.; Validation, W.H.; Visualization, J.L.; Writing—original draft, W.H.; Writing—review and editing, W.G.L. All authors have read and agreed to the published version of the manuscript.

Funding: This work was supported by the National Research Foundation of Korea (NRF) grant funded by the Ministry of Science and ICT, Korea (No. 2020R1A2C1006842).

Conflicts of Interest: The authors declare no conflict of interest.

Nomenclature

FMI	Food mass and intake
EGG	Electroglottography
PET	Polyethylene terephthalate
PC	Polycarbonate
PMMA	Poly(methyl methacrylate)
PSA	Pressure-sensitive adhesive
FPGA	Field-programmable gate array
L_{FA}	Length of the food arm
L_{SA}	Length of the sensor arm
TP	True positive
FN	False negatives
FP	False positive
TN	True negative

References

1. Flegal, K.M.; Carroll, M.D.; Kit, B.K.; Ogden, C.L. Prevalence of obesity and trends in the distribution of Body Mass Index among US adults, 1999–2010. *JAMA* **2012**, *307*, 491–497. [CrossRef]
2. Linderman, G.C.; Lu, J.; Lu, Y.; Sun, X.; Xu, W.; Nasir, K.; Schulz, W.; Jiang, L.; Krumholz, H.M. Association of Body Mass Index with blood pressure among 1.7 million Chinese adults. *JAMA Netw. Open* **2018**, *1*, e181271. [CrossRef] [PubMed]

3. Lloyd, L.J.; Langley-Evans, S.C.; McMullen, S.; Langley-Evans, S.C. Childhood obesity and adult cardiovascular disease risk: A systematic review. *Int. J. Obes.* **2009**, *34*, 18–28. [CrossRef] [PubMed]
4. World Health Organization. *Noncommunicable Diseases Progress Monitor.* 2020. Available online: https://www.who.int/publications/i/item/ncd-progress-monitor-2020 (accessed on 1 October 2020).
5. Weihrauch-Blüher, S.; Schwarz, P.; Klusmann, J.-H. Childhood obesity: Increased risk for cardiometabolic disease and cancer in adulthood. *Metabolism* **2019**, *92*, 147–152. [CrossRef] [PubMed]
6. Li, C.-Y.; Chen, Y.-C.; Chen, W.-J.; Huang, P.; Chu, H.-H. Proceedings of the 2013 International Symposium on Wearable Computers, ISWC '13, Zurich, Switzerland, 9–12 September 2013; pp. 41–44.
7. Roh, E.; Hwang, B.-U.; Kim, D.; Kim, B.-Y.; Lee, N.-E. Stretchable, transparent, ultrasensitive, and patchable strain sensor for human–machine interfaces comprising a nanohybrid of carbon nanotubes and conductive elastomers. *ACS Nano* **2015**, *9*, 6252–6261. [CrossRef] [PubMed]
8. Tseng, P.; Napier, B.; Garbarini, L.; Kaplan, D.L.; Omenetto, F.G. Functional, RF-trilayer sensors for tooth-mounted, wireless monitoring of the oral cavity and food consumption. *Adv. Mater.* **2018**, *30*, 1703257. [CrossRef] [PubMed]
9. Parate, K.; Pola, C.C.; Rangnekar, S.V.; Mendivelso-Perez, D.L.; Smith, E.A.; Hersam, M.C.; Gomes, C.L.; Claussen, J.C. Aerosol-jet-printed graphene electrochemical histamine sensors for food safety monitoring. *2D Mater.* **2020**, *7*, 034002. [CrossRef]
10. Passler, S.; Fischer, W.-J. Food intake monitoring: Automated chew event detection in chewing sounds. *IEEE J. Biomed. Heal. Inform.* **2014**, *18*, 278–289. [CrossRef] [PubMed]
11. Gao, Y.; Zhang, N.; Wang, H.; Ding, X.; Ye, X.; Chen, G.; Cao, Y. iHear food: Eating detection using commodity bluetooth headsets. In Proceedings of the 2016 IEEE First International Conference on Connected Health: Applications, Systems and Engineering Technologies (CHASE), Washington, DC, USA, 27–29 June 2016; Institute of Electrical and Electronics Engineers (IEEE): Piscataway, NJ, USA, 2016; pp. 163–172.
12. Kalantarian, H.; Alshurafa, N.; Sarrafzadeh, M. A wearable nutrition monitoring system. In Proceedings of the 2014 11th International Conference on Wearable and Implantable Body Sensor Networks, Zurich, Switzerland, 16–19 June 2014; pp. 75–80.
13. Farooq, M.; Fontana, J.M.; Sazonov, E. A novel approach for food intake detection using electroglottography. *Physiol. Meas.* **2014**, *35*, 739–751. [CrossRef] [PubMed]
14. Choe, E.K.; Abdullah, S.; Rabbi, M.; Thomaz, E.; Epstein, D.A.; Cordeiro, F.; Kay, M.; Abowd, G.D.; Choudhury, T.; Fogarty, J.; et al. Semi-automated tracking: A balanced approach for self-monitoring applications. *IEEE Pervasive Comput.* **2017**, *16*, 74–84. [CrossRef]
15. Kawano, Y.; Yanai, K. FoodCam: A real-time food recognition system on a smartphone. *Multimed. Tools Appl.* **2014**, *74*, 5263–5287. [CrossRef]
16. Bettadapura, V.; Thomaz, E.; Parnami, A.; Abowd, G.D.; Essa, I. Leveraging context to support automated food recognition in restaurants. In Proceedings of the 2015 IEEE Winter Conference on Applications of Computer Vision, Waikoala, HI, USA, 5–9 January 2015; pp. 580–587.
17. Zhu, F.; Bosch, M.; Woo, I.; Kim, S.; Boushey, C.J.; Ebert, D.S.; Delp, E.J. The use of mobile devices in aiding dietary assessment and evaluation. *IEEE J. Sel. Top. Signal. Process.* **2010**, *4*, 756–766. [CrossRef] [PubMed]
18. Liang, Y.; Li, J. Computer vision-based food calorie estimation: Dataset, method, and experiment. *arXiv* **2017**, arXiv:1705.07632.
19. Gao, J.; Tan, W.; Ma, L.; Wang, Y.; Tang, W. MUSEFood: Multi-Sensor-based food volume estimation on smartphones. In Proceedings of the 2019 IEEE SmartWorld, Ubiquitous Intelligence & Computing, Advanced & Trusted Computing, Scalable Computing & Communications, Cloud & Big Data Computing, Internet of People and Smart City Innovation (SmartWorld/SCALCOM/UIC/ATC/CBDCom/IOP/SCI), Leicester, UK, 19–23 August 2019; pp. 899–906.
20. Yang, X.; Doulah, A.; Farooq, M.; Parton, J.; McCrory, M.A.; Higgins, J.A.; Sazonov, E. Statistical models for meal-level estimation of mass and energy intake using features derived from video observation and a chewing sensor. *Sci. Rep.* **2019**, *9*, 45. [CrossRef] [PubMed]
21. Thomaz, E.; Essa, I.; Abowd, G.D. A practical approach for recognizing eating moments with wrist-mounted inertial sensing. In Proceedings of the 2015 ACM International Joint Conference on Pervasive and Ubiquitous Computing, Osaka, Japan, 7–11 September 2015; pp. 1029–1040.
22. Farooq, M.; Sazonov, E. A novel wearable device for food intake and physical activity recognition. *Sensors* **2016**, *16*, 1067. [CrossRef] [PubMed]

23. Farooq, M.; Sazonov, E. Accelerometer-based detection of food intake in free-living individuals. *IEEE Sens. J.* **2018**, *18*, 3752–3758. [CrossRef] [PubMed]
24. Chung, J.; Oh, W.; Baek, D.; Ryu, S.; Lee, W.G.; Bang, H. Design and evaluation of smart glasses for food intake and physical activity classification. *J. Vis. Exp.* **2018**, e56633. [CrossRef] [PubMed]
25. Chung, J.; Chung, J.; Oh, W.; Yoo, Y.; Lee, W.G.; Bang, H. A glasses-type wearable device for monitoring the patterns of food intake and facial activity. *Sci. Rep.* **2017**, *7*, 41690. [CrossRef] [PubMed]
26. Han, D.Y.; Park, B.O.; Kim, J.W.; Lee, J.H.; Lee, W.G. Non-verbal communication and touchless activation of a radio-controlled car via facial activity recognition. *Int. J. Precis. Eng. Manuf.* **2020**, *21*, 1035–1046. [CrossRef]

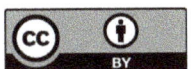

© 2020 by the authors. Licensee MDPI, Basel, Switzerland. This article is an open access article distributed under the terms and conditions of the Creative Commons Attribution (CC BY) license (http://creativecommons.org/licenses/by/4.0/).

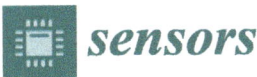

Article
Development of a Sensor to Measure Physician Consultation Times

Roman Gabl [1,*] and Florian Stummer [2,*]

1. School of Engineering, Institute for Energy Systems, FloWave Ocean Energy Research Facility, The University of Edinburgh, Max Born Crescent, Edinburgh EH9 3BF, UK
2. Deanery of Molecular, Genetic and Population Health Sciences, Usher Institute, The University of Edinburgh, Old Medical School, Teviot Place, Edinburgh EH8 9AG, UK
* Correspondence: Roman.Gabl@ed.ac.uk (R.G.); F.O.Stummer@sms.ed.ac.uk (F.S.)

Received: 2 October 2019; Accepted: 30 November 2019; Published: 5 December 2019

Abstract: The duration of patient–physician contact is an important factor for the optimisation of treatment processes in healthcare systems. Available methods can be labour-intensive and the quality is, in many cases, poor. A part of this research project is to develop a sensor system, which allows the detection of people passing through a door, including the direction. For this purpose, two time of flight sensors are combined with a door sensor and a motion detection sensor (for redundancy) on one single side of the door frame. The period between two single measurements could be reduced to 50 ms, which allows the measurement of walking speed up to 2 ms^{-1}. The accuracy of the time stamp for each event is less than one second and ensures a precise documentation of the consultation time. This paper presents the development of the sensor system, the miniaturisation of the installation and first measurement results, as well as the measurement's concept of quality analysis, including multiple door applications. In future steps, the sensor system will be deployed at different medical practices to determine the exact duration of the patient–physician interaction over a longer time period.

Keywords: people counting; bi-directional; motion detection; time of flight sensor

1. Introduction

Demographic changes around the world bring new challenges to healthcare systems. People now live longer and their healthy years increase, especially in higher- and middle-income countries. However, a longer life expectancy can also mean that individuals have to live longer with illness [1]. The treatment of chronic illnesses and accompanying comorbidities is a primary healthcare system issue, as it leads to continuous public health monitoring through healthcare professionals and an increase of patient–physician contacts.

In 2017, Irving et al. [2] presented the results of an international survey on variations in primary care physicians' consultation times. The results show a wide range of consultation periods: from 48 s in Bangladesh, through 15 min in Australia, to 22.5 min in Sweden. Eighteen countries, which hold more than 50 percent of the world's population, needed less than 5 min to treat a patient. However, the main finding was the lack of continuous data collection. A majority of countries were not able to provide adequate data on measurement methods, the person measuring time, the study design, the general duration in min, the number of consultations, and the quality of data sets. The paper at hand introduces actual standard measurement methods and presents a possible new solution for direct and automated gross patient–physician interaction duration measurement. This new sensor-led collection method aims to exclude biased data collection and the feared "Hawthorne"-effect to a certain extent.

The primarily used measurement methods can be categorised as (a) self-reported, (b) video, (c) audio, (d) stopwatch, (e) SMS (short message service), (f) International Network for the Rational Use of Drugs (INRUD), and (g) calculation-centred. Each method is introduced and discussed below:

(a) Self-reported means that a member of the healthcare staff (mostly the treating physician) answered a survey or provided a collection of duration times. These self-reported figures can, however, be categorised as biased.
(b) Video means that a video recording of the activities in the treatment room were evaluated. This approach needs the patient's recruitment and consent and is highly problematic regarding the General Data Protection Regulation (GDPR).
(c) Audio recordings are used to verify the duration of patient–physician interactions; however, similarly to the video method, audio recordings are problematic regarding GDPR.
(d) As part of the stopwatch method, a member of the healthcare staff (mostly the treating physician) timed the consultation period. This method is more reliable, as the net results can be evaluated. However, a comparison to gross results is not possible.
(e) A short message (SMS) is sent by a member of the healthcare staff or the physician to a certain phone number, deriving the consultation duration time from the received message.
(f) World Health Organisation/International Network for the Rational Use of Drugs (WHO/INRUD) means using data provided by the drug use indicators for health facilities, which contain a set of patient care indicators including the average consultation time. The number is evaluated by "dividing the total time for a series of consultations by the number of consultations".
(g) Calculation means that certain time parameters were collected and average consultation duration times were derived. Most of the data sets used to do the calculations cannot be verified.

Irving et al. [2] found that the quality of studies using these methods were good in 40%, poor in 36%, and fair in 24%, leaving a ratio of 40% to 60% with regard to trustworthiness (good) versus dubiousness (poor/fair).

Knowing how long a patient–physician consultation lasts is not only a matter of improving the patient's journey, but also a business administration factor. Taking the project management triangle (time, costs, scope, and quality) into account, time is the only factor that can neither be regained nor changed. However, costs can be derived from time. Scope and quality are functions of cost and time. A direct, automated time measurement method that excludes biases as far as possible, therefore allows a more substantial and sustaining documentation of treatment processes and the development of lean organisational systems for business administration, human resource departments, and healthcare staff interaction.

The paper presents a novel sensor system to automatically measure the interaction time between patient and physician in a single and multi-room configuration. Especially the latter requires a documentation of the time period individuals take to pass through a door and in which direction they are headed. Existing methods are often either strongly dependent on possibly biased, sometimes imprecise self-reporting, or they are problematic in regard to GDPR (video and/or audio recordings), and are also likely to be very labour-intensive. The novel sensors system aims to overcome those weaknesses, and allows the combination of the individual treatment period with anonymous patient data to verify the provided services, and additionally develop optimised operation methods in medical practices. The development of the proposed solution is summarised and discussed. Exemplary results are presented and a long term deployment of five sensors is currently ongoing.

2. Materials and Methods

2.1. Overview and Objectives

Sensors that count and track people are commercially available and deliver a wide range of applications in airports, museums, libraries, or any other type of (public) buildings. Possible applications are crowd management, transport systems, heating as well as air conditioning, and optimisation of evacuation planning [3]. Significant user groups are retailers and shopping centres. These can deploy available products to track the behaviour of costumers in different zones, identify specific targeted groups (children, families, and adults) and also combine those data with further available sales information. This helps to allocate staff and optimise marketing tools. An advanced application such as this requires stereo/video capturing, covering a wider area and specific analysis methods [4–6]. Li et al. [7] added a near-infrared stereo camera system for application in low light levels. Consequently, this method is available for nearly every condition but raises significant privacy issues.

The deployment of such a sensor system in a medical practice includes specific restrictions and ethical considerations. Patients and the content of the consultation with the physician need to stay fully anonymous. Each analysis based on video, which would be used in the previously mentioned commercially available solutions, can be stored and is subject to a potentially unauthorised access. Nevertheless, a video system can be used under specific conditions. An example is presented by Mousavi et al. [8], who recorded an operating room. Based on a manual analysis, he tracked how long and why the door was opened in relation to the different stages of the operation. The main objective of the presented development of a novel sensor system is to reduce risks regarding GDPR as well as the potential risk of abuse. The aim is to reduce these concerns in order to increase the patient's as well as the physician's trust and acceptance.

Hence, the instrumentation should only be capable of recording specific data needed for the research project. This restriction has to be included in the design and should not depend on filters, processing, or storing. Consequently, all video surveillance solutions are excluded and the choice of commercially available solutions are limited to light barrier. Various available products also include detection of direction (leaving or entering the door), but all found solutions are limited regarding the time resolutions. The internal data processing in the device sums up the detection and only adds up values for a time period of typically 15 min. This is absolutely sufficient for the above mentioned applications but is not enough for the detailed analysis of the time the patient interacts with the physician. Those interactions are typically in the range of minutes [2]. An extended search and the contact with various manufacturers and service providers brought the authors to the conclusion that no product allows access to the raw data or the needed resolution time. Consequently, the development of a specific instrumentation is required. An additional benefit is that it can be custom-made for the specific needs of the research project.

Door sensors, based on a magnetic contact, can deliver a basic evaluation of the time in which the patient or the physician enters the room. Each closing and opening of the door can be captured with a time stamp. However, there is no specification regarding the number of people passing through a door at once or whether they are entering or leaving a room. This results in an uncertainty and makes it hard to analyse the captured data. The deployment of a single beam switch improves the situation significantly and allows for counting of the number of individuals entering or leaving. A double beam approach is needed to determine the direction of motion as it is used in commercially available products. Alternative methods would have to face the motion direction, which can potentially distract from the movement of the person through the door. Bi-directional detection and the limitation to the door frame are key objectives for the development.

In addition to the mentioned requirements concerning ethical aspects, as well as the time resolution (a few seconds), the installation should be straightforward, unobtrusive, and not limited to specific conditions. This includes the requirement to contain the entire instrumentation in one unit and the elimination of a mirror, a reflector, or a (light) source on the other side of the door. The utilisation and combination of standardised components allow the minimisation of costs and ensure the durability of the system. A redundant documentation based on different methods helps to validate the results and reduces uncertainties. Furthermore, both temporary observation (a few days to weeks) and also the potential for a long time observation over months should be given. The developed sensor combination meets all those objectives and based on the presented analysis method an objective documentation of the duration of patient and physician interaction can be delivered.

2.2. Combination of the Sensors

Based on the objectives (Section 2.1) a combination of three different sensors was chosen for the final design: (a) magnetic door sensor (DS), (b) one additional motion detection (MD) sensor (RCWL 0516), and (c) two time of flight (ToF) sensors (VL53L0X). All three different components are available from various suppliers and in a wide range of options (size, colour, and connections). The first tests were conducted with an Arduino Uno (Figure 1a), which has been replaced by an Arduino Nano for the final version due to the smaller dimensions (Figure 1d,e).

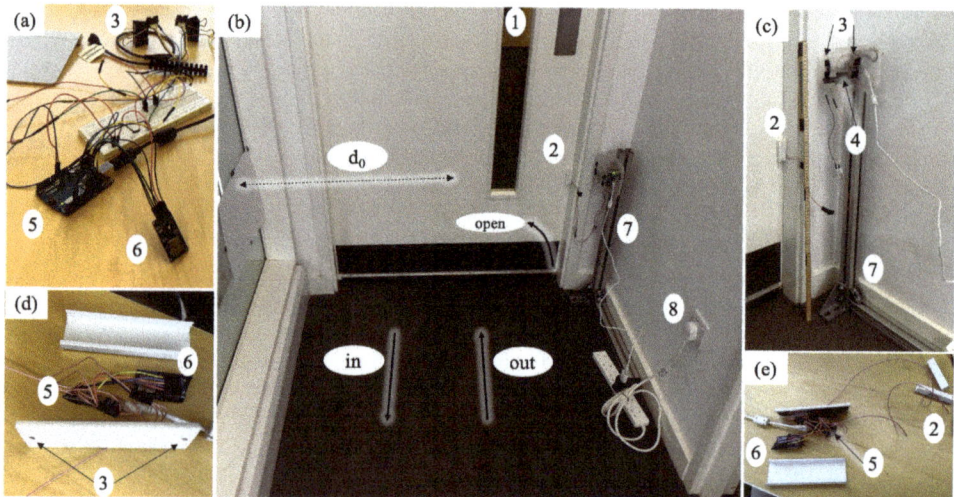

Figure 1. Development of the sensor system (**a**) desk version; (**b,c**) prototype installation to test the concept; (**d,e**) final design. Door (1), door sensor (2), time of flight (3), motion detection (4), Arduino (5), Micro SD card module (6), support structure (7), and power supply (8).

The door sensor is a magnetic surface contact. For the presented application a product was chosen, which is commonly used in alarm circuits (supplier CQR Security). This guarantees a high reliability and durability. It would also include a tamper alarm, which is unused. The operation distance between the switch and the magnet housing is dependant on the direction as well as the mounting position. It ranges from 5 mm to 35 mm for non-ferrous surfaces and is reduced in combination with ferrous components (door frame or panel). This information is provided in the operation and installation instructions by the supplier [9]. The DS delivers the basic information of if the door is open or closed and the Arduino logs the time stamp as soon as a change in the status occurs.

Initially different passive infrared sensors (PIR) were tested, which also allowed sensitivity and delay adjustments. Those motion sensors are commonly used as a light switch and typically deliver an output signal as long as motion is detected (including a further delay). The exact limitation of the activation range was not easy to achieve and the sensor system did not trigger precisely. Issues in collecting precise data are encountered if a person just steps into the room and immediately walks out again or if a person passes by on the door. An approach based on a line observation is more sensible and precise in comparison to a comparable big region, in which the sensor is the trigger. Consequently, PIR sensors were discarded in an early design state. Nevertheless, one single radar module RCWL 0516 [10] is still used in the presented instrumentation. This sensor detects motion with comparable accuracy to a PIR system but works through plastic. Hence, it can be very easy added to the systems and allows an additional independent motion detection as validation for the other systems.

Both previously mentioned methods are not capable of detecting the direction of motion. Therefore a delay between two lines (vertical planes) has to be measured. Huang et al. [11] showed a successful installation of a bi-directional system, which provides additional inputs for the building automation system. Therefore, infrared sources are mounted on one side of the door and the detector is mounted on the other side. An exact alignment is needed as well as devices on both sides of the door. Alternatively, the emitter and detector can be installed on one side and only a reflector is added opposite to the instrument. The previously mentioned objectives of the research include that the installation effort should be reduced. Different range finding devices are available, which allow the measurement of the distance without a specific arrangement on the target. As part of the discovery phase, commercially available small ultrasonic sensors and infrared distance meters were investigated. They were tested to determine if they are suitable to work in a pair and in close range. The investigated lower price devices did not deliver the needed quality nor reliability and those techniques were not further studied.

Far better results could be reached with a time of flight (ToF) distance sensor, which is typically used as a scanning device [12–15] rang finder [16–18] and gesture detection sensor [19]. The used VL53L0X module is capable of capturing distances up to a maximum range of 2 m with a very high accuracy. This specific device includes a Class 1 laser, which is integrated with the collector on the chip. The beam is invisible to the human eye and the spreading is comparatively small [20]. The communication with the Arduino is based on the I2C (Inter-Integrated Circuit) interface. For the current application, two devices are installed in parallel. This requires that as part of every power up the XSHUT pin (Rest or interrupt the communication) is activated to change the default address of the device. Two parallel distance measurements are captured, which allow us to identify the direction of the motion. Further details are presented in Section 3.1.

The motion detector as well as the two ToF sensors allow a clear identification, even when the door is kept open—if, for example, the physician switches between two rooms (Section 3.2). Under regular conditions, the combination of all three different types of sensors delivers an exact recording of the door state, an additional motion detection and two distances, which allows us to determine the motion direction of the person passing through the door.

2.3. Prototype Development

The development of the sensor system was done in three phases. For the initial desk version (Figure 1a), different sensor types and combinations were tested. Based on this, it was decided to use the final combination of sensors, which are installed (Section 2.2). Furthermore, the Arduino code was developed and tested (Section 3.1).

In a second step, a realistic configuration was built up and tested. Figure 1 b,c shows the set-up at one door at FloWave Ocean Energy Research Facility (University of Edinburgh). It is a fire door with a door closer, which connects the main office with the wave tank area. A piece of paper is used to limit the distance measurement of the ToF sensors on the opposing side as there is a big window. This construction provides a high flexibility of heights for the ToF sensors and the location is ideal to deploy a generously designed box. The presented results in Section 3 are captured with this set-up.

Finally, an additional step in the development is made to further miniaturise the instrumentation (Figure 1). A vital part of this is the change from an Arduino Uno SMD R3 to a Nano (HiLetgo Mini USB Nano V3.0 ATmega328P CH340G), which has nearly the same capability but is far smaller in size. Figure 2 shows the circuit and how the sensors are connected to the Arduino. In the final design, the magnetic door contact remains as a separate unit and is connected via cable to the main unit. Thus, an independent installation as well as an optimal usage of the available space in the door frame is possible. It was noticed that the distance from the door to a wall socket is in the range of a few meters for all the physicians' offices, where the sensor will be deployed in the next project phase. Hence, the power supply based on batteries was considered, however a direct power supply is preferred. This decision was made to secure a long term deployment of the system.

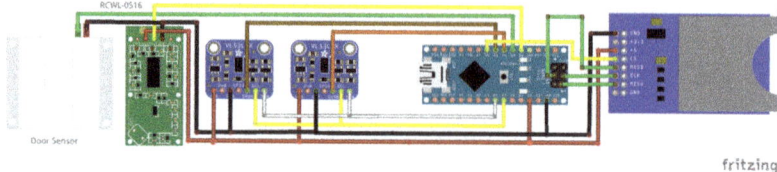

Figure 2. Shematic representation of the circuit including the Arduino Nano: power (red), ground (black) and all further colours mark connections to input/output pins.

Different cases and boxes were investigated to enclose the system. The best fit and usability could be gained with a cable trunking as shown in Figure 1d,e. This provides protection of the electrical parts and a good accessibility. The distance between the two holes for the ToF sensor is 100 mm and all sensors are mounted to the cover piece. The needed cable feed-through can be included in the other part, which is attached to the door frame with double sided adhesive tape. This back part can be easily replaced and custom-made for each specific location. The dimensions are 38 mm by 16 mm and 120 mm in length. Both ends are closed with caps and can further be sealed with tape. Only a weak extraction-proof could be included in the casing and the cables have to be further secured with tape.

The captured data is stored for each individual sensor in one txt-file on a Micro SD card, which is included in the case. A wide range of different applications successfully included a real-time transmission of the measurement data ranging from traffic systems [21], displacement sensors of piles and columns [22], or weather stations [23]. For the current research project, reliable storage is more important than immediate transmission hence the analyses are conducted after the test. This also gives the opportunity to eventually combine the findings with anonymous treatment categories, which include factors like a patient's age, gender, and main diagnosis. Consequently, a transmission of the data is not needed but is considered for future applications, hence the device also allows for remote management. The simultaneous observation of more than one door requires a synchronisation of several installed sensor systems. This is conducted as part of the installation and the possible time offset is acceptable.

3. Results

3.1. Single Door

In this first section, the data capturing of the sensor system is described in general as well as the processing for one door. Figure 3 presents the exemplary set-up, which is similar to the one presented in Figure 1b. For the following consideration, it is assumed that the door solely gives access to one single room, in which the time of the interaction between physician and patient has to be measured. Therefore, the full data set is captured and the analysis is conducted as a post processing. Section 3.2 expands this to further doors and more than one room.

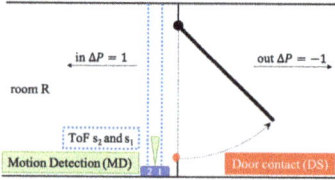

Figure 3. Exemplary sketch of the set-up of sensors and definition of the motion direction.

The processing tasks done on the Arduino are tried to keep as low as possible. This allows to go through the loops efficiently and to reduce the time step between two readings. Status changes of the motion detector (MD) as well as the door sensors (DS) are simplified to 0 and 1. This coded information is written in separate files including a time stamp. In this process, the time values for changes of the MD and DS are rounded to full seconds.

A different approach is implemented for the time of flight (ToF) sensors. In an initial step the distance between the sensors and the opposing wall is adapted. This allows us to define a location-specific criterion (it includes the measurements of both sensors) to trigger the recording of the two sensors. Each device measures the distance between the sensor and the next object individually, and the results is only stored when the criterion is fulfilled. Finally, the analysis method for the ToF data is presented.

The first 10 s after the initialisation of the Arduino (power is switched on) are used to adapt the code to the specific circumstances of the deployment location. An initial distance d_0 is defined in the code (typically 900 mm for the door width) and is adapted to the specific locations as follows:

$$d_{j+1} = (d_j + s_1 + s_2)/3 \text{ with } d_j = d_0 \text{ for } j = 1. \tag{1}$$

Based on Equation (1), the measured distance of each sensor s_1 and s_2 is average with the distance to define the suitable distance d_0, which is set equal to d_j at the end of the 10 s. The index j indicates one loop and each step of this iteration is documented in a separate text file. For the test deployment shown in Figure 1b the distance d_0 was 1110 mm. After this adaptation, the results of both ToF sensors are written in a further file only if the following criterion is fulfilled:

$$s_1 + s_2 < d_0 \cdot 2 - 200 \text{ mm}. \tag{2}$$

This allows us to limit the file size by not recording the ToF sensor data if nothing happens. The 200 mm are based on the first tests and allow us to introduce a certain threshold before the values are written into the file so that the file size is not unnecessarily increased. Each line further includes the time in milliseconds. A typical time difference between two measurements is close to 50 ms (milliseconds). It can vary depending what else has to be done in the specific loop (for example the documentation of a change at the MD or DS). Theoretically, a walking speed of up to 2 m s^{-1} (=10 cm/50 ms) or 7.2 km h^{-1} can be captured. This is in an acceptable range [24–28], especially as the operation of the door reduces the walking speed.

The durability of the measurement system was proven with a continuous deployment over three weeks under comparable high traffic (approximately 10 people working in the office). The detected errors could be clearly associated with deliberate behaviour of colleagues. In a future step of the research project, the sensor system will be installed in different healthcare settings and tested under those specific conditions. Each installation will initially be paired with a further validation by observation (using the stopwatch method).

As part of the post processing, the file is imported into Matlab and the difference between both measured values is calculated:

$$\Delta s = s_2 - s_1. \tag{3}$$

Significant for the analysis of the direction is the algebraic sign of the Δs value. Figure 4 presents exemplary single events of only one person passing (a and b) as well as more complex events (c to e). In those cases, Δs was standardised by the adapted distance d_0, but this could be further extracted with a sign function. The presented time was set individually to 0 for the first found result based on the ToF sensor. This allows a direct comparison of the duration of the event. Depending on the speed of the person, the first two to five values of Δs define the direction. Further quality controls are possible, based on the availability of the full measurements of both sensors. An obvious check is to look for the zero crossing of Δs and the following changed algebraic sign when a person leaves the sensor area. Errors caused by person standing in front of the sensor can be detected and have to be either manually corrected or when it happens more, the algorithm can adapt. Passing of more than one person can also be detected as presented in Figure 4c, which can also be in different directions (Figure 4e).

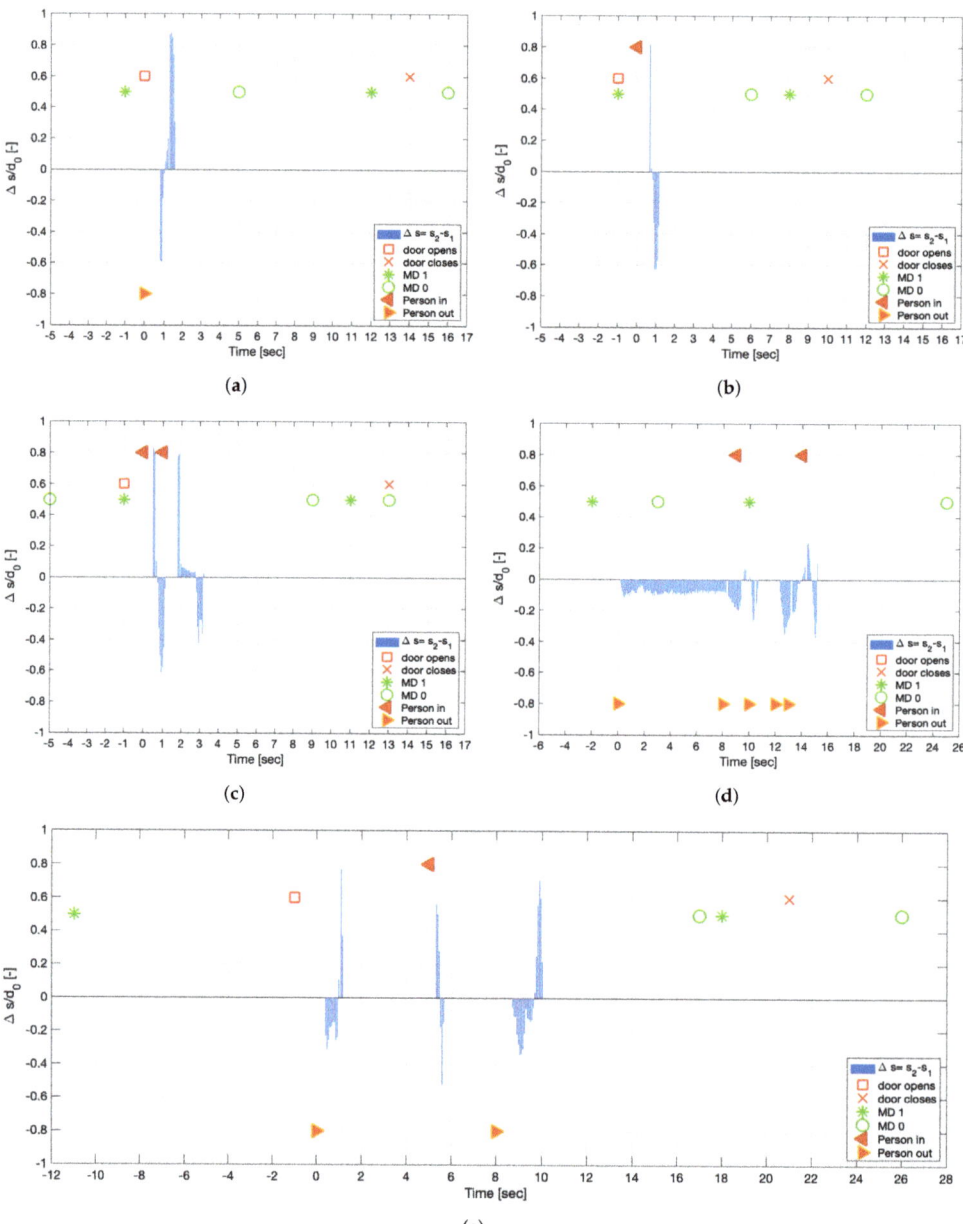

Figure 4. Exemplary result for different events. Results of MD and DS as well as the direction arrow are plotted with a constant offset (0.5, 0.6, and ± 0.8) for a better visualisation. (**a**) Outgoing event. (**b**) Incoming event. (**c**) Detection of two person entering the room. (**d**) Error detection caused by waiting person. (**e**) Outgoing person opens the door, which keeps open for an incoming and following outgoing event—MD stays up as long as motion happens and reacts again caused by the closing door.

The conducted test showed a very high reliability of this measurement concept and especially of the ToF sensors. Based on this experience, the hierarchy of the analysis is chosen as following: (1) ToF sensor as main indicator and (2) door contact as well as (3) motion detector to further validate the event detection.

The first event detection is based on the analysis of the ToF sensors. The time stamp of the first trigger measurement is stored in a vector t_i as well as ΔP_i for the direction (values ± 1). The index i represents the number of events in the total observation time. A new event is defined, when the previous documented value is more than Δt_{event} apart (typically 150 milliseconds, depending on the specific location). Those events are filters in a first step based on the difference between each event. Therefore, the time difference is calculated based on $\Delta t = t_{i-1} - t_i$. All events in which Δt is smaller a location specific threshold $\Delta t_{multiPers}$ (for example 2 s) is interpreted as multiple persons. The comparison between the two events presented in Figure 4c,d show potential problems. Those examples represent a real event and an error measurement caused by a person standing in front of the sensor. In the current version of the analysis algorithm such multi events are simplified and analysed assuming that up to three people moving close to each other go through the door shortly after each other. The event presented in Figure 4d was flagged for an additional check and had to be interpreted separately. The exact analysis method will be further developed based on the initial tests under real conditions, which will not contain such a slow automatic door closer. An additional value $\Delta t_{assistant}$ can be introduced, which allows to filter short-term stays of assisting personnel, additional physicians, or a patient's attendants.

Those filtered events are further checked for plausibility. Firstly, the door has to be opened or be still open in a time window of $\pm \Delta t_{door}$. Furthermore should the motion detector indicate a movement, however, this is not mandatory hence an error in this sensor is comparably more likely. Based on this, an actual event with a moving person is stated and a ΔP with $\pm$ the number of moving persons—depending on the direction shown in Figure 3—defined. After those checks, the value of t_i is similar to the other sensors rounded to full seconds.

The exemplary results in Figure 4 also clearly show that the closing door also indicates the motion sensor (door is closed by an automatic closer). An additional plausibility check is conducted for all door opening events, which are not connected to a motion detection based on the ToF sensors in the previous step. Those are manually checked. Further combinations of results and the conclusions are presented in Table 1.

Table 1. Decision matrix for time of flight measurement (ToF), door sensor (DS) and motion detector (MD), motion detection (mD), no detection (nD), opening (o) and closing (c) of the door, open (O) and closed (C) door. * Depending on the exact location of the sensor.

ToF	DS	MD	ΔP	Conclusion Event
mD	o + c	mD	±1	incoming or outgoing person
mD	O	mD	±1	incoming or outgoing person (open door)
mD	o + c	nD	±1	incoming or outgoing person (MD error)
mD	O	nD	±1	incoming or outgoing person (MD error)
mD	C	mD	0	passing by inside * or error
nD	O or C	mD	0	passing by outside * or error
nD	c	mD	0	door closed only (typical for automatic door closer)
nD	o	mD	0	door is opend but nobody comes in
nD	o + c	nD	0	error DS

The full data set is further split into separate days and the number of people in the room R is calculated by adding up the vector ΔP after each event. An obvious control is to find cases in which R is smaller than 0. Such an error can be caused for example by the following occurrence: Two persons enter the room together side by side (due to the support of a walking impediment) or one person enters directly behind the other (wheelchair). In those cases, the sensor system cannot detect a clear difference from a single (slow walking) person. When they leave separately, which will be correctly detected, such a problem can occur. The solution is to check the previous event manually or refine the algorithm depending on the specific location of the sensor. It is further advisable to match the total number of patient–physician interactions with the records of the day. The involved physicians are also asked to document unexpected circumstances, which could influence the measurements. They further note down the time and if they are currently talking to a patient or not (in a range of 1 or 2 h). This allows validation of the record of the sensors, as well as, in extreme cases, a reset of R.

3.2. Multi Door and Room Set-Up

In the previous section only the scenario of one single door into one room was covered. If there are two doors, obviously an additional sensor is needed. The more interesting case is a multi room set-up, as it is shown for example in Figure 5. This allows either to host two physicians or to give the opportunity of one physician switching between two rooms. In this case, the door D4 connects both rooms and does not necessarily have to be closed. If the person leaves one room, he or she enters the other room. The calculation can be either done for each event, which includes changing the length of the vectors, or based on a fixed time resolution. In the latter case, the vectors R and ΔP for each door are initially zero vector. The specific values of the detected event are added to the entry of the vector closest to t_i. The evaluation for each time step can be calculated as following:

$$R_{1,t+1} = R_{1,t} + \Delta P_1^{D1} + \Delta P_1^{D3} + \Delta P_1^{D4} \qquad (4)$$

$$R_{2,t+1} = R_{2,t} + \Delta P_1^{D2} + \Delta P_2^{D4} \qquad (5)$$

$$\text{with } \Delta P_1^{D4} = \Delta P_2^{D4} \cdot -1. \qquad (6)$$

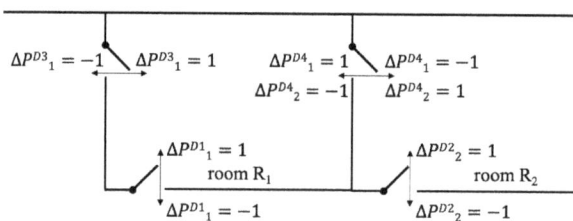

Figure 5. Example of a multiroom set-up. ΔP indicates the changes of the number of people in the room R.

It has to be assumed that only the physicians use the door D3 and D4 and the patients enter and leave through the same door. All cases in which R is bigger than two persons have to be checked, hence it is possible that a patient and an accompanying person enter the room separately and the physician enters later. It is inevitable that the specific analysis has to be adapted to each setting and the given circumstances.

There is also the possibility of installing a sensor at the main entrance door to the medical practice. This allows for evaluation of the total traffic, however, it has to be mentioned that the usage of these values is limited. With the current sensor system it is not possible to identify the person and so the calculation of the individual waiting time until the patient enters the physician's room is not possible. More suitable is the comparison of the predicted appointment to the actual entering of the patient into the room. This evaluation can be used to optimise the appointment allocation. Further applications are evaluated in the following project phase for which five of the presented sensors systems are installed in different medical practices.

4. Discussion

As part of the initial desk model, different measurement methods were investigated. The tested ultrasonic range finders needed too large a spacing and the infrared light sensor was not as fast and accurate as needed. Both types are comparably large in relation to the time of flight (ToF) sensor.

A further significant advantage of the ToF is that it can operate through a single small hole and has a very small observation footprint. In contrast to this, motion sensors based on the PIR technology are more suitable to observe a larger area/volume. Nevertheless, the chosen radar based MD allows independent verification of the motion detection, and in combination with the magnetic door switch, a workable combination was found.

In the literature, further detection approaches based on impulse radio ultra-wideband radar sensors are available. Choi et al. [29] showed that using this technique, a complete passage at a subway station in Seoul with a counting accuracy of less than 10% can be covered. Specific arrangements with WiFi signals can be also used to detect bi-directional motion [30,31]. Very promising is the expansion from a single point measurement to a scanning range [17,18], which also includes an increased effort in the post processing. Nevertheless, the inclusion of a further sensor type will be considered as part of the future work.

The distance of 10 cm between the two ToF sensors was chosen as similar to the commercially available products with infrared light sensors. Based on the prototype testing, the choice was proven functional and no further iteration was needed. A bigger distance would be desirable in principle. This would make the measurement clearer and would allow it to capture even faster movements. However, this would subsequently make it harder or even impossible to fit the device into the door frame, which increases the risk of the device being damaged or being a potential safety hazard. For locations, in which a mounting on the door frame is not possible, temporary boxes or other structures can be placed close to the door. It has to be ensured that the opposing side is rigid to avoid errors. Furthermore, the sensor is limited to 2 m and it is highly recommended not to make use of the full range. It should also be kept in mind that the area should be kept clear—objects such as umbrella stands or coat hooks can potentially trigger the measurement.

Two different heights of the ToF sensors were tested, namely 60 cm and 75 cm from the ground. Both installations showed good results but the lower one delivered slightly better results. The main concern is that the location is high enough to detect the body of the passing person but not too close to the doorknob, which could potentially lead to an incorrect measurement of a hand. For usage of this sensors in settings with mainly children the exact positioning should be evaluated.

The door contacts are at the moment only used opposite of the door hinges (Figures 1 and 3). In this location the needed distance for releasing the magnetic contact is reached with a small opening angle. A mounting of the sensors on the same side as the hinges brings the advantage that the sensor is better protected as the persons are more likely to move closer to the doorknob through the door. This has to be tested as part of the further installation of the final version of the sensor.

The presented analysis is focused on the detection of one person passing through the door. It is not possible to detect the entrance of two people side by side or to distinguish between two people in direct physical contact at the height of the sensor system. The latter can occur for wheelchair users. Those cases can lead to a misinterpretation of the sensor readings if the supporting person leaves the room for the consultation. The involved physician will be informed of this and a manual correction will be needed, which can further be used to refine the analysis. Nevertheless, multiple persons can be registered separately if the time between them is larger than a defined threshold as shown in Figure 4c. The exact value for this threshold will be evaluated in the next step of the research project, however, delivered good results with the current setting. In the actual application this is more likely to be used in a multi-room setting in which the physician is switching between two rooms.

At state of the current project, each individual unit operates separately and no time module is included. Consequently, only a relative time beginning with the initialisation of the Arduino is available. The synchronisation is done manually, which is sufficient for the current applications. An additional time module would allow the exclusion of out-of-office time periods, in which the current sensors continues to observe. The data is currently stored only locally, which ensures that a potential interference with medical instruments is negligible but has the disadvantage that the operation cannot be controlled as long as the sensor is deployed. In a future step of the project, the final version of the sensor system will be installed in medical practices under authentic conditions. In the course of this, a direct comparison of the sensor system with an observation (similar to the stopwatch method) will be conducted. The recordings will be further checked with the total number of patients per day. Also, the acceptance and the need for a real time data transmission will be evaluated as well as the need for the integration of a battery.

5. Conclusions

Based on the specific requirements of healthcare applications, a novel sensor system was developed. The paper discusses the different investigated approaches which led to the final combination of three different types: (a) time of flight, (b) door sensor, and (c) motion detection. This combination allows the documentation of motion, including the direction of the person passing through the door, as well as a high reliability based on the different sensor types. The time resolution of the output has an accuracy of less than one second and allows the capture of the duration of the interaction between patient and physician. The limitation to one side of the door frame is an achieved goal and reduces the effort for the installation, as well as possible errors throughout a longer deployment, significantly.

The paper includes exemplary results based on the initial test and the developed concept for the quality control of the measurement. An expansion of the system for multiple doors, as well as rooms, is described. In a next step of the project, the sensor system is installed at different medical practices to measure the duration of patient–physician interactions. This will also include a direct comparison to an observation outside the door and also focus on possible problems with simultaneously entering persons (wheelchairs). The gained experiences will allow us to optimise the analysis and further reduce the needed manual work.

Author Contributions: R.G. and F.S. designed the measurement concept, R.G. built the prototype, R.G. and F.S. conducted the measurements, analysed the data and wrote the initial draft.

Funding: This research was funded by Austrian Science Fund (FWF) grant number J3918. Open Access Funding by the Austrian Science Fund (FWF).

Conflicts of Interest: The authors declare no conflict of interest. The funders had no role in the design of the study; in the collection, analyses, or interpretation of data; in the writing of the manuscript, or in the decision to publish the results.

Notation

d	distance sensor to opposing wall (mm)
i	index numbering of detected events at the door (-)
j	index numbering the loops (-)
$s_{1,2}$	measured value of the ToF sensor (mm)
Δs	difference (mm)
t	time (sec)
Δt	time step (sec)
ΔP	change (Person)
R	persons in the room (Person)
D	door
DS	door sensor
GDPR	General Data Protection Regulation
INRUD	International Network for the Rational Use of Drugs
MD	motion detector
PIR	passive infrared sensor
ToF	Time of Flight
WHO	World Health Organisation

References

1. Government—Office of Science: Future of an Ageing Population 2016. Available online: https://assets.publishing.service.gov.uk/government/uploads/system/uploads/attachment_data/file/816458/future-of-an-ageing-population.pdf (accessed on 24 October 2019).
2. Irving, G.; Neves, A.L.; Dambha-Miller, H.; Oishi, A.; Tagashira, H.; Verho, A.; Holden, J. International variations in primary care physician consultation time: A systematic review of 67 countries. *BMJ Open* **2017**, *7*, e017902. [CrossRef]
3. Al-Zaydi, Z.Q.H.; Ndzi, D.L.; Kamarudin, M.L.; Zakaria, A.; Shakaff, A.Y.M. A robust multimedia surveillance system for people. *Multimed. Tools Appl.* **2017**, *76*, 23777–23804. [CrossRef]
4. Wang, W.; Liu, P.; Ying, R.; Wang, J.; Qian, J.; Jia, J.; Gao, J. A High-Computational Efficiency Human Detection and Flow Estimation Method Based on TOF Measurements. *Sensors* **2019**, *19*, 729. [CrossRef]
5. Xia, T.; Fan, H.; Yu, S.; Zhang, L.; Wen, J. An improved multi-target tracking algorithm for pedestrian counting. *J. Phys. Conf. Ser.* **2018**, *1069*, 012113. [CrossRef]
6. Lee, G.-C.; Lee, S.-H.; Yoo, J. 3-D People Counting with a Stereo Camera on GPU Embedded Board. *Appl. Sci.* **2018**, *8*, 2017. [CrossRef]
7. Li, J.; Zhang, F.; Wei, L.; Yang, T.; Lu, Z. Nighttime Foreground Pedestrian Detection Based on Three-Dimensional Voxel Surface Model. *Sensors* **2017**, *17*, 2354. [CrossRef]
8. Mousavi, E.S.; Jafarifiroozabadi, R.; Bayramzadeh, S.; Joseph, A.; San, D. An observational study of door motion in operating rooms. *Build. Environ.* **2018**, *144*, 502–507. [CrossRef]
9. CQR Surface Contacts. Available online: https://cqr.co.uk/contacts/surface-contact/ (accessed on 1 October 2019).
10. GitHub jdesbonnet/RCWL-0516. Available online: https://github.com/jdesbonnet/RCWL-0516/ (accessed on 1 October 2019).
11. Huang, Q.; Rodriguez, K.; Whetstone, N.; Habel, S. Rapid Internet of Things (IoT) prototype for accurate people counting towards energy efficient buildings. *J. Inf. Technol. Constr.* **2019**, *24*, 1–13. [CrossRef]
12. Kim, B.H.; Khan, D.; Bohak, C.; Choi, W.; Lee, H.J.; Kim, M.Y. V-RBNN Based Small Drone Detection in Augmented Datasets for 3D LADAR System. *Sensors* **2018**, *18*, 3825. [CrossRef]
13. Beer, M.; Haase, J.F.; Ruskowski, J.; Kokozinski, R. Background Light Rejection in SPAD-Based LiDAR Sensors by Adaptive Photon Coincidence Detection. *Sensors* **2018**, *18*, 4338. [CrossRef]
14. Li, X.; Yang, B.; Xie, X.; Li, D.; Xu, L. Influence of Waveform Characteristics on LiDAR Ranging Accuracy and Precision. *Sensors* **2018**, *18*, 1156. [CrossRef]
15. Suh, Y.S. Laser Sensors for Displacement, Distance and Position. *Sensors* **2019**, *19*, 1924. [CrossRef]
16. Yin, D.; Liu, J.; Wu, T.; Liu, K.; Hyyppä, J.; Chen, R. Extrinsic Calibration of 2D Laser Rangefinders Using an Existing Cuboid-Shaped Corridor as the Reference. *Sensors* **2018**, *18*, 4371. [CrossRef]
17. Carballo, A.; Ohaya, A.; Yuta, S. Reliable People Detection Using Range and Intensity Data from Multiple Layers of Laser Range Finders on a Mobile Robot. *Int. J. Soc. Robot.* **2011**, *3*, 167–186. [CrossRef]
18. Lee, J.H.; Kim, Y.S.; Kim, B.K.; Ohba, K.; Kawata, H.; Ohya, A.; Yuta, S. Security door system using human tracking method with laser range finders. In Proceedings of the 2007 IEEE International Conference on Mechatronics and Automation, Harbin, China, 5–8 August 2007.
19. Zengeler, N.; Kopinski, T.; Handmann, U. Hand Gesture Recognition in Automotive Human–Machine Interaction Using Depth Cameras. *Sensors* **2019**, *19*, 59. [CrossRef]
20. CPC Technical Datasheet VL53L0X. Available online: http://www.farnell.com/datasheets/2703141.pdf (accessed on 1 October 2019).
21. Handscombe, J.; Yu, H.Q. Low-Cost and Data Anonymised City Traffic Flow Data Collection to Support Intelligent Traffic System. *Sensors* **2019**, *19*, 347. [CrossRef]
22. Aguero, M.; Ozdagli, A.; Moreu, F. Measuring Reference-Free Total Displacements of Piles and Columns Using Low-Cost, Battery-Powered, Efficient Wireless Intelligent Sensors (LEWIS2). *Sensors* **2019**, *19*, 1549. [CrossRef]
23. Strigaro, D.; Cannata, M.; Antonovic, M. Boosting a Weather Monitoring System in Low Income Economies Using Open and Non-Conventional Systems: Data Quality Analysis. *Sensors* **2019**, *19*, 1185. [CrossRef]

24. Steffen, T.M.; Hacker, T.A.; Mollinger, L. Age- and gender-related test performance in community-dwelling elderly people: Six-Minute Walk Test, Berg Balance Scale, Timed up & Go Test, and gait speeds. *Phys. Ther.* **2002**, *82*, 128–137.
25. Kretz, T.; Grünebohm, A.; Kessel, A.; Klüpfel, H.; Meyer-König, T.; Schreckenberg, M. Upstairs walking speed distributions on a long stairway. *Saf. Sci.* **2008**, *46*, 72–78. [CrossRef]
26. Lindemann, U.; Schwenk, M.; Klenk, J.; Kessler, M.; Weyrich, M.; Kurz, F.; Becker, C. Problems of older persons using a wheeled walker. *Aging Clin. Exp. Res.* **2016**, *28*, 215–220. [CrossRef] [PubMed]
27. Kesler, R.M.; Klieger, A.E.; Boes, M.K.; Hsiao-Wecksler, E.T.; Klaren, R.E.; Learmonth, Y.; Motl, R.W.; Horn, G.P. Egress Efficacy of Persons with Multiple Sclerosis During Simulated Evacuations. *Fire Technol.* **2017**, *53*, 2007–2021. [CrossRef]
28. Crozara, L.F.; Marques, N.R.; LaRoche, D.P.; Pereira, A.J.; Silva, F.C.C.; Flores, R.C.; Payao, S.L.M. Hip extension power and abduction power asymmetry as independent predictors of walking speed in individuals with unilateral lower-limb amputation. *Gait Posture* **2019**, *70*, 383–388. [CrossRef]
29. Choi, J.W.; Quan, X.; Cho, S.H. Bi-Directional Passing People Counting System Based on IR-UWB Radar Sensors. *IEEE Internet Things J.* **2018**, *5*, 512–522. [CrossRef]
30. Kura, S.; Yamaguchi, H.; Shiraishi, Y. Low-cost pedestrian counter using Wi-Fi APs for smart building applications. *Proc. Int. Comput. Softw. Appl. Conf.* **2018**, *2*, 640–645.
31. Yang, Y.; Cao, J.; Liu, X.; Liu, X. Wi-Count: Passing People Counting with COTS WiFi Devices. In Proceedings of the 2018 27th International Conference on Computer Communication and Networks (ICCCN), Hangzhou, China, 30 July–2 August 2018; pp. 1–9.

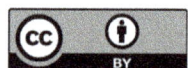

© 2019 by the authors. Licensee MDPI, Basel, Switzerland. This article is an open access article distributed under the terms and conditions of the Creative Commons Attribution (CC BY) license (http://creativecommons.org/licenses/by/4.0/).

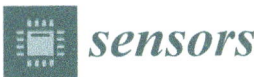

Article

A Mechatronic Platform for Computer Aided Detection of Nodules in Anatomopathological Analyses via Stiffness and Ultrasound Measurements

Luca Massari [1,*], Andrea Bulletti [2,†], Sahana Prasanna [1,†], Marina Mazzoni [2,3], Francesco Frosini [4], Elena Vicari [1], Marcello Pantano [1], Fabio Staderini [4], Gastone Ciuti [1], Fabio Cianchi [4], Luca Messerini [4], Lorenzo Capineri [2], Arianna Menciassi [1] and Calogero Maria Oddo [1,*]

1. Sant'Anna School of Advanced Studies, The BioRobotics Institute, 56025 Pisa, Italy; sahana.prasanna@santannapisa.it (S.P.); elenavicari.ev@gmail.com (E.V.); marcello.pantano03@gmail.com (M.P.); gastone.ciuti@santannapisa.it (G.C.); arianna.menciassi@santannapisa.it (A.M.)
2. Department of Information Engineering, Università Degli Studi di Firenze, 50139 Florence, Italy; andrea.bulletti@unifi.it (A.B.); m.mazzoni@ifac.cnr.it (M.M.); lorenzo.capineri@unifi.it (L.C.)
3. Consiglio Nazionale delle Ricerche of Italy, Istituto di Fisica Applicata "Nello Carrara", 50121 Florence, Italy
4. Azienda Ospedaliera Careggi University Hospital of Florence and University of Florence, 50134 Florence, Italy; francesco.frosini@unifi.it (F.F.); staderini.fabio@gmail.com (F.S.); fabio.cianchi@unifi.it (F.C.); luca.messerini@unifi.it (L.M.)
* Correspondence: luca.massari@santannapisa.it (L.M.); calogero.oddo@santannapisa.it (C.M.O.)
† These authors share second authorship based on equal contribution.

Received: 30 March 2019; Accepted: 29 May 2019; Published: 31 May 2019

Abstract: This study presents a platform for ex-vivo detection of cancer nodules, addressing automation of medical diagnoses in surgery and associated histological analyses. The proposed approach takes advantage of the property of cancer to alter the mechanical and acoustical properties of tissues, because of changes in stiffness and density. A force sensor and an ultrasound probe were combined to detect such alterations during force-regulated indentations. To explore the specimens, regardless of their orientation and shape, a scanned area of the test sample was defined using shape recognition applying optical background subtraction to the images captured by a camera. The motorized platform was validated using seven phantom tissues, simulating the mechanical and acoustical properties of ex-vivo diseased tissues, including stiffer nodules that can be encountered in pathological conditions during histological analyses. Results demonstrated the platform's ability to automatically explore and identify the inclusions in the phantom. Overall, the system was able to correctly identify up to 90.3% of the inclusions by means of stiffness in combination with ultrasound measurements, paving pathways towards robotic palpation during intraoperative examinations.

Keywords: cancer nodules detection; phantom; stiffness analysis; ultrasound analysis; visual analysis; automatic robotic platform; remote support for pathologists

1. Introduction

Cancer is an abnormal and uncontrolled cell growth that invades healthy tissues, and that can spread via metastases to other locations in the body [1]. Various cancer treatments involve chemical and radiation therapies or surgery [2–4]. Following surgical intervention, biopsy is performed on the lymph nodes excised from the tissue to properly characterize cancer spread and examine whether it has developed the ability to spread to other lymph nodules or organs too. The accuracy in estimating the amount of spread of cancer is extremely important to avoid complications caused by an extensive resection of healthy lymph nodes and tissues. Accurate localization of tumors in tissues resected during surgery can also allow the surgeon to decide and modify in itinere the planned intervention so to remove malignant tissues missed in pre-operative imaging. Stiffness of human tissue is higher for tumor nodules with respect to healthy tissues [5–10]. Hence, inspecting the mechanical properties of cancerous tissues can contribute to the detection of nodules. Intraoperative palpations of the resected malignant tissue provide essential information about the presence of abnormalities [11]. Indeed, such investigation is part of the general practice performed by a specialist through manual palpation to retrieve several information about cancer nodules [12]. The reliable confidence of medical practitioners to detect tumors is achieved with rigorous training before they reach proper expertise in examining various organs and detecting abnormalities [13]. The human capability to detect lumps in the tissues, however, degrades with increasing lump depth, decreased compliance of the tissue, deformation of the finger pad induced by the lump itself, and the finger indentation velocity [14,15]. Ultrasound analysis [16] can complement stiffness data because of the different acoustic properties of cancer nodules, as demonstrated by intraoperative ultrasonography recordings having reported influence (varying from 2.7% up to 73%) on the surgical procedures that were preoperatively planned [17–20]. Elastography is also used for the investigation of many diseases in tissues (liver, breast, thyroid, kidney, prostate, and lymph nodes) [21]. The elastographic equipment is of two types depending on the US sensors arrangement: Strain imaging and shear wave imaging. In both cases a US array probe is gel coupled to tissues; the latter requirement represents a limiting factor for the anatomo-pathology examinations for which any contamination of tissue samples must be avoided and only the natural wetness of excised tissues is allowed.

In this study, we combined stiffness and ultrasound data to aid the intraoperative histological exams performed on tissues excised during surgery by the identification of regions with different stiffness and US impedance characteristics. Such an examination is crucial in case of misdiagnosis or in case of unforeseeable diagnostic queries that might arise during surgery. Results from the examination may be used as a guide for surgical resection and decision-making to modify the common surgical procedure (see Figure 1). Initially, the surgeon gets a small tissue specimen (2–3 cm) from patient in order to get information about the presence of pathological patterns. Then, this specimen is placed on an automated system able to move and scan the material in order to get the data. The system proposed in this work is based on a precision mechanical scanner that provides a map of the tissue sample with inclusions. Data were derived from a sensor designed with a load cell for stiffness measurements, which also ensures the contact force on the sample to a vertically supported needle-type ultrasonic transducer provided for US measurements. In this way, two types of data (mechanical stiffness and US impedance) are measured at the same time in each position providing in practice two maps with well-correlated information regarding the positions of inclusions within the scanned area. Finally, with the position of the inclusion the pathology lab technician is able to sample the material and create a precise number of slices for microscopy analysis. Directly from the operating theatre the images are sent to the pathologist for the remote diagnosis. The time between the initial part of the process (excision) and the final part (medical report) should be contained within 20–30 min.

With instrumented tools, automatic classification of tumors in tissues can be addressed by machine learning techniques: Supervised–unsupervised classification, clustering and learnt neural networks [22,23]. The proposed system aims at reproducing the activity of pathologists in intraoperative tumor identification using feedback from vision, stiffness [24] and ultrasound measurements [25]. Using a robotic platform, and machine learning techniques for classification, the focus of this work is to detect and localize nodules buried in phantoms mimicking the elastic and ultrasound properties of excised human tissues. Specifically, the experimental evaluation was carried out by means of Agar-based phantoms suited to mimic liver, cardiac, brain and soft tissues [26–28], either in their acoustic and mechanical properties and temperature dependency [29,30].

The paper is organized as follows. Section 2 describes the experimental setup, the technical specifications of the used phantoms, the experimental protocol and data analysis methods. Results are presented in Section 3, showing the results of stiffness and ultrasound data analyses both separately and merging them together. The last section concludes with the discussion of the entire work and presents potential future investigations.

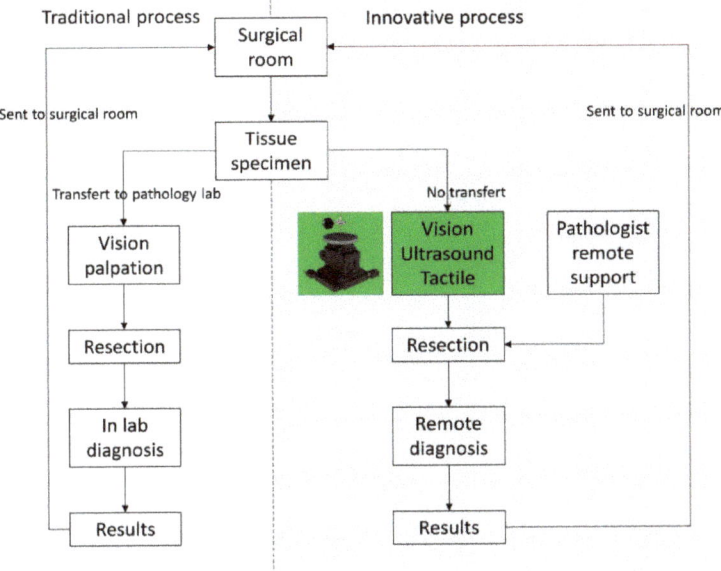

Figure 1. Block diagram of the histological procedure. On the left the traditional process is shown, whereas the proposed process is depicted on the right.

2. Materials and Methods

2.1. Platform Design

A platform was developed to detect embedded rigid inclusions surrounded by a soft matrix. The automated system consists of the following components (Figure 2):

(i) Three motorized translational stages and one rotational stage allowing to move the sample. A commercial stage (8MTF-102LS05, STANDA, Vilnius, Lithuania) with 10 cm of travel range and a resolution of 2.5 μm was used for the X and Y axes, while another translational stage (8MVT120-25-4247, STANDA, Vilnius, Lithuania) was used to indent the sample along the Z axis, having a travel range of 2.5 cm and a resolution of 5 μm. Additionally, a fourth stage was mounted on the mechatronic platform (8MR190-2-28, STANDA, Vilnius, Lithuania) in order to enable the rotation of the sample. Such stage had 360° rotation range with 0.01° resolution.

(ii) An ultrasound probe (Sonomed, mod. 2014059, Warsaw, Poland) with 16 MHz central frequency and a fractional bandwidth equal to 0.25 at −6 dB used in pulse-echo mode. The needle-type probe, 3 mm in diameter, was selected for directly contacting and indenting the sample. A 30 Vpp pulsed excitation was delivered to the probe via a transmitter (US-Key, Lecoeur-Electronique, Chuelles, France) connected to a PC via USB2. The experimental setup was completed with the ultrasound data acquisition device, NI FlexRIO (National Instruments Corp., Austin, TX, USA), for acquisitions at high frequency (1.6 GHz).

(iii) A load cell (Nano 43, ATI Industrial Automation, Apex, NC, USA) to collect interaction forces, up to 18 N with 0.004 N resolution along normal axis, arising at the interface between the ultrasound probe and the sample, also used in the control loop of the translation stages in order to operate force-controlled indentations. The developed software used this force data to calculate the stiffness and to trigger the high frequency US data collection at the threshold point of contact (0.2 N).

(iv) A waterproof HD-camera (Hero5 Session, GoPro, San Mateo, CA, USA) with 10 MP and 4 K resolution, integrated to perform the sample shape recognition and to create a matrix of points to be indented.

(v) A stainless-steel disk fixed on the top of the motorized stages for the positioning of the sample, but also to permit the reflection of the ultrasound signal back to the probe. The disk had a diameter of 16 cm and a thickness of 1 cm.

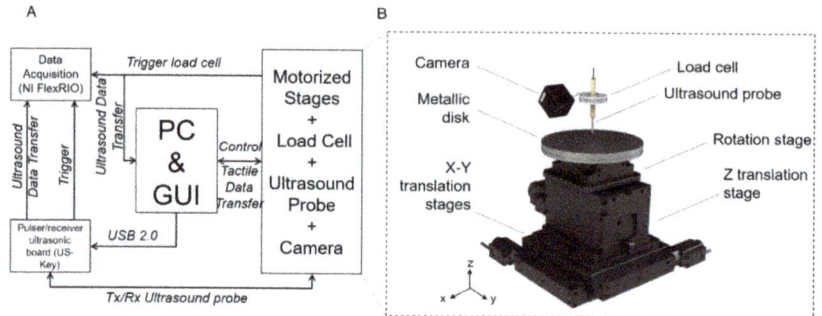

Figure 2. (**A**) Block diagram of the experimental setup. (**B**) Experimental setup showing the different components.

The software routines for controlling the platform and the automatic scan of the samples and for performing data acquisition, as well as the graphical user interfaces were developed in LabVIEW, LabVIEW Real-Time and LabVIEW FPGA (National Instruments Corp., Austin, TX, USA), while the data analyses were performed using MATLAB (The MathWorks, Inc., Natick, MA, USA).

2.2. Phantom of Healthy Tissue and Inclusions

Tests were performed on seven Agar block-shaped phantoms, realized to mimic both the mechanical and the acoustic properties of diseased human tissues. Each phantom had a soft surrounding matrix representing the human healthy tissue and hard inclusions embedded inside to represent tumor nodules. Each fabricated phantom was nominally 60 mm wide, 100 mm long and 15 mm thick, while the buried spherical inclusions had different diameters ranging from 3 mm to 12 mm. The volume of the phantom was large enough to introduce up to 8 inclusions, 2 per each diameter, in different X–Y positions with adequate separation distance (Figure 3) in order to execute computer-aided detection trials. It is worth to mention that the Agar phantom did not need any pre-treating before performing the automatic scan process. However, also in case of biological tissues, it is not necessary any further pre-treatments apart from the one required within custom histological evaluations.

Agar-based phantoms were prepared using a predefined concentration of Agar in distilled water. Changing the concentration of Agar resulted in a variation of both the mechanical and acoustic properties. A concentration of 2 g of Agar in 100 mL of water was used to represent a healthy human tissue (fabricating a phantom entirely with this concentration results in 1.59 MRayl acoustic impedance, 1457 m/s speed of sound and 0.33 N/mm mechanical impedance). A concentration of 8 g of Agar in 100 mL of water was used for simulating a tumor tissue (fabricating a phantom entirely with this concentration results in 1.92 MRayl acoustic impedance, 1534 m/s speed of sound and 4.6 N/mm mechanical impedance) [28,30–32].

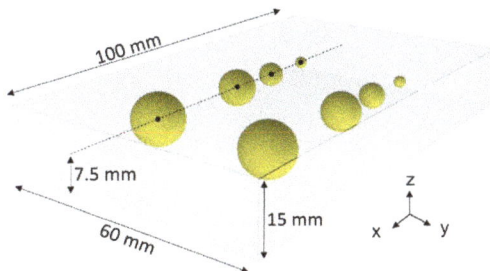

Figure 3. Rendering of the Agar phantom used during the experimental acquisition. The spherical inclusions are marked in yellow (⌀ 12–9–6–3 mm). The volume of the phantom is $100 \times 60 \times 15$ mm^3.

2.3. Experimental Protocol

The experimental protocol consisted in an automatic scan of the sample. The procedure was divided in two steps:

(i) Visual analysis;
(ii) Stiffness and ultrasound analysis.

The purpose of the automatic visual analysis was to recognize the shape of the sample by acquiring its boundaries and to create the indentation matrix, namely the points to be analyzed. Such analysis is crucial when dealing with real tissues, where the shape and size is unknown or irregular, so that the scan can be defined automatically. The visual part (Figure 4) consisted in subtracting the background image from the sample image, thus obtaining the shape, the size and the orientation. Starting from this new image (Figure 4C), a set of indentation points was created with a 2 mm step along the X and Y-axes.

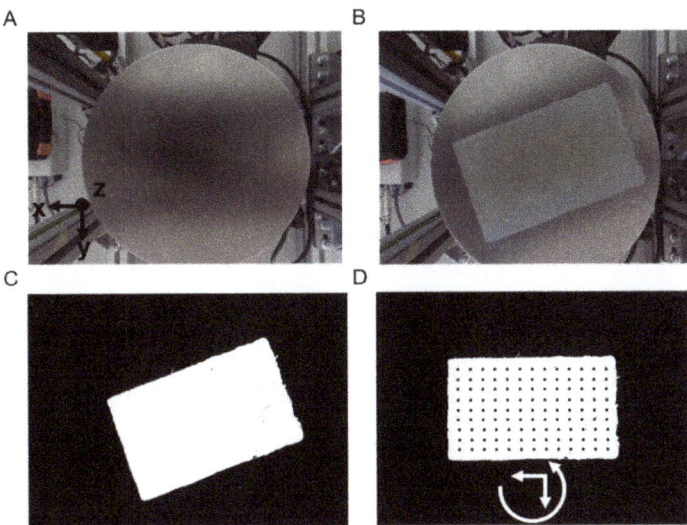

Figure 4. Visual part: Positioning of the sample, boundary detection and creation of the indentation matrix. (**A**) Background. (**B**) Sample in an arbitrary position. (**C**) Background subtraction. (**D**) Positioning by rotation of the sample and creation of the indentation matrix.

Once the visual analysis was completed, it was possible to start the acquisition of the compression force and ultrasound signals. Per each X–Y point of the indentation matrix, the phantom was indented along the Z-axis at constant speed (0.5 mm/s). The compression force was recorded and, at a low threshold (0.2 N, to avoid damaging the phantom), a trigger signal was generated for ultrasonic pulse transmission and reflected signal reception for recording (Figure 5). In a nutshell, the robotic platform control was fully automatic from the placement of the tissue onto the platform up to the localization of the inclusions. However, the system provided the user interface for an operator to supervise the scan according to the physician's requirements.

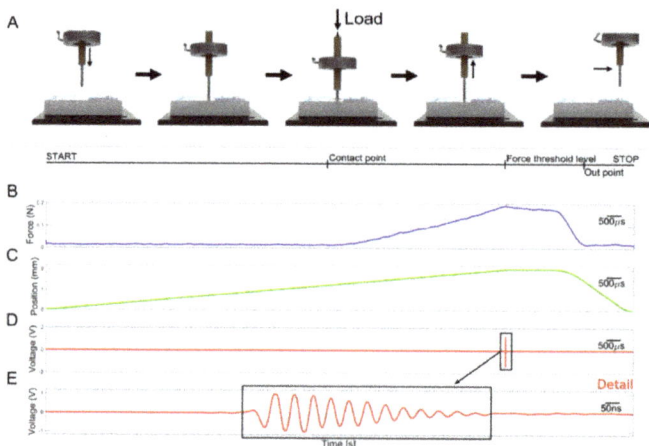

Figure 5. (**A**) Experimental protocol involving indentation of the ultrasound probe under regulation of the contact force. (**B**) Normal force. (**C**) Position along Z-axis. (**D**) Ultrasound signal reflected from the steel metal plate. (**E**) Zoom of the ultrasonic signal shown in panel D reflected at the tissue sample bottom in contact with the steel plate.

2.4. Data Analysis

The detection and localization of the different inclusions was based on the elaboration of indentation force (F_Z), vertical position (Z) and ultrasound signals. The stiffness parameter k is the ratio between the change in force and the change in Z displacement and for each indentation was calculated according to Equation (1). Here, $F_{z_{max}}$ refers to the force threshold of the indentation and F_{z_0} refers to force measured by the load cell following the first contact.

$$k = \frac{\Delta F_z}{\Delta Z} = \frac{F_{z_{max}} - F_{z_0}}{Z_{F_{z_{max}}} - Z_{F_{z_0}}} \qquad (1)$$

The ultrasound technique used for the detection of the inclusions was based on the reflectometric method. In fact, we considered more reliable to work with the variation of the signal reflected from the interface created by the bottom of the phantom and the steel plate. This signal has a higher amplitude than the back scattered or reflected signal from the inclusion embedded into the tissue-like matrix. For our phantoms, according to the selected acoustic parameters mimicking healthy and cancerous tissues [31], we can estimate a reflection coefficient generated by the acoustic impedance difference at a planar interface less than 1%. The ultrasonic analysis consisted in the processing of the signal detected in each point of the indentation matrix defining a Correlation Index Amplitude (*CIA*) parameter derived from [33], as reported in Equation (2):

$$CIA = 1 - \left(\frac{min\left(\sqrt{\sum S_{ref}^2}, \sqrt{\sum S_i^2} \right)}{max\left(\sqrt{\sum S_{ref}^2}, \sqrt{\sum S_i^2} \right)} \right) \qquad (2)$$

In Equation (2), S_i is the signal acquired in each point and S_{ref} is the reference signal. The *CIA* assumed values between 0 and 1: For two identical signals the *CIA* is zero, while for very different amplitude signals the *CIA* approaches to 1. We assume that a reference signal can be acquired in a position where neither inclusions nor other inhomogeneity have been detected; under this assumption the transmitted signal from the US probe is only attenuated by the two-way travel path defined by the steel plate interface. Due to low tissue sample thickness (typically from 5 mm to 20 mm) and moderate attenuation of the US at the operating frequency (1.25 dB/cm @16 MHz) this signal has an amplitude that is greater than the amplitude of the echo signals obtained in the probe positions over an inclusion; in our test samples, we found an amplitude variation of about 10% and 60% for the echo signal at the steel plate interface over and outside the inclusions, respectively. A high *CIA* indicates the detection of an inclusion since the two signals become poorly correlated.

For each indented point, a colour map was created both for stiffness and for correlation index amplitude. An unsupervised classifier, called Fuzzy C-mean (FCM) clustering [34], was used to classify each indentation of the scan on the phantom. Such unsupervised classification system, starting from the elaborated data, enabled the categorization of the point and the subsequent organization into different clusters. In this way, it was possible to divide the data into two classes: (a) Tumor class, which were the sites classified as inclusions, and (b) healthy class, which were the sites classified as non-inclusions. From the wrong classification prediction, we obtained the number of false positive, i.e., soft matrix points classified as inclusions, and the false negative number, i.e., inclusions classified as soft matrix. Furthermore, new datasets were obtained and classified by merging the stiffness and the ultrasound data using AND–OR logics. In the AND case, we considered tumor only the points identified as inclusion in both the datasets simultaneously, thus we expected an increase in the total number of false negatives. In the OR case, we considered tumor all the points classified as inclusion in either the stiffness dataset or the ultrasound dataset, thus we expected an increase of the number of false positives and reduced false negatives. The results of the OR logics are crucial to include all of the cancerous tissues. Through a confusion matrix, the accuracy and the misclassification rate were calculated for all the datasets and methods.

3. Results

All the experimental results presented in this section have been repeated over seven replicas of the developed phantoms.

3.1. Results from Stiffness Measurements

An elaboration example of the stiffness analysis, for one of the seven phantoms, is shown in the top parts of Figure 6. The bottom part of Figure 6A shows the positions of the inclusions inside the indentation matrix. Since the inclusions were embedded into a soft matrix, their stiffness was depending not only on the materials properties, like the elasticity, but also on their dimensions. The stiffness parameter recorded at the location of indentation is the complex homogenized combination of the inclusion below and the surrounding soft "healthy" tissue. Hence, the stiffness parameter, *k* from Equation (1), was found to increase with the dimension. Stiffness analysis was clearly capable to detect the bigger inclusions, namely 12 mm and 9 mm. Figure 6B, showing the results for the whole indentation matrix, confirmed this trend. A visual inspection of the image allows discriminating big inclusions compared to the soft surrounding matrix.

The results of the identification based on stiffness measurements are shown in Figure 7A, obtained by the Fuzzy C-mean (FCM) clustering. The results of this unsupervised classification system confirmed the ability of the stiffness measurement system to recognize all the points belonging to the big inclusions, thus without false negatives. Such performances were evident from the high number of true positive (green points) for 12 mm and 9 mm inclusions. However, stiffness analysis was not able to reliably identify the smallest inclusions, as pointed out by the high number of false negatives (red points) for 6 mm and 3 mm inclusions (Figure 7A).

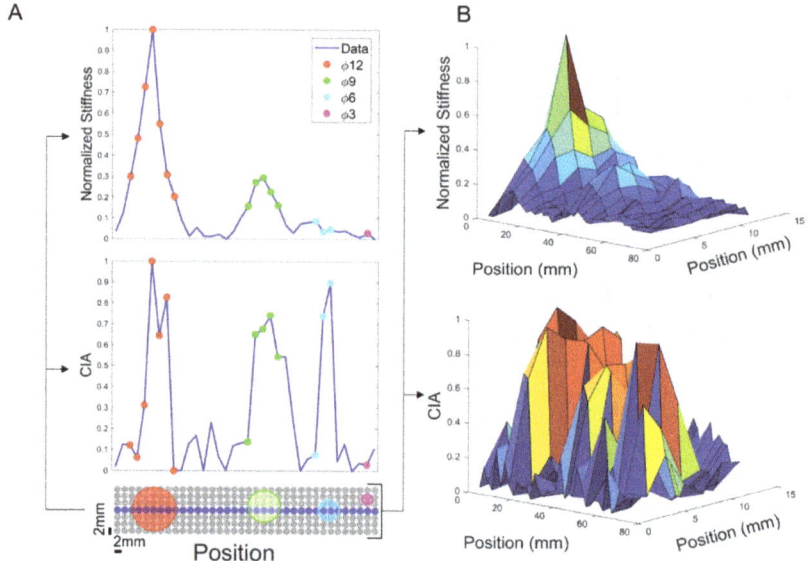

Figure 6. (**A**) (**top**) graph showing stiffness as a function of position, calculated as $\Delta Fz/\Delta Z$, for the central row; (**bottom**) graph showing ultrasound signal processing of CIA index. (**B**) (**top**) 3D graph showing stiffness across the whole indentation matrix; (**bottom**) 3D graph showing ultrasound signal processing of Correlation Index Amplitude (CIA) index.

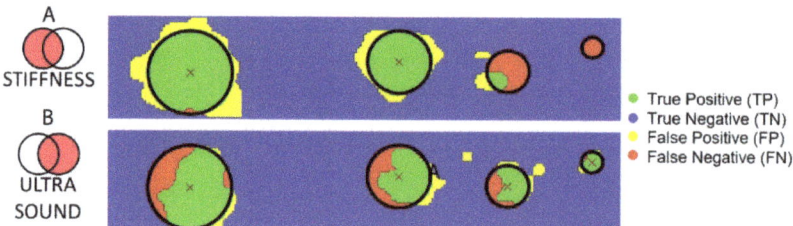

Figure 7. Classification (TP–TN–FP–FN) of all the points of the indentation matrix for the analyses with stiffness (**A**) and ultrasound (**B**) measurements.

3.2. Results from Ultrasound Measurements

According to the ultrasound data analysis, shown in Figure 6 (bottom part), we can observe in Figure 6A that the CIA index increases consistently in correspondence of the inclusions. However, unlike the stiffness measurements, higher CIA values were observed also for the smaller inclusions. Thanks to the high CIA peak recorded for each inclusion, this approach led to the detection of all the inclusions buried in the phantom. Figure 6B, showing the results for the whole indentation matrix, confirmed this trend. As for the stiffness measurement part, Figure 7B shows the results of the FCM clustering, highlighting the ability of the ultrasound system to detect each inclusion. The trend is visible in Figure 7B where true positives (in green) are present in each inclusion. Remarkably, false positives (in yellow) and false negatives (in red) were obtained in the area at the boundary between the inclusion and the soft matrix, confirming the high specificity in identifying the area to focus on for histological analyses. At such boundaries, the ultrasonic beam, coming from the source and returning to the source upon reflection on the stainless steel plate, could have experienced diffraction effects that produced an apparent enlargement of the real dimensions of the spherical inclusions thus giving origin to false positives.

3.3. AND–OR Logics to Merge Stiffness and Ultrasound Measurements

With the aim to improve the detection performance (true positives vs. false negatives), new datasets were obtained and classified by merging stiffness and ultrasound measurements using AND–OR logics and the corresponding results are shown in Figure 8. The AND logics (Figure 8A) turned out in an increase of false negatives and decrease of false positives. The growth of false negative predictions can lead to the worst-case scenario, since might bring to a loss of identified tumors. Instead, the OR logics demonstrated to be a safer approach since it turned out in an acceptable increase of false positives and a consistent decrease of false negatives. As shown in Figure 8B, the OR logics between stiffness and ultrasound measurements was able to correctly discriminate all the inclusions, even the smaller ones. Such results were achieved thanks to the complementarity of the two systems. It was observed that the stiffness analysis was better in localizing bigger inclusions, whereas the ultrasound analysis was better for the detection of smaller inclusions (compare Figure 7A,B).

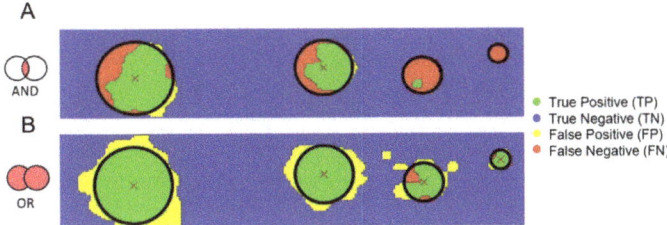

Figure 8. Classification (TP–TN–FP–FN) for all the points of the indentation matrix following the AND (**A**) and OR (**B**) logics of stiffness- and ultrasound-based classifications shown in Figure 7.

This behavior was further confirmed by the confusion matrices obtained with the seven experimented phantoms and with all the identification techniques, i.e., based on just stiffness measurements, just ultrasound, and with the AND–OR logics (Figure 9).

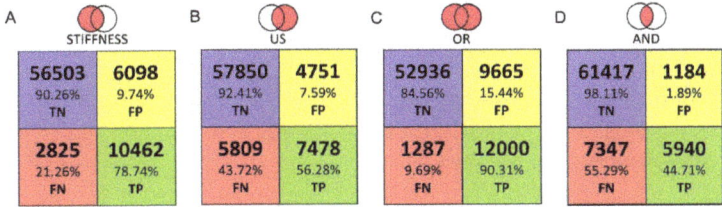

Figure 9. Confusion Matrix with classification based on (**A**) stiffness measurements; (**B**) ultrasound measurements; (**C**) stiffness or ultrasound measurements; (**D**) stiffness and ultrasound measurements.

4. Discussion

In this work we present a platform aiming at identifying cancer nodules in ex-vivo tissues. Such tool, oriented towards the automation of diagnostic procedures during surgery, has the scope of increasing the effectiveness of histopathological evaluations. Such exams need to be performed as correctly as possible because the report may lead in a modification of the surgical procedure. The human capability to detect these lumps with characteristic dimension of few mm, depends on the pathologist expertise and tactile capabilities. To achieve this goal, the presented platform combines three different measurements, such as camera vision, stiffness calculations via force-position sensing and ultrasound recordings to perform an automatic scan and evaluation of the indented tissue. In this paper the tests were performed in a laboratory environment using seven Agar phantoms that mimicked the mechanical and acoustic properties of human ex-vivo tissues. The phantoms integrated eight spherical inclusions with different diameters (from 3 mm up to 12 mm) to reproduce tumors inside healthy tissues. The results, for all phantoms, summarized in the confusion matrices, demonstrated the ability of the platform to automatically identify the inclusions, particularly when complementing stiffness with ultrasound measurements via OR logics. In particular, as reported in the confusion matrix, the tactile analysis presents valuable classification results in detecting the inclusions as reflected from the 78.73% of TP and 90.26% of TN. Moreover, it shows a low percentage of FP and FN, 9.74% and 21.27%, respectively. We observe that the tactile analysis provides satisfactory shape recognition and tumor detection for inclusions above 6 mm in diameter. On the other hand, it missed the smaller inclusions that were buried deeper into the softer matrix. The ultrasound analysis can be a very good guiding tool for localization and detection of tumors, including the smaller ones, because the ultrasound resolution is much higher than the size of the inclusion and the difference in the acoustic impedance along the z-axis is sufficient to generate an amplitude variation than can be detected from noise. The ultrasound data presents high amount of TN of 92.41% and a low FP of 7.59%. However, the ultrasound alone shows a high number of FN of 43.72%. To improve the performance, the classified datasets were logically merged using the OR and AND logics. As expected, the results of OR logics gave evidence of a higher rate of inclusions recognition (i.e., 90.3% of TP and 84.56% TN), while maintaining low error rates (i.e., 9.68% FN and 15.44% FP). Such a result is a direct consequence of the implementation of this logics, since we considered all the points classified as inclusion, in either the stiffness dataset or the ultrasound dataset, as tumor. This entails a better localization and reconstruction of the buried inclusions. Interestingly, the AND logics localizes the bigger inclusions with an increased TN rate of 98.10%and reduced the FP rate to 1.90%, but the TP rate of 44.70% and FN rate of 55.30% missed the correct shape and smaller tumors entirely.

In addition, we found that the ultrasound method was also sensitive to the presence of air bubbles formed in the agar inclusions as the surface of such bubbles might introduce a significant impedance contrast for the ultrasound signals. This could create amplitude variation in the reflected signal that resembled to the "healthy tissue". Thanks to the good spatial resolution of our system, the positions around the air bubbles provide faithful data that can reduce the impact of this constraint; moreover, the biological tissues are expected to not have air bubbles. However, the tactile data were not sensitive to these air bubbles inside the inclusions, reproducing their shape a more faithfully in the OR logics. Within the present work, we adopted a scan resolution with step of 2 mm inspired by the 16 MHz needle probe diameter (i.e., 3 mm). To keep a balance between the scan speed and area, we decided to scan with step of 2 mm. Lesser resolution values lead to insufficient data points in the scanned area, while higher values would introduce unaffordable scan time and oversampling.

The phantoms we used were the simplistic versions of the biological tissues. Hence, further developments will address the experimentation of the robotic platform on ex-vivo tissues. After this validation step, we can envisage that the sensorized platform placed in the operating theatre will enable the pathologist to access data remotely with the purpose of assisting the surgeon in adapting the procedures during surgery. Information obtained from the platform can also be used to provide haptic feedback to the pathologist by means of wearable interfaces [35–38]. The analysis of vision data, now used only for detecting the boundary of the tissue and thus to define the indentation matrix, can be improved to provide a visual report too. Such a new procedure will target the extraction of several features from the pictures of both healthy and tumorous tissues to learn their differences via artificial intelligence methods and thus complement stiffness and ultrasound measurements. Finally, the results will be translated in an electronic report and integrated with the management software (e.g., HL7) of the healthcare system.

Author Contributions: L.M. (Luca Massari) developed the mechatronic platform, integrated the experimental setup, co-designed the experimental protocol, performed the experimental protocol, analyzed the data, discussed the results and edited the paper; A.B. realized the phantom, co-designed the experimental protocol, performed the experimental protocol, analyzed the data, discussed the results and edited the paper; S.P. realized the phantom, co-designed the experimental protocol, performed the experimental protocol, analyzed the data, discussed the results and edited the paper; M.M. realized the phantom, co-designed the experimental protocol, performed the experimental protocol, discussed the results; F.F. handled the project administration, discussed the results and revised the paper; E.V. analyzed the data and discussed the results; M.P. developed the visual analysis and discussed the results; F.S., F.C., L.M. (Luca Messerini), provided medical background, co-designed the experimental protocol, contributed to perform the experimental protocol and revised the paper; G.C. co-supervised the development of the mechatronic platform, co-designed the experimental protocol and revised the paper; L.C. and A.M. co-supervised the development of the mechatronic platform, co-designed the experimental protocol, contributed to data analysis, discussed the results and revised the paper; C.M.O. designed and supervised the study, supervised the development of the mechatronic platform, co-designed the experimental protocol, contributed to data analysis, discussed the results and revised the paper.

Funding: This work was supported in part by the Tuscany Region within the FAS-Salute call, via the IMEROS project (CUPD66D16000120002).

Acknowledgments: This paper is a result of a collaborative project involving different institutes and entities. The authors thank all the collaborators for their valuable contributions.

Conflicts of Interest: The authors submitted a patent on the platform presented in the present study. The funders had no role in the design of the study; in the collection, analyses, or interpretation for data; in the writing of the manuscript, or in the decision to publish the results.

References

1. Pierangelo, A.; Benali, A.; Antonelli, M.-R.; Novikova, T.; Validire, P.; Gayet, B.; Martino, A. De Ex-vivo characterization of human colon cancer by Mueller polarimetric imaging. *Opt. Express* **2011**, *19*, 1582. [CrossRef] [PubMed]
2. Adam, R. Chemotherapy and surgery: New perspectives on the treatment of unresectable liver metastases. *Ann. Oncol.* **2003**, *14*, ii13–ii16. [CrossRef] [PubMed]
3. Nagai, T.; Niikura, H.; Okamoto, S.; Nakabayashi, K.; Matoda, M.; Utsunomiya, H.; Nagase, S.; Watanabe, M.; Takeshima, N.; Yaegashi, N. A new diagnostic method for rapid detection of lymph node metastases using a one-step nucleic acid amplification (OSNA) assay in endometrial cancer. *Ann. Surg. Oncol.* **2015**, *22*, 980–986. [CrossRef] [PubMed]
4. Candefjord, S.; Ramser, K.; Lindahl, O.A. Technologies for localization and diagnosis of prostate cancer. *J. Med. Eng. Technol.* **2009**, *33*, 585–603. [CrossRef] [PubMed]
5. Krouskop, T.A.; Wheeler, T.M.; Kallel, F.; Garra, B.S.; Hall, T. Elastic moduli of breast and prostate tissues under compression. *Ultrason. Imaging* **1998**, *20*, 260–274. [CrossRef] [PubMed]
6. Samani, A.; Zubovits, J.; Plewes, D. Elastic moduli of normal and pathological human breast tissues: An inversion-technique-based investigation of 169 samples. *Phys. Med. Biol.* **2007**, *52*, 1565. [CrossRef] [PubMed]
7. Zhang, M.; Nigwekar, P.; Castaneda, B.; Hoyt, K.; Joseph, J.V.; di Sant'Agnese, A.; Messing, E.M.; Strang, J.G.; Rubens, D.J.; Parker, K.J. Quantitative characterization of viscoelastic properties of human prostate correlated with histology. *Ultrasound Med. Biol.* **2008**, *34*, 1033–1042. [CrossRef]
8. Raveh Tilleman, T.; Tilleman, M.M.; Neumann, H.A.M. The elastic properties of cancerous skin: Poisson's ratio and Young's modulus. *Isr. Med. J.* **2004**, *6*, 753–755.
9. Winstone, B.; Melhuish, C.; Pipe, T.; Callaway, M.; Dogramadzi, S. Toward Bio-Inspired Tactile Sensing Capsule Endoscopy for Detection of Submucosal Tumors. *IEEE Sens. J.* **2017**, *17*, 848–857. [CrossRef]
10. Carter, F.J.; Frank, T.G.; Davies, P.J.; McLean, D.; Cuschieri, A. Measurements and modelling of the compliance of human and porcine organs. *Med. Image Anal.* **2001**, *5*, 231–236. [CrossRef]
11. Konstantinova, J.; Li, M.; Mehra, G.; Dasgupta, P.; Althoefer, K.; Nanayakkara, T. Behavioral characteristics of manual palpation to localize hard nodules in soft tissues. *IEEE Trans. Biomed. Eng.* **2014**, *61*, 1651–1659. [CrossRef] [PubMed]
12. Wells, P.N.T.; Liang, H.H.-D. Medical ultrasound: Imaging of soft tissue strain and elasticity. *J. R. Soc. Interface* **2011**, *8*, 1521–1549. [CrossRef] [PubMed]

13. Carson, W.C.; Gerling, G.J.; Krupski, T.L.; Association Kowalik, C.G.; Harper, J.C.; Moskaluk, C.A. Material characterization of ex vivo prostate tissue via spherical indentation in the clinic. *Med. Eng. Phys.* **2011**, *33*, 302–309. [CrossRef] [PubMed]
14. Gwilliam, J.C.; Yoshioka, T.; Okamura, A.M.; Hsiao, S.S. Neural coding of passive lump detection in compliant artificial tissue. *J. Neurophysiol.* **2014**, *112*, 1131–1141. [CrossRef] [PubMed]
15. Yau, J.M.; Kim, S.S.; Thakur, P.H.; Bensmaia, S.J. Feeling form: The neural basis of haptic shape perception. *J. Neurophysiol.* **2016**, *115*, 631–642. [CrossRef] [PubMed]
16. Nam, K.; Rosado-Mendez, I.M.; Wirtzfeld, L.A.; Pawlicki, A.D.; Kumar, V.; Madsen, E.L.; Ghoshal, G.; Lavarello, R.J.; Oelze, M.L.; Bigelow, T.A. Ultrasonic attenuation and backscatter coefficient estimates of rodent-tumor-mimicking structures: Comparison of results among clinical scanners. *Ultrason. Imaging* **2011**, *33*, 233–250. [CrossRef]
17. Hoch, G.; Croise-Laurent, V.; Germain, A.; Brunaud, L.; Bresler, L.; Ayav, A. Is intraoperative ultrasound still useful for the detection of colorectal cancer liver metastases? *Int. Hepato Pancreato Biliary Assoc.* **2015**, *17*, 514–519. [CrossRef] [PubMed]
18. Hata, S.; Imamura, H.; Aoki, T.; Hashimoto, T.; Akahane, M.; Hasegawa, K.; Bekku, Y.; Sugawara, Y.; Makuuchi, M.; Kokudo, N. Value of visual inspection, bimanual palpation, and intraoperative ultrasonography during hepatic resection for liver metastases of colorectal carcinoma. *World J. Surg.* **2011**, *35*, 2779–2787. [CrossRef]
19. Ferrero, A.; Langella, S.; Giuliante, F.; Viganò, L.; Vellone, M.; Zimmitti, G.; Ardito, F.; Nuzzo, G.; Capussotti, L. Intraoperative liver ultrasound still affects surgical strategy for patients with colorectal metastases in the modern era. *World J. Surg.* **2013**, *37*, 2655–2663. [CrossRef] [PubMed]
20. Chou, R.; Cuevas, C.; Fu, R.; Devine, B.; Wasson, N.; Ginsburg, A.; Zakher, B.; Pappas, M.; Graham, E.; Sullivan, S.D. Imaging techniques for the diagnosis of hepatocellular carcinoma: A systematic review and meta-analysis. *Ann. Intern. Med.* **2015**, *162*, 697–711. [CrossRef] [PubMed]
21. Sigrist, R.M.S.; Liau, J.; El Kaffas, A.; Chammas, M.C.; Willmann, J.K. Ultrasound elastography: Review of techniques and clinical applications. *Theranostics* **2017**, *7*, 1303. [CrossRef] [PubMed]
22. Baker, A.R.; Windsor, C.G. The classification of defects from ultrasonic data using neural networks: The Hopfield method. *NDT Int.* **1989**, *22*, 97–105. [CrossRef]
23. Jain, A.K. Data clustering: 50 years beyond K-means. *Pattern Recognit. Lett.* **2010**, *31*, 651–666. [CrossRef]
24. Ahn, B.M.; Kim, J.; Ian, L.; Rha, K.H.; Kim, H.J. Mechanical property characterization of prostate cancer using a minimally motorized indenter in an ex vivo indentation experiment. *Urology* **2010**, *76*, 1007–1011. [CrossRef] [PubMed]
25. Barr, R.G.; Ferraioli, G.; Palmeri, M.L.; Goodman, Z.D.; Garcia-Tsao, G.; Rubin, J.; Garra, B.; Myers, R.P.; Wilson, S.R.; Rubens, D. Elastography assessment of liver fibrosis: Society of radiologists in ultrasound consensus conference statement. *Radiology* **2015**, *276*, 845–861. [CrossRef] [PubMed]
26. Li, W.; Belmont, B.; Greve, J.M.; Manders, A.B.; Downey, B.C.; Zhang, X.; Xu, Z.; Guo, D.; Shih, A. Polyvinyl chloride as a multimodal tissue-mimicking material with tuned mechanical and medical imaging properties. *Med. Phys.* **2016**, *43*, 5577–5592. [CrossRef]
27. Culjat, M.O.; Goldenberg, D.; Tewari, P.; Singh, R.S. A review of tissue substitutes for ultrasound imaging. *Ultrasound Med. Biol.* **2010**, *36*, 861–873. [CrossRef] [PubMed]
28. Cafarelli, A.; Verbeni, A.; Poliziani, A.; Dario, P.; Menciassi, A.; Ricotti, L. Tuning acoustic and mechanical properties of materials for ultrasound phantoms and smart substrates for cell cultures. *Acta Biomater.* **2017**, *49*, 368–378. [CrossRef] [PubMed]
29. Cao, R.; Huang, Z.; Varghese, T.; Nabi, G. Tissue mimicking materials for the detection of prostate cancer using shear wave elastography: A validation study. *Med. Phys.* **2013**, *40*, 022903. [CrossRef] [PubMed]
30. Manickam, K.; Machireddy, R.R.; Seshadri, S. Study of ultrasound stiffness imaging methods using tissue mimicking phantoms. *Ultrasonics* **2014**, *54*, 621–631. [CrossRef]
31. Bamber, J.C.; Hill, C.R. Acoustic properties of normal and cancerous human liver—I. Dependence on pathological condition. *Ultrasound Med. Biol.* **1981**, *7*, 121–133. [CrossRef]
32. Azhari, H. *Basics of Biomedical Ultrasound for Engineers*; John Wiley & Sons: Hoboken, NJ, USA, 2010.
33. Bulletti, A.; Giannelli, P.; Calzolai, M.; Capineri, L. An integrated acousto/ultrasonic structural health monitoring system for composite pressure vessels. *IEEE Trans. Ultrason. Ferroelectr. Freq. Control* **2016**, *63*, 864–873. [CrossRef] [PubMed]

34. Bezdek, J.C.; Ehrlich, R.; Full, W. FCM: The fuzzy c-means clustering algorithm. *Comput. Geosci.* **1984**, *10*, 191–203. [CrossRef]
35. Sorgini, F.; Massari, L.; D'Abbraccio, J.; Palermo, E.; Menciassi, A.; Petrovic, P.; Mazzoni, A.; Carrozza, M.; Newell, F.; Oddo, C. Neuromorphic Vibrotactile Stimulation of Fingertips for Encoding Object Stiffness in Telepresence Sensory Substitution and Augmentation Applications. *Sensors* **2018**, *18*, 261. [CrossRef] [PubMed]
36. Massari, L.; D'Abbraccio, J.; Baldini, L.; Sorgini, F.; Farulla, G.A.; Petrovic, P.; Palermo, E.; Oddo, C.M. Neuromorphic haptic glove and platform with gestural control for tactile sensory feedback in medical telepresence applications. In Proceedings of the 2018 IEEE International Symposium on Medical Measurements and Applications (MeMeA), Rome, Italy, 11–13 June 2018; pp. 1–6.
37. Sorgini, F.; Mazzoni, A.; Massari, L.; Caliò, R.; Galassi, C.; Kukreja, S.; Sinibaldi, E.; Carrozza, M.; Oddo, C. Encapsulation of Piezoelectric Transducers for Sensory Augmentation and Substitution with Wearable Haptic Devices. *Micromachines* **2017**, *8*, 270. [CrossRef] [PubMed]
38. D'Abbraccio, J.; Massari, L.; Prasanna, S.; Baldini, L.; Sorgini, F.; Airò Farulla, G.; Bulletti, A.; Mazzoni, M.; Capineri, L.; Menciassi, A. Haptic Glove and Platform with Gestural Control For Neuromorphic Tactile Sensory Feedback In Medical Telepresence. *Sensors* **2019**, *19*, 641. [CrossRef] [PubMed]

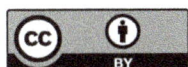

© 2019 by the authors. Licensee MDPI, Basel, Switzerland. This article is an open access article distributed under the terms and conditions of the Creative Commons Attribution (CC BY) license (http://creativecommons.org/licenses/by/4.0/).

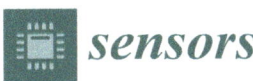

Article

Investigation of Regression Methods for Reduction of Errors Caused by Bending of FSR-Based Pressure Sensing Systems Used for Prosthetic Applications

Chakaveh Ahmadizadehand Carlo Menon *

Menrva Research Group, Schools of Mechatronic Systems Engineering and Engineering Science, Simon Fraser University, Metro Vancouver, BC V3T 0A3, Canada; cahmadiz@sfu.ca
* Correspondence: cmenon@sfu.ca

Received: 14 November 2019; Accepted: 10 December 2019; Published: 13 December 2019

Abstract: The pressure map at the interface of a prosthetic socket and a residual limb contains information that can be used in various prosthetic applications including prosthetic control and prosthetic fitting. The interface pressure is often obtained using force sensitive resistors (FSRs). However, as reported by multiple studies, accuracies of the FSR-based pressure sensing systems decrease when sensors are bent to be positioned on a limb. This study proposes the use of regression-based methods for sensor calibration to address this problem. A sensor matrix was placed in a pressure chamber as the pressure was increased and decreased in a cyclic manner. Sensors' responses were assessed when the matrix was placed on a flat surface or on one of five curved surfaces with various curvatures. Three regression algorithms, namely linear regression (LR), general regression neural network (GRNN), and random forest (RF), were assessed. GRNN was selected due to its performance. Various error compensation methods using GRNN were investigated and compared to improve instability of sensors' responses. All methods showed improvements in results compared to the baseline. Developing a different model for each of the curvatures yielded the best results. This study proved the feasibility of using regression-based error compensation methods to improve the accuracy of mapping sensor readings to pressure values. This can improve the overall accuracy of FSR-based sensory systems used in prosthetic applications.

Keywords: force myography; prosthetic fitting; regression; calibration; error reduction; linear regression; random forest; general regression neural network; cross-talk; force sensitive resistor

1. Introduction

The pressure profile at the interface of the prosthetic socket and the residual limb contains important information that can be used for various applications in the field of prostheses. Some of the most common prosthetic applications for which the use of this pressure map has been explored include control of powered prostheses using Force Myography (FMG) [1–3] and prosthetic fitting [4–6].

FMG for prosthetic control has been explored for both upper extremity and lower extremity prostheses [7,8]. For the upper limb, FMG has been mostly used for gesture classification to control externally-powered prosthetic hands [9,10]. The feasibility of using FMG for continuous finger movement control has also been investigated [8,11]. In lower limb prostheses, the use of FMG has been mainly focused on locomotion mode detection. Information about the mode of locomotion can be used for the ankle's angle correction as the user walks over ramps, flat surfaces, or stairs [7,12]. Moreover, studies have shown promising results using FMG for gait phase detection [13] which can potentially be used for lower limb prostheses control [14].

Another application for which the interface pressure can be used is prosthetic fitting. Correct shaping of the socket is a critical and complex part of the prostheses design process [15]. Poor socket fit can cause various problems such as pain and discomfort [16], skin problems such as edema, dermatitis and ulcer [17] which can lead to abandonment of the prosthesis or even further surgery. These problems may also drive users to put more load on their intact limb which can cause other problems such as osteoarthritis of the knee and/or the hip joints of the intact limb [18]. Moreover, insufficient loading of the residual limb may lead to osteopenia and subsequent osteoporosis [18]. Using the aforementioned interface pressure, location of high pressure areas and the value of pressure in these areas can be determined. This information can enhance the accuracy of the prosthetic fitting process and prevent some of the problems associated with a poor socket fit.

Various force/pressure measurement techniques are used in biomedical applications. Strain gauges and load cells are used in different forms and for various applications such as measurement of ground reaction forces for gait analysis using instrumented shoes [19] and prosthetic interface pressure measurement [17]. Force plates are also commonly used in such applications due to their accuracy of measurement [19–21]. Other force/pressure measurement methods for biomedical applications include the use of piezoelectric sensors for measurement of normal forces in shoe insoles [19], instrumented implants for telemetric measurement of forces [22], dynamometers [23], and electromyography for measurement of muscle activation forces [21].

The measurement method is determined based on the application for which the results are to be used. For example, despite the high accuracy of measurements by a shoe insole instrumented with strain gauge transducers, it is not a suitable measurement system for gait analysis due to the interference of the thickness of the sensors with parameters of the experiment [19]. For pressure measurement within prosthetic sockets, various techniques are investigated including the use of strain gauge transducers, capacitive sensors, and piezoresistive sensors [6]. The use of strain gauge-based sensors are amongst the most accurate methods that can measure both normal and shear forces. However, factors such as the high cost of these sensors and their dimensions limit their practicality for the real use case of the applications considered in this study. The use of such sensors for prosthetic pressure measurement requires modification of the prosthetic socket to make embedment of the sensors possible. Such alterations to the prosthetic socket may affect the interface pressure distribution [24–26].

Capacitive sensors are used both in single point form and as sensor arrays for prosthetic pressure measurement. The rigid substrates of the single point capacitive sensors prevented them from complying with the geometry of the socket, which in addition to their costly fabrication prevented them from being an optimal technique for prosthetic pressure measurement [6]. The Pliance system by Novel Electronics (Minneapolis, MN, USA) uses capacitive sensor arrays for this application, however, the measurements are limited to direct pressure and are uni-directional [27,28].

Design and development of sensors that are thin, less costly, and can measure shear forces have been investigated in the research community. Chase et al. fabricated and tested a flexible capacitive force sensor that was able to measure normal and shear forces [29]. Razian et al. designed and developed a miniature triaxial piezoelectric copolymer film pressure transducer with thickness of 2.7 mm that can be embedded in shoe insoles [30]. Although these sensory systems can potentially be used for prosthetic pressure map registration, their development methods are still in their early stages and are bound to the research laboratories.

FSR-based pressure measurement systems are amongst the most common methods for prosthetic pressure map registration as well as a multitude of other biomedical application [31]. Despite their inability to measure shear forces which is undesirable for some prosthetic applications, their thin profile, flexibility, cost effectiveness, computationally affordable signal pre-processing [17,27,32] , and commercially established development have made them a practical solution for prosthetic pressure measurement. The F-scoket system by Tekscan (Boston, MA, USA) has been one of the most commonly preferred solutions for pressure measurement inside prosthetic sockets [5,6,17,26,28,32].

Despite availability of FSR-based prosthetic pressure measurement systems in the market and their wide use in research communities, when these systems are evaluated in practical situations, higher errors are reported compared to their performance in constrained environments of the labs.

In prostheses control using FMG, higher errors are reported for inter-subject and inter-trial cases [13,33]. In prosthetic fitting systems, higher errors are reported when FSR sensors are placed on moulds of the limbs [4,27,28].

Factors affecting stability of FSR responses have been investigated in multiple studies. Chegani et al. assessed the effect of sensor placement and spatial coverage on stability of FMG signals used for gesture classification through studying their effect on obtained classification accuracy. It was determined that increasing spatial coverage improved accuracy when two custom FMG bands were used instead of one. However, increasing spatial coverage beyond that did not further improve the results. They also reported that optimal placement of sensors can potentially compensate for the lower spatial coverage [8]. Delva et al. investigated the effect of anthropometry and grip strength on stability of FMG signals and determined that these factors do not contribute to variability in FMG signals. They also demonstrated that FMG signal's stability was not decreased in non-stationary tasks [34].

Another factor that can decrease the stability of FSR signals is the curvature of sensors. In the use of FSR-based pressure sensing systems for prosthetic applications, as sensors are embedded inside a prosthetic socket, they are inevitably bent. When FSRs are bent, their neutral value changes and as the sensor responses are usually non-linear, this could considerably affect sensors' responses.

Multiple studies have assessed the effect of bending on stability of FSR readings by studying the effect of placement of FSR sensor arrays on moulds of the limb on the sensors' error compared with when they were laid flat [4,28]. These assessments showed that when the sensors were placed on moulds of residual limbs, their errors increased significantly compared with when they were laid flat. Three off-the-shelf FSR-based pressure sensing systems were assessed in these studies: the Rincoe SFS system, the F-Socket, and the Pliance system. Their reported accuracy error increased from 24.7% to 32.9% for the Rincoe SFS system [4], 8.5% to 11.2% for the F-Socket [4], and from 2.42% to 9.96% for the Pliance system [28].

To the best of authors' knowledge, no study has been conducted to solve the problem of instability of FSR-based pressure sensing systems due to bending. The objective of this study is to determine feasibility of reducing errors introduced in sensor matrix readings due to the matrix being bent using information about the values of curvature of the sensors. This is a preliminary study using an off-the-shelf matrix of FSRs and five values of curvature that are uniform across the matrix. Proposed methods in this study can be applied to any system of sensor matrices that are prone to decreased accuracy when bent, including pressure measurement systems for prosthetic fitting that are available in the market. Since sensor bending affects the physical characteristic of the sensors, it could also affect other aspects of sensors' response in addition to what was assessed in this study such as creep and hysteresis. Moreover, when sensors are placed on a residual limb, they might be bent in multiple planes. This study assessed the effect of bending in one plane. The effect of bending on creep and hysteresis in addition to multi-plane curvature of sensors should be investigated in future work.

The proposed approach for this study was to test sensor readings in a chamber with varying pressure when sensors were laid flat or when they were bent with known curvatures. Recorded data was then analyzed offline. In order to reduce the error due to bending, four regression-based error compensation methods were investigated. These error compensation methods required the use of a regression algorithm to form a model for pressure prediction based on FSR data and sensors' curvatures. To determine which regression algorithm to use in these error compensation methods, three algorithms, namely linear regression (LR), general regression neural network (GRNN), and random forest (RF), were assessed on the data collected from the sensors in the pressure chamber. The data that were used for assessment of the three regression algorithms was the combination of sensor data in all curved conditions in addition to the flat condition. Data were split to 5 repetitions and Leave-one-out cross validation was used to chose one of the regression algorithms be used in the four regression-based error compensation methods proposed in this study. The assessment was performed based on two outcome measures: R^2 and $RMSE\%$.

The three regression algorithms that were assessed for this study are amongst the most vastly used for regression purposes for FSR signals used in biomedical applications [8,35–37]. Linear machine learning algorithms are commonly used for various types of signals for a multitude of applications due to their capability of prediction and their computational efficiency [9,35,38,39]. These characteristics make LR suitable for applications that are sensitive to processing time such as the ones that require repetitions of data processing, and the applications that require real-time data processing.

GRNN is a probabilistic, memory-based neural network with a highly parallel structure. This algorithm learns in a single pass through available data and converges to the optimal regression surfaces with availability of more samples. It is capable of forming acceptable regression surfaces based on limited data and is known to work with sparse data in real-time environments. GRNN is fast learning and computationally efficient as it does not need back propagation. Moreover, its implementation is relatively simple and easy to use [36,40]. These characteristics of GRNN make it suitable for the analysis of this study, especially considering sparsity of curvature values.

RF is a non-conventional machine learning algorithm that is commonly used for classification and regression of FSR signals. It improves on individual decision trees by using an aggregation of weakly pruned trees to prevent over-fitting to training data. This enhances generalization of the models created by RF [41]. These characteristics of the three aforementioned algorithms, common application of them to FSR signals, and their performance for the baseline condition of this study, which is when data from the flat condition and various curved conditions were combined, are the reasons they were chosen for assessment of the dataset of this study.

The selected regression algorithm was used in the four regression-based error compensation methods that were investigated. The objective of the error compensation methods was to take into account the variability introduced in the sensors' responses due to their bending. A common method to account for such variability in different conditions is to calibrate sensors separately for each condition [31]. Method1 does so by separating data based on the curvature of the sensors and making a separate model for each condition using the selected regression algorithm. To predict pressure for test data using this method, the model associated with the curvature of test data would be used. Method2 uses the selected regression algorithm to make a single model for all data. In this method, the value of curvature is used as an input channel for model training and pressure prediction. Findings of method2 motivated implementation of method3 and method4. More explanation on this is provided in the "Discussion" section. Method3 splits the data to flat and curved. It then uses the selected regression algorithm to make a separate model for each of these two conditions. Pressure prediction for test data using this method is similar to the first method. Method4 is similar to method2 except that the curvature input channel in this method has binary values of 0 and 1 representing whether the sensor is curved or flat. For comparison of performance of these methods, data were split to 5 partitions and Leave-one-out cross validation was used with the two aforementioned outcome measures (R^2 and $RMSE\%$).

2. Materials and Methods

To assess the effect of bending on accuracy of the response of FSRs, sensors' responses to known pressure values were examined as they were placed on structures that were flat or were curved with various curvatures. Regression methods were used to map sensor responses to pressure values. To assess whether bending the sensors significantly affected their response accuracy, two conditions were first compared: sensors' responses when only the flat condition was considered and sensors' responses when all six conditions were considered. Multiple error compensation methods were then used to decrease the errors introduced due to the bending of the sensors and their performances were compared.

To collect required data for this study, a test setup was needed that could apply pressure on sensors in the matrix while measuring the value of the applied pressure, that is, true pressure value. The measured value would then be used to produce the regression model.

For all statistical tests, normality of data was determined using the Shapiro-Wilk test. When data were from a normal distribution, depending on the number of populations being compared, either the Student's paired *t*-test at significance level of 5% or a repeated measures ANOVA was employed. For these tests, 70 samples were used, each representing the outcome measure for one of the sensors in the matrix.

For cases where the assumption of normality was violated, non-parametric tests were used. When more than two populations were being compared, the Friedman test was used. For post hoc analysis in these cases, or in cases where two populations were being compared, depending on symmetry of the distribution of differences between paired variables, either the Wilcoxon signed-rank test or the paired-samples sign test with a Bonferroni correction was used. All tests were conducted with the IBM SPSS Statistics v24 software.

2.1. Sensor Matrices

To explore the extent of the effect of bending on accuracy of the response of FSRs, an off-the-shelf sensor matrix of FSRs was chosen for this study: the TPE-900 Series multi-touch resistive evaluation sensor by Tangio Printed Electronics. This sensor matrix was chosen due to its independence on specific hardware or electronics. The FSR matrix used in this study was comprised of 7 rows and 10 columns of individual FSR sensors and its dimensions were approximately 7 cm × 10 cm. The sensor matrix is shown in Figure 1. For this experiment, the sensor matrix was sealed using Polydimethylsiloxane (PDMS) to prevent the pressurized air inside the chamber from filling the air channel that was integrated in the design of the matrix. If the air channel was filled with pressurized air, the pressure difference between the environment and the sensor matrix's air channel would be zero. This would prevent the sensors from sensing the air pressure in their surrounding environment.

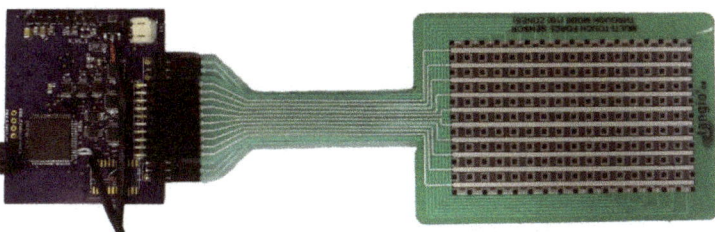

Figure 1. FSR matrix and the data acquisition printed circuit board (PCB) used in this study.

2.2. Data Acquisition

Two-dimensional (2D) networks of matrices are used in variety of applications such as tactile sensing, pressure distribution measurements, temperature sensing, gas detection, and so forth [42]. Shared signal and power lines between sensors in a row and sensors in a column allow for smaller number of traces which simplifies hardware and electronics. However, an inherent problem with the row-column fashion of these matrices is the cross-talk between adjacent elements of the matrix.

Various circuits are proposed and used in the literature for the scanning of piezoresistive sensor arrays that reduce the interference of unwanted paths [42–44]. Two of the commonly used cross-talk suppression circuits are based on the Voltage Feedback method and the Zero-potential method [43].

In this study, a printed circuit board (PCB) was designed for data acquisition that used the Zero-potential circuitry shown in Figure 2. The data acquisition PCB used a Cypress PSoC 4 (model CY8C4247AXI-M485) microcontroller, op-amps, switches, a voltage regulator chip, a voltage reference chip, and multiplexers. Outputs of the circuit were transferred to a computer using universal asynchronous receiver-transmitter (UART) communication and were then saved on the computer for offline data analysis. The PCB could acquire data from sensor matrices of up to 10 columns and 16 rows. The PCB is shown in Figure 1.

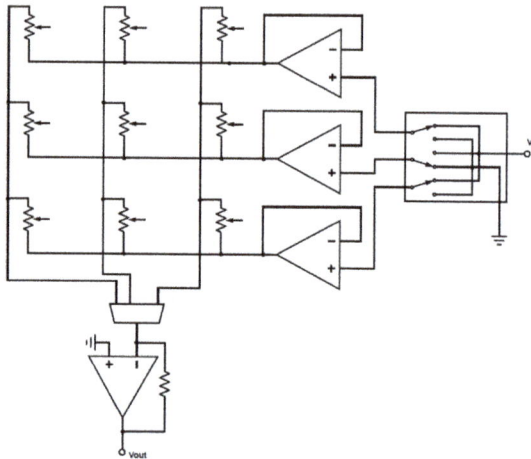

Figure 2. Cross talk compensation circuit used in this study.

True pressure values also needed to be measured and recorded. This was done using a digital pressure transducer by Omega Engineering (model PX309) whose data was acquired using a National Instrument (NI) Data Acquisition Unit (DAQ)(model USB-6001). Recordings of sensor readings and pressure sensor values were synchronized using NI LabVIEW software.

2.3. Test Setup

Sensors' responses were assessed in six conditions—when sensors were laid flat and when they were placed on each of the five structures that were designed with varying curvatures. The curved structures were 3D printed and are shown in Figure 3. Each structure was part of a cylinder with a different radius, namely 5, 7, 9, 11, and 13 cm, with corresponding curvatures of approximately 0.20, 0.14, 0.11, 0.091, and 0.077 m^{-1}, respectively. As transtibial amputations account for majority of the major lower limb amputations [45,46], and transhumeral amputations account for majority of the upper limb amputations [45], chosen curvatures are based on measurements of the lower transtibial residual limb reported by Persson et al. [47] and the average circumference of the arm reported by Holzbaur et al. [48].

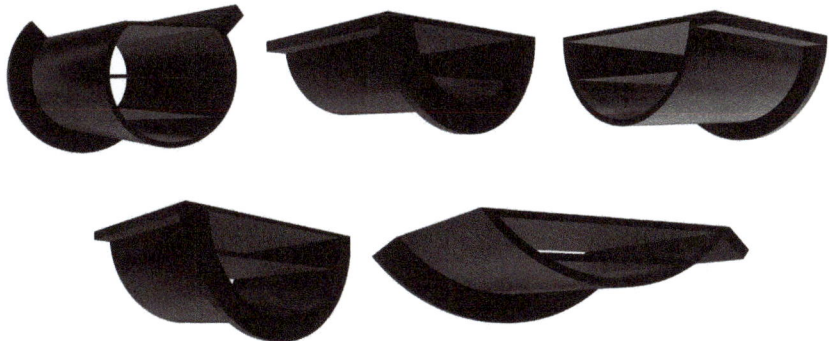

Figure 3. Curved structured used to bend sensor matrix with known curvatures. From left to right, top to bottom, 5, 7, 9, 11, 13 cm.

Persson et al. studied dimensions of 93 lower residual limbs to construct a standard formula of their classification into cylindrical (ordinary), conical, and club-shaped as well as short, ordinary ($breadth < length < 2 * breadth$), or long. In this study, they tested the constructed classification formula on 96 residual limbs of 86 volunteers in 135 examinations and determined that 80% of them were ordinary in both size and shape. Measurements of the breadth of the residual limbs were not reported, however, considering the ordinary length of the majority of the residual limbs and the range reported for their length, breadth of the stump of majority of participants can be approximated to be larger than 9 cm which corresponds to the curvature of about 0.2 m^{-1} [47].

Holzbaur et al. used magnetic resonance imaging for measurement of the features of 32 upper limbs and reported an average of approximately 31 cm for the circumference of the arm which corresponds to the curvature of about 0.2 m^{-1}. Based on the measurements reported by the aforementioned studies, the highest curvature used in this study was 0.2 m^{-1}. The rest of the curvatures were chosen with 2 cm variations in the radius of the cylinders up to the radius of 13 cm. The reason lower curvatures were not considered is that they were not expected to have considerable effects on sensors' responses [48]. As this was a preliminary study, it did not consider double curvatures which would be more important for the conical and club-shaped stumps which account for about 20% of the stumps according to the above study [47]. This should be considered in future work.

Design of the curved structures included fixtures to assure fixed placement of sensor matrices that was normal to the horizontal cross section of the cylinders. Fixtures were also added to the structures to ensure their mechanical stability under pressure. For the experiments in this study, to bend sensor matrices to specific, known curvatures, they were placed on these structures.

A test setup was required to apply and measure known values of pressure to the sensor matrix as it was bent. The setup included an air pressure chamber rated at 793 kPa built to American Society of Mechanical Engineers' specifications, a pressure transducer with ±0.25% best straight-line accuracy and range of approximately −103 to 1034 kPa, and an electrical feed-through to allow for powering the system and reading output values. This setup was similar to the one used in literature to evaluate sensory systems for prosthetic fitting [4,28]. The test setup is shown in Figure 4.

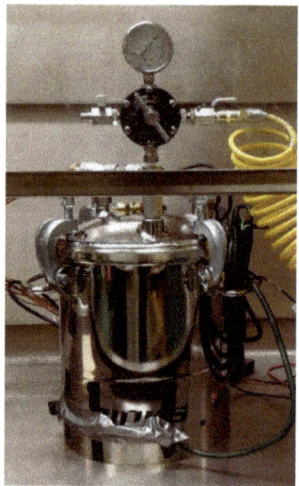

Figure 4. Experimental setup using a pressure chamber.

2.4. Data Collection

The sensor matrix was placed on a flat or curved surface and was placed inside the chamber. Sensors were then tested by increasing air pressure inside the chamber up to about 620 kPa and decreasing it back to room pressure in a cyclic manner. This was repeated for each condition (five curved surfaces and the flat surface) for up to 10 cycles. This method was similar to what has been done in literature for assessment of accuracy of similar systems [4].

Frequency of data collection was 10 Hz. At each frame, both sensor values and the pressure inside the chamber were recorded. Total number of data samples (observations) for the 6 sets combined was about 45,000.

2.5. Regression Methods

To determine which regression algorithm to use in this study, three algorithms, GRNN, LR, and RF, were applied to collected data and their performance was compared using two outcome measures.

Linear regression uses a linear combination of input data to create the regression model as shown in the equation below [49]:

$$y = \omega_0 + \sum_{i=1}^{N} \omega_i x_i, \tag{1}$$

where ω_i represents the weight of input feature i, x_is are the input features, N is the number of features, y is the predicted value, and ω_0 is the intercept of the linear model. In this study Matlab's implementation of LR was used. No parameter turning was required.

GRNN functions based on two layers other than the input and output layers: a pattern layer and a summation layer. First, the pattern layer assesses the relationship between each input feature and the corresponding prediction value. Then, the summation layer performs a dot product of a vector containing produced signals in the previous layer and a weight vector. This layer consists of two neurons: a numerator neuron that is the summation of weighted target values; and the denominator neuron which is the summation of weight values. The mathematical representation is the following [36,40]:

$$Y(x) = \frac{\sum_{j=1}^{N} Y_j L(x, x_j)}{\sum_{j=1}^{N} L(x, x_j)} \qquad (2)$$

$$L(x, x_j) = exp[\frac{-D_j^2}{2\sigma^2}],$$

where $Y(x)$ is the prediction value, x is the new input, x_js are the training samples, D_j^2 is the Euclidean distance between x and x_j, and σ is the spread constant that was tuned to 2^{-7} using a grid search. The smaller the distance between new test data x and the training sample X_j is, the larger the value of $L(x, x_j)$ becomes. This makes the effect of training samples that are more similar to the new test data greater on its predicted value.

The RF algorithm functions based on a modified version of decision trees. It creates an ensemble of weakly pruned trees. In a standard decision tree, each split is based on all available features while in RF trees, decision splits are based on comparisons of guesses among randomly selected input features. To perform prediction on a data point after the RF model is learned, the aggregation of prediction of all decision trees are used. In the implementation used in this study, the mean of prediction of trees are used as the predicted pressure [8,41]. Matlab's implementation of RF was used in this study. A grid search was performed to tune the number of trees to 150. The default option was used for the number of features used for each decision split which is one third of the number of variables.

The two outcome measures used in this study were: coefficient of determination (R^2) and Root Mean Square Error Percentage ($RMSE\%$) that are calculated using the following formulas:

$$R^2 = 1 - \frac{\sum_{k=1}^{n}(y_k - y_k')^2}{\sum_{k=1}^{n}(y_k - \overline{y_k})^2} \qquad (3)$$

$$RMSE\% = \frac{\sqrt{\frac{1}{n}\sum_{k=1}^{n}(y_k - y_k')^2}}{range_y} * 100, \qquad (4)$$

where y_k is the expected value of the reading, y_k' is the predicted value, $\overline{y_k}$ is the mean of expected values, n is the number of observations, and $range_y$ is the range of values in observations of expected values. R^2 and $RMSE\%$ are commonly used for assessment of performance of regression methods [50]. Based on these outcome measures, one of the regression algorithms was chosen to be used in this study.

Four different regression-based error compensation methods were examined to reduce the error caused in sensors' responses due to their bending. These methods were compared with each other and the baseline results based on the two aforementioned outcome measures. Baseline values were obtained by combining data from all 6 conditions (flat and curved). In the baseline method, one regression model was created and used for the combined data. In order to eliminate any bias based on the number of samples used in different regression methods, data were down-sampled in any of the methods that were using data from multiple conditions. The four error compensation methods are described in Table 1:

Table 1. Regression-based error compensation methods used to reduce the errors introduced due to bending of the sensors.

Method1	A separate model was made for each curvature and data for each curve was assessed separately. A total of 6 models were used in this method.
Method2	The value of curvature for each of the curved or flat structures was inputted as an extra channel to the model. Data was down sampled to 1/6 of total observations so that the number of observations was comparable to the one for Method1.
Method3	All curved structures were grouped together, and two models were made in total: one for when the matrix was laid flat, and one for all the curved conditions. Data was down sampled so that the total amount of data for each of the two groups was comparable to the one in method1.
Method4	Similar to method2, an input was added for curvature values. However, value of curvature was set to 0 for flat, and 1 for all the curved conditions. Data was down sampled similar to method3.

In all methods data were normalized based on the mean and the standard deviation of training data before model was made. This was done since in practice, test data is unknown and cannot affect these factors. Each sensor was analyzed separately in all methods and the means of outcome measures for the 70 sensors were reported to represent the outcome measures for each method.

Leave-one-out cross validation method was used for all assessments done in this study. Data were split to 5 sections. Five repetitions of the assessment were done, in each, one of the 5 sections of data was held out as test data and the rest was used as training data. Obtained values of the outcome measures for each sensor was the average of the five repetitions.

3. Results

Figure 5 illustrates how the curvature of an FSR sensor affects its response to applied force or pressure. Since such variations can negatively impact the stability of sensor readings in practical situations, we propose a regression-based calibration system that takes into account the information about the curvature of a sensor in addition to its pressure measurements. In this section, results of our proposed method are explained in detail.

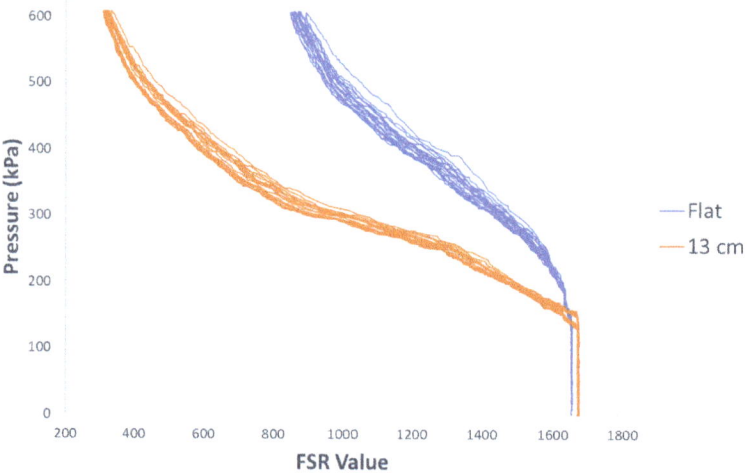

Figure 5. Comparison of the response of one of the FSRs when sensor was laid flat vs. when it was placed on the curved structure with radius of 13 cm.

3.1. Algorithm Selection

Results of the two outcome measures using the three regression algorithms assessed in this study are shown in Figure 6.

Statistical analysis showed significant differences between results of the three algorithms in terms of both R^2 ($\chi^2(2) = 107.31, p < 0.001$) and $RMSE\%$ ($\chi^2(2) = 109.83, p < 0.001$). Post hoc analysis determined that LR had significantly worse performance in terms of both outcome measures. Means of R^2 values obtained using GRNN and RF were also significantly different. However, significance of the difference between GRNN's and RF's performances in terms of $RMSE\%$ was not determined.

GRNN was chosen as the regression algorithm to be used moving forward due to its better performance, lower standard deviations of errors and ease of use.

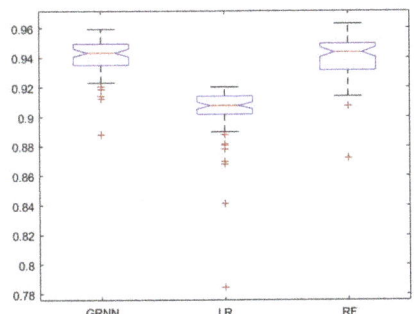 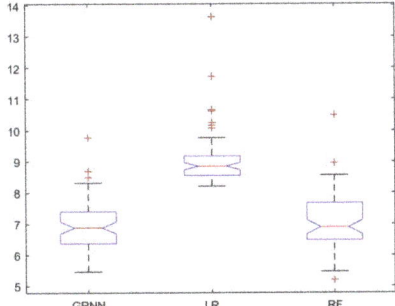

Figure 6. Comparison of performance of three regression algorithms: general regression neural network (GRNN), linear regression (LR), and random forest (RF). The results of the two outcome measures are shown in this figure: R^2 in the right figure and $RMSE\%$ in the left one.

3.2. Method Selection

The comparison of when only the flat condition was considered versus when data from all six conditions were combined yielded results shown in Table 2.

Table 2. Comparison of when sensors were laid flat vs. when all 6 conditions were considered.

Method	R^2	$RMSE\%$
Flat	0.99 ± 0.0012	3.51 ± 0.19
All Curvatures	0.94 ± 0.013	6.93 ± 0.81

These results determined that inclusion of varying curvatures statistically reduced accuracy of prediction based on both outcome measures. To compensate for this effect, the four error compensation methods explained in Table 1 were used. Results obtained using these methods are shown in Figure 7 and Table 3.

Table 3. Results of method selection.

Method	R^2	$RMSE\%$
Baseline	0.94 ± 0.013	6.93 ± 0.81
Method1	0.98 ± 0.0014	4.26 ± 0.18
Method2	0.96 ± 0.0027	5.03 ± 0.20
Method3	0.97 ± 0.0055	4.66 ± 0.40
Method4	0.98 ± 0.0060	4.96 ± 0.64

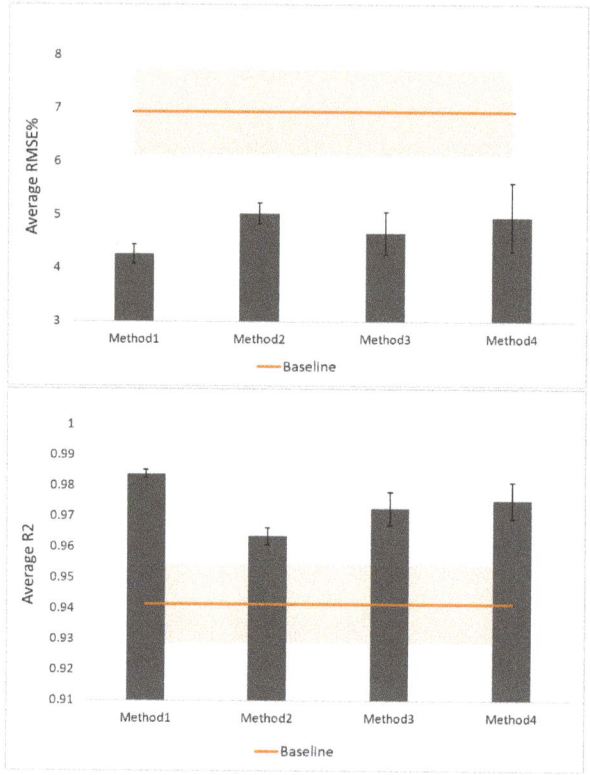

Figure 7. Outcome measures for the four proposed methods. The results of the two outcome measures are shown in this figure: $RMSE\%$ in the top figure and R^2 in the bottom one.

The baseline method had the worst performance compared to all the other methods. Method1 yielded the best results. Method2 made significant improvement compared to the baseline results, however, its performance was significantly worse than method1. Method3 showed improvement over both the baseline and method2 with significant difference for both R^2 and $RMSE\%$ outcome measures. Yet it did not achieve as much improvement as method1. Method4 also showed improvement over method2 but could not reach the amount of improvement obtained using method1. Means of the average values for both outcome measures for this method were statistically significantly different from both method2 and method3. This method performed better in terms of R^2 but worse in terms of $RMSE\%$ compared with method3 with significant difference.

Statistical analysis using the Friedman test determined significant differences between results of all methods including the baseline in terms of both R^2 ($\chi^2(4) = 270.09, p < 0.001$) and $RMSE\%$ ($\chi^2(4) = 246.83, p < 0.001$). Post hoc analysis of means of both outcome measures showed significant differences between all methods.

4. Discussion

As mentioned in the 'Introduction' section, bending FSR sensors can affect their neutral state value which is their response in the minimum pressure of the system. The effect of bending on the neutral state value of sensors is shown in Figure 8 by comparing the response of one of the sensors in a low range of pressure when the sensor matrix was laid flat versus when it was placed on the structure with the radius of 13 cm. This phenomenon, in addition to other factors such as the non-linearity of sensors' response to applied pressure, can considerably affect the response of FSRs when they are positioned with various curvatures. To better highlight this point, Figure 9 shows how applied pressure can be inaccurately interpreted from FSR readings if the sensor's curvature is not taken into account. Figure 9 also shows how a regression-based calibration method can resolve this issue.

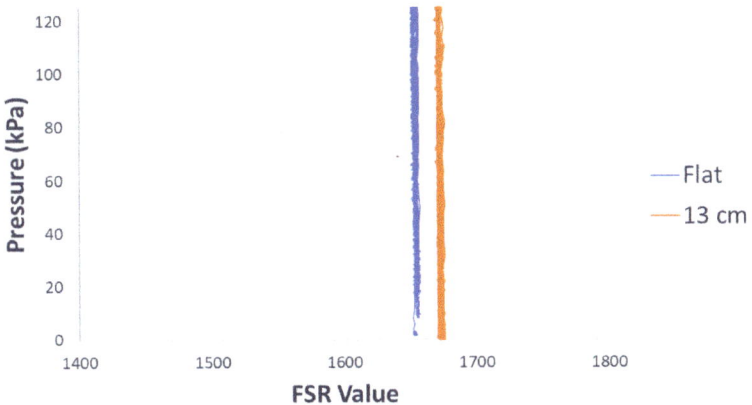

Figure 8. Comparison of the response of one of the FSRs when sensors were laid flat vs. when they were placed on the curved structure with radius of 13 cm. Response of the sensors in low pressure values is shown.

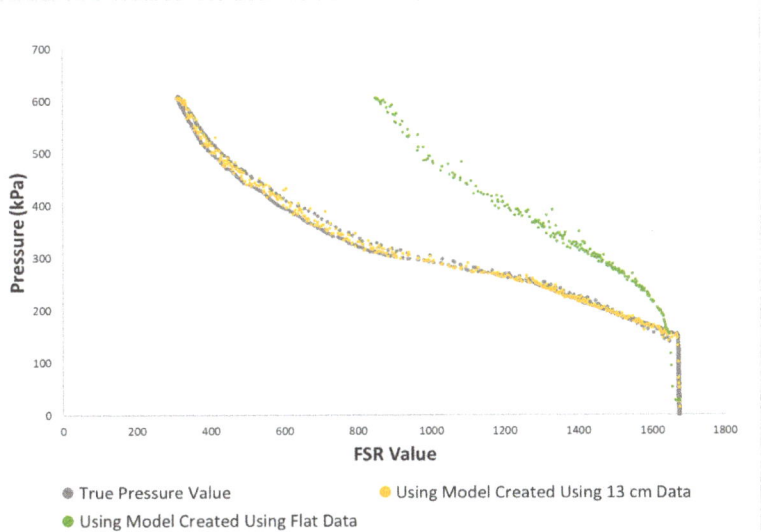

Figure 9. Comparison of predicting pressure from output of one of the sensors without and with considering sensor's curvature information. Sensor was curved with a curvature of approximately 0.77 m^{-1}. GRNN regression algorithm was applied to predict pressure values from the measurements of one of the sensors.

The goodness of fit of the regression models was compared in two cases—when only the flat condition was considered versus when varying curvatures were also included. This comparison determined that the effect of variation in curvatures of the sensors on their responses was statistically significant. In this step of the experiment, statistical significance was determined using the Student's paired t-test.

Four regression-based error compensation methods were used to compensate for this effect. These methods were compared with the baseline. The baseline method yielded values for errors without any attempt to compensate for the bending errors in the sensor matrix. As expected, this method had the worst performance compared to all the other methods.

Method1 classified data to six classes of matrix positioning: one for flat and five for bent with different curvatures and created a separate model for each class. This method resulted in the best accuracy of prediction based on both of the outcome measures used in this study. This was likely because in this method, data from each condition was considered separately without any effect from data from other conditions. In this method, variation of data used for training and testing of each model was minimal compared to other methods. The main disadvantage of this method was its difficulty of implementation in practice. This is because, in practice, curvature values are continuous while this method requires classification of data into discrete curvature conditions. A solution for this is to classify data based on ranges of curvatures and to use separate models for each of the classes of curvature range.

Method2 used values of curvatures of the sensor matrix as an added input channel to the regression algorithm. Compared to method1, this method performed significantly worse. A closer look at the data indicated that similarities between the data when sensors were curved with different curvatures was much more than similarity of the data between any of the curved conditions and the flat condition. This can be seen in Figure 10.

Looking at the physics and operation of FSRs may help in understanding why their behaviour changes when they are curved. It may also clarify the reason for similarity of sensors' responses when curved with various curvatures. Force sensitive resistors are resistive polymer-thick-film (RPTF) sensors comprised of multiple layers including semi-conductive layers and electrode layers. These sensors often employ a spacer mechanism such as spacer layers or air channels to control the spacing between the substrates of the sensors. This layer ensures high resistance of the sensors in the absence of external forces. When force is applied to the sensors, their resistance decreases due to two main factors. The first factor is the comprising layers of the sensors becoming in contact with each other. The other factor is variation in the geometry of the semi-conductive layer in a way that reduces sensors' resistance [35].

When sensors are bent, their physics that play an important role in their responses to pressure also change. Curving FSRs causes their comprising layers to become closer to each other which can be considered similar to pre-loading the sensors. Moreover, since the forces due to bending are not distributed evenly across the sensors [40], their curvature affects their responses not only by pre-loading the sensors, but also by changing the rate of the change of their responses to increasing pressure. It is likely that the similarity of the responses of curved sensors regardless of the value of their curvatures is because of the similarity in distribution of bending forces across sensors in these conditions compared to when they are laid flat.

The reason method2 did not make as much improvement as expected is likely that the differences between curvature values are not good representatives of the variation in data in corresponding conditions. The model likely assumes that the difference between the value of the curvatures of two conditions determines the difference between the sensors' responses in those conditions. However, this is not the case according to the data collected for this study. For example, the difference between the curvatures of the flat condition and the curved condition with the radius of 13 cm is about 0.08 m^{-1} and the difference between the curvatures of the curved condition with the radius of 13 cm and the one with the radius of 7 cm is about 0.07 m^{-1}. The differences between the value of curvatures in these cases are comparable, so the model likely assumes that the variations of the sensors' responses in these cases would also be similar. However, looking at the graph in Figure 10, it can be seen that the sensors' responses are much more different in the former case compared to the latter one.

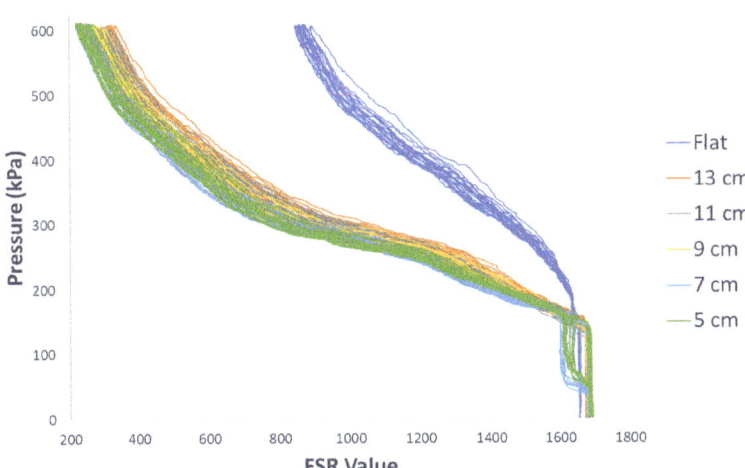

Figure 10. Comparison of the response of one of FSRs when sensors are positioned on structures with varying curvatures.

A solution for this could be to use binary inputs for curvatures. This would imply using 6 extra input channels for model creation. In each of the 6 conditions, a unique binary sequence consisting of a single 1 and five 0s would be used. This solution was implemented for the dataset of this experiment. Obtained results were 0.96 ± 0.003 and $5.05\% \pm 0.19\%$ for the R^2 and $RMSE\%$ respectively. Both outcome measures were improved compared to method2, however, significant improvement was not determined using the Student's t-test for either of the outcome measures. To further improve on this, categorical inputs could be used for curvature. However, in that case, curvature values would need to be classified to curvature ranges which would entail similar problems as the ones explained for method1.

Another solution to improve on method2 would be to determine a mapping of curvatures to continuous values that would be able to accurately represent the extent of their effect on variation of FSR responses. This should be investigated in future work.

The similarity between all curved conditions compared to the flat condition brought up the possibility of grouping all curved data and simply separating the two situations when the sensor matrix was laid flat and when it was curved, regardless of the amount of its curvature. This led to method3 and method4. Both method3 and method4 improved on the results obtained using method2 significantly.

Method3 made two different models, one for flat and one for curved. This method yielded improvement over method2 with significant statistical difference for both R2 and RMSE% outcome measures. This is likely because the error caused by ignoring variations in data when sensors were bent with various curvatures is smaller than the error caused by assuming that the value of curvatures were accurate representatives of the amount of variation introduced in data as sensors were bent. This was expected as discussed before. Method3 did not achieve as much improvement as method1 since, in method1 the error caused by assuming no variation in data from various curvatures was also omitted.

Method3 is easier to implement in practical situations compared to both previous methods. This is because there is no need to know the exact or even approximate value of curvatures, as long as it is known that the matrix is curved. It is reasonable to assume that sensors are bent in most locations when the matrix is embedded in a prosthetic socket.

Method4 inputted an extra channel to the algorithm. The value of this channel was 0 when the sensors were laid flat, and it was 1 when they were curved regardless of the amount of bend. This method, similar to method3 groups all curved data together. Method4 also showed improvement over method2 but could not reach the amount of improvement obtained using method1 for the same reasons explained for method3.

It is worth noting that, since only two values, 0 and 1, were used as the second input for method4, this method is similar to binary curvature inputs that was discussed for method2. This is likely the reason why method3 and method4 have comparable performances (each outperforms the other based on one of the outcome measures). Method3 performed significantly better than method4 in terms of $RMSE\%$, however, it performed significantly worse than method4 in terms of R^2. In comparison of the last two methods, that is, method3 and method4, it was determined that method3 outperformed method4 based in $RMSE\%$ while method4 outperformed method3 based on the other outcome measure (R^2). Because we only considered two outcome measures in this study, neither of which was considered more important than the other, and due to the fact that each of these methods performed better that the other based on one of these outcome measures, we cannot conclude superiority of one of these methods compared with the other. As a result, we cannot consider one of them to have had better overall performance for the dataset of this study.

In terms of computing power and running time, variations for testing using these methods are not considerable. This is because in all methods, the model is produced using offline data. In online testing, at each sample and for each sensor, one prediction is performed using the pre-built model. The main difference among different methods would be in the training time. However, this is not an important factor in applications considered in this study since model production would be performed offline.

In order to use the proposed methods of this study, information about curvature of the limb is required. Various methods are used for geometric assessments of a residual limb that can be used for this purpose. Some possible methods include circumferential measurements and contacting methods utilizing digitizing methods of the cast of the limb or the residual limb itself [51,52]. Since, in common practice for the fabrication of prosthetic sockets, casts are made in one of the initial steps, cast of the limb is available and can be used for geometric assessment of the limb [53]. Three-dimensional (3D) scanning is another method that has recently gained attention in the field of prosthesis for various applications. 3D scans of the limb can be used for extraction of information required for the methods proposed in this study. Another option would be to place sensors on the cast of the limb and calibrate them as they are curved and placed on the location of the limb that they would later be positioned on for measurements.

Bend sensors can also potentially be used to measure the value of curvature of sensors. Compared to the aforementioned methods, the use of bend sensors can be faster and easier but less accurate. Another method that could be valuable for this purpose in the settings similar to the one used in this study, is to use the value of FSRs in specific states to determine their curvature value. To achieve this, values of sensors in room pressure or another known state could be considered. Another option would be to determine the curvature value based on the response of sensors to cyclic variations of pressure. In either of these cases, features should be extracted from time windows with optimized lengths. For more reliable prediction of curvatures, values of multiple adjacent sensors can be considered. This method should be investigated in future work.

5. Conclusions

In this study, it was determined that when FSR sensors were bent, the error in their mapping to pressure values significantly increased compared to when they were laid flat.

Four regression-based error compensation methods were proposed to solve the problem of instability of FSR sensor matrices when placed on a curved structure. All proposed methods significantly improved the accuracy of mapping of sensor readings to pressure values. It was determined that by just knowing when the sensor was curved without any knowledge about the value of its curvature, results could be improved using proposed methods in this study.

The best performance was achieved by making separate models based on the value of curvature of sensors. The second best performance was obtained by grouping all curved conditions and separating them from the flat condition. The former method would require classifying curvature values to pre-defined ranges. This is to be investigated in future work. The latter method is simpler and more practical since no knowledge about the value of the curvature is required, however, the amount of improvement obtained using this method is significantly less than the former method.

Based on findings of this study, for practical use of the proposed methods, method1 is recommended due to its better performance in terms of both outcome measures. To use this method with continuous curvature values, curvatures would be grouped into classes of different ranges and a model would be made for each group. Then, depending on the range that the sensor's curvature falls into when placed on the limb, the regression model for its calibration would be selected. More investigation is required to determine the optimum ranges of curvatures.

6. Limitations and Future Work

This was a preliminary study that demonstrated feasibility of using the proposed methods to increase robustness of FSR-based systems for prosthetic applications. Some of the limitations of this study and future work are explained in this section.

Experimental conditions such as sensor sealing with PDMS may have affected the reported results. This reduces generality of the findings of this study. Various types of FSR sensors, for example sensors that do not need to be sealed, should be tested in different experimental conditions to confirm findings of this study in future work.

In order to fully control the experiments carried out in this study, the sensors were not removed in between tests. Next steps in future work, should assess the effect of removing and re-positioning sensors between multiple repetitions of data collection. This would be to assess the effect of variability of data due to re-positioning on accuracy of pressure prediction using the methods proposed in this study. The use of proposed methods for sensors incorporated into prosthetic systems should also be investigated and clinical tests of these systems should be conducted.

In future studies, more curvature values need to be tested to determine whether even with very low values of curvature, these methods would prove useful. Continuous curvatures need to be examined to obtain a more generalized dataset. Moreover, more complex shapes need to be tested in future work that would cause different sensors in a matrix to have different amounts of bend. This would be to mimic the scenario when sensor matrices are placed on a residual limb. An experiment should be conducted in which sensors are placed on a mould of the residual limb inside the pressure chamber and models are built according to data recorded in this situation. Moreover, these methods should be examined using a variety of sensor matrices and single FSRs.

To further build on findings of this study, the effect of hysteresis and creep on FSRs should also be investigated. Compensation methods should be proposed to enhance stability of these sensors in practical and prolonged prosthetic applications.

Author Contributions: Conceptualization, C.A. and C.M.; methodology, C.A.; validation, C.A. and C.M.; formal analysis, C.A.; investigation, C.A.; writing—original draft preparation, C.A.; writing—review and editing, C.M.; visualization, C.A.; supervision, C.M.; project administration, C.M.; funding acquisition, C.M.

Funding: Research supported by the Natural Sciences and Engineering Research Council of Canada (NSERC), the Canadian Institutes of Health Research (CIHR), and the Canada Research Chair (CRC) program.

Conflicts of Interest: The authors declare no conflict of interest.

Abbreviations

The following abbreviations are used in this manuscript:

FSR	Force Sensitive Resistor
FMG	Force Myography
PDMS	Polydimethylsiloxane
GRNN	General Regression neural network
LR	Linear Regression
RF	Random Forest
RMSE	Root Mean Square Error
PCB	Printed Circuit Board
UART	Universal Asynchronous Receiver-transmitter

References

1. Ferigo, D.; Merhi, L.K.; Pousett, B.; Xiao, Z.G.; Menon, C. A Case Study of a Force-myography Controlled Bionic Hand Mitigating Limb Position Effect. *J. Bionic Eng.* **2017**, *14*, 692–705. [CrossRef]
2. Ahmadizadeh, C.; Merhi, L.K.; Pousett, B.; Sangha, S.; Menon, C. Toward Intuitive Prosthetic Control: Solving Common Issues Using Force Myography, Surface Electromyography, and Pattern Recognition in a Pilot Case Study. *IEEE Robot. Autom. Mag.* **2017**, *24*, 102–111. [CrossRef]
3. Godiyal, A.K.; Singh, U.; Anand, S.; Joshi, D. Analysis of force myography based locomotion patterns. *Meas. J. Int. Meas. Confed.* **2019**, *140*, 497–503. [CrossRef]
4. Polliack, A.A.; Sieh, R.C.; Craig, D.D.; Landsberger, S.; McNeil, D.R.; Ayyappa, E. Scientific validation of two commercial pressure sensor systems for prosthetic socket fit. *Prosthetics Orthot. Int.* **2000**, *24*, 63–73. [CrossRef]
5. Buis, A.W.; Convery, P. Calibration problems encountered while monitoring stump/socket interface pressures with force sensing resistors: Techniques adopted to minimise inaccuracies. *Prosthetics Orthot. Int.* **1997**, *21*, 179–182. [CrossRef]
6. Al-Fakih, E.A.; Abu Osman, N.A.; Mahmad Adikan, F.R. Techniques for interface stress measurements within prosthetic sockets of transtibial amputees: A review of the past 50 years of research. *Sensors* **2016**, *16*, 1119. [CrossRef]
7. Godiyal, A.K.; Verma, H.K.; Khanna, N.; Joshi, D. A force myography-based system for gait event detection in overground and ramp walking. *IEEE Trans. Instrum. Meas.* **2018**, *67*, 2314–2323. [CrossRef]
8. Chengani, R.; Delva, M.L.; Sakr, M.; Menon, C. Pilot study on strategies in sensor placement for robust hand/wrist gesture classification based on movement related changes in forearm volume. In Proceedings of the 2016 IEEE Healthcare Innovation Point-of-Care Technologies Conference, HI-POCT 2016, Cancun, Mexico, 9–11 November 2016; pp. 46–49. [CrossRef]
9. Radmand, A.; Scheme, E.; Englehart, K. High-density force myography: A possible alternative for upper-limb prosthetic control. *J. Rehabil. Res. Dev.* **2016**, *53*, 443–456. [CrossRef]
10. Rasouli, M.; Ghosh, R.; Lee, W.W.; Thakor, N.V.; Kukreja, S. Stable force-myographic control of a prosthetic hand using incremental learning. In Proceedings of the 37th Annual International Conference of the IEEE Engineering in Medicine and Biology Society (EMBC), Milano, Italy, 25–29 August 2015; pp. 4828–4831. [CrossRef]
11. Li, N.; Yang, D.; Jiang, L.; Liu, H.; Cai, H. Combined use of FSR sensor array and SVM classifier for finger motion recognition based on pressure distribution map. *J. Bionic Eng.* **2012**, *9*, 39–47. [CrossRef]
12. Varol, H.A.; Sup, F.; Goldfarb, M. Multiclass Real-Time Intent Recognition of a powered Lower Limb Prosthesis. *IEEE Trans. Biomed. Eng.* **2010**, *57*, 542–551. [CrossRef]
13. Jiang, X.; Tory, L.; Khoshnam, M.; Chu, K.H.; Menon, C. Exploration of Gait Parameters Affecting the Accuracy of Force Myography-Based Gait Phase Detection. In Proceedings of the IEEE RAS and EMBS International Conference on Biomedical Robotics and Biomechatronics, Enschede, The Netherlands, 26–29 August 2018; pp. 1205–1210. [CrossRef]
14. Cherelle, P.; Grosu, V.; Flynn, L.; Junius, K.; Moltedo, M.; Vanderborght, B.; Lefeber, D. The Ankle Mimicking Prosthetic Foot 3—Locking mechanisms, actuator design, control and experiments with an amputee. *Robot. Auton. Syst.* **2017**, *91*, 327–336. [CrossRef]
15. Zachariah, S.G.; Sanders, J.E. Interface mechanics in lower-limb external prosthetics: A review of finite element models. *IEEE Trans. Rehabil. Eng.* **1996**, *4*, 288–302. [CrossRef] [PubMed]

16. Nielsen, C.C. A survey of amputees: Functional level and life satisfaction, information needs, and the prosthetist's role. *JPO J. Prosthetics Orthot.* **1991**, *3*, 125–129. [CrossRef]
17. Mak, A.F.; Zhang, M.; Boone, D.A. State-of-the-art research in lower-limb prosthetic biomechanics-socket interface: A review. *J. Rehabil. Res. Dev.* **2001**, *38*, 161–74. [PubMed]
18. Gailey, R.; Allen, K.; Castles, J.; Kucharik, J.; Roeder, M. Review of secondary physical conditions associated with lower-limb amputation and long-term prosthesis use. *J. Rehabil. Res. Dev.* **2008**, *45*, 15–29. [CrossRef]
19. Ancillao, A.; Tedesco, S.; Barton, J.; O'Flynn, B. Indirect measurement of ground reaction forces and moments by means of wearable inertial sensors: A systematic review. *Sensors* **2018**, *18*, 2564. [CrossRef]
20. Schütz, P.; Taylor, W.R.; Postolka, B.; Fucentese, S.F.; Koch, P.P.; Freeman, M.A.; Pinskerova, V.; List, R. Kinematic evaluation of the GMK sphere implant during gait activities: A dynamic videofluoroscopy study. *J. Orthop. Res.* **2019**, *37*, 2337–2347. [CrossRef]
21. Kumar, D.; Manal, K.T.; Rudolph, K.S. Knee joint loading during gait in healthy controls and individuals with knee osteoarthritis. *Osteoarthr. Cartil.* **2013**, *21*, 298–305. [CrossRef]
22. Bergmann, G.; Bender, A.; Dymke, J.; Duda, G.N.; Damm, P. Physical activities that cause high friction moments at the cup in hip implants. *JBJS* **2018**, *100*, 1637–1644. [CrossRef]
23. Ancillao, A.; Rossi, S.; Cappa, P. Analysis of knee strength measurements performed by a hand-held multicomponent dynamometer and optoelectronic system. *IEEE Trans. Instrum. Meas.* **2016**, *66*, 85–92. [CrossRef]
24. Zhang, M.; Turner-Smith, A.R.; Tanner, A.; Roberts, V.C. Clinical investigation of the pressure and shear stress on the trans-tibial stump with a prosthesis. *Med Eng. Phys.* **1998**, *20*, 188–198. [CrossRef]
25. Williams, R.; Porter, D.; Roberts, V.; Regan, J. Triaxial force transducer for investigating stresses at the stump/socket interface. *Med Biol. Eng. Comput.* **1992**, *30*, 89–96. [CrossRef] [PubMed]
26. Hachisuka, K.; Takahashi, M.; Ogata, H.; Ohmine, S.; Shitama, H.; Shinkoda, K. Properties of the flexible pressure sensor under laboratory conditions simulating the internal environment of the total surface bearing socket. *Prosthetics Orthot. Int.* **1998**, *22*, 186–192. [CrossRef]
27. Lai, C.H.; Li-Tsang, C.W. Validation of the Pliance X System in measuring interface pressure generated by pressure garment. *Burns* **2009**, *35*, 845–851. [CrossRef]
28. Polliack, A.; Craig, D.; Sieh, R.C.; Landsberger, S.; McNeil, D.R. Laboratory and clinical tests of a prototype pressure sensor for clinical assessment of prothetic socket fit. *Prosthetics Orthot. Int.* **2002**, *26*, 23–34. [CrossRef]
29. Chase, T.A.; Luo, R.C. A thin-film flexible capacitive tactile normal/shear force array sensor. In Proceedings of the IECON'95-21st Annual Conference on IEEE Industrial Electronics, Orlando, FL, USA, 6–10 November 1995; Volume 2, pp. 1196–1201.
30. Razian, M.A.; Pepper, M.G. Design, development, and characteristics of an in-shoe triaxial pressure measurement transducer utilizing a single element of piezoelectric copolymer film. *IEEE Trans. Neural Syst. Rehabil. Eng.* **2003**, *11*, 288–293. [CrossRef]
31. Schofield, J.S.; Evans, K.R.; Hebert, J.S.; Marasco, P.D.; Carey, J.P. The effect of biomechanical variables on force sensitive resistor error: Implications for calibration and improved accuracy. *J. Biomech.* **2016**, *49*, 786–792. [CrossRef]
32. Luo, Z.P.; Berglund, L.J.; An, K.N. Validation of F-Scan pressure sensor system: A technical note. *J. Rehabil. Res. Dev.* **1998**, *35*, 186–191.
33. Wang, Z.; Fang, Y.; Li, G.; Liu, H. Facilitate sEMG-based human-machine interaction through channel optimization. *Int. J. Hum. Robot.* **2019**, *16*, 1941001. [CrossRef]
34. Delva, M.L.; Menon, C. FSR based Force Myography (FMG) Stability Throughout Non-Stationary Upper Extremity Tasks. In Proceedings of the Future Technologies Conference, Vancouver, BC, Canada, 29–30 November 2017; pp. 29–30.
35. Xiao, Z.G.; Menon, C. A Review of Force Myography Research and Development. *Sensors* **2019**, *19*, 4557. [CrossRef]
36. Sakr, M.; Menon, C. Exploratory Evaluation of the Force Myography (FMG) Signals Usage for Admittance Control of a Linear Actuator. In Proceedings of the 2018 7th IEEE International Conference on Biomedical Robotics and Biomechatronics (Biorob), Enschede, The Netherlands, 26–29 August 2018; pp. 903–908.

37. Sakr, M.; Menon, C. Study on the force myography sensors placement for robust hand force estimation. In Proceedings of the 2017 IEEE International Conference on Systems, Man, and Cybernetics (SMC), Banff, AB, Canada, 5–8 October 2017; pp. 1387–1392.
38. Xiao, Z.G.; Menon, C. Counting Grasping Action Using Force Myography: An Exploratory Study With Healthy Individuals. *JMIR Rehabil. Assist. Technol.* **2017**, *4*, e5. [CrossRef] [PubMed]
39. Ahmadizadeh, C.; Menon, C.; Pousett, B. Investigation of Channel Selection for Gesture Classification for Prosthesis Control Using Force Myography: A Case Study. *Front. Bioeng. Biotechnol.* **2019**, *7*, 331. [CrossRef]
40. Specht, D.F. A general regression neural network. *IEEE Trans. Neural Netw.* **1991**, *2*, 568–576. [CrossRef] [PubMed]
41. Breiman, L. Random forests. *Mach. Learn.* **2001**, *45*, 5–32. [CrossRef]
42. Wu, J.; Wang, L.; Li, J. Design and crosstalk error analysis of the circuit for the 2-D networked resistive sensor array. *IEEE Sensors J.* **2015**, *15*, 1020–1026. [CrossRef]
43. D'Alessio, T. Measurement errors in the scanning of piezoresistive sensors arrays. *Sens. Actuators A Phys.* **1999**, *72*, 71–76. [CrossRef]
44. Vidal-Verd, F.; Oballe-Peinado, O.; Sanchez-Duran, J.A.; Castellanos-Ramos, J.; Navas-Gonzalez, R. Three realizations and comparison of hardware for piezoresistive tactile sensors. *Sensors* **2011**, *11*, 3249–3266. [CrossRef]
45. Raichle, K.A.; Hanley, M.A.; Molton, I.; Kadel, N.J.; Campbell, K.; Phelps, E.; Ehde, D.; Smith, D.G. Prosthesis use in persons with lower-and upper-limb amputation. *J. Rehabil. Res. Dev.* **2008**, *45*, 961. [CrossRef]
46. Dillon, M.P.; Fortington, L.V.; Akram, M.; Erbas, B.; Kohler, F. Geographic variation of the incidence rate of lower limb amputation in Australia from 2007-12. *PLoS ONE* **2017**, *12*, e0170705. [CrossRef]
47. Persson, B.; Liedberg, E. A clinical standard of stump measurement and classification in lower limb amputees. *Prosthetics Orthot. Int.* **1983**, *7*, 17–24.
48. Holzbaur, K.R.; Murray, W.M.; Gold, G.E.; Delp, S.L. Upper limb muscle volumes in adult subjects. *J. Biomech.* **2007**, *40*, 742–749. [CrossRef] [PubMed]
49. Bishop, C.M. *Pattern Recognition and Machine Learning*; Springer Science + Business Media: New York, NY, USA, 2006.
50. Sadeghi Chegani, R.; Menon, C. Regressing grasping using force myography: An exploratory study. *BioMedical Eng. Online* **2018**, *17*, 159. [CrossRef] [PubMed]
51. Krouskop, T.; Yalcinkaya, M.; Muilenberg, A.; Holland, K.; Zuniga, E. A measurement technique to assess residual limb volume. *Orthop Rev.* **1979**, *8*, 69–77.
52. Saunders, C.G.; Bannon, M.; Sabiston, R.M.; Panych, L.; Jenks, S.L.; Wood, I.R.; Raschke, S. The CANFIT system: Shape management technology for prosthetic and orthotic applications. *JPO J. Prosthetics Orthot.* **1989**, *1*, 122–130. [CrossRef]
53. Zheng, Y.P.; Mak, A.F.; Leung, A.K. State-of-the-art methods for geometric and biomechanical assessments of residual limbs: A review. *J. Rehabil. Res. Dev.* **2001**, *38*, 487–504.

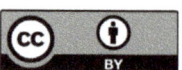

© 2019 by the authors. Licensee MDPI, Basel, Switzerland. This article is an open access article distributed under the terms and conditions of the Creative Commons Attribution (CC BY) license (http://creativecommons.org/licenses/by/4.0/).

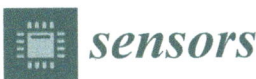

Article

Simulating Arbitrary Electrode Reversals in Standard 12-Lead ECG

Vessela Krasteva [1,*], Irena Jekova [1] and Ramun Schmid [2]

[1] Institute of Biophysics and Biomedical Engineering, Bulgarian Academy of Sciences, Acad. G. Bonchev Str. Bl 105, 1113 Sofia, Bulgaria; irena@biomed.bas.bg
[2] Signal Processing, Schiller AG, Altgasse 68, CH-6341 Baar, Switzerland; ramun.schmid@schiller.ch
* Correspondence: vessika@biomed.bas.bg

Received: 24 May 2019; Accepted: 29 June 2019; Published: 1 July 2019

Abstract: Electrode reversal errors in standard 12-lead electrocardiograms (ECG) can produce significant ECG changes and, in turn, misleading diagnoses. Their detection is important but mostly limited to the design of criteria using ECG databases with simulated reversals, without Wilson's central terminal (WCT) potential change. This is, to the best of our knowledge, the first study that presents an algebraic transformation for simulation of all possible ECG cable reversals, including those with displaced WCT, where most of the leads appear with distorted morphology. The simulation model of ECG electrode swaps and the resultant WCT potential change is derived in the standard 12-lead ECG setup. The transformation formulas are theoretically compared to known limb lead reversals and experimentally proven for unknown limb–chest electrode swaps using a 12-lead ECG database from 25 healthy volunteers (recordings without electrode swaps and with 5 unicolor pairs swaps, including red (right arm—C1), yellow (left arm—C2), green (left leg (LL) —C3), black (right leg (RL)—C5), all unicolor pairs). Two applications of the transformation are shown to be feasible: 'Forward' (simulation of reordered leads from correct leads) and 'Inverse' (reconstruction of correct leads from an ECG recorded with known electrode reversals). Deficiencies are found only when the ground RL electrode is swapped as this case requires guessing the unknown RL electrode potential. We suggest assuming that potential to be equal to that of the LL electrode. The 'Forward' transformation is important for comprehensive training platforms of humans and machines to reliably recognize simulated electrode swaps using the available resources of correctly recorded ECG databases. The 'Inverse' transformation can save time and costs for repeated ECG recordings by reconstructing the correct lead set if a lead swap is detected after the end of the recording. In cases when the electrode reversal is unknown but a prior correct ECG recording of the same patient is available, the 'Inverse' transformation is tested to detect the exact swapping of the electrodes with an accuracy of (96% to 100%).

Keywords: ECG electrode swaps; ECG electrode potentials; WCT potential change; reconstructing correct ECG leads; MSMinv transformation; unicolor limb–chest electrodes

1. Introduction

The routine use of the standard 12-lead electrocardiogram (ECG) for noninvasive clinical investigation of acute and chronic cardiovascular diseases makes it very important to ensure the generation of diagnostically interpretable ECG leads [1]. An essential problem in the recording of multilead ECGs is the improper placing of the electrodes on the patient's body [2], reported to be as frequent as 0.8% and 7.5% for limb lead reversals in 12-lead ECG and Holter devices, respectively [3]; 0.4% and 4% for 12-lead ECG interchanges in clinical and intensive care settings, respectively [4]. Errors in electrode placement can lead to significant ECG changes that could confuse physicians and affect the clinical diagnosis. Studies and case reports dedicated to this problem are further grouped in the following three categories according to the affected ECG electrodes:

- *Reversals between limb electrodes* are reported to provoke deep QS complexes and inverted T waves in leads (II, III, aVF) that could be misdiagnosed as old myocardial infarctions (MI) involving the inferior heart wall [5]. Right arm (RA) and left arm (LA) interchange is associated with inverted T waves in leads (I, aVL) suggestive of lateral wall MI [6] as well as indicative of ECG features of dextrocardia [7]. RA and right leg (RL) swap results in low-amplitude QRS complexes in lead II [7,8] and all other frontal leads resembling scaled variations of lead III and changed QRS axes in the frontal plane [8]. LA and left leg (LL) reversal creates suspicions of inferior-wall MI [7]. RA and LL swap could be confused for the combined features of lateral wall MI and low atrial rhythm [7].

- *Reversals between chest electrodes* have been found to provoke erroneous diagnosis in 17% to 24% of cases involving wrongly placed C1 electrodes [9]. Generally, when another precordial lead is substituted for V1, the result is a tall R wave in V1, which could be taken as a sign of right bundle branch block, left ventricular ectopy, right ventricular hypertrophy, acute right ventricular dilation, Type A Wolff-Parkinson-White syndrome, posterior MI, hypertrophic cardiomyopathy, progressive muscular dystrophy or dextrocardia [10].

- *Reversals between limb and chest electrodes* are a possible scenario due to the matching colors of the two ECG cables [11] or the incorrect attachment of the cable connectors to the junction box of the ECG machine [12]. C2/LA (yellow) cable interchange is described in two case reports [13,14] to have produced right axis deviation and Q waves in (III, aVF), accompanied by an inverted T wave in both leads, together with a quick transition in V2 with qR complex and an inverted T wave. The ECGs are interpreted as an inferior MI with residual ischemia in [13] or recent inferior and a posterior MI [14]. Limb/precordial cable interchange has been observed to result in tall R waves in aVR, negative QRS complexes in the other five limb leads and inverted ST elevation/depression in some of the leads. Thus, inferior, anterior, and lateral MI could be erroneously diagnosed [12]. In another study [15], the authors suspect the same interchange to have resulted in ST-segment elevation in the inferior leads; however, their thesis has been impugned by [16], who have explained the wandering ST elevation with medical reasons.

Such studies indicate that special measures should be taken to ensure the correct placement of ECG electrodes, e.g., staff training has been reported to improve electrode placement by 50% [17], while combined training and technical improvements have succeeded to reduce the rate of electrode cable reversals from 4.8 % down to 1.2 % [18]. ECG changes induced by ECG cable reversals have been analyzed in a number of studies [19–24]. Methods for the automatic detection of ECG electrode reversals within the limb and precordial set have been proposed, such as:

- *Limb leads:* LA and LL reversal is indicated by P wave amplitude [25] and QRS, P-axes [26]; RA and RL interchange is detected when lead II presents as a flat line [27] or with peak-to-peak amplitude less than 185 µV [8]; LA-RA and RA-LL swaps are recognized by analysis of P and QRS frontal axes and clockwise vector loop rotation direction, R and T wave amplitudes in leads (I, II) [28]; various LA/RA/LL/RL combinations are detected by a number of analytical approaches based on the assessment of the QRS axis [29,30], together with P wave amplitudes [31], direction of P-loop inscription and/or frontal P-axis [32]; lead reconstruction using redundancy of information in eight independent leads [33]; morphological measurements of QRS, P-wave amplitudes, frontal axis and clockwise vector loop rotation, combined with redundancy features [34]; maximal and minimal QRS, T-wave amplitudes in leads (I, II, III) [35]; correlation coefficients of limb leads vs. V6 [36,37]; combining the features described in [26] and [33] for a more robust and accurate performance [36].

- *Chest leads:* Different reversal sets have been examined, such as five reversals of adjacent leads (V1/V2, V2/V3, V3/V4, V4/V5, V5/V6), analyzed by P, QRS and ST-T measurements [26] and PQ-RS

amplitude distances [31]; nine reversals (five adjacent leads, V1/V3, V4/V6, V4/V5/V6/V1/V2/V3, V6/V5/V4/V3/V2/V1) are evaluated via correlations between measured and reconstructed leads [33]; seven reversals (five adjacent leads, V1/V3, V4/V6) are handled by processing of both morphology and redundancy features [34]; 15 reversals, including all possible pairwise V1–V6 swaps, have been tested in our previous study by applying analysis of inter-lead correlation coefficients [38].
- *Limb and chest leads:* Interchanges between limb and C2 precordial electrodes specific for a telemonitoring system are detected by correlation to a previously recorded ECG [39]. This early work, together with our recent publication on the unicolor electrode interchange detection [11], are the only studies dealing with recognition of reversals between limb and precordial leads.

The methods for the detection of ECG cable reversals should be designed/tested using dedicated databases. Only a few of the mentioned studies [7,19,27,35,39,40] use real ECG recordings with erroneous electrode placements, which are, however, small-sized and proprietary. Typically, reversal detection algorithms are trained and validated using databases with correctly recorded 12-lead ECGs and simulated reversals within the limb lead set [11,26,28–34,36,38] or the precordial lead set [11,26,31,33,34,38], where the Wilson's central terminal (WCT) is not changed. All other reversals modifying the WCT, such as swaps between the limb and precordial electrodes, have not been simulated, although they are quite possible and should be detected due to the distorted morphology of most leads [6,8,21]. For example, the interactive web-based tool [41] for the rendering of ECG leads from body surface potential maps (BSPM) separately simulates two effects—precordial lead misplacement (by linear interpolation from neighboring BSPM leads) or limb lead interchange. However, considering that this tool uses bulky BSPM data and does not allow for electrode misplacements that change WCT potential, it has restricted application for machine learning on large arrhythmia datasets with arbitrary ECG electrode reversals.

We have not found in the literature an algebraic transformation that can simulate all possible ECG electrode reversals. This paper presents the formula of such a transformation and its application in the standard 12-lead ECG setup, computing reordered leads and the WCT potential change from the correctly recorded leads. Additionally, we show the applicability of this method for reconstructing the correct leads from an ECG recorded with known electrode reversals, as well as for detection of the exact electrodes that were swapped, provided there are at least two ECGs from the same patient.

2. Methods

2.1. Derivation of the Transformation Formula

The presented transformation formula can be used to simulate reversals between arbitrary ECG electrodes in the standard 12-lead ECG, although the final transformation formula can be extended to an arbitrary number of leads.

According to the fundamental principles of electrocardiography [42], standard 12-lead ECG systems (Figure 1) use 10 electrodes on the LA, RA, LL, RL and 6 precordial positions (C1-C6), and acquire 8 independent signals (e.g. leads I, II, V1-V6):

$$\left| \begin{array}{l} I = P_E(LA) - P_E(RA) \\ II = P_E(LL) - P_E(RA) \\ V_X = P_E(C_X) - P_{WCT} = P_E(C_X) - \frac{P_E(LL) + P_E(RA) + P_E(LA)}{3} \end{array} \right. \quad (1)$$

where:

- P_E denotes the electrical potential of the respective electrodes, also referred to as the raw electrode biopotential.
- (I, II) are the bipolar leads measuring the potential differences between limbs (LA-RA, LL-RA), forming the Einthoven's triangle.

- V_X represents any of the unipolar chest leads (V1-V6) measuring the potential of the chest electrodes against the reference WCT potential (P_{WCT}), which is defined to be the average of the RA, LA and LL electrodes.
- Note that the ground electrode placed on the RL is used for technical reasons (driven right leg) and does not have direct influence on any ECG leads.

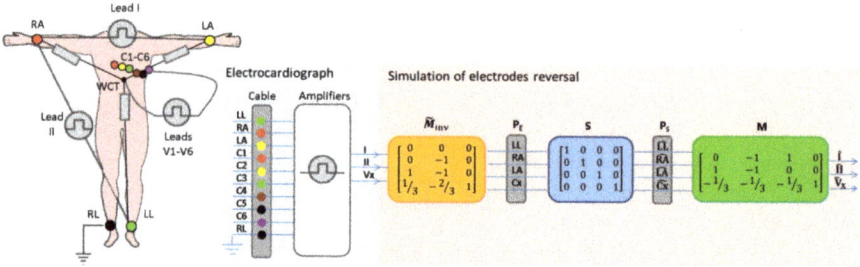

Figure 1. Acquisition of 12-lead ECG via a 10-electrode cable with standard IEC color coding, recording 8 independent leads I, II, V1-V6 (denoted as Vx) in the ECG device. The flow diagram shows the simulation of reversals between LL, RA, LA and one chest electrode (denoted as Cx) by conversion of the recorded leads (I, II, Vx) to reordered leads ($\hat{I}, \hat{II}, \hat{V}_X$) using the matrix transformations $\widetilde{\mathbf{M}}_{inv}$, $\mathbf{S}$, $\mathbf{M}$. The specific example shows an identity $\mathbf{S}$ matrix that corresponds to the correct order of LL, RA, LA, Cx electrodes. Other estimates of the $\mathbf{S}$ matrix are presented on Figure 2 and Section 4.1 in the description of different examples for electrode reversals.

The calculations in (1) are usually performed by the input circuits in ECG devices. As soon as an electrode swap can lead to a change in the WCT potential, it becomes difficult to imagine the changes in the standard 12-lead ECG. Therefore, the derivation and handling of the electrode potentials corresponding to the nine active ECG electrodes with respect to a common reference point is the main target of further mathematical transformations.

The basic 12-lead ECG computations (1) can also be presented using the matrix notation:

$$\begin{bmatrix} I \\ II \\ V_X \end{bmatrix} = \begin{bmatrix} 0 & -1 & 1 & 0 \\ 1 & -1 & 0 & 0 \\ -\frac{1}{3} & -\frac{1}{3} & -\frac{1}{3} & 1 \end{bmatrix} \begin{bmatrix} P_E(LL) \\ P_E(RA) \\ P_E(LA) \\ P_E(C_X) \end{bmatrix} = \mathbf{M} \begin{bmatrix} 0 \\ P_E(RA) \\ P_E(LA) \\ P_E(C_X) \end{bmatrix}, \quad (2)$$

where $\mathbf{M}$ is the matrix that converts the raw electrode potentials $P_E(LL)$, $P_E(RA)$, $P_E(LA)$ and $P_E(C_X)$ into leads I, II, Vx. Formula (2) shows the setting ($P_E(LL) = 0$), which defines our choice that $P_E(LL)$ is the reference potential. This is an arbitrary choice because we can set any electrode as the reference one without changing the final outcome of our derivations. We can further simplify (2):

$$\begin{bmatrix} I \\ II \\ V_X \end{bmatrix} = \begin{bmatrix} -1 & 1 & 0 \\ -1 & 0 & 0 \\ -\frac{1}{3} & -\frac{1}{3} & 1 \end{bmatrix} \begin{bmatrix} P_E(RA) \\ P_E(LA) \\ P_E(C_X) \end{bmatrix} = \mathbf{M}_F \begin{bmatrix} P_E(RA) \\ P_E(LA) \\ P_E(C_X) \end{bmatrix}, \quad (3)$$

where $\mathbf{M}_F$ is a full-rank matrix that is further inverted ($\mathbf{M}_F^{-1}$) for solving of the opposite task for the conversion of leads into body electrode potentials:

$$\begin{bmatrix} P_E(RA) \\ P_E(LA) \\ P_E(C_X) \end{bmatrix} = \mathbf{M}_F^{-1} \begin{bmatrix} I \\ II \\ V_X \end{bmatrix} = \begin{bmatrix} 0 & -1 & 0 \\ 1 & -1 & 0 \\ \frac{1}{3} & -\frac{2}{3} & 1 \end{bmatrix} \begin{bmatrix} I \\ II \\ V_X \end{bmatrix}. \quad (4)$$

Further, $\mathbf{M}_F^{-1}$ is extended so that (4) is able to reproduce the electrical potential of the left leg, using the definition ($P_E(LL) = 0$):

$$\begin{bmatrix} P_E(LL) \\ P_E(RA) \\ P_E(LA) \\ P_E(C_X) \end{bmatrix} = \begin{bmatrix} 0 & 0 & 0 \\ & \mathbf{M}_F^{-1} & \end{bmatrix} \begin{bmatrix} I \\ II \\ V_X \end{bmatrix} = \begin{bmatrix} 0 & 0 & 0 \\ 0 & -1 & 0 \\ 1 & -1 & 0 \\ \frac{1}{3} & -\frac{2}{3} & 1 \end{bmatrix} \begin{bmatrix} I \\ II \\ V_X \end{bmatrix} = \tilde{\mathbf{M}}_{inv} \begin{bmatrix} I \\ II \\ V_X \end{bmatrix}, \quad (5)$$

where $\tilde{\mathbf{M}}_{inv}$ is the matrix that allows the computation of the raw body electrode potentials in the order $\{P_E(LL), P_E(RA), P_E(LA), P_E(C_X)\}$ using the recorded leads $\{I, II, V_X\}$. Once the body electrode potentials are known, they can be reordered to simulate an arbitrary reversal between ECG electrodes. The simulated electrode order can be algebraically described by a binary swap matrix (**S**), which equals an identity matrix for the correct order:

$$\begin{bmatrix} P_S(\widehat{LL}) \\ P_S(\widehat{RA}) \\ P_S(\widehat{LA}) \\ P_S(\widehat{C_X}) \end{bmatrix} = \begin{bmatrix} 1 & 0 & 0 & 0 \\ 0 & 1 & 0 & 0 \\ 0 & 0 & 1 & 0 \\ 0 & 0 & 0 & 1 \end{bmatrix} \begin{bmatrix} P_E(LL) \\ P_E(RA) \\ P_E(LA) \\ P_E(C_X) \end{bmatrix} = \mathbf{S} \begin{bmatrix} P_E(LL) \\ P_E(RA) \\ P_E(LA) \\ P_E(C_X) \end{bmatrix} \quad (6)$$

where P_S denotes the simulated electrical potential at the respective electrode $\{\widehat{LL}, \widehat{RA}, \widehat{LA}, \widehat{C_X}\}$. Different examples of matrix **S** are further given in Section 4.1 upon the description of the performed theoretical simulations of electrode reversals.

The correspondence between the leads recorded by the ECG device (I, II, V_X) and the reordered leads ($\hat{I}, \hat{II}, \hat{V}_X$) after the simulation of ECG electrode reversals can be calculated by substituting successively (6) and (5) into (2):

$$\begin{bmatrix} \hat{I} \\ \hat{II} \\ \hat{V}_X \end{bmatrix} = \mathbf{M} \begin{bmatrix} P_S(\widehat{LL}) \\ P_S(\widehat{RA}) \\ P_S(\widehat{LA}) \\ P_S(\widehat{C_X}) \end{bmatrix} = \mathbf{MS}\tilde{\mathbf{M}}_{inv} \begin{bmatrix} I \\ II \\ V_X \end{bmatrix}. \quad (7)$$

The flow diagram of (7), further denoted as 'MSMinv' transformation, which is presented on Figure 1, clearly indicates the embedded logic of matrix operations that have a general applicability to simulate arbitrary configurations of electrode swaps. It is just necessary to adapt the values of the matrices **M**, **S**, $\tilde{\mathbf{M}}_{inv}$ to the specific lead configuration, assuming that the derived mathematical proof shows the full set of two independent bipolar limb leads in 12-lead ECG (can be reduced) and one unipolar lead (can be deleted or extended to multiple unipolar leads by copy of the row (C_X) in **M**, $\tilde{\mathbf{M}}_{inv}$ and expand S accordingly).

Note that the matrices in the 'MSMinv' transformation (7) take into account only the potentials of the active input electrodes, excluding the grounded RL. The result of a swap of an arbitrary active electrode with RL can be, however, approximated by setting the potential of the swapped active electrode equal to the LL potential in the matrix **S** (6):

$$P_S(\text{swapped electrode to RL}) = P_E(RL) \approx P_E(LL) \quad (8)$$

The assumption for equipotential legs can be considered from an anatomical perspective because the leg recording sites are sufficiently distant and similarly oriented to the heart, thus attaining the same electrical signal generated by the myocardium [24]. Generally, both (RL, LL) potentials are essentially very similar that is typically adopted in the known ECG lead transformations of rotated RL with other peripheral electrodes [7,8,21,22].

Another application of the derived mathematical transformations is the calculation of the WCT potential change due to ECG electrode swaps:

$$\Delta P_{WCT} = \hat{P}_{WCT} - P_{WCT}, \qquad (9)$$

where P_{WCT} and $\hat{P}_{WCT}$ are the WCT potentials before and after the electrode swap, respectively. Both can be derived as a function of the recorded leads (I, II, V_X) with a reference to a zero LL potential $(P_E(LL) = 0)$, as assumed in Equations (2) and (5):

$$P_{WCT} = \mathbf{W} \begin{bmatrix} P_E(LL) \\ P_E(RA) \\ P_E(LA) \\ P_E(C_X) \end{bmatrix} = \mathbf{W}\tilde{\mathbf{M}}_{inv} \begin{bmatrix} I \\ II \\ V_X \end{bmatrix} \qquad (10)$$

$$\hat{P}_{WCT} = \mathbf{W} \begin{bmatrix} P_S(\widehat{LL}) \\ P_S(\widehat{RA}) \\ P_S(\widehat{LA}) \\ P_S(\widehat{C_X}) \end{bmatrix} = \mathbf{WS}\tilde{\mathbf{M}}_{inv} \begin{bmatrix} I \\ II \\ V_X \end{bmatrix}, \qquad (11)$$

where $\mathbf{W} = \begin{bmatrix} 1/3 & 1/3 & 1/3 & 0 \end{bmatrix}$ is the matrix that transforms electrode potentials into WCT potential, taking the potentials for the correct electrode position $\{P_E(LL), P_E(RA), P_E(LA), P_E(C_X)\}$ from (5) and for the swapped position $\{P_S(\widehat{LL}), P_S(\widehat{RA}), P_S(\widehat{LA}), P_S(\widehat{C_X})\}$ from (6) and (5). Although WCT potential is calculated only from the potentials of the three limb electrodes $(\widehat{LL}, \widehat{RA}, \widehat{LA})$, Equation (11) covers the general option for a swap between some of them and the unipolar electrode $(\widehat{C_X})$.

Substituting (10) and (11) in (9) gives the generalized notation of the 'WSMinv' transformation that is further used for estimating of the relative WCT potential change during different simulated swaps:

$$\Delta P_{WCT} = (\mathbf{WS} - \mathbf{W})\tilde{\mathbf{M}}_{inv} \begin{bmatrix} I \\ II \\ V_X \end{bmatrix}. \qquad (12)$$

2.2. Verification of 'MSMinv' Transformation

The correctness of the 'MSMinv' transformation (7) is verified by two approaches, depending on the kind of simulated ECG electrode reversals:

- *ECG electrode reversals with known lead transforms* are theoretically studied. For this purpose, the formula for computation of the reordered leads $(\hat{I}, \hat{II}, \hat{V}_X)$ is directly compared to the published lead transformations. This simple approach is applicable only to reversals between peripheral electrodes, widely analyzed in the literature [5,7,12,21,24,36–38,43].
- *ECG electrode reversals with unknown lead transformations* (such as reversals between limb and chest electrodes) are experimentally studied with a dedicated database (described in Section 3). For this purpose, the 8 independent leads $L_R = (I_R, II_R, V1_R - V6_R)$ of 2 recordings from the same person (RC, taken with correct electrode position; RS, taken with real electrode swap) are compared in three different scenarios:

    ○ (L_{RC} vs. L_{RS}): *No transformation* is applied to study the lead-specific differences between recordings with correct vs. swapped electrodes.
    ○ ($\widehat{L_{RC}}$ vs. L_{RS}): *Forward 'MSMinv' transformation* is applied on the recording with correct lead set to simulate lead swap $\left(\widehat{L_{RC}} = \mathbf{MSM}_{inv}L_{RC}\right)$ and to study the lead-specific differences of simulated vs. recorded electrode reversals (L_{RS}).

○ (L_{RC} vs. $\widetilde{L_{RS}}$): Inverse 'MSMinv' transformation is applied on the recording with reversed lead set to simulate correct electrode positions ($\widetilde{L_{RS}} = \widetilde{\mathbf{MSM}}_{inv}L_{RS}$) and to study the lead-specific differences of simulated vs. recorded, correctly placed electrodes (L_{RC}).

The lead-specific differences in each of the above 3 scenarios (denoted as $\widetilde{L_{RC}}$ vs. $\widetilde{L_{RS}}$) are estimated for the average beat ($BEAT_i$), indexed within a window of 500ms ($i = QRS_f - 150ms$ to $QRS_f + 350ms$, where QRS_f denotes the QRS fiducial point), using three quantitative measures:

○ Root-mean-square error:

$$RMS\ Error = \sqrt{\frac{1}{500ms * Fs} \sum \left(BEAT_i\left(\widetilde{L_{RC}}\right) - BEAT_i\left(\widetilde{L_{RS}}\right)\right)^2}, \quad (13)$$

where Fs denotes the sampling frequency of the average beat.

○ Peak error:

$$Peak\ Error = \max\left(\left|BEAT_i\left(\widetilde{L_{RC}}\right) - BEAT_i\left(\widetilde{L_{RS}}\right)\right|\right). \quad (14)$$

○ Correlation coefficient:

$$CorCoef = \frac{\sum BEAT_i\left(\widetilde{L_{RC}}\right).BEAT_i\left(\widetilde{L_{RS}}\right)}{\sqrt{\sum BEAT_i^2\left(\widetilde{L_{RC}}\right). \sum BEAT_i^2\left(\widetilde{L_{RS}}\right)}} \quad (15)$$

Statistical results of all quantitative measurements over the whole ECG database are reported as a mean value and standard deviation (std). The level of significant differences between different scenarios is measured with paired Student's t-test and one-tailed p-value < 0.05.

3. Database

The database used for verification of the 'MSMinv' transformation contains 10s recordings of standard 12-lead resting ECGs taken from 25 volunteers with no history of heart diseases—gender: 28% (male), age: 49 ± 11 years (mean value ± standard deviation), 28–67 years (range). The ECGs are acquired via a 10-electrode cable with standard IEC color coding [44]. Six ECG recordings per subject are collected, applying prospective electrode cable reversals at the time of the recording, including:

- Correct positions of the electrodes (no electrode is swapped);
- Swap of red electrodes (RA-C1);
- Swap of yellow electrodes (LA-C2);
- Swap of green electrodes (LL-C3);
- Swap of black electrodes (RL-C5);
- Swap of all unicolor electrodes (RA-C1, LA-C2, LL-C3, RL-C5).

The ECG signals are recorded at 1 kHz sampling rate, 1 μV resolution, and pre-filtered in a bandwidth (0.5 to 25 Hz). Each 10s ECG recording is processed by a commercial ECG measurement and interpretation module (ETM, Schiller AG, Switzerland) for the extraction of a 12-lead average beat [45]. The average beats are commonly used for the measurement of ECG features with diagnostic precision because they provide higher signal-to-noise ratio and are more robust to respiration induced morphology changes than the single beats.

4. Results and Discussion

4.1. Theoretical Simulations of Electrode Reversals

This section simulates three major types of ECG electrode reversals (reversals of peripheral electrodes involving RL; not involving RL; reversals of peripheral and chest electrodes), applying

'WSMinv' transformation (12) for the calculation of WCT potential change (Table 1) and 'MSMinv' transformation (7) for the calculation of the reordered leads (Tables 2–4). Several general examples are shown on Figure 2. Details will be further discussed in Sections 4.1.1–4.1.3

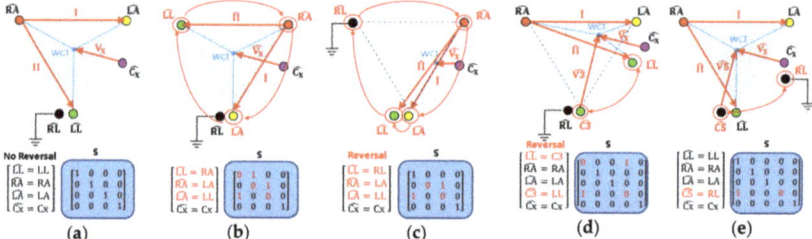

Figure 2. Classic depiction of the Einthoven's triangle, WCT and lead vectors (I, II, Vx), projected in the frontal plane for correct electrode position (**a**) and their displacement ($\hat{I}, \hat{II}, \hat{V}_X$) in case of four types of limb electrode reversals: (**b**) CW rotation of 3 active limb electrodes ($\widehat{RA} \to \widehat{LA} \to \widehat{LL} \to \widehat{RA}$); (**c**) CW rotation of 4 limb electrodes, including RL ($\widehat{RL} \to \widehat{RA} \to \widehat{LA} \to \widehat{LL} \to \widehat{RL}$); (**d**) swap of an active limb electrode and chest electrode, illustrated for the green couple ($\widehat{LL} \leftrightarrow \widehat{C3}$); (**e**) swap of the grounded and chest electrode, illustrated for the black couple ($\widehat{RL} \leftrightarrow \widehat{C5}$). The text with red font color highlights the electrodes in wrong geometrical positions, and the swap matrix entries different from the identity matrix in (**a**).

Table 1. Calculation of the WCT potential change from the recorded leads via the 'WSMinv' transformation (12), applying the swap matrices **S** in Tables 2–4.

Reversed Electrodes		ΔP_{WCT}
Reversals of peripheral electrodes not involving RL	RA↔LA	0 *
	RA↔LL	0 *
	LA↔LL	0 *
	CW rotation RA→LA→LL→RA	0 *
	CCW rotation RA→LL→LA→RA	0 *
Reversals of peripheral electrodes involving RL	RL↔RA	$1/3 II$
	RL↔LA	$1/3(II - I)$
	RL↔LL	0 *
	CW rotation with RL RL→RA→LA→LL→RL	$1/3 II$
	CCW rotation with RL RL→LL→LA→RA→RL	0 *
	Bilateral arm-leg rotation RL↔RA, LA↔LL	$1/3 II$
	Cross rotation RL→RA→LL→LA→RL	$1/3(II - I)$
Reversals of unicolor peripheral and chest electrodes	Red electrodes RA↔C1	$1/9 I + 1/9 II + 1/3 V_1$
	Yellow electrodes LA↔C2	$-2/9 I + 1/9 II + 1/3 V_2$
	Green electrodes LL↔C3	$1/9 I - 2/9 II + 1/3 V_3$
	Black electrodes RL↔C5	0 *
	All unicolor electrodes RA↔C1, LA↔C2, LL↔C3, RL↔C5	$1/3(V_1 + V_2 + V_3)$

Note: For comprehension purposes of various electrode combinations, the reversed electrodes are depicted with their respective colors according to the IEC color coding [44]. * $\Delta P_{WCT} = 0$ corresponds to the correct position of the active limb electrodes ($\widehat{LL}, \widehat{RA}, \widehat{LA}$).

4.1.1. Reversals of Peripheral Electrodes Not Involving RL

All 5 possible rotations of the 3 active limb electrodes ($\widehat{LL}, \widehat{RA}, \widehat{LA}$) are simulated (Table 2) and none of them is related to the displacement of WCT, as illustrated in the example of clockwise (CW) electrode rotation (Figure 2b), where the Einthoven's triangle remains geometrically unaffected. This is theoretically proven by the 'WSMinv' transformation (12), where all swap matrices **S** (Table 2) are consequently applied, and zero WCT potential differences to the correct electrode position ($\Delta P_{WCT} = 0$)

are detected (Table 1). The rearranged limb leads ($\hat{I}$, $\hat{II}$) obtained by the 'MSMinv' transformation (Table 2) match the expressions in other studies, applying geometrical perspectives between leads (I, II, III) [5,12,21,24,36–38]. Furthermore, the unipolar chest lead $\hat{V}_X$ is unchanged for all simulated swap matrices **S** that corresponds to the real case scenario of unchanged WCT (Figure 2a,b).

Table 2. Reversals of peripheral electrodes not involving RL.

Reversed Electrodes	S	$\mathbf{MS\widetilde{M}_{inv}}$	Reordered Leads
		$\widehat{RA} \leftrightarrow \widehat{LA}$	
$\begin{bmatrix} \widehat{LL} = LL \\ \widehat{RA} = LA \\ \widehat{LA} = RA \\ \widehat{C_X} = C_X \end{bmatrix}$	$\begin{bmatrix} 1 & 0 & 0 & 0 \\ 0 & 0 & 1 & 0 \\ 0 & 1 & 0 & 0 \\ 0 & 0 & 0 & 1 \end{bmatrix}$	$\begin{bmatrix} -1 & 0 & 0 \\ -1 & 1 & 0 \\ 0 & 0 & 1 \end{bmatrix}$	$\hat{I} = -I$ $\hat{II} = -I + II = III$ $\hat{V}_X = V_X$
		$\widehat{RA} \leftrightarrow \widehat{LL}$	
$\begin{bmatrix} \widehat{LL} = RA \\ \widehat{RA} = LL \\ \widehat{LA} = LA \\ \widehat{C_X} = C_X \end{bmatrix}$	$\begin{bmatrix} 0 & 1 & 0 & 0 \\ 1 & 0 & 0 & 0 \\ 0 & 0 & 1 & 0 \\ 0 & 0 & 0 & 1 \end{bmatrix}$	$\begin{bmatrix} 1 & -1 & 0 \\ 0 & -1 & 0 \\ 0 & 0 & 1 \end{bmatrix}$	$\hat{I} = I - II = -III$ $\hat{II} = -II$ $\hat{V}_X = V_X$
		$\widehat{LA} \leftrightarrow \widehat{LL}$	
$\begin{bmatrix} \widehat{LL} = LA \\ \widehat{RA} = RA \\ \widehat{LA} = LL \\ \widehat{C_X} = C_X \end{bmatrix}$	$\begin{bmatrix} 0 & 0 & 1 & 0 \\ 0 & 1 & 0 & 0 \\ 1 & 0 & 0 & 0 \\ 0 & 0 & 0 & 1 \end{bmatrix}$	$\begin{bmatrix} 0 & 1 & 0 \\ 1 & 0 & 0 \\ 0 & 0 & 1 \end{bmatrix}$	$\hat{I} = II$ $\hat{II} = I$ $\hat{V}_X = V_X$
		CW rotation $\widehat{RA} \to \widehat{LA} \to \widehat{LL} \to \widehat{RA}$	
$\begin{bmatrix} \widehat{LL} = RA \\ \widehat{RA} = LA \\ \widehat{LA} = LL \\ \widehat{C_X} = C_X \end{bmatrix}$	$\begin{bmatrix} 0 & 1 & 0 & 0 \\ 0 & 0 & 1 & 0 \\ 1 & 0 & 0 & 0 \\ 0 & 0 & 0 & 1 \end{bmatrix}$	$\begin{bmatrix} -1 & 1 & 0 \\ -1 & 0 & 0 \\ 0 & 0 & 1 \end{bmatrix}$	$\hat{I} = -I + II = III$ $\hat{II} = -I$ $\hat{V}_X = V_X$
		CCWrotation $\widehat{RA} \to \widehat{LL} \to \widehat{LA} \to \widehat{RA}$	
$\begin{bmatrix} \widehat{LL} = LA \\ \widehat{RA} = LL \\ \widehat{LA} = RA \\ \widehat{C_X} = C_X \end{bmatrix}$	$\begin{bmatrix} 0 & 0 & 1 & 0 \\ 1 & 0 & 0 & 0 \\ 0 & 1 & 0 & 0 \\ 0 & 0 & 0 & 1 \end{bmatrix}$	$\begin{bmatrix} 0 & -1 & 0 \\ 1 & -1 & 0 \\ 0 & 0 & 1 \end{bmatrix}$	$\hat{I} = -II$ $\hat{II} = I - II = -III$ $\hat{V}_X = V_X$

Note: For comprehension purposes of various electrode combinations, the reversed electrodes are depicted with their respective colors according to the IEC color coding [44], - *1st column:* The simulated placement of ECG electrodes $\{\widehat{LL}, \widehat{RA}, \widehat{LA}, \widehat{C_X}\}$ referring to their geometrical positions $\{LL, RA, LA, C_X\}$. The electrodes which are assumed to be in the wrong geometrical positions are indicated with red font color as being reversed. - *2nd column:* The values of the swap matrix **S**, where red font colored entries indicate the difference to the identity matrix as defined in (6) for the correct electrode placement. - *3rd column:* The result of matrix multiplication $\mathbf{MS\widetilde{M}_{inv}}$, considering **M** and $\widetilde{\mathbf{M}}_{inv}$ equal to their definitions in (2) and (5), respectively. - *4th column:* The formula for calculation of the reordered leads ($\hat{I}$, $\hat{II}$, $\hat{V}_X$) using the recorded leads (I, II, Vx) that is obtained after substituting $\mathbf{MS\widetilde{M}_{inv}}$ in (7). For simplification, the substitution ($III = II - I$) is applied in some formulas.

4.1.2. Reversals of Peripheral Electrodes Involving RL

Seven rotations of the 4 limb electrodes ($\widehat{LL}$, $\widehat{RA}$, $\widehat{LA}$, $\widehat{RL}$) are simulated (Table 3) and normally they should be related to the displacement of WCT, as illustrated in the example (Figure 2c), where the Einthoven's triangle is transformed to a thin 'slice'.

Table 1 shows that all electrode reversals present WCT potential change, depending only on the position of the neutral electrode RL, such that:

- RL is in the position of RA: $\Delta P_{WCT} = 1/3 II$
- RL is in the position of LA: $\Delta P_{WCT} = -1/3 I + 1/3 II$
- RL is in the position of LL: $\Delta P_{WCT} = 0$, where P_{WCT} is equal to the correct electrode placement.

Table 3. Reversals of peripheral electrodes involving RL.

Reversed Electrodes	S	MS$\widehat{M}_{inv}$	Reordered Leads
		RL↔RA	
$\begin{bmatrix} \widehat{LL} = LL \\ \widehat{RA} = RL \\ \widehat{LA} = RA \\ \widehat{C_X} = C_X \end{bmatrix}$	$\begin{bmatrix} 1 & 0 & 0 & 0 \\ 1 & 0 & 0 & 0 \\ 0 & 0 & 1 & 0 \\ 0 & 0 & 0 & 1 \end{bmatrix}$	$\begin{bmatrix} 1 & -1 & 0 \\ 0 & 0 & 0 \\ 0 & -1/3 & 1 \end{bmatrix}$	$\hat{I} = I - II = -III$ $\hat{II} = 0$ $\hat{V}_X = V_X - 1/3 II$
		RL↔LA	
$\begin{bmatrix} \widehat{LL} = LL \\ \widehat{RA} = RA \\ \widehat{LA} = RL \\ \widehat{C_X} = C_X \end{bmatrix}$	$\begin{bmatrix} 1 & 0 & 0 & 0 \\ 0 & 1 & 0 & 0 \\ 1 & 0 & 0 & 0 \\ 0 & 0 & 0 & 1 \end{bmatrix}$	$\begin{bmatrix} 0 & 1 & 0 \\ 0 & 1 & 0 \\ 1/3 & -1/3 & 1 \end{bmatrix}$	$\hat{I} = II$ $\hat{II} = II$ $\hat{V}_X = V_X - 1/3(II - I)$
		RL↔LL	
$\begin{bmatrix} \widehat{LL} = RL \\ \widehat{RA} = RA \\ \widehat{LA} = LA \\ \widehat{C_X} = C_X \end{bmatrix}$	$\begin{bmatrix} 1 & 0 & 0 & 0 \\ 0 & 1 & 0 & 0 \\ 0 & 0 & 1 & 0 \\ 0 & 0 & 0 & 1 \end{bmatrix}$	$\begin{bmatrix} 1 & 0 & 0 \\ 0 & 1 & 0 \\ 0 & 0 & 1 \end{bmatrix}$	$\hat{I} = I$ $\hat{II} = II$ $\hat{V}_X = V_X$
	CW rotation with RL	RL→RA→LA→LL→RL	
$\begin{bmatrix} \widehat{LL} = RL \\ \widehat{RA} = LA \\ \widehat{LA} = LL \\ \widehat{C_X} = C_X \end{bmatrix}$	$\begin{bmatrix} 1 & 0 & 0 & 0 \\ 0 & 0 & 1 & 0 \\ 1 & 0 & 0 & 0 \\ 0 & 0 & 0 & 1 \end{bmatrix}$	$\begin{bmatrix} -1 & 1 & 0 \\ -1 & 1 & 0 \\ 0 & -1/3 & 1 \end{bmatrix}$	$\hat{I} = -I + II = III$ $\hat{II} = -I + II = III$ $\hat{V}_X = V_X - 1/3 II$
	CCW rotation with RL	RL→LL→LA→RA→RL	
$\begin{bmatrix} \widehat{LL} = LA \\ \widehat{RA} = RL \\ \widehat{LA} = RA \\ \widehat{C_X} = C_X \end{bmatrix}$	$\begin{bmatrix} 0 & 0 & 1 & 0 \\ 1 & 0 & 0 & 0 \\ 0 & 1 & 0 & 0 \\ 0 & 0 & 0 & 1 \end{bmatrix}$	$\begin{bmatrix} 0 & -1 & 0 \\ 1 & -1 & 0 \\ 0 & 0 & 1 \end{bmatrix}$	$\hat{I} = -II$ $\hat{II} = I - II = -III$ $\hat{V}_X = V_X$
	Bilateral arm–leg rotation	RL↔RA, LA↔LL	
$\begin{bmatrix} \widehat{LL} = LA \\ \widehat{RA} = RL \\ \widehat{LA} = LL \\ \widehat{C_X} = C_X \end{bmatrix}$	$\begin{bmatrix} 0 & 0 & 1 & 0 \\ 1 & 0 & 0 & 0 \\ 1 & 0 & 0 & 0 \\ 0 & 0 & 0 & 1 \end{bmatrix}$	$\begin{bmatrix} 0 & 0 & 0 \\ 1 & -1 & 0 \\ 0 & -1/3 & 1 \end{bmatrix}$	$\hat{I} = 0$ $\hat{II} = I - II = -III$ $\hat{V}_X = V_X - 1/3 II$
	Cross rotation	RL→RA→LL→LA→RL	
$\begin{bmatrix} \widehat{LL} = RA \\ \widehat{RA} = RL \\ \widehat{LA} = LL \\ \widehat{C_X} = C_X \end{bmatrix}$	$\begin{bmatrix} 0 & 1 & 0 & 0 \\ 1 & 0 & 0 & 0 \\ 1 & 0 & 0 & 0 \\ 0 & 0 & 0 & 1 \end{bmatrix}$	$\begin{bmatrix} 0 & 0 & 0 \\ 0 & -1 & 0 \\ 1/3 & -1/3 & 1 \end{bmatrix}$	$\hat{I} = 0$ $\hat{II} = -II$ $\hat{V}_X = V_X - 1/3(II - I)$

Note: All columns correspond to the description in the footer of Table 2.

These results and the 'MSMinv' transformation (Table 3) are obtained with the general approximation for equipotential legs that is coded in the swap matrix **S** with an entry of '1' in the position of LL (first column) for both cases: $\{\hat{X} = LL, \hat{X} = RL\}$, whereas $\hat{X}$ denotes an arbitrary ECG electrode. Thus, all electrode reversals leading to a 'sliced' Einthoven's triangle with two tips on both legs appear with two '1' entries in the first column of matrix **S** (Table 3), while '1' is deficient in the second (RA) or third (LA) columns (equal to '0'). Only two reversals (RL-LL and the counter-clockwise (CCW) rotation with RL) have '1' entries in each of the first three columns of matrix **S** (corresponding to the three active limb electrodes in the Einthoven's triangle tips). Just for them, the WCT potential is correctly found to be unchanged (Table 1), although the reordered limb leads ($\hat{I}$, $\hat{II}$) in CCW rotation appear to be different (Table 3). Generally, all simulated reversals show that ($\hat{I}$, $\hat{II}$) leads, resulting from the 'MSMinv' transformation, are matching the expressions in other studies that have been derived by geometrical analysis of the leads, assuming "0" [6,12,19,21,22,24,35,36] or "near zero" signal <100 μV [5,7,8,38] for the lead between the active electrodes on both legs.

Considering the chest lead V_X, we find a correspondence between 'MSMinv' and 'WSMinv' transformations so that the reordered lead $\hat{V}_X = V_X - \Delta P_{WCT}$ (Table 3) is corrected exactly with the term ΔP_{WCT} (Table 1). Generally, no chest lead V_X is considered in case of limb leads reversals, so we cannot compare the derived $\hat{V}_X$ expressions to published studies. We can justify the unchanged $\hat{V}_X$ in both aforementioned reversals with WCT not being displaced (RL-LL and CCW rotation), as well as $\hat{V}_X = V_X - 1/3 II$ for the RL-RA reversal. This reversal has been analytically described in Haisty et al. [8], who explained that WCT potential difference is equal to one third of the difference between RA and RL potentials that approximates one third of the standard lead II.

Table 4. Reversals of unicolor chest and peripheral electrodes.

Reversed Electrodes	S	$\widetilde{MSM}_{inv}$	Reordered Leads
		Red electrodes RA↔C1	
$\begin{bmatrix}\widehat{LL}=LL\\\widehat{RA}=C_1\\\widehat{LA}=LA\\\widehat{C_1}=RA\\\widehat{C_x}=C_x\end{bmatrix}$	$\begin{bmatrix}1&0&0&0&0\\0&0&0&1&0\\0&0&1&0&0\\0&1&0&0&0\\0&0&0&0&1\end{bmatrix}$	$\begin{bmatrix}2/3&-1/3&-1&0\\-1/3&2/3&-1&0\\-4/9&-4/9&-1/3&0\\-1/9&-1/9&-1/3&1\end{bmatrix}$	$\hat{I}=(I-III)/3-V_1$ $\hat{II}=(II+III)/3-V_1$ $\hat{V}_1=-\frac{4}{9}(I+II)-\frac{1}{3}V_1$ $\hat{V}_x=V_x-\frac{1}{9}(I+II)-\frac{1}{3}V_1$
		Yellow electrodes LA↔C2	
$\begin{bmatrix}\widehat{LL}=LL\\\widehat{RA}=RA\\\widehat{LA}=C_2\\\widehat{C_2}=LA\\\widehat{C_x}=C_x\end{bmatrix}$	$\begin{bmatrix}1&0&0&0&0\\0&1&0&0&0\\0&0&0&1&0\\0&0&1&0&0\\0&0&0&0&1\end{bmatrix}$	$\begin{bmatrix}1/3&1/3&1&0\\0&1&0&0\\8/9&-4/9&-1/3&0\\2/9&-1/9&-1/3&1\end{bmatrix}$	$\hat{I}=\frac{1}{3}(I+II)+V_2$ $\hat{II}=II$ $\hat{V}_2=\frac{4}{9}(I-III)-\frac{1}{3}V_2$ $\hat{V}_x=V_x+\frac{1}{9}(I-III)-\frac{1}{3}V_1$
		Green electrodes LL↔C3	
$\begin{bmatrix}\widehat{LL}=C_3\\\widehat{RA}=RA\\\widehat{LA}=LA\\\widehat{C_3}=LL\\\widehat{C_x}=C_x\end{bmatrix}$	$\begin{bmatrix}0&0&0&1&0\\0&1&0&0&0\\0&0&1&0&0\\1&0&0&0&0\\0&0&0&0&1\end{bmatrix}$	$\begin{bmatrix}1&0&0&0\\1/3&1/3&1&0\\-4/9&8/9&-1/3&0\\-1/9&2/9&-1/3&1\end{bmatrix}$	$\hat{I}=I$ $\hat{II}=\frac{1}{3}(I+II)+V_3$ $\hat{V}_3=\frac{4}{9}(II+III)-\frac{1}{3}V_3$ $\hat{V}_x=V_x+\frac{1}{9}(II+III)-\frac{1}{3}V_1$
		Black electrodes RL↔C5	
$\begin{bmatrix}\widehat{LL}=LL\\\widehat{RA}=RA\\\widehat{LA}=LA\\\widehat{C_5}=RL\\\widehat{C_x}=C_x\end{bmatrix}$	$\begin{bmatrix}1&0&0&0&0\\0&1&0&0&0\\0&0&1&0&0\\1&0&0&0&0\\0&0&0&0&1\end{bmatrix}$	$\begin{bmatrix}1&0&0&0\\0&1&0&0\\-1/3&2/3&0&0\\0&0&0&1\end{bmatrix}$	$\hat{I}=I$ $\hat{II}=II$ $\hat{V}_5=(II+III)/3$ $\hat{V}_x=V_x$
		All unicolor electrode pairs RA↔C1, LA↔C2, LL↔C3, RL↔C5	
$\begin{bmatrix}\widehat{LL}=C_3\\\widehat{RA}=C_1\\\widehat{LA}=C_2\\\widehat{C_1}=RA\\\widehat{C_2}=LA\\\widehat{C_3}=LL\\\widehat{C_4}=C_4\\\widehat{C_5}=RL\\\widehat{C_6}=C_6\end{bmatrix}$	$\begin{bmatrix}0&0&0&0&1&0&0&0\\0&0&0&1&0&0&0&0\\0&0&0&0&1&0&0&0&0\\0&1&0&0&0&0&0&0\\0&0&1&0&0&0&0&0\\1&0&0&0&0&0&0&0\\0&0&0&0&0&0&1&0&0\\1&0&0&0&0&0&0&0\\0&0&0&0&0&0&0&0&1\end{bmatrix}$	$\begin{bmatrix}0&0&-1&1&0&0&0\\0&0&-1&0&1&0&0&0\\\frac{1}{3}&\frac{1}{3}&\frac{1}{3}&-\frac{1}{3}&\frac{1}{3}&0&0&0\\\frac{2}{3}&-\frac{1}{3}&\frac{1}{3}&\frac{1}{3}&-\frac{1}{3}&0&0&0\\-\frac{1}{3}&\frac{2}{3}&\frac{1}{3}&\frac{1}{3}&-\frac{1}{3}&0&0&0\\0&0&-\frac{1}{3}&\frac{1}{3}&-\frac{1}{3}&1&0&0\\-\frac{1}{3}&\frac{2}{3}&\frac{1}{3}&\frac{1}{3}&-\frac{1}{3}&0&0&0\\0&0&-\frac{1}{3}&\frac{1}{3}&-\frac{1}{3}&0&0&1\end{bmatrix}$	$\hat{I}=V_2-V_1$ $\hat{II}=V_3-V_1$ $\hat{V}_1=-\frac{I+II}{3}-\frac{V_1+V_2+V_3}{3}$ $\hat{V}_2=\frac{I-III}{3}-\frac{V_1+V_2+V_3}{3}$ $\hat{V}_3=\frac{II+III}{3}-\frac{V_1+V_2+V_3}{3}$ $\hat{V}_4=V_4-\frac{V_1+V_2+V_3}{3}$ $\hat{V}_5=\frac{II+III}{3}-\frac{V_1+V_2+V_3}{3}$ $\hat{V}_6=V_6-\frac{V_1+V_2+V_3}{3}$

Note: All columns correspond to the description in the footer of Table 2. Cx represents all chest electrodes with unchanged positions, Vx denotes their unipolar leads.

4.1.3. Reversals of Chest and Peripheral Electrodes

Five swaps are simulated (Table 4) involving the matching-color electrode pairs in the peripheral and precordial cables (IEC color coding standard [44]), i.e., red (RA-C1), yellow (LA-C2), green (LL-C3), black (RL-C5) and all pairs (RA-C1, LA-C2, LL-C3, RL-C5).

Figure 2d,e illustrates the two principal types of reversals where the unipolar chest electrode is swapped either with an active limb electrode (WCT is displaced in Figure 2d) or with the grounded electrode (WCT is not displaced in Figure 2e). In both cases, we highlight two types of unipolar leads:

- $\hat{V}x$ for the precordial electrodes $\hat{C}x$, which keep their position unchanged on the chest;
- $\hat{V}n$ for the precordial electrodes $\hat{C}n$, where n = 1,2,3,5 is substituting the chest electrode number, which changes its position to some of the limbs.

The calculation of two different unipolar leads is achieved by an extension of the swap matrix **S** (4×4) to (5×5) to include 3 limb electrodes and 2 chest electrodes ($\widehat{LL}, \widehat{RA}, \widehat{LA}, \hat{C}n, \hat{C}x$), as shown in Table 4 and Figure 2d,e. The last row of Table 4 presents the most complex example for simulation of swaps between all unicolor electrode pairs, which requires the use of a swap matrix **S** (9×9), configured for the full set of electrodes ($\widehat{LL}, \widehat{RA}, \widehat{LA}, \hat{C}1 - \hat{C}6$). All expressions of the rearranged leads ($\hat{I}, \hat{II}, \hat{V}x, \hat{V}n$) in Table 4 are further verified in the experimental study of Section 4.2 because they have not been investigated in any other study. The respective WCT potential changes (Table 1) cannot be compared to examples in the literature either. We can only justify the result for the RL-C5 reversal, which corresponds to non-displaced WCT, exactly as shown in the example (Figure 2e).

4.2. Experimental Verification of Simulated Swaps Between Unicolor Chest and Peripheral Electrodes

The experimental study is used to verify the 'MSMinv' transformation for simulation of reversals between unicolor chest and peripheral electrodes (using the expressions in Table 4), according to the concept in Section 2.2 (*ECG electrode reversals with unknown lead transformations*). For this purpose, all ECG recordings in the database are analyzed and the three measurements (RMS Error, Peak Error, CorCoef) are calculated to estimate the average beat waveform differences in 3 scenarios (Table 5):

- *No transformation*, showing the largest differences between correct vs. swapped electrode recordings for all leads because WCT is considerably displaced in most chest-limb reversals (except RL-C5). We note the greatest mean value differences for the unipolar lead with a chest electrode placed on the limbs:

    - V1 (120 µV, 529 µV, 0.832) for RA-C1,
    - V2 (246 µV, 1121 µV, 0.456) for LA-C2,
    - V3 (206 µV, 868 µV, 0.512) for LL-C3,
    - V5 (131 µV, 639 µV, 0.785) for RL-C5,
    - V1-V3 (225-289 µV, 967-1235 µV, 0.365-0.652) for all unicolor pairs.

- *Forward 'MSMinv' transformation*, simulating electrode reversals which have significantly reduced differences when compared to the recordings with really swapped electrodes ($p < 0.05$). We measure mean values (RMS Error, Peak Error, CorCoef) in the range (<20 µV, <60 µV, ≥0.995), assuming they represent negligible average beat differences mainly due to rhythm variation and signal acquisition noises in the compared recordings. We have noticed one exception for both reversals involving RL (RL-C5, all unicolor pairs), where the Forward 'MSMinv' transformation introduces a slight error in the calculation of the swapped lead V5 (≤26 µV, ≤104 µV, ≥0.986), assuming the C5 potential to be equal to LL, while C5 is placed on the RL (approximation error from the equipotential legs).

- *Inverse 'MSMinv' transformation*, recovering the correct electrode order, which has significantly reduced differences when compared to the recordings with really correct electrodes ($p < 0.05$), estimated within the above outlined range of negligible errors (<20 µV, <60 µV, ≥0.995). We have again found an exception for both reversals involving RL (RL-C5, all unicolor pairs), where the Inverse 'MSMinv' transformation fails to reconstruct the correct lead V5 (<142 µV, <660 µV, ≥0.792) from a recording with RL electrode in the position of C5 electrode. As soon as RL stops being an input to the ECG device, the potential of V5 electrode is lost and not reproduced by any active electrode in the swap matrix **S** (Table 4, all **S** entries are equal to '0' for the column, corresponding to C5).

Table 5. Statistical analysis (mean value ± standard deviation) of measures (RMS Error, Peak Error, CorCoef) calculated for the average beat in 8 independent leads (I, II, V1-V6), quantifying the lead-specific differences between experimentally recorded ECGs – raw leads vs. reordered leads (based on the expressions in Table 4) for 3 different scenarios:. No transformation; Forward 'MSMinv' transformation applied on the recording with correct electrodes; Inverse 'MSMinv' transformation applied on the recording with swapped electrodes.

Unicolor Reversals		RMS Error (μV)			Peak Error (μV)			Cor. Coef. (0-1)		
		Transf. None	Transf. MSMinv Forward	Transf. MSMinv Inverse	Transf. None	Transf. MSMinv Forward	Transf. MSMinv Inverse	Transf. None	Transf. MSMinv Forward	Transf. MSMinv Inverse
RA-C1	I	81 ± 40	14 ± 5 *	15 ± 5 *	351 ± 162	48 ± 19 *	53 ± 20 *	0.921 ± 0.093	0.997 ± 0.004 *	0.995 ± 0.006 *
	II	81 ± 38	13 ± 5 *	13 ± 4 *	356 ± 163	48 ± 19 *	46 ± 16 *	0.909 ± 0.172	0.998 ± 0.002 *	0.996 ± 0.005 *
	V1	120 ± 52	11 ± 4 *	11 ± 4 *	529 ± 227	38 ± 15 *	38 ± 13 *	0.832 ± 0.136	0.996 ± 0.002 *	0.998 ± 0.002 *
	Vx	27 ± 13	11 ± 5 *	12 ± 5 *	116 ± 61	44 ± 9 *	42 ± 18 *	0.989 ± 0.029	0.998 ± 0.003 *	0.998 ± 0.003 *
LA-C2	I	197 ± 80	16 ± 5 *	15 ± 5 *	924 ± 336	55 ± 20 *	54 ± 20 *	0.746 ± 0.144	0.997 ± 0.004 *	0.995 ± 0.005 *
	II	18 ± 5	13 ± 3 *	13 ± 3 *	78 ± 37	44 ± 12 *	46 ± 13 *	0.994 ± 0.013	0.995 ± 0.011 *	0.995 ± 0.009 *
	V2	246 ± 102	13 ± 6 *	13 ± 5 *	1121 ± 396	50 ± 25 *	54 ± 26 *	0.456 ± 0.180	0.990 ± 0.010 *	0.998 ± 0.002 *
	Vx	58 ± 5	12 ± 4 *	12 ± 5 *	264 ± 103	41 ± 16 *	47 ± 19 *	0.956 ± 0.073	0.998 ± 0.003 *	0.997 ± 0.003 *
LL-C3	I	15 ± 5	15 ± 5	15 ± 6	56 ± 27	54 ± 23	56 ± 26	0.996 ± 0.006	0.995 ± 0.006 *	0.995 ± 0.006 *
	II	154 ± 50	18 ± 5 *	15 ± 4 *	644 ± 228	59 ± 22 *	53 ± 20 *	0.869 ± 0.146	0.998 ± 0.001 *	0.995 ± 0.008 *
	V3	206 ± 65	12 ± 5 *	14 ± 5 *	868 ± 296	47 ± 25 *	53 ± 21 *	0.512 ± 0.197	0.988 ± 0.012 *	0.997 ± 0.004 *
	Vx	52 ± 18	12 ± 5 *	13 ± 5 *	219 ± 80	45 ± 23 *	46 ± 20 *	0.970 ± 0.051	0.997 ± 0.004 *	0.997 ± 0.003 *
RL-C5	I	16 ± 5	15 ± 5	15 ± 5	57 ± 24	54 ± 20	54 ± 20	0.995 ± 0.008	0.995 ± 0.008	0.995 ± 0.009
	II	14 ± 4	14 ± 4	14 ± 4	47 ± 15	48 ± 18	48 ± 17	0.995 ± 0.009	0.995 ± 0.009	0.995 ± 0.010
	V5	131 ± 60	24 ± 12 *$	136 ± 54 #	639 ± 287	102 ± 54 *$	660 ± 268 #	0.785 ± 0.210	0.957 ± 0.047 *$	0.792 ± 0.144 #
	Vx	14 ± 5	14 ± 5	14 ± 5	51 ± 25	51 ± 25	51 ± 25	0.998 ± 0.002	0.998 ± 0.002	0.997 ± 0.002
RA-C1 LA-C2 LL-C3 RL-C5	I	143 ± 72	17 ± 9 *	18 ± 8 *	726 ± 361	59 ± 33 *	69 ± 35 *	0.836 ± 0.100	0.994 ± 0.006 *	0.994 ± 0.005 *
	II	138 ± 45	19 ± 5 *	18 ± 9 *	631 ± 275	71 ± 26 *	60 ± 27 *	0.925 ± 0.062	0.997 ± 0.002 *	0.993 ± 0.009 *
	V1	225 ± 97	16 ± 5 *	14 ± 5 *	967 ± 445	50 ± 17 *	57 ± 18 *	0.652 ± 0.195	0.996 ± 0.003 *	0.997 ± 0.003 *
	V2	289 ± 125	16 ± 7 *	18 ± 8 *	1235 ± 487	62 ± 35 *	69 ± 30 *	0.365 ± 0.133	0.993 ± 0.007 *	0.996 ± 0.004 *
	V3	248 ± 92	15 ± 5 *	16 ± 4 *	1003 ± 378	55 ± 19 *	58 ± 23 *	0.494 ± 0.184	0.994 ± 0.010 *	0.997 ± 0.003 *
	V4	110 ± 56	14 ± 4 *	16 ± 4 *	443 ± 258	54 ± 20 *	58 ± 25 *	0.835 ± 0.204	0.997 ± 0.003 *	0.997 ± 0.002 *
	V5	161 ± 63	26 ± 10 *$	142 ± 75 #	615 ± 285	104 ± 50 *$	659 ± 368 #	0.705 ± 0.230	0.986 ± 0.019 *$	0.859 ± 0.106 #
	V6	113 ± 53	13 ± 5 *	13 ± 5 *	472 ± 231	50 ± 23 *	45 ± 16 *	0.886 ± 0.135	0.998 ± 0.002 *	0.996 ± 0.005 *

Note: Vx denotes the unipolar chest leads without electrode swaps; Color of electrodes follows IEC standard [44]; Gray columns highlight the baseline measurements without transformation ('None' transformation). * $p < 0.05$: Significant reduction of (RMS Error, Peak Error) and increment of (CorCoef) for the reordered leads after applying 'MSMinv' transformation (Forward or Inverse) compared to 'None' transformation. $: Approximation effect of the Forward 'MSMinv' transformation to simulate a swapped lead V5, while C5 is placed on the RL and its potential is assumed equal to the LL. #: Deficiency of the Inverse 'MSMinv' transformation to reconstruct the correct lead V5 from a recording with RL electrode in the position of C5 electrode.

Figure 3 illustrates the average ECG beats in leads (I, II, V1-V6) recorded with all types of swapped unicolor chest and peripheral electrodes. This ECG trace is almost fully overlapping with the simulated electrode reversals from the ECG raw data with correct electrode positions, applying Forward 'MSMinv' transformation. This once again validates the derived algebraic transformations in Table 4, which are able to exactly reproduce the diversity of lead-specific morphologies (amplitudes, polarities and durations) that each swap introduces to any lead via change of its electrode position and/or WCT potential.

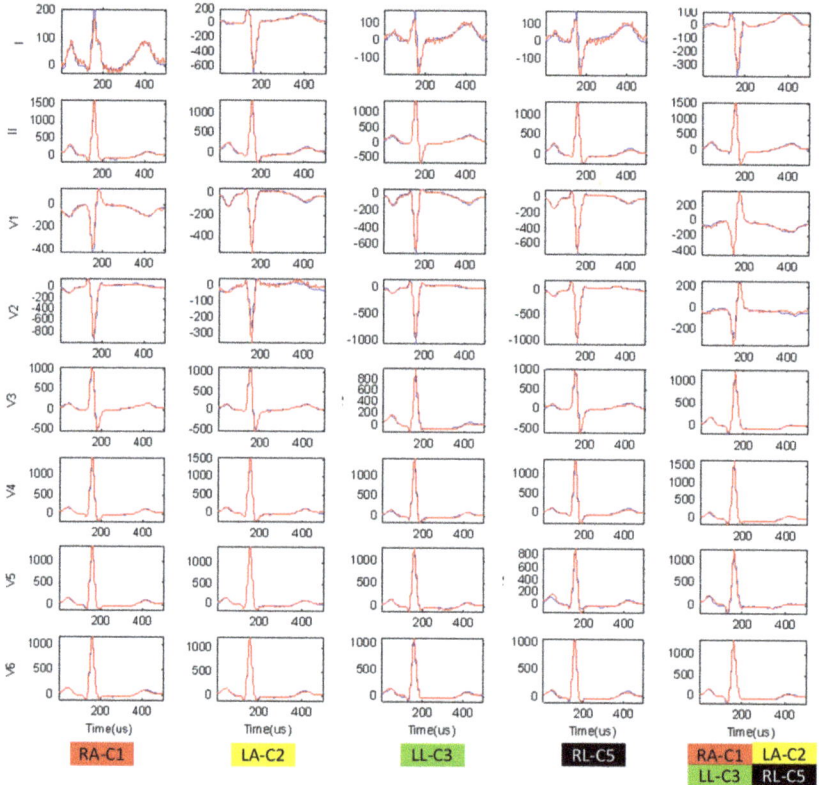

Figure 3. The average beat of 8 independent leads (I, II, V1-V6) taken from the same subject in two scenarios: (1) Red trace: Recorded ECG with swapped unicolor electrodes; (2) Blue trace: Simulated ECG with swapped unicolor electrodes, applying Forward 'MSMinv' transformation on the ECG recorded with the correct lead set.

4.3. Application of the 'MSMinv' Transformation for Automatic Detection of the Exact ECG Electrode Reversals

We further show an important practical application of the Inverse 'MSMinv' transformation for the detection of the exact reversals between ECG electrodes. This application is relevant to the case when two ECG recordings in a patient are available:

(1) an ECG recording with correct lead set (L_{RC});
(2) an ECG recording with an unknown/suspected lead swap (L_{RS}).

The 'MSMinv' transformation is applied to the swapped ECG recording, iteratively simulating all possible permutations of the nine active ECG electrodes (i = 9! = 362 880):

$$\widehat{L_{RS}}(i) = \mathbf{MSi\tilde{M}}_{inv}L_{RS} \tag{16}$$

The swap matrix $\mathbf{S}_i$, which produces the lead set reconstruction $\widehat{L_{RS}}(i)$ with the minimal difference $d(\cdot)$ to the correct lead set can indicate the true lead swap (TLS):

$$TLS = \arg\min_{1 \leq i \leq 9!} \left(d\left(\widehat{L_{RS}}(i) - L_{RC} \right) \right) \tag{17}$$

We test this swap detection criterion using our ECG database under the following conditions:

- All 25 patients are considered, comparing the available pairs of recordings (L_{RC}, L_{RS}) per patient, where L_{RC} is the recording without electrode reversals, and L_{RS} represents one of the recorded 3 lead swaps (RA-C1, LA-C2, LL-C3), not involving the RL.
- The minimal difference rule (17) is applied on the average beat of each recording.
- The minimal difference rule (17) is evaluated with 3 distance metrics $d(\cdot)$ – min(RMS Error) (Equation (13)), min(Peak Error) (Equation (14)), max(CorCoef) (Equation (15)).
- The accuracy for detection of the TLS is evaluated as the true positive (TP) rate, considering the tested population of N subjects:

$$\text{Accuracy} = \sum_{p=1}^{N} \frac{TP_p}{N}, \tag{18}$$

where $TP = f(x) = \begin{cases} 1, & \text{correct lead swap detected} \\ 0, & \text{otherwise} \end{cases}$

Table 6 presents the experimental verification of the Inverse 'MSMinv' transformation, applied for automatic detection of the exact ECG electrode reversals. We have achieved 100% accuracy in the detection of (RA-C1) and (LL-C3) reversals, and 96% for the detection of (LA-C2) reversal when the decision rule (17) uses a minimal difference metric equal to the minimal RMS Error or the maximal correlation between the reconstructed swap and the correct recording. All false negatives are observed to present TLS with either the 2nd or the 3rd ranked minimal differences, while the decision rule (17) is presently adjusted to simply report the exact lead swap with the 1st ranked minimal difference. For example, the lowest LA-C2 accuracy is due to one case, where the true LA-C2 is 2nd ranked, while the true LA-C2 in combination with RA-C1 is 1st ranked. Obviously, the detection of the exact electrode swap among many electrodes with close geometrical positions might include a portion of uncertainty due to indistinguishable geometrical perspectives of the heart vector in neighboring leads. Further updates of the decision rule (17) could potentially improve the accuracy for TLS detection, e.g., by majority voting of many distance metrics after exclusion of those with the lowest accuracy (i.e., the peak Error with 88% to 96%).

Table 6. Accuracy for the detection of the exact lead swaps, applying the 'MSMinv' transformation on 3 swapped recordings (RA-C1), (LA-C2), (LL-C3) from 25 patients in our database. Color of electrodes follows IEC standard [44];

Unicolor Lead Swaps	Accuracy		
	RMS Error (%)	Peak Error (%)	Cor Coef (%)
RA-C1	100	96 *	100
LA-C2	96 *	88 #	96 *
LL-C3	100	88 #	100

* 1 false negative case due to TLS with the 2nd ranked minimal difference in the decision rule (17). # 3 false negative cases due to TLS with either the 2nd or the 3rd ranked minimal differences in (17).

The presented rules are easily applicable in a warning system that can alert the medical staff to check the electrodes suggested for reversal within the first seconds of 12-lead ECG acquisition.

Principally, the analysis is not fixed exactly to 10 s but can take a single beat or an average beat over ECGs with an arbitrary duration. It is important to note that the results reported in this section represent the best-case results, because they are based on resting ECG recordings that were taken within a short window of time and with exactly the same electrode positions (only the electrode cables were swapped). In a clinically relevant application, the ECGs under question will most likely have a substantially different recording date (leading to possible physiological changes in the ECG), and they will most likely be recorded with slightly different electrode positions. Although the average beat pattern of the same individual has been shown to have a long-term stability independent of recording sessions and physiological factors (age, gender, heart rate) [46,47], the reliable clinical application should always consider a final approval of the alarmed electrode reversals by the medical staff and electrode correction at the time of the recording.

5. Conclusions

This study derives a novel algebraic transformation which converts the standard 12-lead ECG leads from a correct to reordered set in case of arbitrary reversals between ECG electrodes. The formula of the 'MSMinv' transformation (7) is generalized to the calculation of all kinds of electrode reversals, giving the exact lead reordering for:

- Limb electrode swaps that have been previously drawn from anatomical perspectives (Tables 2 and 3);
- Limb–chest electrode swaps with WCT potential change which, to the best of our knowledge, have never been simulated in the literature (Table 4). The formulas are exhibited for the most probable reversals of unicolor electrode pairs in the peripheral and precordial ECG cables.

The validity of the 'MSMinv' transformation is proven in our experimental study for two bilateral applications with a certain practical significance:

- *The 'Forward' application* computing the reordered lead set from an ECG recorded with correctly placed electrodes is important for educational purposes of both humans and machines to reliably recognize and warn of electrode swaps before potentially erroneous diagnostic interpretation has been made. In this respect, 'MSMinv' transformation is applicable to the available immense databases of correctly recorded ECGs (from normal and abnormal heart conditions) for reproducing the vast diversity of distorted ECG leads that can be observed in arbitrary swaps within the limb and precordial electrode set (such as the examples in Figure 3). This is an indispensable tool for the comprehensive training platforms to visualize and study the effects of electrode swaps (e.g. online cardiology courses for physicians, researchers, and instructors) or software design platforms (training the automatic detection algorithms) on abundant ECG electrode reversals.
- *The 'Inverse' application* reconstructing the correct lead set from an ECG recorded with known electrode reversals can save time and the cost of having to repeat ECG recordings in case of follow-up detection of electrode reversals and error-screening of clinical databases. The possibility for straightforward visualization of the correct lead set and its interpretation can easily uncover diagnostic errors or answer dilemmas for suspected or mistrusted electrode swaps (such as the dispute between [15] and [16]). In the general case when the electrode reversal is unknown but a prior correct ECG recording of the same patient is available, the Inverse 'MSMinv' transformation is able to solve the non-trivial task of detecting which electrodes have been exactly swapped. For this purpose, all possible swapped reconstructions can be simulated to ultimately determine the one which yields the minimal RMS difference or the highest correlation with the known recording. We have achieved a detection accuracy of 96% to 100% for this simple criterion, which has been tested with available recordings of three electrode swaps (RA-C1, LA-C2, LL-C3, not involving the RL) from 25 healthy persons. One should consider, however, the limitations for the validation of such an application which should be tested against the functional and physiological ECG instability between the two ECG sessions (e.g., the criterion validated on a

specific population with "normal" ECG during rest could fail on cardiac patients or patients under environmental stress with lead-wise ECG morphology change). As this work is focused only on the problem of simulating all possible ECG cable reversals, the design and validation of criteria for a self-consistency check for detection of the ECG cable reversals is an extensive problem for a future study.

Another important derivation of the present study is the 'WSMinv' transformation (12), which computes WCT potential change for all kinds of electrode reversals. It quantifies the common distortion that all unipolar leads would meet while their reference potential is changed, regardless of whether or not they maintain their correct position. Table 1 shows that WCT distortion is proportional to leads I, II, and the displaced unipolar leads (V1-V3 in the simulation) with fractions, which are hardly envisaged without the derived transformation. The overall influence of WCT change on all unipolar leads is also reproduced by the 'MSMinv' transformation in Tables 3 and 4.

This study provides the means for calculation of the potentials of the ECG electrodes and WCT toward a common reference potential using Equations (5) and (10), respectively. These mathematical transformations can be applied to any standard 12-lead ECG for deriving the 'true' unipolar ECG leads and WCT measurements that have recently been experimentally acquired via special ECG machines [43,47]. The experimental studies have considered the position of the reference potential on the right leg, while this study shows the values of the matrix $\tilde{M}_{inv}$ for the reference left leg leading to the same global observations (WCT measured with respect to the left leg does not have a stable voltage and is correlated to the limb leads (I, II), exhibiting all ECG waves). Although both legs have essentially insignificant potential difference, its value is the only unknown and approximated to be a zero measurement while applying our transformation equations.

Author Contributions: Conceptualization, R.S.; data curation, V.K. and I.J.; formal analysis, V.K. and I.J.; investigation, V.K. and I.J.; methodology, V.K., I.J., and R.S.; project administration, R.S.; resources, V.K. and I.J.; software, V.K. and I.J.; supervision, R.S.; validation, V.K., I.J., and R.S.; visualization, V.K.; writing – original draft, V.K.; writing – review and editing, I.J. and R.S.

Funding: This research received no external funding.

Conflicts of Interest: The authors declare no conflicts of interest.

References

1. Kligfield, P.; Gettes, L.S.; Bailey, J.J.; Childers, R.; Deal, B.J.; Hancock, E.W.; van Herpen, G.; Kors, J.A.; Macfarlane, P.; Mirvis, D.M.; et al. Recommendations for the standardization and interpretation of the electrocardiogram: part I: The electrocardiogram and its technology: a scientific statement from the American Heart Association Electrocardiography and Arrhythmias Committee, Council on Clinical Cardiology; the American College of Cardiology Foundation; and the Heart Rhythm Society: endorsed by the International Society for Computerized Electrocardiology. *J. Am. ColL. Cardiol.* **2007**, *115*, 1306–1324. [CrossRef]
2. Rajaganeshan, R.; Ludlam, C.L.; Francis, D.P.; Parasramka, S.V.; Sutton, R. Accuracy in ECG lead placement among technicians, nurses, general physicians and cardiologists. *Int. J. Clin. Pract.* **2008**, *62*, 65–70. [CrossRef] [PubMed]
3. Salvi, V.; Karnad, D.R.; Panicker, G.K.; Kothari, S.; Hingorani, P.; Natekar, M.; Mahajan, V.; Narula, D. Limb lead interchange in thorough QT/QTc studies. *J. Clin. Pharmacol.* **2011**, *51*, 1468–1473. [CrossRef] [PubMed]
4. Rudiger, A.; Hellermann, J.; Mukherjee, R.; Follath, F.; Turina, J. Electrocardiographic artifacts due to electrode misplacement and their frequency in different clinical settings. *Am. J. Emer. Med.* **2007**, *25*, 174–178. [CrossRef] [PubMed]
5. Amin, M.; Chowdhury, A.; Ahmed, M.; Sabah, K.; Haque, H.; Kabir, S.; Islam, K.N.; Saleh, M.A.D. Lead-Reversal ECG Simulating Myocardial Infarction—A Case Report and Literature Review. *Bangladesh Heart J.* **2016**, *31*, 104–108. [CrossRef]
6. Raut, M.; Maheshwari, A. Know the errors in ECG recording. *Curr. Med. Res. Pract.* **2015**, *5*, 81–91. [CrossRef]

7. Vardan, S.; Mookherjee, D.; Sarkar, T.; Mehrotra, K.; Fruehan, T.; Mookherjee, S. Guidelines for the Detection of ECG Limb Lead Misplacements. *Resid. Staff* **2008**, *54*. Available online: https://www.mdmag.com/journals/resident-and-staff/2008/2008-01/2008-01_05 (accessed on 24 February 2019).
8. Haisty, W.K.; Pahlm, O.; Edenbrandt, L.; Newman, K. Recognition of Electrocardiographic Electrode Misplacements Involving the Ground (Right Leg) Electrode. *Am. J. Cardiol.* **1993**, *71*, 1490–1495. [CrossRef]
9. Bond, R.; Finlay, D.; Nugent, C.; Breen, C.; Guldenring, D.; Daly, M. The effects of electrode misplacement on clinicians' interpretation of the standard 12-lead electrocardiogram. *Eur. J. Int. Med.* **2012**, *23*, 610–615. [CrossRef]
10. Mattu, A.; Brady, W.; Perron, A.; Robinson, D. Prominent R Wave in Lead V1: Electrocardiographic Differential Diagnosis. *Am. J. Emerg. Med.* **2001**, *19*, 504–513. [CrossRef]
11. Jekova, I.; Leber, R.; Krasteva, V.; Schmid, R. Detection of Unicolor ECG Electrode Reversals in Standard 12-Lead ECG. *Comput. Cardiol.* **2018**, *45*. [CrossRef]
12. Lynch, R. ECG lead misplacement: A brief review of limb lead misplacement. *African J. Emerg. Med.* **2014**, *4*, 130–139. [CrossRef]
13. García-Niebla, J.; García, P.L. An unusual case of electrode misplacement: left arm and V2 electrode reversal. *J. Electrocardiol.* **2008**, *41*, 380–381. [CrossRef] [PubMed]
14. Vanninen, S.U.; Nikus, K.C. Electrocardiogram Acquisition Errors or Myocardial Infarct. *Case Rep. Cardiol.* **2011**, *2011*, 605874. [CrossRef] [PubMed]
15. Joshi, K.R.; Morris, D.L.; Figueredo, V.M. Wandering acute myocardial infarction. *Am. J. Med.* **2014**, *127*, e5–e6. [CrossRef]
16. Givens, P.M.; Goldonowicz, J.M.; Littmann, L. The electrocardiogram of chest and limb lead reversal. *Am. J. Med.* **2014**, *127*, e29–e30. [CrossRef] [PubMed]
17. Medani, S.A.; Hensey, M.; Caples, N.; Owens, P. Accuracy in precordial ECG lead placement: Improving performance through a peer-led educational intervention. *J. Electrocardiol.* **2018**, *51*, 50–54. [CrossRef]
18. Thaler, T.; Tempelmann, V.; Maggiorini, M.; Rudiger, A. The frequency of electrocardiographic errors due to electrode cable switches: A before and after study. *J. Electrocardiol.* **2010**, *43*, 676–681. [CrossRef]
19. Mond, H.G.; Garcia, J.; Visagathilagar, T. Twisted Leads: The Footprints of Malpositioned Electrocardiographic Leads. *Heart Lung Circ.* **2016**, *25*, 61–67. [CrossRef]
20. Baranchuk, A.; Shaw, C.; Alanazi, H.; Campbell, D.; Bally, K.; Redfearn, D.P.; Simpson, C.S.; Abdollah, H. Electrocardiography Pitfalls and Artifacts: The 10 Commandments. *Crit. Care Nurse* **2009**, *29*, 67–73. [CrossRef]
21. Batchvarov, V.N.; Malik, M.; Camm, A.J. Incorrect electrode cable connection during electrocardiographic recording. *Europace* **2007**, *9*, 1081–1090. [CrossRef] [PubMed]
22. Rosen, A.V.; Koppikar, S.; Shaw, C.; Baranchuk, A. Common ECG Lead Placement Errors. Part I: Limb lead Reversals. *Int. J. Med. Stud.* **2014**, *2*, 92–98.
23. Rosen, A.V.; Koppikar, S.; Shaw, C.; Baranchuk, A. Common ECG Lead Placement Errors. Part II: Precordial Misplacements. *Int. J. Med. Stud.* **2014**, *2*, 99–103.
24. Sakaguchi, S.; Sandberg, J.; Benditt, D. ECG Electrode Reversals: An Opportunity to Learn from Mistakes. *J. Cardiovasc. Electrophysiol.* **2018**, *29*, 806–815. [CrossRef] [PubMed]
25. Abdollah, H.; Milliken, J.A. Recognition of electrocardiographic left arm/left leg lead reversal. *Am. J. Cardiol.* **1997**, *80*, 1247–1249. [CrossRef]
26. Hedén, B.; Ohlsson, M.; Holst, H.; Mjöman, M.; Rittner, R.; Pahlm, O.; Peterson, C.; Edenbrandt, L. Detection of frequently overlooked electrocardiographic lead reversals using artificial neural networks. *Am. J. Cardiol.* **1996**, *78*, 600–604. [CrossRef]
27. Hoffman, I. A flatline electrocardiogram in lead II is a marker for right arm/right leg electrode switch. *J. Electrocardiol.* **2007**, *40*, 226–227. [CrossRef] [PubMed]
28. Han, C.; Gregg, R.; Babaeizadeh, S. Automatic Detection of ECG Lead-wire Interchange for Conventional and Mason-Likar Lead Systems. *Comput. Cardiol.* **2014**, *41*, 145–148.
29. Krishnan, R.; Ramesh, M. QRS axis based classification of electrode interchange in wearable ECG devices. *EAI Endorsed Trans. Future Intell. Educ. Env.* **2015**, *2*. [CrossRef]
30. Ho, R.T.; Mukherji, L.; Evans, G.T.Jr. Simple diagnosis of limb-lead reversals by predictable changes in QRS axis. *Pacing Clin. Electrophysiol.* **2006**, *29*, 272–277. [CrossRef]

31. De Bie, J.; Mortara, D.W.; Clark, T.F. The development and validation of an early warning system to prevent the acquisition of 12-lead resting ECGs with interchanged electrode positions. *J. Electrocardiol.* **2014**, *47*, 794–797. [CrossRef] [PubMed]
32. Ho, K.K.L.; Ho, S.K. Use of the sinus P wave in diagnosing electrocardiographic limb lead misplacement not involving the right leg (ground) lead. *J. Electrocardiol.* **2001**, *34*, 161–171. [CrossRef] [PubMed]
33. Kors, J.A.; van Herpen, G. Accurate automatic detection of electrode interchange in the electrocardiogram. *Am. J. Cardiol.* **2001**, *88*, 396–399. [CrossRef]
34. Han, C.; Gregg, R.E.; Field, D.Q.; Babaeizadeh, S. Automatic detection of ECG cable interchange by analyzing both morphology and interlead relations. *J. Electrocardiol.* **2014**, *47*, 781–787. [CrossRef] [PubMed]
35. Gregg, R.; Hancock, E.W.; Babaeizadeh, S. Detecting ECG limb lead-wire interchanges involving the right leg lead-wire. *Comput. Cardiol.* **2017**, *44*. [CrossRef]
36. Xia, H.; Garcia, G.A.; Zhao, X. Automatic detection of ECG electrode misplacement: A tale of two algorithms. *Physiol. Meas.* **2012**, *33*, 1549–1561. [CrossRef] [PubMed]
37. Dotsinsky, I.; Daskalov, I.; Iliev, I. Detection of peripheral ECG electrodes misplacement. *Proc. 7th Int. Conf. Electronics ET'98, Sozopol, Bulgaria* **1998**, *S2*, 21–26. Available online: http://ecad.tu-sofia.bg/et/1998/Statii%20ET98-II/Detection%20of%20Peripheral%20ECG%20Electrodes%20Misplacement.pdf (accessed on 24 February 2019).
38. Jekova, I.; Krasteva, V.; Leber, R.; Schmid, R.; Twerenbold, R.; Müller, C.; Reichlin, T.; Abächerli, R. Inter-lead correlation analysis for automated detection of cable reversals in 12/16-lead ECG. *Comput. Methods Programs Biomed.* **2016**, *134*, 31–41. [CrossRef]
39. Végső, B.; Balázs, G.; Gaál, B.; Kozmann, G. Electrode reversal detection in ECG remote monitoring. *Meas. Sci. Rev.* **2005**, *5*, 45–48. Available online: http://www.measurement.sk/2005/S2/Vegso.pdf (accessed on 24 February 2019).
40. Cooper, C.; Clark, E.; Macfarlane, P.W. Enhanced Detection of Electrode Placement/Connection Errors. *Comput. Cardiol.* **2008**, *35*, 89–92. [CrossRef]
41. Bond, R.; Finlay, D.; Nugent, C.; Moore, G.; Guldenring, D. A simulation tool for visualizing and studying the effects of electrode misplacement on the 12-lead electrocardiogram. *J. Electrocardiol.* **2011**, *44*, 439–444. [CrossRef]
42. Macfarlane, P.W.; Van Oosterom, A.; Pahlm, O.; Kligfield, P.; Janse, M.; Camm, J. *Comprehensive Electrocardiography*, 2nd ed.; Springer-Verlag: London, UK, 2010; ISBN 978-1-84882-047-0.
43. Gargiulo, G.D. True Unipolar ECG Machine for Wilson Central Terminal Measurements. *BioMed Res. Int.* **2015**, *586397*, 1–7. [CrossRef] [PubMed]
44. IEC 60601-2-25 International Standard. *Medical electrical equipment—Part 2-25: Particular requirements for the basic safety and essential performance of electrocardiographs*, 2nd ed.; International Electrotechnical Commission: Geneva, Switzerland, 2011.
45. Kligfield, P.; Badilini, F.; Denjoy, I.; Babaeizadeh, S.; Clark, E.M.A.; de Bie, J.; Devine, B.; Extramiana, F.; Generali, G.; Gregg, R.; et al. Comparison of automated interval measurements by widely used algorithms in digital electrocardiographs. *Am. Heart J.* **2018**, *200*, 1–10. [CrossRef]
46. Krasteva, V.; Jekova, I.; Schmid, R. Perspectives of human verification via binary QRS template matching of single-lead and 12-lead electrocardiogram. *Plos ONE* **2018**, *13*, e0197240. [CrossRef] [PubMed]
47. Gargiulo, G.D.; Bifulco, P.; Cesarelli, M.; McEwan, A.; Moeinzadeh, H.; O'Loughlin, A.; Shugman, I.M.; Tapson, J.C.; Thiagalingam, A. On the Zero of Potential of the Electric Field Produced by the Heart Beat. A Machine Capable of Estimating this Underlying Persistent Error in Electrocardiography. *Machines* **2016**, *4*, 18. [CrossRef]

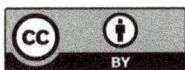

© 2019 by the authors. Licensee MDPI, Basel, Switzerland. This article is an open access article distributed under the terms and conditions of the Creative Commons Attribution (CC BY) license (http://creativecommons.org/licenses/by/4.0/).

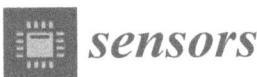

Article

A Novel Fetal Movement Simulator for the Performance Evaluation of Vibration Sensors for Wearable Fetal Movement Monitors

Abhishek Kumar Ghosh [1], Sonny F. Burniston [2], Daniel Krentzel [2], Abhishek Roy [2], Adil Shoaib Sheikh [2], Talha Siddiq [2], Paula Mai Phuong Trinh [2], Marta Mambrilla Velazquez [2], Hei-Ting Vielle [2], Niamh C. Nowlan [2,†] and Ravi Vaidyanathan [1,*,†]

1. Department of Mechanical Engineering, Imperial College London, London SW7 2AZ, UK; a.ghosh18@imperial.ac.uk
2. Department of Bioengineering, Imperial College London, London SW7 2AZ, UK; sonnyburniston@yahoo.co.uk (S.F.B.); daniel.krentzel16@imperial.ac.uk (D.K.); royabhishek77@gmail.com (A.R.); adil.sheikh15@imperial.ac.uk (A.S.S.); talha.siddiq15@imperial.ac.uk (T.S.); mai.trinh16@imperial.ac.uk (P.M.P.T.); martamamvel@hotmail.com (M.M.V.); hei-ting.vielle16@imperial.ac.uk (H.-T.V.); n.nowlan@imperial.ac.uk (N.C.N.)
* Correspondence: r.vaidyanathan@imperial.ac.uk
† These authors contributed equally to this work.

Received: 21 September 2020; Accepted: 15 October 2020; Published: 23 October 2020

Abstract: Fetal movements (FM) are an important factor in the assessment of fetal health. However, there is currently no reliable way to monitor FM outside clinical environs. While extensive research has been carried out using accelerometer-based systems to monitor FM, the desired accuracy of detection is yet to be achieved. A major challenge has been the difficulty of testing and calibrating sensors at the pre-clinical stage. Little is known about fetal movement features, and clinical trials involving pregnant women can be expensive and ethically stringent. To address these issues, we introduce a novel FM simulator, which can be used to test responses of sensor arrays in a laboratory environment. The design uses a silicon-based membrane with material properties similar to that of a gravid abdomen to mimic the vibrations due to fetal kicks. The simulator incorporates mechanisms to pre-stretch the membrane and to produce kicks similar to that of a fetus. As a case study, we present results from a comparative study of an acoustic sensor, an accelerometer, and a piezoelectric diaphragm as candidate vibration sensors for a wearable FM monitor. We find that the acoustic sensor and the piezoelectric diaphragm are better equipped than the accelerometer to determine durations, intensities, and locations of kicks, as they have a significantly greater response to changes in these conditions than the accelerometer. Additionally, we demonstrate that the acoustic sensor and the piezoelectric diaphragm can detect weaker fetal movements (threshold wall displacements are less than 0.5 mm) compared to the accelerometer (threshold wall displacement is 1.5 mm) with a trade-off of higher power signal artefacts. Finally, we find that the piezoelectric diaphragm produces better signal-to-noise ratios compared to the other two sensors in most of the cases, making it a promising new candidate sensor for wearable FM monitors. We believe that the FM simulator represents a key development towards enabling the eventual translation of wearable FM monitoring garments.

Keywords: fetal movement simulator; fetal movement monitor; maternal abdomen model; acoustic sensor; accelerometer; piezoelectric diaphragm

1. Introduction

Monitoring of fetal movements (FM) has long been a subject of interest to medical and research communities due to the association between reduced FM and several fetal health conditions, such as fetal distress, placental dysfunction, fetal growth restriction, and hypoxia [1–6]. A reduction in FM often provides an early warning of fetal health complications [7–10]. For example, in a study on 305 pregnant volunteers with reduced FM after 28 weeks of gestation, 22.1% reported poor outcomes at birth, such as preterm or small-for-gestational-age births [9]. Another study on 161 singleton pregnancies resulting in stillbirths at Nottingham City Hospital from 1991 to 1997 stated that reductions in FM were reported in 54.7% of the cases [10]. A recent study on 409,175 pregnancies in the UK and Ireland found that the awareness of reduced FM through maternal sensation does not significantly reduce the risk of stillbirth [11], but this does not negate the value and impact of a method for objectively quantifying FM.

The oldest and most commonly used method of quantifying FM is through maternal sensation. Despite being a very common screening method followed by a large portion of pregnant women around the world, this method has largely been set aside by medical professionals [12]. Studies have shown that this method is highly patient dependent, especially with subtle or gentle movements [13]. Results from recent studies propose that only around 40% of the movements observed in ultrasonography are detected by maternal sensation [14,15]. While pregnant women are always counseled to report any perceived decrease in fetal movements, formal "kick counting" is actively discouraged in many contemporary guidelines for antenatal care [16,17]. Additionally, there is a lack of clear guidance on a "safe" number of perceived movements [12]. Other common methods of quantifying fetal activity include ultrasonography [18,19], MRI scanning [20], and cardiotocography [21]. Such methods need expert operators and can only be performed for short periods in clinical environments. Additionally, ultrasonography (and especially MRI) may not be available in the majority of the rural areas in low-income countries. Current clinical methods are, therefore, unsuitable for regular monitoring of fetuses and have failed to determine a reliable quantitative guideline for a normal or safe level or frequency of FM.

Building upon advances in electronics and sensor technology, several attempts to develop a low-cost, wearable, non-transmitting system for detecting FM have been reported in recent years. Most of these attempts have used accelerometer-based systems to detect low-frequency vibrations of maternal abdomens created by fetal movements. For example, Thomas et al. [22] used a single accelerometer to record FM from 27 pregnant women and achieved average true and false detection rates of 62% and 40%, respectively, compared to concurrent ultrasound scans. Using two custom-made capacitive acceleration sensors, Roy et al. [23] found 79% positive agreement with concurrent ultrasound recordings from 14 pregnant women for gross movement of fetal trunks. However, their positive detection rates for the isolated limb and breathing movements were only 36% and 21%, respectively. Mesbah et al. [24] presented a fetal activity monitor that uses three accelerometers to detect fetal activities and an additional accelerometer, placed on the mother's chest, to detect artefacts from maternal activities. Considering the data recorded by one of the accelerometers only, they obtained positive agreements of 50%, 52%, and 76% with concurrent ultrasound detections for three different recordings. A complete analysis of the data obtained from all four accelerometers was presented by Boashash et al. [15], where special time-frequency based techniques were used to improve the detection rate by removing signal artefacts. Analyzing the data from six pregnant women, they reported overall true detection rates of 78% and 72% for two different methods; the corresponding false detection rates were 17% and 15%, respectively. By experimenting with six accelerometers, Altini et al. [25] reported that the addition of accelerometers after two does not improve the detection accuracy significantly, while the addition of a reference accelerometer to remove artefacts due to maternal activity consistently improves the detection accuracy for any number and arrangement of sensors. In a recent work from our group, Lai et al. [26] presented a new design of FM monitor based on a combination of six acoustic sensors and an inertial measurement unit (IMU). The IMU mainly consisted of an accelerometer, which was used to detect maternal body movements. The system was validated against concurrent ultrasound tests on a cohort of 44 pregnant women. It achieved a promising true positive detection rate of 78% in detecting startle movements (vigorous, whole-body movements) but performed poorly in the cases of general and breathing movements (true positive detection rates were 53% and 41%, respectively). Additionally, the average ratio of sensor-detected movements to ultrasound-detected movements was 2.4, which demonstrates a high number of false-positive detections by this system.

Although extensive efforts have been made to design FM monitors using accelerometers, the desired accuracy of detection has not been achieved and translation remains negligible. Our recent study indicates that while acoustic sensing is promising, the false-positive detection remains unacceptably high [26]. Therefore, it is important now to quantify the limitations of these sensors, look for new candidate sensors, and consider a combination of different types of sensors to further improve the accuracy of detection. This is very challenging to achieve through clinical studies on pregnant women. The "ground truth" for FM can only be provided (partially) with ultrasound testing, and repeated testing of multiple sensors against ultrasound is not feasible ethically or logistically in human studies. We, therefore, approach this problem by enabling extensive testing of sensors and their combinations, prior to a clinical testing phase, through the development of an FM simulator. The only effort towards the development of an FM simulator to date has been reported by Sazali et al. [27], who proposed a very simple design consisting of a servo-controlled kicking mechanism and a flat rubber sheet as a maternal abdomen model. However, to be able to test sensors for an FM monitor, the vibration characteristics of a maternal abdomen due to fetal kicks need to be replicated by the simulator.

In the present study, we design and fabricate a novel FM simulator considering the geometrical and material properties of a maternal abdomen to imitate its vibration characteristics. The design also includes a stretching mechanism to simulate the pre-stress present in a gravid uterus and a kicking mechanism to replicate fetal kicks in terms of the speed, duration, and reaction force from the abdomen wall. To run the simulator, we develop a software application that allows the design of simulated kicks using wide-ranging features. Finally, as a case study, we investigate performances of three vibration sensors, namely an accelerometer, an acoustic sensor, and a piezoelectric diaphragm, analyzing their relative performances when used on the simulator under various input conditions.

2. Design of the Fetal Movement Simulator

The mechanical design of the FM simulator consists of three main components—maternal abdomen model, support structure and stretching mechanism, and kicking mechanism (Figure 1). Detailed descriptions of these components along with the data acquisition and software systems used in the simulator are provided in this section.

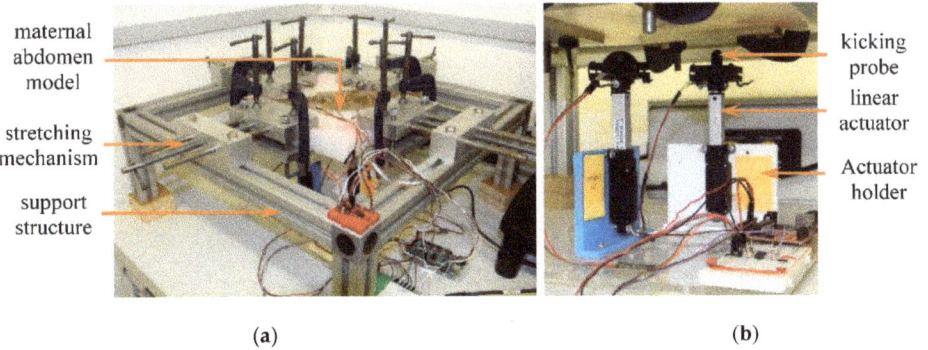

Figure 1. Fully assembled fetal movement (FM) simulator: (**a**) maternal abdomen model, and support structure and stretching mechanism, (**b**) kicking mechanism beneath the abdomen membrane.

2.1. Design of the Maternal Abdomen Model

A single layer membrane with clamped edges was assumed to model the vibrations of the gravid abdomen due to fetal kicks. To understand which material and geometrical properties influence vibration characteristics, a mathematical model of the membrane vibration was studied. The approximate analytical formula for the natural frequency of vibration of a curved rectangular membrane with clamped edges (Figure 2), as derived by P. J. Palmer [28] using the Rayleigh's method, is given as follows:

$$f_n = \frac{1}{2\pi}\sqrt{\frac{D}{\rho h}\left\{72\left(\frac{7}{a^4}+\frac{7}{b^4}+\frac{4}{a^2 b^2}\right)+\frac{12}{h^2}\left(\frac{1}{A^2}+\frac{1}{B^2}+\frac{2\mu}{AB}\right)\right\}}, \qquad (1)$$

where
f_n = natural frequency of vibration (Hz)
A, B = radii of curvature (m)
a, b = length of sides (m)
h = membrane thickness (m)

$D = \frac{Eh^3}{12(1-\mu^2)}$ = flexure rigidity (Pa·m^3)
E = modulus of elasticity (Pa)
μ = Poisson's ratio
ρ = density (kg/m^3)

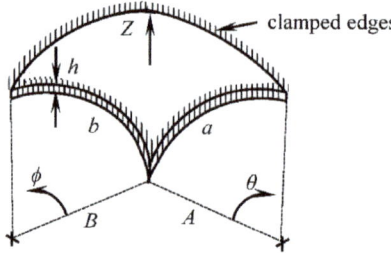

Figure 2. Geometry and boundary conditions of the curved single-layer membrane model of a maternal abdomen.

The region between the fetus and the exterior surface of the maternal abdomen consists of three layers, namely fetal membrane, uterine wall, and abdominal wall. Table 1 lists the previously reported material and geometrical property values of these layers relevant to the formula for the natural frequency of vibration of the membrane (Equation (1)).

Table 1. Previously reported values of material and geometrical properties of maternal abdomens.

Layer	Material Properties, Mean (Min–Max)			Geometrical Properties, Mean (Min–Max)	
	Young's Modulus, (kPa)	Poisson's Ratio	Density (Kg/m^3)	Thickness (mm)	Radius (mm)
Fetal membrane [29–31]	7100 (3200–13,700)	0.40	–	0.19 (0.14–0.28)	–
Uterine wall (30 week gestational age) [30–35]	586	0.40	1052	6.90 (5.0–10.50)	99 (89–117)
Abdominal wall [36–38]	21 (13.6–28.4)	0.50	973.61 (970.13–976.75)	31.40 (7.80–63.0)	–

Table 1. Cont.

Layer	Material Properties, Mean (Min–Max)			Geometrical Properties, Mean (Min–Max)	
	Young's Modulus, (kPa)	Poisson's Ratio	Density (Kg/m^3)	Thickness (mm)	Radius (mm)
Total (mean)	–	–	–	38.49 (12.94–73.78)	–
Weighted average	151.37 (132–224)	0.48	982.86 (980.02–985.42)	–	–

In the cases where explicit mentions of the range of property values were not found, the minimum and maximum values of the properties presented in Table 1 were calculated using "mean ± 2 × standard deviation" formula. The properties of the fetal membrane were obtained from the literature by considering it as a single layer of chorioamniotic material, whose outer surface is attached to the uterine wall. The intrauterine radius was calculated using the previously reported values of intrauterine volume [34] and assuming the spherical shape of the uterus [35]. The thickness of the abdominal wall was calculated by adding the thicknesses of the abdominal muscle and fat tissues [36]. The density of the abdominal muscle was taken from the values reported by Rachel et al. [38]. Using computer tomography images of the abdomen of nearly 2000 subjects, they obtained the density values in the Hounsfield unit (HU), which represents the attenuation of X-ray by the material and is proportional to the physical density of the material. To convert the HU value into Kg/m^3, the linear fitting of the experimental data of the density (Kg/m^3) and the corresponding HU value for soft human tissues presented by Uwe et al. [37] were used. Finally, the weighted average of the abdominal muscle and fat densities [37] with respect to the corresponding mean thicknesses [36] was considered as the abdominal wall density.

Weighted average values of the material properties with respect to the mean thicknesses of the corresponding layers were considered to model the single-layer maternal abdomen. Since the density of the fetal membrane was not found in the literature, only uterine and abdominal walls were considered to calculate the weighted average density of the single-layer abdomen model. For simplicity of modeling, equal radii of curvature and equal lengths of sides in both directions were considered. The inner radius of the fetal membrane was calculated by deducting its thickness from the intrauterine radius. The mean radius of curvature of the abdomen was calculated to be 118.1 mm by adding half of the overall thickness of the fetal membrane, uterine wall, and abdominal wall with the inner radius of the fetal membrane. Finally, the lengths of the sides of the membrane were considered as equal to the circumference of a semicircle with a radius equal to the radius of the abdomen. With the mean values of the above mentioned geometrical and material properties, the natural frequency of undamped free vibration of the single-layer curved model of a maternal abdomen was calculated as 33.46 Hz using Equation (1).

After a preliminary comparison of relevant characteristics of some suitable candidate materials (e.g., silicone, thermoplastic elastomer, alginate gel, etc.) for modeling the maternal abdomen, silicone was selected due to its durability, ease of manufacturing, and availability of variants with required material properties. The uniaxial tensile test was performed on three variants of silicone, namely Dragon skin FX-pro, Dragon Skin 10 NV, and Dragon Skin 10 medium, obtained from the Smooth-on, Inc. (Macungie, PA, USA), following the ASTM D412 standard. The modulus of elasticity was determined from the stress vs. strain curve at 100% elongation (Figure 3a), and the Poisson's ratio was determined by analyzing images of the specimens before and after the elongation (Figure 3b).

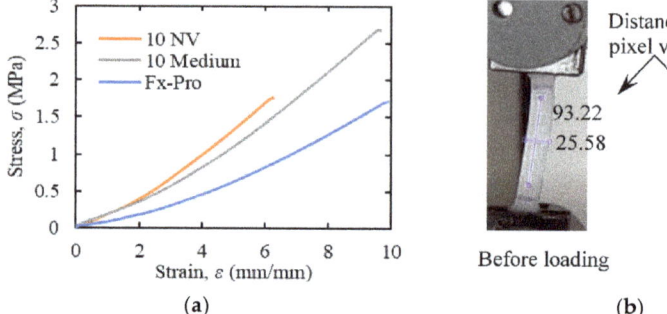

Figure 3. Uniaxial tensile test results for the silicon materials: (**a**) stress-strain diagram, (**b**) pixel values of the longitudinal and lateral dimensions of a specimen before and after applying a tensile load to calculate the Poisson's ratio of the material. ASTM D412 standard was followed to perform the tests.

The uniaxial tensile test was performed on three samples for each of the silicone variants, and the median value was considered as the average property value for that variant (Table 2). Based on the material properties of different variants of silicone (Table 2) and the property requirements for the maternal abdomen model (Table 1), Dragon Skin 10 NV was selected for modeling the abdomen.

Table 2. Material properties of three variants of silicone. Moduli of elasticity and the Poisson's ratios were determined from the uniaxial tensile tests, and the densities were determined by measuring the weights of known volumes of the materials.

Material	Modulus of Elasticity, $E_{100\%}$ (KPa)				Poisson's Ratio, μ				Density, ρ (Kg/m^3)
	Sample 1	Sample 2	Sample 3	Median	Sample 1	Sample 2	Sample 3	Median	
Dragon Skin FX-Pro	81.3	90.9	148.3	90.9	0.47	0.51	0.52	0.51	1120
Dragon Skin 10 NV	207.4	185.5	189.4	185.5	0.45	0.49	0.48	0.48	1030
Dragon Skin 10 Medium	189.4	182.7	196.1	189.4	0.41	0.46	0.46	0.46	1210

For design simplification of the support structure and stretching mechanism, a flat rectangular membrane (Figure 4) with the natural frequency of vibration equal to the natural frequency of vibration of the curved abdomen model (i.e., 33.46 Hz) was used in the simulator. For a flat rectangular membrane with clamped edges, the approximate analytical solution for the natural frequency of free damped vibration, as derived by Milomir M. S. by using the Galerkin's method [39], is given as

$$f_{nd} = \frac{1}{2\pi} \sqrt{\frac{\wedge D}{\rho h a^3 b} - \left(\frac{k}{2\rho h}\right)^2}, \quad (2)$$

where
f_{nd} = natural frequency of free damped vibration (Hz)
$\wedge = 36.11^2$ (square membrane, 1st mode of vibration)
k = coefficient of damping (N·s/m).

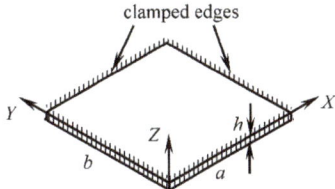

Figure 4. Geometry and boundary conditions of the single-layer flat rectangular model of a maternal abdomen.

Neglecting the effect of damping ($k = 0$), the natural frequency of undamped free vibration of the flat membrane can be obtained from Equation (2) as

$$f_n = \frac{1}{2\pi}\sqrt{\frac{\Lambda D}{\rho h a^3 b}}. \tag{3}$$

For the selected silicone material (Dragon Skin 10 NV), the length of the sides of a square membrane with the natural frequency of vibration equal to the natural frequency of the curved abdomen model (= 33.46 Hz) was calculated to be 171 mm using Equation (3).

Expressions for the damping ratio (ζ) and the time constant (τ) were also derived from the solution of Milomir M. S. [39] to investigate the transient characteristics of the membrane vibration, which are given as follows

$$\zeta = \sqrt{1 - \frac{\rho h a^3 b}{\Lambda D}(2\pi f_{nd})^2}, \tag{4}$$

$$\tau = \frac{2\rho h}{k}. \tag{5}$$

2.2. Design of the Support Structure and Stretching Mechanism

The support structure consists of four clamping mechanisms to hold the silicone membrane from four sides and an aluminum Rexroth frame to support the clamps and provide the required elevation for the kicking mechanism to fit beneath the membrane (Figure 5). To assemble the frame, three-way connectors with self-tapping screws were used at each of the four corners of the frame. Each clamp is attached to the frame using two T-nuts to allow for the clamp attachment piece to slide along the strut and provide added flexibility in the positioning of the clamp. The clamp components are made of aluminum bars and are connected through mild steel rods. The upper jaw of the clamp is connected to the attachment piece through a 10 mm lead screw at the middle and two 10 mm non-threaded stabilizing rods at two sides. G-clamps were used to secure the upper and lower jaws tightly after connecting them through two 8 mm non-threaded vertical rods.

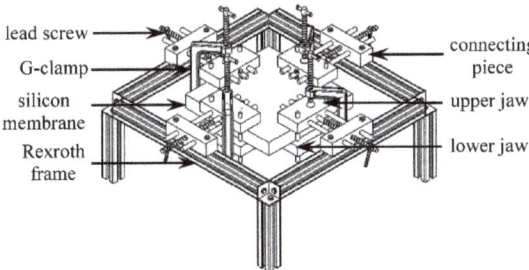

Figure 5. Fully assembled CAD design of the support structure and stretching mechanism.

To simulate the strained condition of a gravid abdomen, the membrane was stretched by rotating the lead screw after clamping. The tensile load was assumed to be uniform throughout the membrane and was calculated from the elongation of the membrane. For this purpose, the relation between the elongation and the tensile stress was derived. Considering isotropic material property and obeyance to Hooke's law, the relationship between stresses and strains for biaxial loading can be given as

$$\epsilon_x = \frac{1}{E}(\sigma_x - \mu\sigma_y), \tag{6a}$$

$$\epsilon_y = \frac{1}{E}(\sigma_y - \mu\sigma_x), \tag{6b}$$

where

ϵ_x, ϵ_y = normal strains along X and Y axes, respectively
σ_x, σ_y = normal stresses along X and Y axes, respectively (Pa).

For a square membrane with the length of side a and equal tensile stress (σ) along both axes, the formula for the elongation (δ) can be derived from Equations (6a) & (6b) as

$$\delta = \frac{a\sigma}{E}(1 - \mu). \tag{7}$$

Uterine wall tensions for different gestational ages (obtained from the literature review) and the elongations of the membrane required to produce the corresponding tensions, which were calculated by using Equation (7) and the material properties of the membrane (Table 2), are listed in Table 3. Applying these elongations, the stretched condition of the maternal abdomen for different gestational ages can be created in the FM simulator.

Table 3. Uterine wall tensions at different gestational ages and the corresponding elongations required along both axes (X, Y) simultaneously to create that tension in the membrane.

Property	Gestational Age (Week)		
	20	25	30
Maximum uterine wall tensile stress, mean (range) (KPa) [34]	11.9 (5.8–19.5)	16.3 (9.5–24.2)	22.8 (14.2–33.3)
Elongation necessary to apply the stress, mean (range) (mm)	0.033 a (0.017–0.059) a	0.046 a (0.017–0.059) a	0.0639 a (0.043–0.1) a

2.3. Design of the Kicking Mechanism

The kicking mechanism consists of two sets of actuators, sensor holders, kicking probes, and actuator holders along with a base to support the whole mechanism (Figure 6a). Actuonix (Victoria, BC, Canada) L16-R linear servo actuator (Model No.: L16-50-63-6-R) was used to simulate the fetal kicks in the simulator. The position of the servo was controlled by 5V pulse-width modulated (PWM) signals from an Arduino Mega board (from Arduino, Torino, Italy). The whole process was automated via MATLAB's "writePosition ()" function, which takes the position of the actuator as a position variable that varies between 0 (fully retracted) and 1 (fully extended). To accurately control the position, the actuators were calibrated by measuring their stroke length for different values of the position variable. When connected to a 5V dc supply, the maximum stroke length and the no-load speed of the actuators were found to be 146 mm and 12.43 mm/s, respectively.

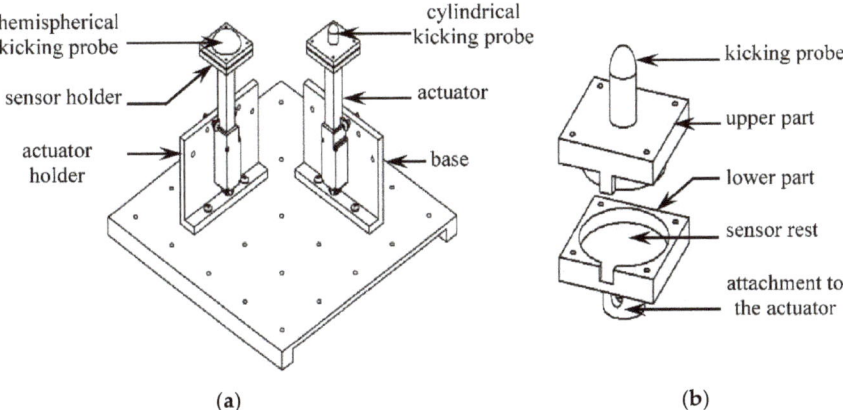

Figure 6. CAD design of the (**a**) fully assembled kicking mechanism, (**b**) sensor holder.

The actuator holder is a 3D-printed structure to hold the actuator in proper position and orientation beneath the silicone membrane (Figure 6a). The holes in the vertical and horizontal planes of the actuator holder serve as the points of attachment for the actuator and the base, respectively. The actuator can be positioned along three different angular orientations in a holder relative to the horizontal plane, namely 90° (perpendicular), 60°, and 55°, to generate kicks with different angles of impact. The base of the kicking mechanism is made of a 250 mm × 250 mm × 5 mm acrylic sheet with 4 mm diameter holes distributed along the whole horizontal plane to ensure multiple arrangements of kicking positions when both the actuators run simultaneously.

The sensor holder consists of a two-part sandwich-like structure that encloses a force sensor in the middle (Figure 6b) to measure the reaction force due to kicking. Piezoresistive force sensor FlexiForce A401 from Tekscan Inc. (South Boston, MA, USA, 2019) was selected to be used for this purpose due to its suitability of dimension (25.4 mm diameter), good repeatability (< ±2.5%), and appropriate range of measurement (0–111 N) [40]. Two force sensors were used with two actuators, and their calibrations were performed using a set of known calibration weights.

The kicking probe is located on the top of the sensor holder and is 3D printed as an integrated structure with the sensor holder (Figure 6b). A 10 mm diameter cylindrical probe was used to represent the geometry of a 20-week old fetal foot [31], and a 30 mm diameter hemispherical probe was used to characterizes the geometry of an older (30 weeks) fetal foot.

2.4. Data Acquisition System

USB 6212, a multifunction I/O device from National Instruments (Austin, TX, USA), was used as the data acquisition (DAQ) system for the FM simulator. It has 16 analog input channels, which can sample data at a maximum rate of 400 kHz for a single channel with a resolution of 16 bit. The output pins of the force sensors were connected to a voltage divider circuit followed by a voltage follower circuit (LM 358 op-amp), and the output from the voltage follower was connected to the analog input channel of the DAQ system as shown in Figure 7. A sampling rate of 2 kHz was used for recording the data during the experiments.

The recorded data from the force sensors were first passed through a low pass filter (4th order zero-phase Butterworth filter, 50 Hz cut-off frequency) and then converted into force values based on the calibration results of the corresponding force sensor. Additionally, the offset error in the sensor output due to the initial compression of the sensor in the sensor holder was subtracted from the readings.

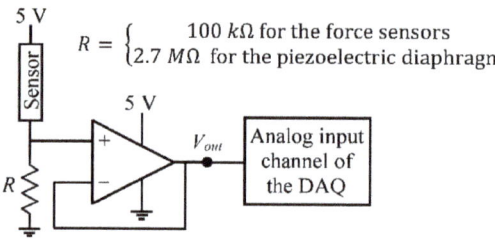

Figure 7. Diagram of the circuit used between the sensor output and the DAQ input in the cases of the force sensors and the piezoelectric diaphragm. LM 358 op-amp was used to design the voltage follower circuit.

2.5. Software for the Simulator

A MATLAB (MathWorks, Natick, MA, USA) -based software application (Fetal Kick Simulator) was developed to run the simulator and record data from the sensors (Figure 8). The application controls the actuators by sending PWM signals from an Arduino Mega board based on a user-defined kick profile. Several parameters, such as the number of kicks, desired wall displacement, pause at the peak, etc., are inputted by the user. Additionally, users can select one of four defined kick modes from a drop-down list in the graphical user interface (GUI) of the software to specify the sequence of movements of the actuators (Table 4).

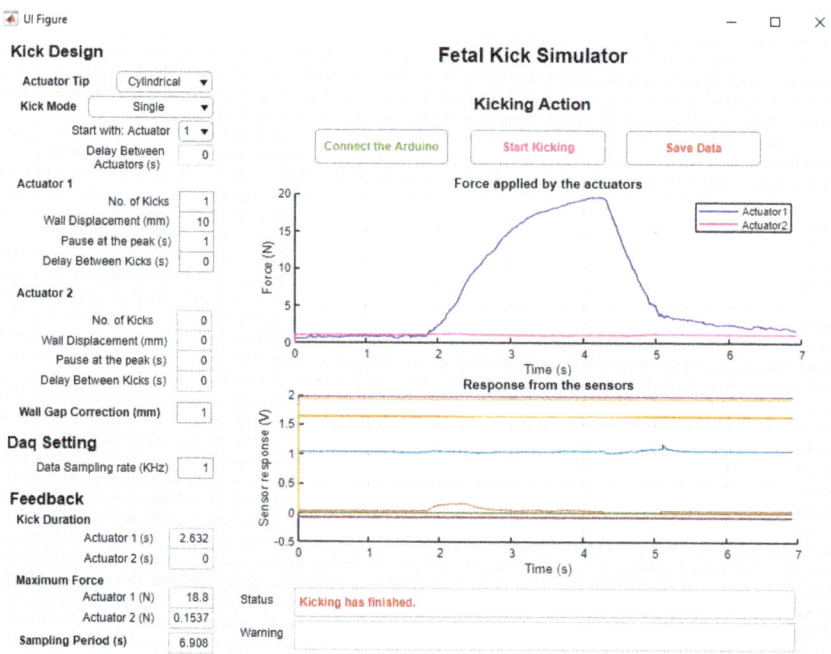

Figure 8. The graphical user interface of the software application developed to run the FM simulator.

Table 4. Description of different "Kick Mode" available in the "Fetal Kick Simulator" software.

Kick Mode	Description
Single	Only one actuator operates in this mode.
Dual: Simultaneous	Two actuators operate simultaneously in this mode. The number of kicks for both the actuators must be equal, and they will start simultaneously at the beginning of each kick.
Dual: Consecutive	Actuators run consecutively one after another.
Dual: Random	Actuators start randomly based on the respective user-defined kick profile.

The sensor data are recorded by the DAQ system in the background and are sent to the computer via serial communication in every 0.25 s. The software updates the data and plots them instantaneously to display almost real-time changes in sensor outputs. At the end of the recording, the user can save the data before starting the next recording. A video recording of the hardware and the software systems running simultaneously is added as Supplementary Material with the paper.

3. Characteristics of the Simulator

After holding the silicone membrane with the gripping mechanism, the area of the flat abdomen model was found as 167 × 167 mm. For simulating the stretched condition of a 30 weeks pregnant abdomen, a bi-axial loading of 22.8 kPa was applied to the membrane through elongations of 11 mm along both axes of the membrane, which was calculated using the formula mentioned in Table 3. The thickness of the membrane was measured as 39 mm. With these geometrical properties and the material properties mentioned in Table 2, the natural frequency of undamped free vibration of the silicone membrane was calculated to be 31.24 Hz (by using Equation (3)), which is very close to the calculated frequency of vibration of the curved abdomen model (33.46 Hz). However, because of the effect of damping, the natural frequency of free vibration of the membrane, as measured by the acoustic sensor and the accelerometer, was found to be 18.7 Hz (Table 5), which is much lower than the calculated natural frequency.

Table 5. Vibration characteristics of the testbed abdomen model. Ten sets of data were used to obtain the natural frequency of the abdomen model.

Property	Value
Natural frequency obtained from the accelerometer, (mean ± SD) (Hz)	18.70 ± 0.10
Natural frequency obtained from the acoustic sensor, (mean ± SD) (Hz)	18.75 ± 0.17
Damping ratio, ζ	0.80
Time constant, τ (ms)	6.40

To understand the transient characteristics of the membrane vibration, the damping ratio was calculated as 0.80 using Equation (4), and the time constant was calculated as 6.4 ms using Equation (5). This value of the damping ratio signifies that the vibration of the abdomen membrane is an underdamped case (as $\zeta < 1$), and it will decay rapidly (as ζ is close to 1). The time constant of 6.4 ms signifies that in the case of free damped vibration, the amplitude will decay by more than 99% of its initial value within a period of 32 ms ($= 5\tau$).

Table 6 shows the comparison of the characteristics of real fetal kicks as reported by Verbruggen et al. [30] with the simulated kicks obtained from the simulator with the cylindrical and the hemispherical kicking probes. For the simulated kicks, the durations presented in this table are the minimum kick durations obtained by running the actuators at their maximum speeds (12.43 mm/s at the no-load condition), which can be easily increased by slowing down the actuators. As the reaction force from the membrane depends on the location of the kick impact point relative to the clamped edges, 40 measurements were taken at different locations of the membrane to calculate the average kick reaction force for each value of the wall displacement. These results demonstrate that for the higher value of the wall displacement (close to the upper limit of the range), the cylindrical kicking probe produces reaction forces similar to 20-week old fetuses, and the hemispherical kicking probe produces reaction forces similar to 30-week old fetuses. However, for the lower value of the wall displacement (close to the lower limit of the range), the hemispherical kicking probe produces reaction forces more similar to 20-week old fetuses.

Table 6. Comparison of the characteristics of real and simulated fetal kicks. Forty sets of measurements at different locations of the membrane were used to calculate the average kick reaction force for each wall displacement.

Kicking Entity	Uterine Wall Displacement, (Mean ± SD) (mm)	Kick Duration, (Mean ± SD) (s)	Kick Reaction, (Mean ± SD) (N)
20-week old fetus [30]	11.78 ± 4.72	2.65 ± 0.35	28.85 ± 1.88
30-week old fetus [30]	11.52 ± 1.47	2.95 ± 0.74	46.64 ± 5.30
Cylindrical probe, 10 mm diameter	10	1.63	14.84 ± 1.76
	15	2.45	33.15 ± 3.92
Hemispherical probe, 30 mm diameter	10	1.69	26.01 ± 1.66
	15	2.53	44.20 ± 2.37

To verify the reliability of the current FM simulator in producing repeatable and consistent simulations of abdominal vibrations due to fetal kicks, multiple measurements were used to obtain the simulator characteristics as reported in Tables 5 and 6. Table 5 shows that the measurements of the natural frequency of vibration of the simulator abdomen model obtained independently from two different sensors (accelerometer and acoustic sensor) are very close to each other (18.70 Hz for the accelerometer and 18.75 Hz for the acoustic sensor), and the standard deviations (SD) (obtained from 10 measurements) are very small (0.10 for the accelerometer and 0.17 for the acoustic sensor). Similarly, the standard deviations of the kick reaction forces (obtained from 40 sets of measurements) are also quite reasonable (ranges from 1.66 to 3.92 N) considering the mean value of the forces (ranges from 14.84 to 44.2 N) and the variation of the membrane resistance due to the location of the kick impact point (Table 6). These results show that the performance of the simulator is consistent and repeatable under the experimental conditions reported in this paper.

4. Testing of the Sensors on the Simulator

The developed FM simulator can be used to test any kind of candidate sensors for FM monitors to evaluate their ability to detect abdominal vibrations due to fetal kicks. In this study, three types of passive vibration sensors, namely an accelerometer, an acoustic sensor, and a piezoelectric diaphragm (Figure 9), were tested, and the outputs from these sensors were stored for post-processing. A sampling rate of 2 kHz was used for recording the data during the experiments.

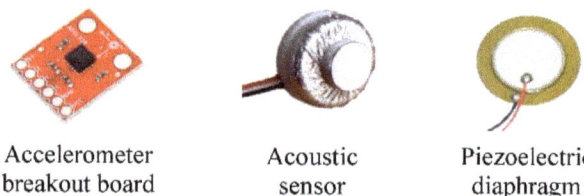

Figure 9. Vibration sensors that were tested on the FM simulator as a case study in this research. The detailed specification of the accelerometer breakout board and the piezoelectric diaphragm can be found in [41,42], respectively. The design of the acoustic sensor is adopted from [43].

4.1. Selection of the Sensors

The breakout board for ADXL335 from SparkFun Electronics (Niwot, CO, USA, 2014) was selected as a suitable accelerometer for testing. ADXL335 is a 3-axis MEMS accelerometer from Analog Devices Inc. (Norwood, MA, USA, 2009), which has a range and sensitivity of ±3 g and 300 mV/g, respectively, with extremely low noise and power consumption rate [41]. The breakout board includes 0.1 µF capacitors connected to the output pins of the sensor axes to limit their bandwidth to 50 Hz [41].

The acoustic sensor tested on the FM simulator is similar to the sensors used by Lai et al. [26] in their wearable FM monitor. The design of this sensor was originally adapted from the design first presented by Posatskiy and Chau [43]. It consists of a diaphragm covering a sealed chamber and a microphone (SPU1410LR5H-QB, Knowles Acoustics, Itasca, IL, USA, 2012). The chamber is a 3D printed structure, which is dimensioned to capture low-frequency vibrations. The microphone is positioned at the opposite end of the chamber to record the pressure changes when the diaphragm is disturbed. A frequency sweep using a custom-made vibration rig has shown that the sensor can detect low-frequency vibrations ranging from 1 Hz to 100 Hz with the peak response lying below 50 Hz [44].

A 20 mm diameter piezoelectric diaphragm from Murata Electronics (manufacturer part no. 7BB-20-6L0, Kyoto, Japan, 2009) was selected as the third type of vibration sensor to be tested on the FM simulator. This sensor consists of a 14 mm diameter piezoelectric ceramic plate glued to a 20 mm diameter brass plate [42]. Two lead wires are soldered to the plates, which are used to measure the voltage difference between them. Similar to the force sensors used in the kicking mechanism, the output from the piezoelectric diaphragm was connected to the analog input channel of the DAQ system through a voltage divider and a voltage follower circuit (LM 358 op-amp), as shown in Figure 7. Output ports of the rest of the sensors were directly connected to the analog input channels of the DAQ system.

4.2. Processing of Sensor Data

Recorded data from the sensors were first passed through a bandpass filter (4th order zero-phase Butterworth filter) with a suitable passband frequency of 1–40 Hz, which was selected based on the expected frequency of vibration of the membrane due to kicking as calculated in Section 2.1. In the case of the accelerometer, further processing of data was done on the magnitude (Euclidian norm) of the acceleration, A, which was calculated as

$$A = \sqrt{A_x^2 + A_y^2 + A_z^2}, \tag{8}$$

where A_x, A_y, and A_z represent the components of acceleration along the X, Y, and Z axes, respectively.

Matrices that were used to compare the performance of different sensors are sensor response, signal energy, signal-to-noise ratio (SNR), and the dominant frequency mode in the output signal. The following steps were performed to calculate the signal energy and the SNR:

1. A noise estimate, e, was determined by taking the average of the absolute value of sensor response (V_i) for a window of time w (=2 s) during a period when no kick action was going on.

$$e = \frac{1}{F_s w} \sum_{i=1}^{F_s w} |V_i|, \tag{9}$$

where F_s is the frequency of data sampling. The time window was taken at a period sufficiently away (= 6 s) from the previous kick action to ensure the complete decay of oscillation due to the previous kick.

2. The signal due to kick, S, was defined as the part of sensor response that exceeds the threshold level $h = me$, where m is a multiplier evaluated from trial and error:

$$S = \{x \in |V| \, | \, x > h\}. \tag{10}$$

$m = 5$ was found to generate the most suitable threshold value for the majority of the cases, and this value was, therefore, used for all the datasets. Figure 10 demonstrates the application of this algorithm in the case of acoustic sensor response due to a simulated kick.

3. The rest of the data were considered as noise N:

$$N = \{x \in V \mid x \leq h\}. \tag{11}$$

4. Energy, E, of the signal and the noise were calculated as

$$E_W = \sum_{x \in W} |x_i|^2, \tag{12}$$

where $W = S$ for signal and $W = N$ for noise.

5. Finally, the SNR was calculated as

$$SNR = 10 \log_{10}\left(\frac{E_S/n_S - E_N/n_N}{E_N/n_N}\right) (dB), \tag{13}$$

where n_S and n_N are the number of elements in the signal and the noise data, respectively. The noise power was assumed to be constant throughout the whole sensor response. It was, therefore, subtracted from the overall signal power to determine the power due to the kick action alone.

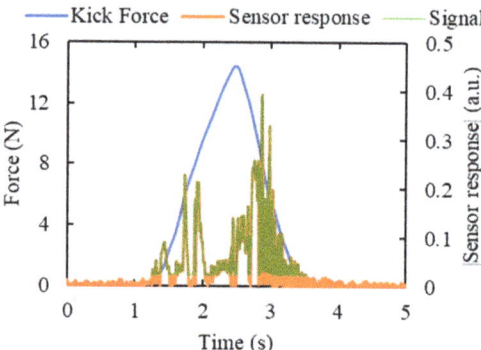

Figure 10. Determination of the part of the sensor response that is considered as the signal due to kicking based on the condition mentioned in Equation (10). Response from the acoustic sensor due to a simulated kick of 10 mm wall displacement using the cylindrical kicking probe is used in this figure. The distance between the sensor and the kick impact point was 5 cm.

5. Results and Discussion

This section describes the results obtained from the performance testing of three vibration sensors, namely an accelerometer, an acoustic sensor, and a piezoelectric diaphragm, using the FM simulator. All the sensors were attached tightly to the exterior surface of the simulator membrane using adhesive tapes, and the center of the membrane was maintained as the middle point between the sensor and the kick impact point. All kicks were produced at the maximum actuator speed.

5.1. Comparative Responses from Different Sensors

To study the comparative responses, all the sensors were placed at a distance of 5 cm from the kick impact point. Simulated kicks of 14 mm wall displacement were applied using the hemispherical probe to replicate kick characteristics of a 30-week old fetus (Table 6). Kicks of a 30-week old fetus were chosen here, because this time point provided the best match between actual and simulated fetal kicks, as shown in Table 6. Sensor performances are displayed in Figure 11 in terms of sensor response, spectrogram, and power spectral density (PSD) distribution. Hann window of length 0.5 s and 80% overlap between the segments were used to obtain the spectrograms, which resulted in frequency and time resolutions of 2 Hz and 100 ms, respectively. The PSD distributions were obtained using the Welch method and a dataset of 10 similar kicks. Hann window of length 1s and 50% overlap between segments were used to generate the PSD distributions.

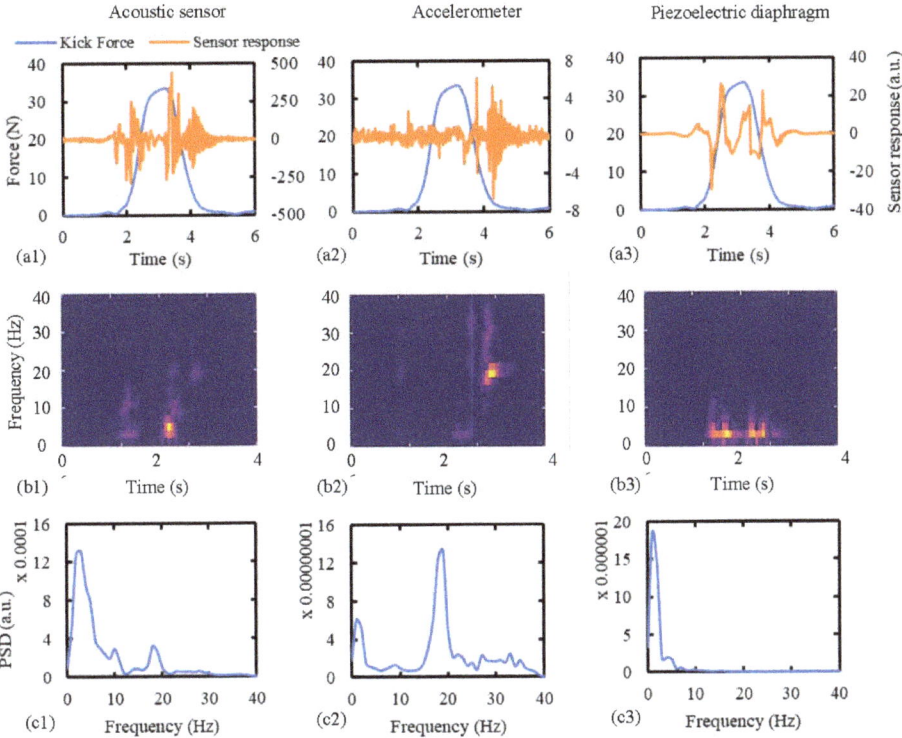

Figure 11. Comparison of signal characteristics of the sensors due to simulated fetal kicks in terms of: (**a1,a2,a3**) sensor response, (**b1,b2,b3**) spectrogram, and (**c1,c2,c3**) power spectral density (PSD) distribution. The abdomen model was subjected to simulated kicks of a 30-week fetus and the sensors were attached to a distance of 5 cm from the kick impact point. Datasets of 10 repeated kicks were used to generate the PSD distributions.

Figure 11a shows that the acoustic sensor and the piezoelectric diaphragm were responsive to the kick during the majority of the kick duration. Though the accelerometer detected the starting of the kick, it was mainly responsive near the end of the return stroke, which is the period when the membrane starts vibrating freely. This demonstrates the accelerometer's inability to detect membrane vibrations during the period of forced movements by the kicking probe. This can also be observed from the spectrograms of the sensor responses (Figure 11b), which show that after the 4th second (near the end of kick) the membrane was vibrating at around 19 Hz, which is equal to the natural frequency of vibration of the membrane. Both the acoustic sensor and the accelerometer picked up this vibration, but the piezoelectric diaphragm did not show any response. This characteristic of the sensors is further observed in the PSD distribution curves (Figure 11c), which show that the power of the piezoelectric signal was completely concentrated below 10 Hz. In the cases of the acoustic sensor and the accelerometer, concentrations of signal power around 2 Hz and 19 Hz were observed. However, the main peak occurred around 2 Hz in the case of the acoustic sensor and around 19 Hz in the case of the accelerometer. This PSD distribution of the acoustic signal also conforms with the PSD distribution obtained from the acoustic signals due to the real fetal kicks, as reported by Lai et al. [26].

5.2. Effect of Wall Displacement and Kick Distance on the Sensor Response

To study the effect of wall displacement on the sensor performance, all sensors were placed 5 cm away from the kick impact point and were subjected to kicks of wall displacements ranging from 2–14 mm using the hemispherical kicking probe. Each kick was repeated 10 times to evaluate the mean and the standard deviation of the output signal parameters, and the obtained results are shown in Figure 12 in terms of SNR, signal energy, and the dominant frequency mode. It can be seen from this figure that in the cases of the acoustic sensor and piezoelectric diaphragm, both SNR and signal energy increased with the increase in wall displacement (Figure 12(a1,c1)). For the accelerometer, SNR decreased with the increase in wall displacement, and signal energy initially decreased and then increased with the increase in wall displacement (Figure 12(b1)). Additionally, changes in these parameters (SNR and signal energy) were comparatively smaller in the case of the accelerometer compared to the other two sensors. This happened because the accelerometer is mainly responsive to the free vibration of the membrane (at around 19 Hz), which is much less affected by the change in wall displacement compared to the vibrations during the forced movement of the membrane. This is also evident from the consistent dominant mode of acceleration signal around 19 Hz (Figure 12(b2)) with the increase in wall displacement. The increase in wall displacement also did not affect the dominant mode in the case of the piezoelectric diaphragm, which maintained a value between 1–2 Hz (Figure 12(c2)). Finally, in the case of the acoustic sensor, the dominant mode changed from around 19 Hz to a lower frequency value below 3 Hz with the increase in wall displacement (Figure 12(a2)), which demonstrates the acoustic sensor's ability to respond effectively to both the frequency ranges and the fact that the duration of the low-frequency vibration increases more with the increase in the wall displacement compared to the duration of the free vibration of the membrane.

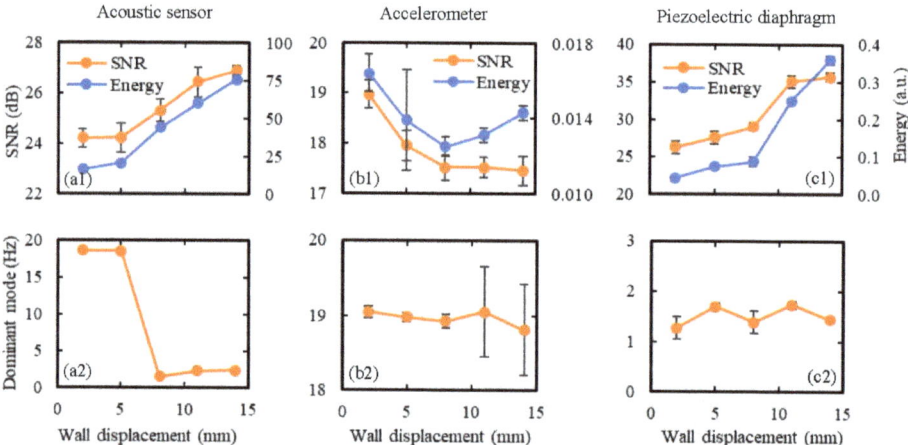

Figure 12. Effect of wall displacement on the sensor performance in terms of: (**a1,b1,c1**) SNR and signal energy, and (**a2,b2,c2**) the dominant frequency mode. The sensors were attached to the model abdomen membrane at 5 cm away from the kick impact point, and the wall displacement due to kicking was varied from 2 to 14 mm using the hemispherical kicking probe. Ten sets of data were taken for each wall displacement and the results are shown in terms of the mean values as the data points on the graph and the standard deviations as the error bars.

To study the effect of the distance between the sensor and the kick impact point (i.e., kick distance) on the sensor performance, the kick distance was varied from 0–15 cm, while keeping the wall displacement fixed at 10 mm. Again, the hemispherical kicking probe was used, and each kick was repeated 10 times to evaluate the mean and the standard deviation of output signal parameters. The results of the tests are shown in Figure 13 in terms of SNR, signal energy, and the dominant frequency mode. As expected, both SNR and signal energy decreased gradually with the increase in kick distance for all three sensors as the vibration of the membrane becomes weaker with the increase in the sensor's distance from the kick impact point. There was no significant effect of the kick distance on the dominant signal mode for any of the sensors. Again, changes in SNR and signal energy were much smaller in the case of the accelerometer compared to the acoustic sensor and the piezoelectric diaphragm.

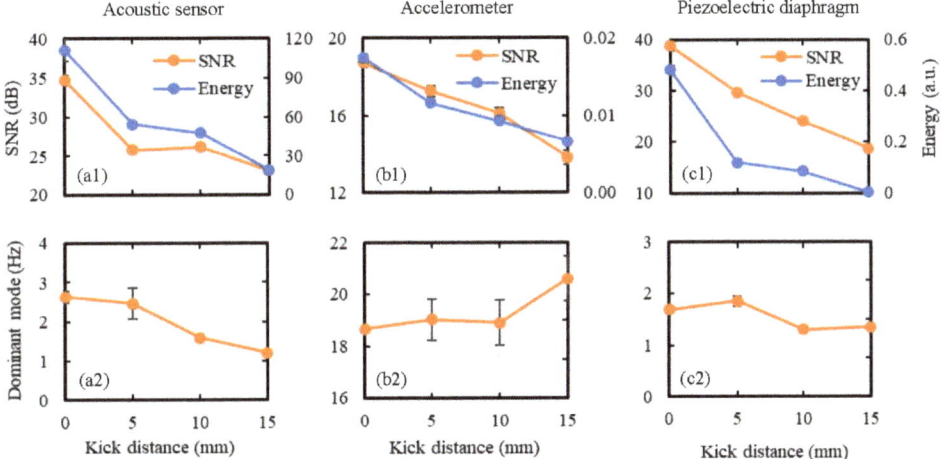

Figure 13. Effect of kick distance (i.e., the distance between the sensor and the kick impact point) on the sensor performance in terms of: (**a1,b1,c1**) SNR and signal energy, and (**a2,b2,c2**) the dominant frequency mode. The kick distance was varied from 0–15 cm while the abdomen was subjected to kicks of 10 mm wall displacement using the hemispherical kicking probe. Ten sets of data were taken for each kick distance, and the results are shown in terms of the mean values as the data points on the graph and the standard deviations as the error bars.

Finally, the best SNR was achieved from the piezoelectric diaphragm in most of the cases, as shown in both Figures 12 and 13, meaning that the piezoelectrical diaphragm produced better signal quality compared to the other two sensors. The accelerometer signal was found to be least affected by the changes in wall displacement and kick distance, which indicates that it will be difficult to predict the location and intensity of kicks accurately using a fully accelerometer-based FM monitor.

5.3. The Input Thresholds for the Sensors

The input threshold values of the sensors, i.e., the minimum input value recognized by the sensors, are expressed in terms of the minimum wall displacements due to kicking required by the sensors to recognize the kick. These values were determined by placing the sensors at the maximum possible kick distance (for the simulator) and subjecting them to the minimum possible wall displacement (for the simulator) by the weakest (in terms of the produced kick impact) available kicking probe for the current FM simulator. A length of 20 cm was the maximum possible consistent distance between the sensor and the kick impact point for the simulator to avoid attaching sensors close to the gripping mechanisms at the boundaries. Due to the 0.4 mm repeatability of the actuators [45], 0.5 mm was considered as the lowest reliable wall displacement that can be produced by the current kicking mechanism. The cylindrical kicking probe was considered as the weaker kicking probe as it produces less kick reaction force for any specific wall displacement compared to the hemispherical kicking probe (Table 6). All the sensors were, therefore, attached to a distance of 20 cm away from the kick impact point along a diagonal of the membrane and were subjected to a kick of 0.5 mm wall displacement using the cylindrical kicking probe. The obtained results are shown in Figure 14a, which shows that, while the acoustic sensor and the piezoelectric diaphragm recognized the kick clearly, the accelerometer did not have any noticeable change in its response. By gradually increasing the wall displacement by the steps of 0.5 mm, the threshold wall displacement for the accelerometer was found to be 1.5 mm (Figure 14c). The significance of this finding is that, while the smaller input threshold values of the acoustic sensor and the piezoelectric diaphragm make them more suitable for detecting weaker fetal activities compared to the accelerometer, they also make the acoustic sensor and the piezoelectric diaphragm more prone to signal artefacts compared to the accelerometer.

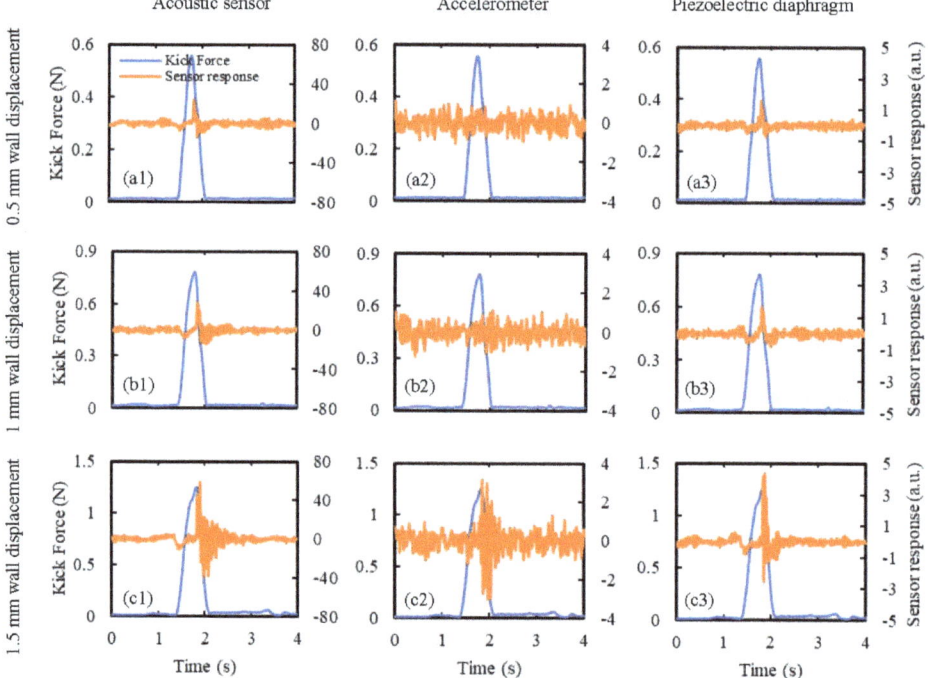

Figure 14. Determination of the minimum input threshold wall displacements for the sensors. Sensor responses were determined for kicks of wall displacements of: (**a1,a2,a3**) 0.5 mm, (**b1,b2,b3**) 1 mm, and (**c1,c2,c3**) 1.5 mm using the cylindrical kicking probe. The sensors were attached to a distance of 20 cm away (maximum possible for the current simulator) from the kick impact point.

The input threshold values may change based on the size of the maternal abdomen. In the case of a larger maternal abdomen, or later in gestation, two sensors on two sides of the abdomen may be needed to reduce the maximum possible distance between the sensor and the kick impact point. The results presented by Altini et al. [25] showed that using two accelerometers instead of one led to substantial improvement in the detection accuracy. In their case, any further increase in the number of sensors did not lead to any significant improvement in the detection accuracy.

5.4. Summary of Results

The main results can be summarized into four key findings regarding the response characteristics of the sensors when subjected to simulated fetal kicks. The first key finding is the differences between the sensors in terms of their responsiveness to different frequency ranges of membrane vibrations during the simulated kicks. While the acoustic sensor and the piezoelectric diaphragm responded strongly to low-frequency vibrations below 10 Hz, the accelerometer mainly responded to the free vibration of the membrane at around 19 Hz. This characteristic makes the acoustic sensor and the piezoelectric diaphragm better equipped to determine the kick duration compared to the accelerometer. Additionally, the acoustic sensor also responded effectively to the free vibration of the membrane. The second key finding is the differences between the sensors in terms of their responses to the changes in the wall displacement (or the reaction force) due to kicking, and the distance between the sensor and the kick impact point. The accelerometer output was found to be significantly less affected by alterations to these parameters compared to the acoustic sensor and the piezoelectric diaphragm, which makes the accelerometer relatively less capable of determining the intensity and location of a kick compared to the other two sensors. The third key finding is the differences between the sensors in terms of their minimum input threshold wall displacement values. The acoustic sensor and the piezoelectric diaphragm had a lower input threshold value compared to the accelerometer, which makes the acoustic sensor and the piezoelectric diaphragm more capable of detecting weaker fetal movements and more prone to signal artefacts compared to the accelerometer. Finally, the piezoelectric diaphragm had the best SNR for most of the input conditions, which signifies its superiority in terms of the signal quality and makes it a promising candidate sensor for fetal movement monitors. While these results establish the baseline performance of these sensors, more tests are needed to statistically compare the performance of the sensors.

6. Conclusions

This paper presents the most comprehensive attempt to simulate vibrations of a maternal abdomen due to fetal kicks in a laboratory set-up to date, fulfilling the unmet need for a pre-clinical facility for testing and calibration of vibration sensors for fetal movement (FM) monitors. We have designed the membrane (representing a gravid abdomen) of the simulator by incorporating relevant material and geometrical properties of gravid abdomens. We have analytically calculated the natural frequency of undamped free vibration of a curved model of gravid abdomens as 33.5 Hz and experimentally determined the actual natural frequency of an equivalent flat model of the abdomen in our simulator as 19 Hz, due to damping effects. The simulator imitates the stretched condition of a gravid abdomen by applying a biaxial tensile load on the membrane. By comparing with the available data for real fetal kicks, we have demonstrated that the designed kicking mechanism can replicate the kicks of 20 and 30-week old fetuses by using 10 mm diameter cylindrical and 30 mm diameter hemispherical kicking probes, respectively, in terms of wall displacement, kicking force, and kick duration.

As a case study, we have tested three candidate sensors for wearable FM monitors, namely an accelerometer, an acoustic sensor, and a piezoelectric diaphragm, on the simulator to investigate their performance. Analysis of the responses has revealed some novel characteristics of these sensors. For example, the acoustic sensor and the piezoelectric diaphragm were responsive to kicks during the whole kick duration because of their ability to respond to the low-frequency vibrations (<10 Hz) due to the forced movement of the membrane. Additionally, the acoustic sensor also effectively detected the free vibration of the membrane (at 19 Hz), which mainly happened at the end of the kick. However, the piezoelectric diaphragm was not responsive to the free vibration of the membrane at all. Conversely, the accelerometer was mainly responsive to the free vibration of the membrane, and therefore, although it recognized the start of the kicks, it mainly responded to inputs near the end of the kicks. These findings have also been supported by their respective spectrograms and PSD distributions. The accelerometer was significantly less responsive to the changes in wall displacement and kick distance than the other two sensors. These results indicate that it will be easier to obtain the duration, intensity, and location of the kicks from FM monitoring systems based on acoustic sensors and piezoelectric diaphragms compared to a fully accelerometer-based system. The piezoelectric diaphragm was found to produce the best SNR for most of the input conditions, which signifies its superiority in terms of the signal quality. Finally, the threshold wall displacements for the acoustic sensor and the piezoelectric diaphragm were found to be smaller compared to the acoustic sensor. This signifies that the acoustic sensor and the piezoelectric diaphragm have better abilities to detect weaker fetal activities compared to the accelerometer, but they are more prone to signal artefacts compared to the accelerometer. All these findings indicate that a combination of different types of sensing modalities will be more suitable to detect and characterize fetal activities compared to systems based on a single type of sensor.

In summary, we have created a facility for preclinical testing of sensors for FM monitors for the first time and demonstrated its capability. We have revealed novel characteristics of the responses of acoustic sensors, accelerometers, and piezoelectric diaphragm sensors to simulated fetal movements, providing valuable insights into optimally designing novel FM monitors. Future studies will involve the optimization of the number and arrangement of sensors and the study of the effect of other input conditions, such as the speed, duration, and simultaneous occurrence of kicks. Once the sensor combination is selected based on the test results from the simulator, they can be embedded in a wearable garment along with a miniaturized DAQ system and used for the clinical testing of the system. We, therefore, believe that the FM simulator presented in this study will be a major addition to the design cycle of the FM monitors.

Supplementary Materials: The following is available online at http://www.mdpi.com/1424-8220/20/21/6020/s1. A video of the FM simulator in action.

Author Contributions: A.K.G. designed the maternal abdomen model, the DAQ system, and the software for the simulator, performed the sensor testing and data analysis, and drafted the manuscript. S.F.B., D.K., A.R., A.S.S., T.S., P.M.P.T., M.M.V., and H.-T.V. designed and manufactured the simulator structure and the kicking mechanism and contributed to the drafting of the manuscript. N.C.N. and R.V. conceived of, designed, and coordinated the study, obtained funding for the study, and reviewed the manuscript. All authors have read and agreed to the published version of the manuscript.

Funding: This research was funded by the Commonwealth Scholarship Commission, UK (Reference No.: BDCS-2018-46), UK-India Education and Research Initiative (UKIERI) (Grant No.: DST-UKIERI-2016-17-0103), and Imperial College London.

Acknowledgments: Authors Sonny F. Burniston, Daniel Krentzel, Abhishek Roy, Adil Shoaib Sheikh, Talha Siddiq, Paula Mai Phuong Trinh, Marta Mambrilla Velazquez, and Hei-Ting Vielle contributed equally to this work.

Conflicts of Interest: The authors declare no conflict of interest.

Data Accessibility: Software for the FM simulator and all the relevant data are available online at https://github.com/IncidentalCoder/Imperial_Kick_Simulator.git.

References

1. Olesen, A.G.; Svare, J.A. Decreased fetal movements: Background, assessment, and clinical management. *Acta Obstet. Gyn. Scan.* **2004**, *83*, 818–826. [CrossRef] [PubMed]
2. Bekedam, D.J.; Visser, G.H.A.; Devries, J.J.; Prechtl, H.F.R. Motor Behavior in the Growth Retarded Fetus. *Early Hum. Dev.* **1985**, *12*, 155–165. [CrossRef]
3. Sival, D.A.; Visser, G.H.A.; Prechtl, H.F.R. The Effect of Intrauterine Growth-Retardation on the Quality of General Movements in the Human Fetus. *Early Hum. Dev.* **1992**, *28*, 119–132. [CrossRef]
4. Velazquez, M.D.; Rayburn, W.F. Antenatal evaluation of the fetus using fetal movement monitoring. *Clin. Obstet. Gynecol.* **2002**, *45*, 993–1004. [CrossRef] [PubMed]
5. Richardson, B.S.; Patrick, J.E.; Abduljabbar, H. Cerebral oxidative metabolism in the fetal lamb: Relationship to electrocortical state. *Am. J. Obstet. Gynecol.* **1985**, *153*, 426–431. [CrossRef]
6. Richardson, B.S.; Carmichael, L.; Homan, J.; Patrick, J.E. Electrocortical activity, electroocular activity, and breathing movements in fetal sheep with prolonged and graded hypoxemia. *Am. J. Obstet. Gynecol.* **1992**, *167*, 553–558. [CrossRef]

7. Pearson, J.F.; Weaver, J.B. Fetal activity and fetal wellbeing: An evaluation. *Br. Med. J.* **1976**, *1*, 1305–1307. [CrossRef]
8. Linde, A.; Pettersson, K.; Radestad, I. Women's Experiences of Fetal Movements before the Confirmation of Fetal DeathContractions Misinterpreted as Fetal Movement. *Birth-Iss. Perinat. Care* **2015**, *42*, 189–194. [CrossRef]
9. Dutton, P.J.; Warrander, L.K.; Roberts, S.A.; Bernatavicius, G.; Byrd, L.M.; Gaze, D.; Kroll, J.; Jones, R.L.; Sibley, C.P.; Froen, J.F.; et al. Predictors of poor perinatal outcome following maternal perception of reduced fetal movements–a prospective cohort study. *PLoS ONE* **2012**, *7*, e39784. [CrossRef]
10. Efkarpidis, S.; Alexopoulos, E.; Kean, L.; Liu, D.; Fay, T. Case-control study of factors associated with intrauterine fetal deaths. *MedGenMed* **2004**, *6*, 53.
11. Norman, J.E.; Heazell, A.E.P.; Rodriguez, A.; Weir, C.J.; Stock, S.J.E.; Calderwood, C.J.; Cunningham Burley, S.; Froen, J.F.; Geary, M.; Breathnach, F.; et al. Awareness of fetal movements and care package to reduce fetal mortality (AFFIRM): A stepped wedge, cluster-randomised trial. *Lancet* **2018**, *392*, 1629–1638. [CrossRef]
12. Froen, J.F.; Heazell, A.E.P.; Tveit, J.V.H.; Saastad, E.; Fretts, R.C.; Flenady, V. Fetal movement assessment. *Semin. Perinatol.* **2008**, *32*, 243–246. [CrossRef] [PubMed]
13. Hertogs, K.; Roberts, A.B.; Cooper, D.; Griffin, D.R.; Campbell, S. Maternal perception of fetal motor activity. *Br. Med. J.* **1979**, *2*, 1183–1185. [CrossRef]
14. Hijazi, Z.R.; Callan, S.E.; East, C.E. Maternal perception of foetal movement compared with movement detected by real-time ultrasound: An exploratory study. *Aust. N. Z. J. Obstet. Gyn.* **2010**, *50*, 144–147. [CrossRef] [PubMed]
15. Boashash, B.; Khlif, M.S.; Ben-Jabeur, T.; East, C.E.; Colditz, P.B. Passive detection of accelerometer-recorded fetal movements using a time-frequency signal processing approach. *Digit. Signal. Process.* **2014**, *25*, 134–155. [CrossRef]
16. Grant, A.; Elbourne, D.; Valentin, L.; Alexander, S. Routine formal fetal movement counting and risk of antepartum late death in normally formed singletons. *Lancet* **1989**, *2*, 345–349. [CrossRef]
17. National Institute for Clinical Excellence. *National Collaborating Centre for Women's and Children's Health. Antenatal Care: Routine Care for the Healthy Pregnant Woman*, 2nd ed.; Welsh, A., Ed.; RCOG Press: London, UK, 2008.
18. de Vries, J.I.P.; Fong, B.F. Normal fetal motility: An overview. *Ultrasound Obst. Gyn.* **2006**, *27*, 701–711. [CrossRef]
19. Andonotopo, W.; Kurjak, A. The assessment of fetal behavior of growth restricted fetuses by 4D sonography. *J. Perinat. Med.* **2006**, *34*, 471–478. [CrossRef]
20. Hayat, T.T.A.; Nihat, A.; Martinez-Biarge, M.; McGuinness, A.; Allsop, J.M.; Hajnal, J.V.; Rutherford, M.A. Optimization and Initial Experience of a Multisection Balanced Steady-State Free Precession Cine Sequence for the Assessment of Fetal Behavior in Utero. *Am. J. Neuroradiol.* **2011**, *32*, 331–338. [CrossRef]
21. Rayburn, W.; Zuspan, F.; Motley, M.E.; Donaldson, M. An Alternative to Antepartum Fetal Heart-Rate Testing. *Am. J. Obstet. Gynecol.* **1980**, *138*, 223–226. [CrossRef]
22. Thomas, G.; Mostefa, M.; Boualem, B.; Ian, C.; Stephen, W.; Miguel, F.; Susan, C.; Christine, E.; Paul, C. Detecting fetal movements using non-invasive accelerometers: A preliminary analysis. In Proceedings of the 10th International Conference on Information Science, Signal Processing and their Applications (ISSPA 2010), Kuala Lumpur, Malaysia, 10–13 May 2010; pp. 508–511.
23. Ryo, E.; Nishihara, K.; Matsumoto, S.; Kamata, H. A new method for long-term home monitoring of fetal movement by pregnant women themselves. *Med Eng. Phys.* **2012**, *34*, 566–572. [CrossRef] [PubMed]
24. Mesbah, M.; Khlif, M.S.; East, C.; Smeathers, J.; Colditz, P.; Boashash, B. Accelerometer-based fetal movement detection. In Proceedings of the 2011 Annual International Conference of the IEEE Engineering in Medicine and Biology Society, Boston, MA, USA, 30 August–3 September 2011; pp. 7877–7880.
25. Altini, M.; Mullan, P.; Rooijakkers, M.; Gradl, S.; Penders, J.; Geusens, N.; Grieten, L.; Eskofier, B. Detection of fetal kicks using body-worn accelerometers during pregnancy: Trade-offs between sensors number and positioning. In Proceedings of the IEEE Eng Med Bio, Orlando, FL, USA, 16–20 August 2016; pp. 5319–5322.
26. Lai, J.; Woodward, R.; Alexandrov, Y.; Ain Munnee, Q.; Lees, C.C.; Vaidyanathan, R.; Nowlan, N.C. Performance of a wearable acoustic system for fetal movement discrimination. *PLoS ONE* **2018**, *13*, e0195728. [CrossRef]

27. Sazali, A.R.; Al-Ashwal, R. Fetal Movement Simulator for Fetal Monitoring System Testing. In Proceedings of the IEEE Embs Conf Bio, Sarawak, Malaysia, 3–6 December 2018; pp. 544–547.
28. Palmer, P.J. The Natural Frequency of Vibration of Curved Rectangular Plates. *Aeronaut. Q.* **1954**, *5*, 101–110. [CrossRef]
29. Helmig, R.; Oxlund, H.; Petersen, L.K.; Uldbjerg, N. Different Biomechanical Properties of Human Fetal Membranes Obtained before and after Delivery. *Eur. J. Obstet. Gyn. Reprod. Biol.* **1993**, *48*, 183–189. [CrossRef]
30. Verbruggen, S.W.; Kainz, B.; Shelmerdine, S.C.; Hajnal, J.V.; Rutherford, M.A.; Arthurs, O.J.; Phillips, A.T.M.; Nowlan, N.C. Stresses and strains on the human fetal skeleton during development. *J. R. Soc. Interface* **2018**, *15*. [CrossRef]
31. Verbruggen, S.W.; Loo, J.H.; Hayat, T.T.; Hajnal, J.V.; Rutherford, M.A.; Phillips, A.T.; Nowlan, N.C. Modeling the biomechanics of fetal movements. *Biomech. Model. Mechanobiol.* **2016**, *15*, 995–1004. [CrossRef]
32. Pearsall, G.W.; Roberts, V.L. Passive Mechanical-Properties of Uterine Muscle (Myometrium) Tested Invitro. *J. Biomech.* **1978**, *11*, 167. [CrossRef]
33. Acar, B.S.; van Lopik, D. Computational pregnant occupant model, 'Expecting', for crash simulations. *Proc. Inst. Mech. Eng. Part D J. Automob. Eng.* **2009**, *223*, 891–902. [CrossRef]
34. Sokolowski, P.; Saison, F.; Giles, W.; McGrath, S.; Smith, D.; Smith, J.; Smith, R. Human uterine wall tension trajectories and the onset of parturition. *PLoS ONE* **2010**, *5*, e11037. [CrossRef]
35. Verbruggen, S.W.; Oyen, M.L.; Phillips, A.T.; Nowlan, N.C. Function and failure of the fetal membrane: Modelling the mechanics of the chorion and amnion. *PLoS ONE* **2017**, *12*, e0171588. [CrossRef]
36. Song, C.; Alijani, A.; Frank, T.; Hanna, G.; Cuschieri, A. Elasticity of the living abdominal wall in laparoscopic surgery. *J. Biomech.* **2006**, *39*, 587–591. [CrossRef] [PubMed]
37. Schneider, U.; Pedroni, E.; Lomax, A. The calibration of CT Hounsfield units for radiotherapy treatment planning. *Phys. Med. Biol.* **1996**, *41*, 111–124. [CrossRef] [PubMed]
38. Van Hollebeke, R.B.; Cushman, M.; Schlueter, E.F.; Allison, M.A. Abdominal Muscle Density Is Inversely Related to Adiposity Inflammatory Mediators. *Med. Sci. Sports Exerc.* **2018**, *50*, 1495–1501. [CrossRef] [PubMed]
39. Stanišić, M.M. Free vibration of a rectangular plate with damping considered. *Q. Appl. Math.* **1955**, *12*, 361–367. [CrossRef]
40. Tekscan Inc. FlexiForce A401 Sensor. Available online: https://www.tekscan.com/products-solutions/force-sensors/a401 (accessed on 12 September 2020).
41. SparkFun Electronics. Sparkfun Triple Axis Accelerometer Breakout-ADXL335. Available online: https://www.sparkfun.com/products/9269 (accessed on 12 September 2020).
42. MMC Ltd. Piezoelectric Sound Components. Available online: https://www.sparkfun.com/products/10293 (accessed on 12 September 2020).
43. Posatskiy, A.O.; Chau, T. Design and evaluation of a novel microphone-based mechanomyography sensor with cylindrical and conical acoustic chambers. *Med Eng. Phys.* **2012**, *34*, 1184–1190. [CrossRef]
44. Woodward, R.B.; Shefelbine, S.J.; Vaidyanathan, R. Pervasive Monitoring of Motion and Muscle Activation: Inertial and Mechanomyography Fusion. *IEEE-ASME Trans. Mechatron.* **2017**, *22*, 2022–2033. [CrossRef]
45. Actuonix Motion Devices Inc. L16-R Miniature Linear Servos for RC & Arduino. Available online: https://www.actuonix.com/L16-R-Miniature-Linear-Servo-For-RC-p/l16-r.htm (accessed on 12 September 2020).

Publisher's Note: MDPI stays neutral with regard to jurisdictional claims in published maps and institutional affiliations.

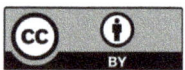

© 2020 by the authors. Licensee MDPI, Basel, Switzerland. This article is an open access article distributed under the terms and conditions of the Creative Commons Attribution (CC BY) license (http://creativecommons.org/licenses/by/4.0/).

MDPI
St. Alban-Anlage 66
4052 Basel
Switzerland
Tel. +41 61 683 77 34
Fax +41 61 302 89 18
www.mdpi.com

Sensors Editorial Office
E-mail: sensors@mdpi.com
www.mdpi.com/journal/sensors

www.ingramcontent.com/pod-product-compliance
Lightning Source LLC
LaVergne TN
LVHW070124100526
838202LV00016B/2225